Textbook of Psychiatric Nursing

Textbook of Psychiatric Nursing

Rajesh G Konnur
MPhil (N) PhD MBA PGDGC PGDCA
Associate Professor
College of Nursing
Kurji Holy Family Hospital
Patna, Bihar, India

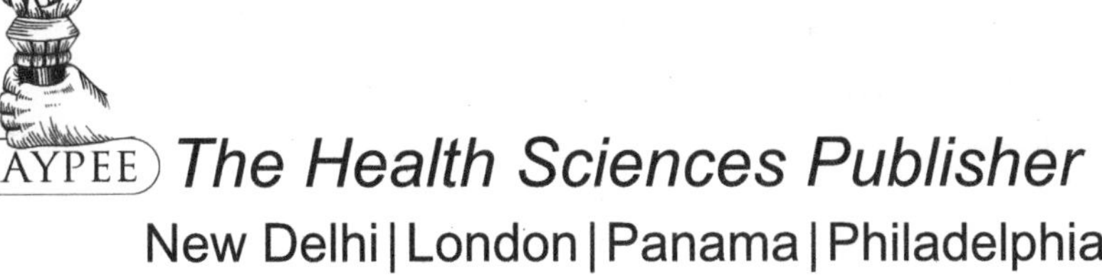

The Health Sciences Publisher
New Delhi | London | Panama | Philadelphia

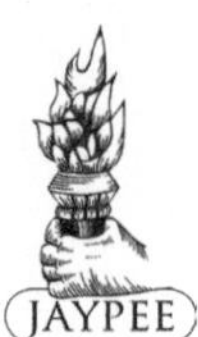

Jaypee Brothers Medical Publishers (P) Ltd

Headquarters

Jaypee Brothers Medical Publishers (P) Ltd.
4838/24, Ansari Road, Daryaganj
New Delhi 110 002, India
Phone: +91-11-43574357
Fax: +91-11-43574314
Email: jaypee@jaypeebrothers.com

Overseas Offices

J.P. Medical Ltd.
83, Victoria Street, London
SW1H 0HW (UK)
Phone: +44-20 3170 8910
Fax: +44-(0)20 3008 6180
Email: info@jpmedpub.com

JP Medical Inc.
325 Chestnut Street, Ste 412
Philadelphia, PA 19106
Phone: +215-713-718
Email: jrusko@jpmedus.com

Jaypee Brothers Medical Publishers (P) Ltd.
Bhotahity, Kathmandu, Nepal
Phone: +977-9741283608
Email: Kathmandu@jaypeebrothers.com

Jaypee-Highlights Medical Publishers Inc.
City of Knowledge, Bld. 237, Clayton
Panama City, Panama
Phone: +1 507-301-0496
Fax: +1 507-301-0499
Email: cservice@jphmedical.com

Jaypee Brothers Medical Publishers (P) Ltd.
17/1-B, Babar Road, Block-B, Shaymali
Mohammadpur, Dhaka-1207, Bangladesh
Mobile: +08801912003485
Email: jaypeedhaka@gmail.com

Website: www.jaypeebrothers.com
Website: www.jaypeedigital.com

Inquiries for bulk sales may be solicited at: jaypee@jaypeebrothers.com

Textbook of Psychiatric Nursing

First Edition: 2016, Reprint: **2024**

ISBN: 978-93-5152-992-7

Printed in India

Dedicated to

My Daughter

Sanjeevini

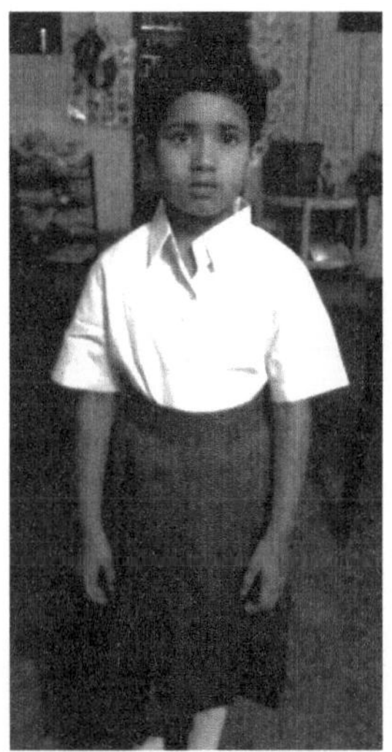

With love and affection

Preface

The plethora of evidence-based practice and research in psychiatry provides a plausible explanation for complex behavior.

The conceptual framework of this book integrates a holistic, developmental and adaptation model that reflects the continuum of mental health throughout lifespan. Modern advances support holistic phenomena. Mental health/illness is a dynamic process, holistic mental health care requires nursing care that synthesizes bio-psycho-socio-spiritual concepts. These concepts have profound impact on human behavior and adaptation primarily by promoting restoration and health maintenance of vital adaptive processes.

This textbook provides the nurse with an extensive discussion of mental health-mental illness continuum. Likewise, the emphasis on holistic nursing care that integrates neurobiological, psychosocial and cultural influences makes this textbook an excellent resource for psychiatric students and others to understand psychiatric disorders and treatment planning including care.

Overall, the unique and iconic feature of this book provides students and clinicians with a pragmatic thought of theory and care. It is immensely helpful for undergraduate and postgraduate scholars who pursue psychiatric/mental health nursing as a 'speciality'.

Rajesh G Konnur

Acknowledgments

I primarily bow to the Almighty for his immense blessings. Sincere thanks are extended to many individuals who contributed to the development of this textbook. I wish to acknowledge those individuals who have been most closely involved in the production of this textbook. Thanks to Jaypee Brothers Medical Publishers (P) Ltd, New Delhi for their patience and support.

Undertaking such a project would have been impossible without the support, help and co-ordination of many family members. I thank my wife, Sangita Singh and daughter, Sanjeevini (Taran) for their immense love and affection. I thank all those who contributed indirectly to this book.

From the Publisher's Desk
We request all the readers to provide us their valuable suggestions/errors (if any) at:

jppgmee@gmail.com

so as to help us in further improvement of this book in the subsequent edition

INC Syllabus

Placement: Third Year

Time: Theory: 90 Hours
Practical: 270 Hours
Internship: 95 hours (2 weeks)

Course description: This course is designed for developing an understanding of the modern approach to mental health, identification, prevention and nursing management of common mental health problems with special emphasis on therapeutic interventions for individuals, family and community.

Unit	Time (hrs)	Learning objective	Contents	Teaching learning activity	Assessment method
I	5	• Describes the historical development and current trends in mental health nursing • Describes the epidemiology of mental health problems • Describes the National Mental Health Act, programs and Mental Health Policy • Discusses the scope of mental health nursing • Describes the concept of normal and abnormal behavior	**Introduction** • Perspectives of mental health and mental health nursing: evolution of mental health services, treatments and nursing practices • Prevalence and incidence of mental health problems and disorders • Mental Health Act • National Mental health policy vis-à-vis National Health Policy • National Mental Health Programme • Mental health team • Nature and scope of mental health nurse in various settings and factors affecting the level of nursing practice • Concepts of normal and abnormal behavior	• Lecture discussion	• Objective-type • Short-answer • Assessment of the field visit reports
II	5	• Defines the various terms used in mental health nursing • Explains the classification of mental disorders	**Principles and Concepts of Mental Health Nursing** • Definition: mental health nursing and terminology used	• Lecture discussion • Explain using charts • Review of personality development	• Essay-type • Short-answer • Objective-type

Contd...

Contd...

Unit	Time (hrs)	Learning objective	Contents	Teaching learning activity	Assessment method
		• Explains psychodynamics of maladaptive behavior • Discusses the etiological factors, psychopathology of mental disorders • Explains the principles and standards of mental health nursing • Describes the conceptual models of mental health nursing	• Classification of mental disorders: ICD • Review of personality development, defense mechanisms • Maladaptive behavior of individuals and groups: stress, crisis and disaster(s) • Etiology: biopsychosocial factors • Psychopathology of mental disorders: review of structure and function of brain, limbic system and abnormal neurotransmission • Principles of mental health nursing • Standards of mental health nursing practice • Conceptual models and the role of nurse: – Existential model – Psychoanalytical models – Behavioral model – Interpersonal model		
III	8	• Describes nature, purpose and process of assessment of mental health status	**Assessment of mental health status** • History-taking • Mental status examination • Minimental status examination • Neurological examination: Review • Investigations: Related blood chemistry, EEG, CT & MRI • Psychological tests, role and responsibilities of a nurse	• Lecture discussion • Demonstration • Practice session • Clinical practice	• Short-answer • Objective-type • Assessment of skills with checklist
IV	6	• Identifies therapeutic communication techniques	**Therapeutic communication and nurse-patient relationship** • Therapeutic communication: Types, techniques, characteristics	• Lecture discussion • Demonstration • Role-play • Process recording	• Short-answer • Objective-type

Contd...

Contd...

Unit	Time (hrs)	Learning objective	Contents	Teaching learning activity	Assessment method
		• Describes therapeutic relationship • Describes therapeutic impasse and its intervention	• Types of relationship • Ethics and responsibilities • Geriatric considerations • Follow-up and home care and rehabilitation • Elements of nurse-patient contract • Review of technique of IPR-Johari Window • Goals, phases, tasks, therapeutic techniques • Therapeutic impasse and its intervention		
V	14	• Explain treatment modalities and therapies used in mental disorders and role of the nurse	**Treatment modalities and therapies used in mental disorders** • Psychopharmacology • Psychological therapies: Therapeutic community, psychotherapy—individual: psychoanalytical, cognitive and supportive, family, group, behavioral, play, psychodrama, music dance, recreational and light therapy, relaxation therapies: Yoga, meditation, biofeedback • Alternative systems of medicine • Occupational therapy • Physical therapy: electroconvulsive therapy • Geriatric considerations Role of a nurse in above therapies	• Lecture discussion • Demonstration • Group work • Practice session • Clinical practice	• Essay-type • Short-answer • Objective-type
VI	5	• Describe the etiology, psychopathology, clinical manifestations, diagnostic criteria and	**Nursing management of a patient with schizophrenia, and other psychotic disorders** • Classification: ICD	• Lecture discussion • Case discussion • Case presentation • Clinical practice	• Essay-type • Short-answer

Contd...

Contd...

Unit	Time (hrs)	Learning objective	Contents	Teaching learning activity	Assessment method
		management of patients with schizophrenia, and other psychotic disorders	• Etiology, psychopathology, types, clinical manifestations, diagnosis • Nursing assessment—history, physical and mental assessment • Treatment modalities and nursing management of patients with schizophrenia and other psychotic disorders		• Assessment of patient management problems
VII	5	• Describes the etiology, psychopathology, clinical manifestations, diagnostic criteria and management of patients with mood disorders	**Nursing management of patient with mood disorders** • Mood disorders: Bipolar affective disorder, Mania depression and dysthamia, etc. • Etiology, psychopathology, clinical manifestations, diagnosis • Nursing assessment: History, physical and mental assessment • Treatment modalities and nursing management of patients with mood disorders • Geriatric considerations • Follow-up and home care and rehabilitation	• Lecture discussion • Case discussion • Case presentation • Clinical practice	• Essay-type • Short-answer • Assessment of patient management problems
VIII	8	• Describes the etiology, psychopathology, clinical manifestations, diagnostic criteria and management of patients with neurotic, stress-related and somatization disorders	**Nursing management of patient with neurotic, stress related and somatization disorders** • Anxiety disorder, phobias, dissociation and conversion disorder, obsessive compulsive disorder, somatoform disorders, post-traumatic stress disorder	• Lecture discussion • Case discussion • Case presentation • Clinical practice	• Essay-type • Short-answer • Assessment of patient management problems

Contd...

Contd...

Unit	Time (hrs)	Learning objective	Contents	Teaching learning activity	Assessment method
			• Etiology, psycho-pathology, clinical manifestations, diagnosis • Nursing assessment: History, physical and mental assessment • Treatment modalities and nursing management of patients with neurotic, stress-related and somatization disorders • Geriatric considerations • Follow-up and home care and rehabilitation		
IX	5	• Describes the etiology, psycho-pathology, clinical manifestations, diagnostic criteria and management of patients with mood disorders	**Nursing management of patient with substance use disorders** • Commonly used psychotropic substance: Classification, forms, routes, action, intoxication and withdrawal • Etiology of dependence: tolerance, psychological and physical dependence, withdrawal syndrome, diagnosis • Nursing assessment: History, physical, mental assessment and drug assay • Treatment (detoxification, antabuse and narcotic antagonist therapy and harm reduction) and nursing management of patients with substance use disorders • Geriatric considerations • Follow-up and home care and rehabilitation	• Lecture discussion • Case discussion • Case presentation • Clinical practice	• Essay-type • Short-answer • Assessment of patient management problems

Contd...

Contd...

Unit	Time (hrs)	Learning objective	Contents	Teaching learning activity	Assessment method
X	4	• Describes the etiology, psychopathology, clinical manifestations, diagnostic criteria and management of patients with personality, sexual and eating disorders	**Nursing management of patient with personality, sexual and eating disorders** • Classification of disorders • Etiology, psychopathology, characteristics, diagnosis, • Nursing assessment: History, physical and mental assessment • Treatment modalities and nursing management of patients with personality, sexual and eating disorders • Geriatric considerations • Follow-up and home care and rehabilitation	• Lecture discussion • Case discussion • Case presentation • Clinical practice	• Essay-type • Short-answer • Assessment of patient management problems
XI	6	• Describes the etiology, psychopathology, clinical manifestations, diagnostic criteria and management of childhood and adolescent disorders including mental deficiency	**Nursing management of childhood and adolescent disorders including mental deficiency** • Classification • Etiology, psycho-pathology, characteristic, diagnosis Nursing Assessment-History, Physical, mental and IQ assessment • Treatment modalities and nursing management of childhood disorders including mental deficiency • Follow-up and home care and rehabilitation	• Lecture discussion • Case discussion • Case presentation • Clinical practice	• Essay-type • Short-answer • Assessment of patient management problems
XII	5	• Describes the etiology, psychopathology, clinical manifestations, diagnostic criteria and management of organic brain disorders	**Nursing management of organic brain disorders** • Classification: ICD • Etiology, psychopathology, clinical features, diagnosis and differential diagnosis (Parkinson's and Alzheimer's)	• Lecture discussion • Case discussion • Case presentation • Clinical practice	• Essay-type • Short-answer • Assessment of patient management problems

Contd...

Contd...

Unit	Time (hrs)	Learning objective	Contents	Teaching learning activity	Assessment method
			• Nursing assessment: History, physical, mental and neurological assessment • Treatment modalities and nursing management of organic brain disorders • Geriatric considerations • Follow-up and home care and rehabilitation		
XIII	6	• Identifies psychiatric emergencies and carry out crisis intervention	**Psychiatric emergencies and crisis intervention** • Types of psychiatric emergencies and thoir management • Stress adaptation model: Stress and stressor, coping, resources and mechanism • Grief: Theories of grieving process, principles, techniques of counseling • Types of crisis • Crisis intervention: Principles, techniques and process • Geriatric considerations: Role and responsibilities of a nurse	• Lecture discussion • Demonstration • Practice session • Clinical practice	• Short-answer • Objective-type
XIV	4	• Explains legal aspects applied in mental health settings and role of the nurse	**Legal issues in mental health nursing** • The Mental Health Act 1987: Act, Sections, Articles and their implications, etc. • Indian Lunacy Act, 1912 • Rights of mentally ill clients • Forensic psychiatry • Acts related to narcotic and psychotropic substances and illegal drug trafficking	• Lecture discussion • Case discussion	• Short-answers • Objective-type

Contd...

Contd...

Unit	Time (hrs)	Learning objective	Contents	Teaching learning activity	Assessment method
			• Admission and discharge procedures • Role and responsibilities of a nurse		
XV	4	• Describes the model of preventive psychiatry • Describes community mental health services and role of the nurse	**Community Mental Health Nursing** • Development of community mental health services • National Mental Health Programme • Institutionalization Versus Deinstitutionalization • Model of preventive psychiatry: Levels of prevention • Mental health services available at the primary, secondary, tertiary levels including rehabilitation and role of nurse • Mental health agencies: Government and voluntary, national and international • Mental health nursing issues for special populations: Children, adolescents, women, elderly, victims of violence and abuse, handicapped, HIV/AIDS, etc.	• Lecture discussion • Clinical/field practice • Field visits to mental health service agencies	• Short-answer • Objective-type • Assessment of the field visit reports

Contents

Introduction

Life is health. Health is a complex word, which contains physical, mental, spiritual, and social domains. The opposite of health is illness. Illness also includes physical, mental, and social domains. To be a healthy individual, he or she has to enjoy the full domain of health. Health and illness are recognized according to the values, beliefs, and philosophies of different society to which an individual belongs. Usually, if a person is able to adjust and adapt to his environment without any biopsychosocial complications he is said to healthy and hale. Like physical health, psychological health is very important at every stage of life, from childhood and adolescence through adulthood.

MENTAL HEALTH

- Mental health and mental illness are the two faces of a same coin. Both are defined on the basis of societal concepts.
- Mental health is defined as a state of well-being in which every individual realizes his or her own potential, can cope with the normal stresses of life, can work productively and fruitfully and is able to make a contribution to her or his community.
- Mental health is also defined as a state of emotional and psychological well-being in which individual is able to use his or her cognitive and emotional capabilities, function in society and meet the ordinary demands of everyday life.
- Mental health is the emotional and spiritual resilience which allows us to enjoy life and to survive pain, disappointment and sadness. It is a positive state of well-being and is underlying belief in our own and others 'dignity and worth'.
- Mental health influences how we think and feel about ourselves, about our future and about others and how we interpret events. It affects our capacity to learn, communicate, and form, sustain and end relationships. It also influences our ability to cope with change, transition, and life events.

Mental Illness

- The American Heritage Dictionary defines Mental Illness as 'Any of various conditions characterized by impairment of an individual's normal cognitive, emotional or behavioral functioning and caused by social, psychological, biochemical, genetic or others factors, such as infection or head trauma'.

- The Dorland's Medical Dictionary defines Mental Illness as 'Any of various psychiatric conditions, usually characterized by impairment of an individual's normal cognitive, emotional or behavioral functioning and caused by physiological or psychosocial factors'.
- Mental illness is a term that describes a broad range of mental and emotional conditions. The term 'psychiatric disability' is used when mental illness significantly interferes with the performance of major life activities, such as learning, working, and communication.

Meaning of Mental Illness

A mental disorder or mental illness is a psychological pattern, potentially reflected in behavior, that is generally associated with distress or disability and which is not considered part of normal development of a person's culture. Mental disorders are generally defined by a combination of how a person feel, acts, thinks or perceives. This maybe associated with particular regions or functions of the brain or rest of the nervous system, often in a social context. The recognitions and understanding of mental health conditions have changed overtime and across culture and there are still variations in definitions, assessment, and classification, although standard guideline criteria are unduly used.

Warning Signs of Mental Illness

- Changes in personality marked by daily lifestyle
- Failure to cope with daily chores
- Strange ideas/illogical thinking
- Excessive anxiety and fear
- Prolonged feeling of sadness
- Extreme highs and lows
- Use and abuse of alcohol and other narcotics
- Inappropriate anger and hostility
- Violent behavior
- Irrational fear and phobias
- Absenteeism
- Frequently being at odds in social life
- Involving in unethical and illegal activities.

Characteristics of a Mentally Healthy Individual

Abraham Maslow (1954), an eminent psychologist and writer developed the following criteria about mentally healthy people:

- They possess the ability to accept themselves, others and nature. It means, they have positive self-concepts and relate well to people and their environment.
- They are able to form close relationships with others and display kindness, patience and comparison for others.
- They perceive the world as it really is and people as they really are. Problem-solving occurs because these people are able to make decisions pertaining to reality rather than fantasy.
- They are able to appreciate and enjoy life at utmost.
- They are independent or autonomous in thought, decisions making and action and rely on personal standards of behavior and values. Such persons are able to face with relative serenity and happiness circumstances that would drive other people to self-destructive behavior.

- They are creative, utilizing a variety of approaches as they perform tasks or solve problems.
- Their behavior is consistent as those appreciates and respect the rights of others, display a willingness to listen and leave from others and show reverence for the uniqueness of and difference in others.

CRITERIA FOR MENTAL HEALTH BY MARIA JAHODA

- Attitude towards self
- Personal growth and self-actualization
- Internal psychological oneness or integrity
- Independence from self-influence the individual is inner directed than directed from outside sources
- Perception of reality without distortion
- Environment mastery

The following is a comparison of some of the characteristics of mental health and mental illness.

Mental health	Mental illness
• Accepts self and others	• Feels inadequate and has poor self-concept
• It is also to cope with or tolerate stress	• It is unable to cope
• Can return to normal work if temporarily disturbed	• Exhibits maladaptive behavior
• It is able to form close and lasting relationships	• It is unable to establish a meaningful relationships
• Uses sound judgment to make decisions	• Displays poor judgment
• Accepts responsibility for actions	• It is irresponsible and unable to accept responsibility for actions
• It is optimistic	• It is pessimistic
• Recognizes limitations	• Does not recognize limitations
• Can function effectively and independently	• Exhibits depending of needs because of feelings of inadequacy.
• It is able to distinguish imagined circumstances from reality	• It is unable to perceive reality
• It is able to develop potential and talents to fullest extent	• Does not recognize potential and talents due to a poor self-concepts
• It is able to solve gratification	• Desires or demands immediate gratification
• Mental health reflects a person's approach to life by communicating emotions, giving and receiving, working above as well as with others, accepting authority displaying a sense of humor and coping successfully and emotional conflict	• Mental illness reflects a person's inability to cope with stress, researching at disruption disorganization, inappropriate and reactions, unacceptable behavior and the mutability to respond according to the person's expectations and the demands of the society.

People who are mentally healthy do not necessarily possess all the characteristics as listed. Under stress they may exhibit transitory traits of mental illness but are able to respond to the stress with automatic, unconscious behavior that serves to satisfy their basic needs in a socially acceptable way.

Misconceptions about Mental Illness

Altrochi (1980) lists several misconceptions about abnormal behavior and mental illness.

These are as follow:
- Abnormal behavior is different or odd, easily recognized
- Abnormal behavior can be predicted and evaluated
- Internal forces are responsible for abnormal behavior
- People who exhibit abnormal behavior are dangerous
- Maladaptive illness is incurable.

Misconceptions about mental illness contribute to the stigma, which leads many people to be ashamed and prevents them from seeking help. Top ten Myths about Mental illness include the following:

- **Myth 1:** Psychiatric disorders are not like medical illness like waterborne disease and diabetes. People who have a mental illness are just 'crazy'.
  Fact: Brain disorders, like heart disease and diabetes, are legitimate medical illness. Current research shows that there are genetic and biological causes for psychiatric disorders and they can be treated effectively.
- **Myth 2:** People with a severe mental illness, such as schizophrenia are usually dangerous and violent.
  Fact: Statistics show that the incident of violence in people who have a brain disorder is not much higher than it is in the general population. Those suffering from a psychiatric such as schizophrenia are more after frightened, confused and despairing than violent.
- **Myth 3:** Mental illness is the result of bad parenting.
  Fact: Most experts agree that a genetic susceptibility, combined with other factors, leads to a psychiatric disorder. In simple terms, mental illness has a physical cause.
- **Myth 4:** Depression results from a personality weakness or character flaw and people who are depressed could just snap out of it if they tried hard enough.
  Fact: Depression has nothing to do with being lazy or weak. It results from changes in brain functions, medication and for psychotherapy often helps people to recover.
- **Myth 5:** Schizophrenia means split personality and there is no way to control it.
  Fact: Schizophrenia is often confused with multiple personality disorder. Actually, schizophrenia is a brain disorder that robs people of their, ability to think clearly and logically.
- **Myth 6:** Depression is a normal part of the aging process.
  Fact: It is normal for older adults to be depressed. Signs of depression in older people include a loss of interest in activities, sleep disturbances and lethargy. Depression in the elderly is often undiagnosed and it is important for senior citizens and their family members to recognize the problem and seek professional help.
- **Myth 7:** Depression and other illness, such as anxiety disorders do not affect children or adolescents. Any problems they have are just a part of growing up.
  Fact: Children and adolescents can develop severe mental illness.
- **Myth 8:** If you have a mental illness, you can will it away. Being treated for a psychiatric disorder means as individual has in some way 'failed' or is weak.
  Fact: A serious mental illness cannot be willed away. Ignoring the problem does not make it go away either it takes courage to seek professional help.

- **Myth 9:** Addiction is a lifestyle choice and shorts a lack of will power. People with a substance abuse problem are morally weak or 'bad'.
  Fact: Addiction is a disease that generally results from changes in brain chemistry. It has nothing to do with being 'bad' persons.
- **Myth 10:** Electroconvulsive therapy (ECT) or shock treatment is painful and barbaric.
  Fact: ECT has given a new lease on life to many people who suffer from severe and debilitating depression. It is used when other treatments such as psychotherapy or medication fail or cannot be used. ECT is administered under authorized so, patients will asleep and they do not feel anything.

The above misconceptions can do irreparable harm to people with legitimate illness who should and can be treated by interdisciplinary and multidisciplinary treated approach.

EVOLUTION OF MENTAL ILLNESS: FROM 'SKULL DRILLS TO HAPPY PILLS'

Attempts to treat mental illness date back as easily as 5000 BC as evidenced by the discovery of trephined skulls in regions that were home to ancient world cultures. Early man widely believed that mental illness was the result of supernatural phenomena such as spiritual and demonic possession, sorcery. The exit eye or an angry deity and so responded with equally mystical and sometimes brutal treatment. Trephining first occurred in Neolithic times. During these procedures, a hole was chipped into the skull using crude store instruments. It was believed that through this opening the evil spirit(s) thought to be inhabiting one's head and causing their psychopathology would be released and the individual would be cured. Pressure on the brain may have also incidentally been relieved. This procedure endured through the centuries to treat various ailments such as skull fractures and migraines as well as mental illness, albeit with more sophisticated tools such as skull saws and drills developed solely for this purpose.

In ancient Mesopotamia, priest-doctors treated the mentally ill with magico religious rituals as mental pathology was believed to mask demonic possession. Exorcisms, incantations, prayer, atonement and other various mystical were used to drive out the evil spirit. Other means attempted to appeal to the spirit with more human devices—threats, bribery, punishment and sometimes submission were hoped to be an effective cure.

Hebrews believed that all illness was inflicted upon humans by God as punishment for committing sin and were demons that were thought to cause some illness were attributed to God's wrath. God was seen as the ultimate healer. Generally, Hebrew physicians were priests who has special ways of appearing to the higher power in order to cure sickness. Along the same spiritual lines, ancient Persians attributed illness to demons and believed that good health could be achieved through proper precautions to prevent and protect one from diseases. These included appropriate hygiene and purity of the mind and body achieved through good deeds and thoughts.

Ancient Egyptians seem to be the most forward thinking in their, treatment of mental illness and they recommended that those afflicted with mental pathology engage in recreational activities such as concerts, dances and painting in order to relieve symptoms and achieve some sense of normalcy. The Egyptians were also advanced in terms of medicines, surgery and knowledge of the human body. Music was used as a therapy to affect emotion to achieve a cure.

Beliefs about mental illness and proper treatments were altered and in some cases advanced, by early European thinkers. Between the 5th and 3rd centuries BC, Greek physicians

Hippocrates denied the long-held belief that mental illness was caused by supernatural forces and instead proposed that it stemmed from natural occurrences in the human body, particularly pathology in the brain. Hippocrates and later the Roman physician Galen introduced the concepts of the four essential fluids of the human body blood, phlegm, bite and neck bite. The combination of which produced the unique personalities of individuals.

Custody and care of the mentally ill were taken by their families. The first mental hospital was established in 1792 CE Baghdad and was soon followed by others in Aleppo and Damascus—mass establishment of asylums and institutionalization folk place much later. The mentally ill in the custody of family were widely abused and restrained. Due to shame and stigma attached to mental illness, many hid their mentally ill family members in cellars, caged them in pigpens or put them under the control of servants. Others were abandoned by their families and left to a life of begging and vagrancy.

Through the middle ages and until the mass establishment of asylums, treatments for mental illness were offered by humanistic physicians, medical astrologers, apothecaries and by folk and traditional healers. Aside from secular exorcisms, prayers, charms and other mystical treatments were available. In the 17th century, astral talismans were popular and were easily made using bars or tin emblems with astrological sign sketched into them and cast at astrologically significant times. These were worn around the neck of the afflicted while they recited prayers.

Ancient Hindu scriptures known as Ramayana and Mahabharata contain fictional descriptions of depression and anxiety states. Mental disorders were generally thought to reflects abstract metaphysical entities, supernatural agents, sorcery or witchcraft. The ancient physician Charaka Samhita from circa 600 BC, part of Hindu Ayurveda (knowledge of life), saw ill health as resulting from an imbalance among three kinds of fluids or forces called Dosha. Different personality types also described, with different propensities to worries or difficulties. The common causes included inappropriate diet, disrespect towards the gods, teachers or others, mental shock due to excessive fear or joy and faulty bodily activity. The management included the use of tasks and ointments, charms and prayers, moral or emotional persuasion and shocking the person.

In 19th century, the influence of industrialization and populations growth saw a massive expansion of the member and size of insane asylums, called ‘asylums era’. Laws were introduced to judge insane by family and hospital superintendents. The concept of moral treatment became more popular. Clear descriptions and schizophrenia have been identified. Numerous classifications of psychiatric disorders and the term psychiatric were coined as the medical specialty.

The turn of the 20th century saw the development of psychoanalysis. Kraepelin classified the diseases and separated mood disorders from schizophrenia. In the US, mental hygiene movement started and aimed to prevent the sanity through public health and clinics. One term ‘mental health’ became were popular. World War I and II influenced for classification and diagnosis of disorders and it has given rise to diagnosis and statistical, manual of mental disorder (DSM) and international classification of diseases (ICD). During 1917 to 1970, lobotomies, Insulin shock therapy, ECT, neurotic, chlorpromazine came into use. In 1960s—Deinstitutionalization gradually occurred and use of lithium, Benzodiazepines, Cognitive behavioral therapy were developed. In 1990s—new SSRI antidepressants became the most widely prescribed drugs.

Milestones in Mental Health and Mental Health Nursing

1. Asciepiades (124 BC) described perceptual disorders.
2. King Asoka (273–232 BC) established mental hospital.
3. Aristotle (384–322 BC) emphasized as referred emotions and thought that hot bite in body is the root cause for psychiatric disorders.
4. Hippocrates (460–375 BC) identified melancholia, depression excitement hysteria and mania.
5. Plato (427–347 BC) identified the relationship between body and mind.
6. Pythagoras (580–570 BC) formulated the concept that the brain is the base for intellectual activities.
7. Charaka (100 AD) considered mental illness as 'Bhuta Vidya'.
8. Shakespeare (1564–1616) described Oedipus complex in his drama.

- **1773**: First mental hospital established in Williamsburg, Virginian.
- **1793**: Philip Pinel introduced humanitarian treatment.
- **1812**: Benjamin Rush written first American Textbook of Psychiatry initiated the provision of Humanistic approach, referred as father of American Psychiatry.
- **1883**: Emil Kraepelin wrote a book on 'Descriptive Psychiatry'.
- **1840**: Demography of mental disorders in and by Dorothea Dix—included the words 'insane' and 'idiotic'.
- **1873**: Linda Richard graduated in 'Mental Health Nursing'.
- **1900**: Movement of Mental Hygiene.
- **1908**: Clifford Beers has written a book 'The Mind that found itself'.
- **1912**: Bluer—a Swiss psychiatrist coined the term 'Schizophrenia'. Indian lunacy Act came with force.
- **1913**: John Hopkins's School of nursing included a fully developed course to prepare psychiatric nurse.
- **1920**: Sullivan emphasized interpersonal relationship for better care.
  - The term lunatic Asylum changed to 'Mental Hospitals'.
  - The first psychiatric nursing textbook, Nursing Mental Diseases was authored by Harriet Bailey.
  - The registration of psychiatric nurses was done in UK and degree course in psychiatric nursing began with USA.
- **1922**: Indian psychoanalytical association was started.
- **1927**: Insulin shock treatment was introduced.
- **1930**: For the first time in India, 11 British members along with are matron were brought from the UK to work in the mental hospital at Ranchi.
  - Short training courses of three to six months were conducted, which were recognized by the Royal Medical psychological Association.
- **1936**: Frontal Lobotomy was introduced.
- **1937**: The first Psychiatric social worker was appointed in Mumbai.
- **1938**: ECT was discovered to treat psychosis.
- **1939**: Sigmund Freud developed psychoanalytical therapy.
- **1946**: The Bhore committee recommended to set up hospitals at Amritsar, Srinagar, Jamnagar and Delhi and NIMHANS.
- **1948-50**: During 1948-50, four nurses were sent to the UK by Govt. of India for Diploma in Psychiatric Nursing Work.

- **1943**: The Chennai Government organized a three months psychiatric nursing course for male nursing students.
- **1947**: The Indian Psychiatric Society was formed.
- **1949**: Lithium therapy was introduced.
- **1950**: The National Association of Mental Health was formed.
- **1952**: The drug chlorpromazine was introduced.
  Hildegard Peplau developed a theory on interpersonal relationship.
- **1953**: Max well Jones emphasized therapeutic Community and Milieu therapy.
- **1960**: The first world wide Mental Health was formed.
- **1963**: The community Health centers Act was passed.
- **1954**: During 1954 Manzil Mental Health Centre, Lucknow gave psychiatric Nursing orientation course of 4–6 weeks duration.
- **1964–65**: INC made is a requirement to integrate psychiatric nursing in the diploma and degree courses.
- **1967**: A separate psychiatric Nursing committee was formed in the TNAI.
- **1972**: William Stake, founded the York Retreat hospital; in England and provided total care without restraints.
- **1981**: Community psychiatric centers were set-up to experiment with primary mental health care approach at Raipur, Ranchi, Chandigarh and Sakalvara at Bangalore, NIMHANS.
- **1982**: The central council of Health, Indian's highest health policy making body accepted the National Mental Health Policy and brought out the National Mental Health Program.
- **1987**: The Indian Mental Health Act was passed in 22nd May, 1987.
- **1991**: Indian Society of Psychiatric Nurses started (ISPN).
- **2002**: 1st National Conference of ISPN at NIMHANS, Bangalore.
- **2003**: 2nd National Conference of ISPN at Mysore, JSSCON.
- **2004**: 3rd National Conference of ISPN at Chennai, Saveetha CON.
- **2005**: 4th International Conference at NIMHANS.
- **2006**: 5th National Conference at Mangalore.
- **2007**: 6th National Conference at CON, Ludhiana (DMC).
- **2012**: 10th National Psychiatric Conference, Dehradun.
- **2014**: National Mental Health Policy.

Current Scenario of Mental Health Services in India

During the past few years, multiple factors brought about major changes in mental health services. Media exposes the drawbacks of mental hospitals has given rise to reformation. This resulted in setting many commissions of enquiring and helped for granting more resources to mental health sector. The Supreme Court also decreed against housing mentally ill persons in jails (Kumar 1993). Now, mental hospitals are steadily acquiring new roles and functions. Many of them opened emergency and ambulatory care services. Rehabilitation services are mostly adopted. The average period of hospitalization is being reduced by several conscious efforts. Hospitals opened, 'short stay' wards, 'open wards' and 'family wards'.

In recent years, there has been a perceptible growth of voluntary and non-governmental organizations taking an active interest in various aspects of programs which include the rehabilitation of patients with chronic mental illness, running day care facilities, half-way homes, quarter-way homes, crisis intervention centers, suicide prevention, treatment and rehabilitation of substance abuse and psychoeducation.

Another visible development during the past few years has been the growth of a private sector in psychiatric services. Private Psychiatric Nursing homes and hospitals have been on the increase contributed for better health services.

The public health consequences of mental and psychosocial disorders are now being realized in India more than ever before. An increasing number of persons with various minor mental disorders are beginning to seek mental health care services. The special needs of certain categories of the population such as children, the aged, women and the underprivileged have been recognized. Although the availability of a variety of mental health services has steadily increased in India, there is still a wide gap between the existing morbidity and the available services. With the current rapid urbanizations and globalization, economic liberalization in the country and the resultant social changes the demand for mental health services is only likely to increase.

Statistics of Mental Disorders

The recent research in the field of epidemiology in psychiatric disorders shows that mental disorders are common throughout the world, affecting tens of millions of people each year and that only a fraction of these affected receive treatment.

Prevalence of mental illness refers to the estimated populations of people who are managing mental illness at any given time. The incidence refers to the annual diagnosis rate or the member of new cases identified each years.

According to WHO (2010) report, globally, 450 million people suffering from different mental disorders/behavioral disorders.

- As many as 450 million people suffer from mental diseases.
- Nearly 1 million people commit suicide every year.
- Four of the leading disorders are depression, alcohol use disorders, schizophrenia and biopolar disorders.
- One in four families has at least are member with a mental disorder.
- The burden of mental disorders is expected to rise significantly over the next 20 years.
- More than 150 million persons suffer from depression at any point in time.
- About 25 million suffer from schizophrenia.
- 38 million suffer from epilepsy and more than 90 million suffer from an alcohol or drug use disorder.
- Neurotic and psychosomatic disorders are 10–20 per 1000 population.
- *Autism*: 1 in 500 to 1 in 2500.
- *Borderline Personality Disorders:* 2% of adults.
- About 20% of all occupational disabilities are stress related.
- *Dysthymic disorder:* 1.6% to 2% in adults.
- *Eating disorders:* 5 million women: 1–4% of young children.
- *Antisocial Personality Disorder:* 2% in adults.
- *Generalized Anxiety Disorder:* 3% of adult total population.
- *Dementia:* 0.1% before 60 years of age and 15–20% in aged 80 years.
- *Insomnia:* Approximately 35 million in adults.
- *Narcolepsy:* 20,0000 Americas; 50,000 diagnosed
- *Obsessive-compulsive Disorders:* 2.3% adults annually.
- *Post-Traumatic stress Disorder:*–3.6% adults annually.

- *Schizophrenia:* 1–2% in total population.
- *Social phobia:* 3–7% adults annually.
- *Tourette syndrome:* Estimated 1–10 per 1000 children.
- Treatment gap in severe Mental Disorders is approximately 50% and in case of common metal disorders is over 90% in India.
- 6% of Kerala's population has mental disorders. One in a 5 has some sort of emotional and behavioral problems.
- Almost 60 to 70 million Indians suffer from severe Mental Disorders and common Mental Disorders.
- Neuropsychiatric disorders account for 12% of the global disease Burden of these disorders is likely to increase to 15% by 2020.

MENTAL HEALTH ACT 1987

An Act to consolidate and amend the law relating to the treatment and care of mentally ill persons, to make better provision with respect to their property and affairs and for matters connected herewith or incidental thereto.

The Mental Health Act, 1987 (No. 14 of 1987) came into prater on dated 22nd May, 1987.

Reasons of Act 14 to 1987

- The attitude of the society towards persons afflicted with mental illness has changed considerably and it is now realized that no stigma should be attached to such illness as it is curable, particularly when diagnosed at an early stage. Thus, the mentally ill persons are to be treated like any other sick persons and the environment around them should be made as normal as possible.
- The experience of the working of Indian Lunacy Act, 1912 has revealed that it has become out molded. With the rapid advance of medical service and the understanding of the nature of malady, it has become necessary to have fresh legislation with provisions for treatment of mentally ill persons in accordance with the new approach.

  It is considered necessary to:

  a. Regulate admission to psychiatric hospitals or psychiatric nursing homes of mentally ill persons who do not have sufficient understanding to scale treatment as a voluntary basis and to protect the rights of such persons while being detained.
  b. To protect society from the presence of mentally ill persons who have become or might become a dance or nuisance to others.
  c. To protect citizens from being detained in psychiatric hospitals or psychiatric nursing homes without sufficient cause.
  d. To regulate responsibilities for maintenance charges of psychiatric nursing homes.
  e. Provide facilities for establishing guardianship or custody of mentally ill persons who are incapable of managing their own affairs.
  f. Provide for the establishment of central authority and state authorities for mental health services.
  g. Regulate the power of the government for establishing, licensing and controlling psychiatric hospitals and psychiatric nursing homes for mentally ill persons.
  h. Provide legal aid to mentally ill persons at state expense in certain cases.
- The main objective of the bill is to implement the aforesaid proposals.

The Mental Health Act 1987, empower the central government to establish central authority for mental health services and the state government to establish a state authority for mental health services. Thus, the central government and state government are given power to establish and maintain psychiatric hospitals and psychiatric nursing homes.

This act prohibits the establishment or maintenance of any person unless he holds a valid license granted to him under the act. Any person or persons who already held a license before the act or intending to start a new facility should apply for license in the prescribed from with required fee. The licensing authority has the power to grant or refuse license for the establishment or maintenance of psychiatric hospital or nursing home, depending upon whether they meet the minimum requirement or not, A license will not be transferable or heritable. A three months period is allowed to renew the license in case of expiry of the license. Every license unless revoked earlier for not meeting the requirement will be valid up to five years from the date of issue. There are specified standards prescribed for establishing and maintaining the facility. License can be revoked by the licensing agency, especially if the maintenance of it is detrimental to the patients. The inspecting officer has the right to inspect and interview patients regarding the condition and treatment facility. Outpatient treatment has to be provided for those patients who do not need admission.

The next section of the act deals with the admission and detention in psychiatric hospital or psychiatric nursing home. Admission of the mentally ill persons to a psychiatric facility can be

- On voluntary basis and
- Under special circumstances.

This type of admission needs a reception order. The special circumstances are on the:

- Application.
- Production of mentally ill persons before a magistrate.
- Admission as in patient after inquisition.
- Admission and retention of mentally ill prisoner.
- Detention of alleged mentally ill.
- Pending examination of the alleged mentally ill.
- Pending examination of the alleged mentally ill by medical officers.

Admission of Client on a Voluntary Basis

Any individual who consider himself to be mentally ill and wishes to be admitted to a psychiatric hospital may make a request to the medical officer and can be admitted as a voluntary client. In case of minors, the guardian may make a request.

The medical officer should make enquiry within 24 hours and would admit the voluntary client. The voluntary client who is admitted is bound to abide by the rules made by the institution. A voluntary client or his guardian in case of a minor can make a request for discharge and within 24 hours after the request he/she maybe discharged. If a minor voluntary patient attains majority during the period of the hospitalization, he/she maybe informed that unless he/she makes a request for voluntary detention within 30 days of attaining the majority, discharge under maybe made of a voluntary patient of mental health status does not seem to be appropriate for discharge, considering the best interest of the client, the medical officer should call a board consulting of two medical officers within 72 hours of expiry of the 30 days and if the board is of the opinion that the individual needs further treatment the medical officer should keep him/her in the hospital for periods not exceeding 90 days at a time.

Admission Under Special Circumstances

If a psychiatric client is not willing to get admitted for treatment, a relative or friend or well-wisher can make a request for admission and on examination, if found but it is the best interest of the mentally ill for whom the is being made, the medical officer may admit the client. Such admissions have to be reviewed within 90 days and he shall be kept in hospital only if found necessary on review. Such admission should be in prescribed form accompanied by two medical certificates from two medical officers, one of whom should be in government service, stating that the individual needs to be treated as an inpatient. Instead of the medical certificate, the medical officer can have the client examined by the medical practitioner, but when any psychiatric ill person is admitted under such conditions, his friend or relative can apply to the magistrate for his discharge. The magistrate may, after enquiring, grant or dismiss the request as deemed appropriate in the light of enquiry.

Admission Through Reception Order

Application for reception order maybe made by the medical officer in-charge of the treatment facility to the magistrate within the local limits. If the patients' condition is in danger to himself or to others, the husband, wife or relative may make such application to the magistrate of the area in which the client normally resides for such an order. If the husband or wife is not the applicant, the reason for that should be stated. No persons who is minor or who had not seen the mentally ill person within the past 14 days should make the application is made the magistrate may use his discretion for the enquiry to his satisfaction that the individual needs treatment. He may issue the order, but if he decides to dismiss the order he should give the reason in black and white to the applicant.

Reception Orders or Production of Mentally Ill Persons before Magistrate

A police officer may detain for protection of any persons wandering unintentionally who in his opinion maybe mentally ill and is liable to harm himself or others. If the relative is available, inform the relative, but produce the ill to the magistrate within 24 hours of taking the wanderer into protection. The magistrate, after proper enquiring, if convinced that the mentally ill needs to be detained for his own protection and from others, shall issue an order for detention in the hospital. If the relative/friend agrees to take the psychiatric client for treatment to any other facility, he may request and sign a bond to pay the expenses of the treatment and if the medical office of that facility agrees to take him, the magistrate may make out a reception order to that facility. If the relative signs a bond and sees that the mentally ill persons is take care of without doing any harm to self or to others, the magistrate may on the basis of that allow the relative to take care.

Admission as Inpatient after Inquisitor

If after the inquisitor it is found that the individual is to be detained in the mental hospital and it is in the best interest of the client. The district court may do so, but the respective court reviews his care from time to time.

Admission of Mentally Ill Prisoner

Reception order maybe carried out for the purpose.
Detention of alleged mentally ill, pending report of the medical officers.

Magistrate may order to keep the psychiatric client or observation for not more than 10 days until the medical examination certificate is made. This maybe extended for 10 days at a time but the total number of days should not exceed more than 30 days.

Detention of Mentally Ill Persons, Pending the Removal to Psychiatric Facility

The magistrate for reason given in writing can direct to retain the individual for not more than 30 days in such a place as he may deem appropriate, pending the removal of the person to the psychiatric facility. The medical examination should have been conducted within two days of application by doctor who signs the application.

If a reception order is given and if the client is not admitted to the place mentioned on expiring of the 30 days after the order is made, the reception order will cease to have effect. A magistrate shall not give a reception order to any institution outside the state or beyond the area of his jurisdiction. In case of reception order, a certified copy of the reception order together with the medical certificate has to be sent to the medical officer in-charge of the institution.

Inspection of the psychiatric facilities: Three visitors appointed by the state government or central government shall visit the institution at least once in every month for joint inspection.

Discharge of the Patient

The medical officer in-charge of the psychiatric hospital or recommendation of two medical practitioners, one of whom preferably a psychiatric, may discharge a client other than the voluntary patient. This discharge cannot be ordered by a medical officer in case of prisoners.

A psychiatric client on reception under maybe discharged, following an application by the relative who originally accepted for the reception order. But the medical officer should classify that the person is not dangerous and is fit to be discharged and is willing to undertake the responsibility of the care of the mentally ill, with respect to this, relative has to sign a bound under the term set up. He is responsible to see that the mentally ill does not harm him or others.

If the individual who was alleged to be mentally ill and was admitted on a reception order finds himself to be of sound mind and thus has recovered from his illness, he/she may make an application to the magistrate for his discharge, but the application should be accompanied by a medical certificate. The magistrate may on satisfactory evidence furnish a discharge order.

If the individual, who had been detained under a reception order, was later found to be of sound mind and capable of taking care of himself, the medical officer should give a discharge order with the clinical findings duly certificated by the district court.

Leave of Absence: The applicant under whose request the reception order was provided for admission and treatment of a mentally ill person, make an application for 'Leave of Absence'. To the medical officer for the said mentally ill person. The medical officer may give permission for 'Leave of Absence'. But the applicant shall be required to sign to a bond with or without surety agreeing to

- To take proper care of the mentally ill person.
- Prevent the mentally ill person from causing harm to himself and others.
- Bring back the mentally ill person to the institution or the date of expiry of the 'Leave of Absence'. In case where the medical officer refuse to provide permission for 'Leave of Absence', an appeal can be made to the magistrate who may after proper enquiring grant in 'Leave of Absence' on bond.

Management of the Property of Alleged Mentally Ill

When a report or application is made with regards to property management of alleged mentally ill, the collector or district court, on enquiry finds that the alleged mentally ill person is unable to manage his financial affairs and the liability is due to his mental illness, may take charge of his property management. This makes the alleged mentally ill persons powerless on his property. The collector or the court their appoints a guardian or manager to manage his affairs and the transactions are made by the manager with the knowledge of the court or by the collector. There cannot be any sale, mortgage or leasing of immovable property without the permission of the court or the collector. The details of the manager's responsibilities and limitations are provided in the act. This law protects the mismanagement of his property and also prevents other people, family or friends, from mishandling their properly for their own benefit.

Protection of Rights of the Mentally Ill

People with mentally illness should receive fair treatment and should be afforded certain rights. These include the right:

- To be treated with respect and dignity
- To have their privacy protected
- To receive age and culturally appropriate services
- To understand available treatment options and alternatives
- To receive care that does not discriminate on the basis of age, race or type of illness.

No mentally ill person shall be subjected during treatment to any indignity. No mentally ill persons under treatment shall be used for research purpose unless

- Such research is of direct benefit to him for the purpose of diagnosis treatment
- Such person is a voluntary client and has given written consent and if he is minor the guardian should be intercepted, detained or destroyed for the purpose other than preventing vexatious or defamatory communication in between others. The act specifics the penalties for improper use of the law related to the mentally ill and also provisions for financial and legal support to all.

National Mental Health Policy

The policy is a system which provides the logical framework and rationality of decision making for the achievement of intended objectives. It sets priorities and guides all resources allocations.

The Ministry of Health and Family Welfare, Government of India has appointed a policy group to prepare a National Mental Health Policy and Plan. The members of the policy group were Keshav Desiraju, Jagdish Prasad, Nirmala Srinivasan, Vikram Gupta, Vikram Patel and others.

Objectives

- To prepare a situational analysis of the need for mental health care in the country and the current promotion of mental health care in the country, including issue of human resources, essential drug procurement and distributor advocacy, prevention of mental illness, rehabilitation and care and promotion of mental health.
- To carry out a systematic review of the evidence base for the policy measures as proposed.

- To take the draft Mental Health care Act into account when drafting the National Mental Health care Policy and Plan and recommend changes to the proposed draft Mental Health care Act, if necessary to support the National Mental Health care Policy and Plan.
- To prepare a National Mental Health care Plan with specific reference to the National Mental Health Programme and the District Mental Health Programme with specific strategies and activities to implement the priority areas of action identified in the National Mental Health care Policy and to further prepare an estimate of financial resources required to implement the plan.
- To conduct broad-based consultations on the above issues with mental health stakeholders in the country before finalizing the situational analysis, the National Mental Health care, Policy and the National Mental Health care Plan.
  - It is estimated that 6–7 percent of population suffers from mental disorders, together these disorders account for 12 percent of the global burden of disease and analysis of trend indicates this will increase 15 percent to 20 percent by 2020. One in four facilities is likely to have at least one member with a behavioral or mental disorder.
  - The major of the mental illness do not require hospitalization and manageable by OPD treatment and follow-up care.
  - There is acute shortage of man power in the field of mental health and this is a major constraint in meeting mental health needs and providing optimal mental health services to the people.
  - The Govt. of India had launched the 'National Mental health Programme' in 1982 keeping in view of the heavy burden of mental illness in the community and the absolute inadequacy of mental health care infrastructure in the country to deal with it. Mental Health Act 1987 is being administered through Ministry of Health and Family Welfare, Govt. of India and State Government.

Epidemiological Data

Major Mental Disorder	1–2% of the population
Major Depression Disorder	5% of the population
Psychological problems among OPD attendees in PHC's	25%
Mental Problem will account by 2020	15% of DALYs.

Approach

- Community based services
- Hospital services
- Special care services
- *National Mental Health Programme:* Implementable at Districts and Rural Area.

The National Mental Health Programme (NMHP) initiated in 1982 attempted to address the vast mental health illness problems in a phased manner. The District Mental Health Programme (DMHP) which constitutes the basic functional component of this plan has been implemented in 25 districts covering twenty states/Union territories over the past several years. Patterned on the 'Bellary Model' developed by NIMHANS the programme comprises.

- Training in basic mental health care for all primary care personnel.
- Provision of essential psychotropic drugs in every peripheral health care institution located in mental areas.
- Resulting and reporting.
- Activities aimed at community participation.
- A continuous support and supervision for trained personnel.

- A district team of mental health professionals to provide support for trained personnel as well as for nursing district level mental health clinics. The district sees patients referred by trained health personnel from the periphery. The district clinic also has inpatient facility for about 10-patients.
- Work with other sectors such as education and social welfare.

Policy Objectives

The National Mental Health Policy outlines the prioritized agenda for extending within a programatic time-frame basic mental health care facilities to all sections of the population across the country by the year 2020. The tactical vehicle for implementing the policy will be the refused National Mental Health Program initially formulated in 1982, with five key thrust areas:

- The District Mental Health Programme (DMHP), redesigned around a Nodal Institution which in most instances will be the Zonal Medical College.
- Strengthening the Medical Colleges with a view to develop psychiatric manpower, improve psychiatric treatment facilities at the secondary level and to promote the development of general hospital psychiatry in order to reduce and eventually to eliminate to a large extent the need for big mental hospitals with huge proportion of long-stay patients.
- Streaming and modernization of Mental Hospitals to transform them from the present mainly custodial mode to tertiary care centers of excellence with a dynamic social orientation providing leadership to research and development (R & D) in the field of community mental health.
- Strengthening of Central and State Mental Health authorities in order that they may effectively fulfill their role of monitoring ongoing mental health programmes, determining priorities at the central/state level and promoting intersectoral collaboration and linkages with other national programs.
- Research and training aimed at building up an extensive database of epidemiological information relating to mental disorders and their course/outcome, therapeutic needs of the community, developed of better and more cost-effective intervention models, promotion of intersectoral research and providing the necessary inputs/conceptual framework for health and policy planning. Focused IEC activities, formulated with the active collaboration of professional agencies such as the National Institute of Mass Communication and diverted towards enhancing public awareness and eradicating the stigma/discrimination related to mental illness, will form an important component of this policy objectives.

Prioritized Goals

Subject to availability of resources the following time-frame is visualized for attainment in a phased manner the policy objectives outlined above:

- District Mental Health Programme (DMHP) will be extended to one district attached to each of the 100–Medical College in country. Thereby covering 100-districts by the end of the plan period including the 27-districts where DMHP is already in place. Thus making a total of 100 districts across the country.
- Strengthening of Medical Colleges with allocation of ₹ 50.00 lakh each to 100 Medical Colleges preferably located in backward areas for upgrading the departments of psychiatry with the aim of instituting post graduate training courses leading to MD (Psychiatric). Infrastructural support to psychiatry departments in all Medical Colleges will be provided as part of the DMHP over the plan period.

- Streamlining and modernization of Mental Hospitals with train of reduction in chronicity through intensive therapeutic intervention using nonconventional antipsychiatric medications, promoting care of chronically mentally ill patients in the community using outreach maintenance modalities and reduction of load/rational downsizing to ensure quality mental health care to a manageable number of patients. The feasibility of disinvesting fixed assets (e.g. 150 acres of land with the Central Institute of Psychiatry, Ranchi) in order to mobilize additional resources for creating state of the art institutions maybe considered, beginning with CIP, Ranchi in the first phase during the 10th plan.
- Strengthening of central and state mental health authorities by facilitating the establishment of permanent secretaries and related machinery and networking of the state authorities with that at the national level to ensure effective coordination in all areas of activity.
- Research and training by sponsoring relevant community based research projects and building up an extensive database which will form the basis for development of intervention models and policy planning. Innovative IEC strategies will be generated through multidisciplinary collaboration and an effective 3 tier monitoring/audit/review machinery will be created to ensure continuous online assessment/course correction.
- *11th Five Year Plan (2007–2012):* The District Mental Health programme will be extended to the remaining 161 districts and the gains made in the previous plans will be consolidated, upgradation of remaining 39. Medical College Psychiatry Departments will be undertaken and 20. Mental Hospitals will be taken up for disinvestments/reconstruction. Nonviable mental hospitals will be closed down or merged with general hospitals to create General Hospital Psychiatry Units (GHPUs). Central and State Mental Health Authorities will be further reinforced and technologically more sophisticated by term research projects will be initiated in selected institutions while continuing support to community based research. IEC activities will be augmented to cover all sections of the population across the whole country. A comprehensive holistic assessment and review of programme performance in the preceding two decades will be undertaken at the national and state levels by an independent agency to identify achievements, areas of non or poor performance, remedial measures, current needs and future requirements.

National Health Policy 1983 (NHP)

The Government of India, Ministry of Health and Family Welfare developed and published the 'National Health Policy' in 1983. NHP was endorsed by the Parliament of India in 1983 and updated in 2002.

Health Policy of a Nation is its strategy for controlling and optimizing the social uses of its health knowledge of health resources.

National Health Policy 2002

Objectives

- Achieving an acceptable standard of good health of Indian population.
- Decentralizing public health system by upgrading infrastructure in existing institutions.
- Ensuring a more equitable access to health service across the social and geographical expanse of India.
- Enhancing the contribution of private sector in providing health service for people who can afford to pay.
- Giving primary importance for prevention and first line creative initiative.

- Emphasizing rational use of drugs.
- Increasing access to traditional systems of medicine.

Goals of NHP 2002

- Eradication of Polio and Yaws 2005
- Elimination of Leprosy 2005
- Elimination of Kala-azar 2010
- Elimination of Lymphatic Filariasis 2015
- Achieve of Zero level growth of HIV/AIDS 2007
- Reduction of mobility by 50% on account of TB, Malaria, other vector waterborne disease 2010
- Reduce prevalence of blindness to 0.5% 2010
- Reduction of IMR to 30/1000 and MMR to 100/lakh 2010
- Increase utilization of public health facilities from current level of 20 to 73%> 2010
- Establishment of an integrated system of surveillance, National Health Accounts and Health Statistics. 2007
- Increase health expenditure by government as a % of GDP from the existing 0.9 to 2.0%. 2010
- Increase state sector health spending from 5.5 to 7% 2005
- Further increase of state sector health spending from 7 to 8%. 2010

NHP–2002 Policy Prescriptions

Financial Resources

- Increase in health sector expenditure to 6% of GDP, with 2% by public health investment by 2010 is recommended by the policy.
- Existing 15% of central government contribution is to be raised to 25% by 2010. This will allow a good rise of current annual per capita public health expenditure of this country from ₹ 200/- by ten-fold say around ₹ 2000/-.

Equity

- NHP 2002 has observed that the attainment of health indices was been very uneven across meal urban divide.
- To overcome the social inequality, NHP 2002 has set an increased allocation of 55% of total public health investment for the primary health sector, 35% of or secondary sector and 10% for tertiary sector.

Delivery of National Health Programme

- NHP 2002 envisages the gradual convergence of all health programme under a single field administration.
- It suggests for a scientific designing of public health projects suited to the local situation.
- Training and reorientation of rural health staff and free hand to district administration to allocate the time of the meal health staff between the various programmes, depending on the local need is stressed.

- NHP 2002 noticed that less than 20% of population which such OPD services and less than 45% of that which seek indoor treatment avail of such service in public hospital.
- In this backdrop, the 2002 NHP envisages kick starting of the revival of public health system by providing some essential drugs through decentralized health system.
- The policy recognizes the need for frequent in-service training.
- The NHP 2002 noted that improvement of public health indices is linked with quantum and quality of investment through public funding in public health sector.
- Expanding the pool of General Practitioners to include a cadres of Licentiates including Indian System of Medicine and Homeopathy is recommended in the policy.
- In order to provide trained manpower in underserved areas it recommends contract employment.

Role of Local Self-Government Institutions

- NHP 2002 emphasizes implementation of health programmes through local self-government institutions by 2005 with financial incentives.
- Norms for Health care Personnel.
- Indian Medical Council Act, Indian Nursing Council Act provide minimal statutory norms for doctors and nurses in medical institutions.
- NHP 2002 suggests for review and making stringent statutory norms for meeting better normative standards.

Suggested Norms of Health Personnel

Category of personnel	Norms suggested	
Doctors	1 per	3,500 population
Nurses	1 per	5000 population
FHW and MHW	1 per	5000 population in plain area and 3000 in tribal/hilly area
Trained Dai	1 per	Village
Health Assistant (M and F)	1 per	30,000 population in plain Area and 20,000 populations in tribals.
Pharmacists	1 per	10,000 population
Lab. Technicians	1 per	10,000 population

Education of Health Care Professionals

- NHP 2002 recommends setting up of a Medical Grant Commission for funding new government medical/dental colleges.
- It suggests for a need based, skill oriented syllabus with a more significant component of practical training.
- The need for inclusion of contemporary medical research and geriatric concern and creation of additional PG seats in deficient specialties are specified.
- For discharging public health responsibilities in the country NHP 2002 recommends specialization in the disciplines of public health and family medicines, where medical doctors. Public health engineers microbiologists and other natural sciences specialist can take up the course.

Nursing Personnel

NHP 2002 recognizes acute shortage of nurses trained in superspecialty disciplines. It recommends increase of nursing personnel in public health delivery centers and establishment of training courses for superspecialty.

Use of Genetic Drugs and Vaccines

- NHP 2002 recommends limited numbers of essential drugs of genetic nature as a requisite for cost effective public health care.

Mental Health

- Decentralized mental health service for diagnosis and treatment by general duty medical staff is recommended.
- It also recommends securing the human rights of mentally sick.

To fulfil, NHP 2002 and Mental Health Policy's objectives, Indian has to go far beyond the miles. Commitment and governance is a prerequisite for the succession of any health policy.

NATIONAL MENTAL HEALTH PROGRAMME (NMHP)

Introduction

Psychiatric symptoms are common in general population in both sides of the globe. These symptoms—worry, tiredness, and sleepless nights affect more than half of the adults at some form of as many as one person in severe experiences come from of diagnosable neuropsychiatric disorder.

Burden of Disease

The World Bank report (1993) revealed that the disability adjusted life year (DALY) loss due to neuropsychiatric disorder in much higher than diarrhea, worm infestations and tuberculosis of taken individually. According to the estimates, DALYs loss due to mental disorders are expected to represent 15% of the global burden of diseases by 2020.

During the last two decades, many epidemiological studies have been conducted in India, which show that the prevalence of major psychiatric disorder is about the same all over the world. The prevalence reported from these studies ranges from the population of 18 to 207 per 1000 with the median 65.4 per 1000 and at any given time, about 2–3% of the population, suffer from seriously, incapacitating mental disorder or epilepsy. Most of these patients live in rural areas remote from any modern health facilities. A large number of adult patients (10.4–53%) coming to the general OPD are diagnosed mentally ill. However, these patients are usually missed because either medical officer or general practitioner at the primary health care unit does not take detail/mental health history. Due to the under diagnosis of these patients, unnecessary investigations and treatments are offered with heavily cost to the health providers.

The Government of India has launched the National Mental Health Programme (NMHP) in 1982, keeping in view the heavy burden of mental illness in the community and the absolute in adequacy of mental health care infrastructure in the country to deal with it.

Aims

- Prevention and treatment of mental and neurological disorders and their associated disabilities.

- Use of mental health technology to improve general health services.
- Application of mental health principles in total national development to improve quality of life.

Objectives

- To ensure availability and accessibility of minimum mental health care for all in the foreseeable future, particularly to the most vulnerable and underprivileged sections of population.
- To encourage application of mental health knowledge in general health care and in social development.
- To promote community participation in the mental health services development and to stimulate efforts towards self-help in the community.

Strategies

- Integration of mental health with primary health care.
- Provision of tertiary care institutions for treatment of neuropsychiatric disorders.
- Eradicating stigmatization of mentally ill patients and protecting their rights through regulatory institutions like the central mental health authority and state mental health authority.

Mental Health Care

- The mental morbidity requires priority in mental health treatment.
- Primary Health care at village and subcentre level.
- At Primary Health Centre level.
- At District Hospital level.
- Mental Hospital and teaching psychiatric units.

District Mental Health Programme

Components

- Training programs of all workers at Nodal Institute in his state.
- Public education in mental health to increase awareness and reduce stigma.
- Early detection and treatment, the OPD and indoor services are provided.
- Providing valuable data and experience at the level of community to the state and centre for future planning, improvement in service and research.

Agencies like World Bank and WHO supports the various components of the programme. Funds are provided by the Govt. of India to the state governments and the nodal institutes to meet the expenditure on staff, equipments, vehicles, medicines, stationary, contingencies, training, etc. Govt. of India has constituted Central Mental Health Authority to oversee the implementation of the Mental Health Act, 1986. It provides for creation of State Mental Health Authority also to carry out the functions.

The National Human Rights Commission also monitors the conditions in the mental hospitals along with the Government of India and the States are currently acting on recommendation of the joint studies conducted to ensure quality in delivery of mental care.

Drawbacks of NMHP

- There is no initiative from the mental health professional to take active part in this programme. Most of them are not aware of the programme.

- There is shortage of professional manpower and training programmes are not able to meet the demand in providing all medical private practitioners and medical officers.
- Appropriate mental health can be provided at the subcenter and village level by minimum training of the health workers that will help in providing comprehensive health care at the most peripheral level.
- The targets set for the programme are not achieved till today after lapse of more than one decade. This shows that there is a poor commitment of the government, psychiatrists, and community at large.
- The programme has given more emphasis on the curative services to the mental disorders and preventive measures are largely ignored. More public awareness programs are required.
- The medical cares in the hospitals are custodial in nature and these needs to be changed to a therapeutic mode.

National Mental Health Policy 2014

In April 2011, the Government of India constituted a Policy Group to recommend a Mental Health Policy for the country. After due deliberations and intense discussions, in accordance with the mandate, the group has submitted recommendations. The suggested mental health policy has been duly considered by Ministry of Health and Family Welfare, Government of India. After minor amendments, additions and changes, the first National Mental Health Policy has been formulated. The policy envisages dynamic engagement and is expected to accommodate future thinking and developments in this field.

The policy is inclusive in nature and incorporates an integrated, participatory, rights and evidence based approach. Mental health issues are addressed in comprehensive manner to address medical-nonmedical aspects of mental health. This policy does not reduce mental health interventions to merely disease and disability prevention and it takes into account the need for all stakeholders to work synergistically and achieve common policy goals.

The strategic areas identified for action are, inter alia, effective governance and accountability, promotion of mental health, prevention of mental disorders and suicide, universal access to mental health services, enhanced availability of human resources for mental health, community participation, research, monitoring and evaluation.

The Government believes that mental health is an integral part of our overall endeavor. A holistic approach that recognizes strong linkage of body, mind, and soul is necessary. Strengthening of health infrastructure must be effected along with addressing the social determinants of health and mental health.

It is significant that the 65th World Health Assembly held in 2013 approved and adopted Resolution WHA 65.4 on global burden of mental disorders and the need for a comprehensive, coordinated response from the health and social sectors at the community level. India was one of the main sponsors of this resolution. This mental health policy is in consonance with the intent of this WHA Resolution.

1. Vision

The vision of the National Mental Health Policy is to promote mental health, prevent mental illness, enable recovery from mental illness, promote destigmatization and desegregation and ensure socioeconomic inclusion of persons affected by mental illness by providing accessible, affordable and quality health and social care to all persons through their life span, within a rights-based framework.

2. Values and Principles

Fundamental values and principles representing the ethos of this policy are discussed below:

2.1 Equity

- Mental Health services should be sensitive and relevant to diverse social and cultural situations and groups and, to the need of remote and rural areas.
- An equitable share of the national health budget should be consistent with the burden of mental health problems and mental illness.
- Nondiscrimination and equal opportunities for education, employment, housing and social welfare should be provided to promote inclusion of persons with mental health problems and mental illness.

2.2 Justice

- The needs of vulnerable and excluded members of the community should receive particular attention.

2.3 Integrated care

- Mental health services should be provided within the existing health care system using the Primary Health care approach.
- Some mental illnesses are chronic in nature. Persons suffering from chronic illness would require provisions for medium and long term, in some cases even life-long the provision of services should keep this requirement in consideration.
- These services should espouse the principles of universal access, equitable distribution, community participation, intersectoral coordination and use of appropriate technology. It is essential to make mental health services universally available and accessible in a time bound manner.
- Mental health services should be comprehensive and address the needs of person with mental illness, their careproviders and health care professionals.

2.4 Evidence-based care

- Evidence-based interventions should inform decisions regarding provision of services.
- Decision making should be based on various evidences for instance: findings from research, practice-based evidence and feedback from clients.

2.5 Quality

- Mental health services should meet quality standards as mandated globally and perceived suitable by local users and caregivers.

2.6 Participatory and rights based approach

- **Service users** and caregivers should be involved in the planning, development, delivery, monitoring and evaluation of mental health services.
- **Human** rights and dignity of persons with mental health problems should be respected, protected and promoted.
- Mental health care should promote and protect the autonomy and liberty of person(s) with mental health problems.
- The rights of the caregiver and service provider should also be respected by ensuring good working conditions, adequate training and support.

2.7 Governance and effective delivery

- The union and state governments, have a major role in actions for promotion of mental health, prevention of mental illness and treatment of mental illness in the country. However, governments alone cannot ensure effective delivery. Other stakeholders such as private care, providers, civil society organizations, user groups, academic and research institutions also have a crucial role in delivery and guiding policy.
- Services and professionals involved in health care planning and delivery whether in public, private or nongovernment sector should at all times display the utmost devotion to duty and be responsible for their actions.
- Services and service providers are ultimately accountable to person(s) with mental illness and their caregivers.

2.8 Value base in all training and teaching programs

- Core values such as quality, integrity, justice, accountability and empathy should be built into all forms of training and academic teaching.

2.9 Holistic approach to mental health

- A holistic approach to health including recognition of the relationship between mind, body and soul is more effective in dealing with mental health problems.
- Cultural ethos, Indian traditions and their impact on behavioral patterns must be recognized and leveraged to achieve policy goals and objectives.

3. Goals and Objectives

Based on vision, goals include the following:

3.1 Goals

3.1.1 To reduce distress, disability, exclusion morbidity and premature mortality associated with mental health problems across life-span of the person.

3.1.2 To enhance understanding of mental health in the country.

3.1.3 To strengthen the leadership in the mental health sector at the national, state and district levels.

3.2 Objectives

3.2.1 To provide universal access to mental health care.

3.2.2 To increase access to and utilization of comprehensive mental health services (including prevention services, treatment and care and support services) by persons with mental health problems.

3.2.3 To increase access to mental health services for vulnerable groups including homeless person(s), person(s) in remote areas, difficult terrains, educationally/socially/economically deprived sections.

3.2.4 To reduce prevalence and impact of six factors associated with mental health problems.

3.2.5 To reduce risk and incidence of suicide and attempted suicide.

3.2.6 To ensure respect for rights and protection from harm of person(s) with mental health problems.

3.2.7 To reduce stigma associated with mental health problems.

3.2.8 To enhance availability and equitable distribution of skilled human resources for mental health.

3.2.9 To progressively enhance financial allocation and improve utilization for mental health promotion and care.

3.2.10 To identify and address the social, biological and psychological determinants of mental health problems and to provide appropriate interventions.

4. Cross Cutting Issues

Mental health is characterized by cross cutting issues that have a far reaching impact on the fulfillment of goals and objectives spelt out as policy strategies and need to be addressed through efforts across society.

4.1 Stigma

- Persons with mental health problems face stigma and discrimination in many ways. Families are frequently unwilling to recognize the presence of illness; even where recognized, families, parents and others care-givers may sometimes be reluctant or afraid to seek professional help. Absence of available, effective and affordable services is a major barrier in large parts of the country. There is a widespread lack of knowledge on the nature and prevalence of mental health problems including mental illness. This lack of knowledge is often accompanied by fear and even hostility towards those with mental health problems, due to which such persons face exclusion from society.
- Government, opinion-makers, media and community leaders should encourage discussions for better understanding of the nature of mental health problems. There is a need for compassion and responsibility in our interaction with persons affected with mental health problems instead of stigmatizing such persons.

4.2 Rights-based approach

- Violation of their rights is a common reality for persons with mental health problems. The design and implementation of policies, programs and services for mental health problems persons with mental health problems should therefore be based on a rights-based perspective. Respecting the rights of persons with mental health problems will reduce stigmatizing and discriminatory behaviors. This policy envisages that there be more discussions in public space on Rights of persons with mental health problems and in design of a system that upholds their rights.

4.3 Vulnerable populations

- Mental health services and related activities should take into account the special condition and needs of vulnerable populations who bear a disproportionate and higher burden of mental health problems. Vulnerable populations may include inter alia, children (both school going and out of school), women, economically and socially deprived, older persons and persons with physical disabilities. It should be ensured that there is no discrimination against vulnerable populations in the provision of services. Conditions that increase vulnerability and need to be addressed to improve mental health are discussed below:

4.3.1 Poverty

Poverty and mental health are inextricably linked in a negative vicious cycle. Persons from lower-socioeconomic groups are more vulnerable to mental health problems. Out-of-pocket health spending to access mental health services and lost productivity due to disability can also lead to poverty.

4.3.2 Homelessness

There are several linkages between homelessness and mental ill health. Homelessness can occur as an adverse consequence of a mental health problem. Persons could either be abandoned by a poorly resourced, helpless or uncaring family or wander away in the absence of accessible and appropriate mental health care. Conversely, the stress of living on the streets and sleeping rough can contribute to the risk of developing mental health problems.

Person(s) with mental health problems with high support needs and no caregivers either due to death or abandonment by family or caregiver) are especially vulnerable. In the absence of existing caregivers, there is almost no provision for care and support for these persons.

4.3.3 Persons Inside Custodial Institutions

Person(s) inside custodial institutions fall into different categories and frequently have multiple vulnerabilities. They include women and children in rescue homes, children in institutions under the Juvenile Justice Act, 2006 (as amended in 2011), people in beggars, homes, long stay homes under the Government and under trails and convicts in prisons. An important aspect to be kept in mind is the issue of deprivation of personal liberty in custodial care.

As with other forms of social disadvantage, the relationship between mental health problems and being in custody is directional. At present mental health services for these vulnerable groups are inadequate.

4.3.4 Orphaned Persons with Mental Illness (OPMI)

It is believed that 70 to 80% of the persons with mental disorders in India live with their families and this is true across all demographic and social variables. Once the existing caregivers are no more, there is no provision for home care and support of these persons. As a result, many of them languish till death due to starvation and lack of critical support systems like monitoring medicines, personal hygiene and food etc. Not all of them fall under category of poor, yet, those with high support needs—irrespective of rich or poor, are highly vulnerable due to their incapacity for self-care. This policy recognizes that needs of this category of persons with mental disorders have been neglected for a long time.

4.3.5 Children of Persons with Mental Health Problems

Children of persons with mental health problems are vulnerable and their needs have not been adequately addressed. They are likely to be exposed to a range of adversities including, but not limited to, poor prenatal care, disruption in parenting and schooling and increasing poverty.

4.3.6 Elderly Caregivers

Elderly caregivers whose own physical and mental health care needs are high vulnerable. Unmet needs have a negative impact on their lives as well as the lives of those for who they provide care. There has been little policy or service delivery action to meet the needs of such elderly caregivers. There could be other vulnerable caregivers such as adolescents, single person responsible for livelihood as well as care giving, and many such others.

MENTAL HEALTH TEAM

Mental health problems can be caused by physical, mental or social conditions. A physical or mental illness past experiences, difficult relationships, stress, unemployment drug and alcohol problems can also play a part. So, a lot of different skills are needed so deal these symptoms. No single professional, however well trained, can possibly exert all these skills. That is why different mental health professionals work in teams. The team members include psychiatrist, general physician, clinical psychologist, psychiatric social workers, mental health nurse, nurse assistant, occupational, educational, art, musical, psychotherapist, play and speech therapist, chaplain, dietician and other support staff.

1. Psychiatrist

Qualification: PG in Psychiatry

- *Role:* Diagnosis and treatment.
  - Serves as a leader.
  - Prescribes various therapies and medications.
  - Counseling and researcher.

2. General Physician

Qualification: MBBS/MD

- *Role:* First point of contact for mental ill patients.
  - Provides advice and support.
  - Follow-up and reference.

3. Clinical Psychologists

Qualification: MA/MSc in Clinical Psychology

- *Role:* Administering/Psychological treatment.
  - Counseling.
  - Research.

4. Mental Health Nurse

Qualification: Dip/BSc/MSc/PhD

- *Role:* Nursing Assessment and diagnosis
  - Providing holistic nursing care.
  - Conducting counseling and psychotherapy and psychodrama.
  - Psychoeducation.
  - Research.

5. Psychiatric Social Workers

Qualification: MSW/PhD

- *Role:* Providing advice, counseling in community.
  - Referral services.
  - Acts as a reference between health team and community.

6. Nurse Assistant/Technician

Qualification: SSLC/PUC/ANM

- *Role:* Assist the mental health team in maintaining therapeutic environment.

7. Occupational Therapist

Qualification: Graduate/PG in Occupational Therapy.

- *Role:* Teaching new coping strategies.
  - Bridging hospital and community setting.
  - Providing different therapies and Rehabilitation.

8. Educational Therapist

Qualification: BA/MA in Education

- *Role:* Assessing and monitoring teaching learning.
  - Conducting continuing education program.
  - Identifying educational problems in learning.

9. Art Therapist

Qualification: BA/MA in Art Therapy.

- *Role:* Use of visual art as a medium for healing.
  - Exploring intense emotion and thoughts of clients.
  - Engagement in a creative personal process.

10. Counseling

Qualification: Graduation in Counseling.

- *Role:* Counseling offers counseling, to those in need.
  - Works in hospital and Community settings.
  - Counselors have people referred to them by GPs, social workers and people themselves.

11. Musical Therapist

Qualification: MA/M Phil/PhD in music.

- *Role:* Focuses on the expression of self through music.
  - Promotes improvement in memory, attention, and concentration and provides an opportunity for the individual to take pride in his achievement.

12. Chaplain

Qualification: Graduation in Theology.

- *Role:* Identification of spiritual needs of mentally ill.
  - Providing spiritual support.
  - Acts as counselors.
  - Providing holistic care.

13. Play Therapist

- *Role:* Observing the patients behavior, offend and communication.
  - Recording and reporting patient's thoughts, feelings, fantasies and resolving emotional conflicts through play.
  - Use of play as a therapy.

14. ECT Technician

Qualification: PUC

- *Role:* Helping the doctor in administrating ECT and post procedure.
  - Identifying and reporting side effects and complications of ECT.

15. Support Workers/Befrienders

- Support workers act as a part of mental health team.
- Supervision and monitoring of mental health activities in community.

Nature and Scope of Mental Health Nursing

- Psychiatric nursing/mental health nursing is the specialty of nursing that cares for people of all ages with mental illness or mental distress. Psychiatric and mental health nurses are trained in psychological therapies, building a therapeutic alliance, dealing with challenging behavior and administration of psychotropic medication. Mental health nursing utilizes nursing models, uses nursing care plans and seeks to care for a whole person in a holistic way. However, the emphasis of mental health nursing is on the development of a therapeutic interpersonal relationship. This involves the nurse and client in care in a positive and collaborative way that will empower the client to draw his or her inner and resources in addition to any other treatment.
- Psychiatric mental health nursing is a specialized area of nursing practice committed to promoting mental health through the assessment, diagnosis and treatment of human responses to mental health problems and psychiatric disorders. Psychiatric mental health nursing, a core mental health profession, employs a purposeful use of self as its art and a wide range of nursing, psychosocial and neurobiological theories and research evidence as its science. Psychiatric mental health nurses provide comprehensive, client-centered mental health and psychiatric care and outcome evaluation in a variety of settings across the entire continuum of care. Essential components of this speciality practice include health and wellness, prevention of mental health problems and care and treatment of persons with psychiatric disorders.
- *Primary Mental Health Nursing Practice:* It is to provide primary mental health care to patients seeking mental health services in a wide range of delivery settings. This involves overall health promotion, universal, selective and preventive interventions, general health teaching, health screening and appropriate referral for treatment of general or complex health problems including psychiatric rehabilitation.

Psychiatric Mental Health Registered Nurse

A psychiatric mental health registered nurse is a registered nurse who demonstrates competence, including specialized knowledge, skills and attitudes, obtained through education or experience, in caring for persons with mental health issues, mental health problems and psychiatric disorders.

Psychiatric mental health registered nursing practice is characterized by the use of the nursing process with persons with actual or potential mental health problems or psychiatric disorders to promote and foster health and safety, assess daily function and assist persons to regain or improve their coping abilities, maximize strength and prevent further disability. Data collection at the point of contact involves observational and investigative activities, which are guided by nursing knowledge of human behavior and the principles of the psychiatric interviewing process.

Psychiatric Mental Health Advanced Practice Registered Nurse

This degrees nurse demonstrates a greater depth and breadth of knowledge, a greater synthesis of data, increased complexity of skills and interventions and significant role of autonomy.

Collaborative Psychiatric Nursing Practice

Psychiatric mental health nurses will collaborate with other health team members for sharing experiences, insights and coordinated care knowledge. This helps for the early recovering of the patient.

Clinical Nurse Specialist

Psychiatric clinical nurse specialist is a postgraduate in specialty. She delivers in the diagnosis and treatment of illness and the delivery of evidence-based nursing interventions by applying theories of human behavior. Other function includes clinical leadership, education to the staff nurses and research.

Psychotherapist

Psychotherapist interventions include all generally accepted methods of brief or long-term therapy. Specifically including individual therapy, group therapy, couple/marital therapy, family therapy being a broad array of therapy models including but not limited to insight oriented, and cognitive, behavioral and interpersonal therapies.

Psychiatric Nurse Case Manager

Case Management involves population specific nursing knowledge coupled with research, knowledge of the social and legal systems related to mental health and expertise to engage a wide range of services for the patient, regardless offsetting. She/he analyzes the barriers to care and intervenes to change or improve systems to mobilize therapeutic resources needed by the patient for maximum positive outcomes. Case management activities maybe with a single client or with a specific population such as the seriously and persistently mentally ill.

Psychiatric Nurse Educator

She is a master degree graduate, mainly focuses on planning and evaluating the curriculum. She involves in teaching–learning activities and research.

Psychiatric Nurse Consultation/Liaison Officer

Consultation–liaison activities take place in general health care arenas such as hospitals, extended care facilities, rehabilitation centers, schools, nursing homes and out-patient clinics. The role of the consultation liaison psychiatric mental health nurse focuses on providing mental health specialist consultation or direct care and psychiatric mental health nursing services.

Psychosocial Rehabilitation Nursing

This includes patient and their family caregivers and care is provided in a comprehensive, holistic way. It involves interdisciplinary as well as multidisciplinary health team.

Psychiatric Emergency Nursing/Crisis Intervention Nursing

Crisis intervention units maybe found in the emergency department of a general or psychiatric hospital or within centers in the community. In crisis, clients demonstrate severe symptoms and require a high intensity of nursing services.

Child Psychiatric Nursing

Child Psychiatric nursing deals with prevention, diagnosis, treatment and rehabilitation of mental and emotional disorders in children. The child psychiatric nurse specialist plays an important role in identifying, treatment and in psychosocial rehabilitation of child.

Community Mental Health Nursing

Community mental health nursing is a treatment philosophy based on social theory of psychiatric care that advocates a comprehensive range of mental health services to be readily accessible to all members of the community. It involves the care of homeless psychiatric client of community living.

Neuropsychiatric Nursing

Neurological disorders influence the behavior of patients either as a result of trauma or due to pathophysiological change of the brain. The neuropsychiatric nurse provides care to patients with severe or usually persistent behavioral manifestations of illness. Neurological, psychiatric, cognitive and functional assessments are done by the neuropsychiatric nurse. Nursing interventions are implemented to improve the functional ability and promote independence.

De-addiction Nursing

The psychiatric nurse with specialization in de-addictions carries out the assessment of deaddicts plans and prepares for nursing therapeutic interventions to make the client independent.

Gerontological and Geriatric Psychiatric Nursing

Geriatric psychiatric nurse provides care to those old people who have been retired from service, who have financial problems and ailing from noncurable diseases. She helps them to cope with life.

Psychiatric Telehealth Nursing

The practice of telehealth is the removal of time and distance barriers for the delivery of health care services and related health care activities through telecommunication technologies. It is an expanded means of communication that promotes access to health care. The psychiatric mental health nurse may utilize electronic means of communication such as telephone consultation, computers, electronic mail, image transmission and interactive video sessions to establish and maintain therapeutic relationships with clients by creating an alternative sense of the nursing presence that may or may not occur in 'real time'. Psychiatric mental health nursing care in telehealth incorporates practice and clinical guidelines that are based on empirical evidence and professional consensus.

Concepts of Normal and Abnormal Behavior

Perceptions of normality and abnormality differ between cultures, subcultures, individuals and change over time. For example, the extreme selfishness of a child is accepted as normal; in an adult such selfishness would be regarded as abnormal.

Normality

From the above context, normality means different things to different people at different times in different settings. If as a soldier, we shoot someone in wartimes we may receive a medal, if we shoot someone in peacetime, we will be put in jail. Therefore, we have to look at emotional/ feelings and behavior in the context in which they occur.

Abnormality

Defining abnormality is as different as defining normality. The following are the criteria often used in defining abnormality.

Deviation from Social Norms

Every society has certain standards (or norms) of behavior that it expects. Such things as the way we dress, politeness, use of language are subject to certain rules (often unwritten). However, social norms are different in different societies. For example, eating in public during the day at Ramadan would be regarded as a deviation in the United Emirates and would be punished. It would not be a deviation in a non-Islamic country. Eye contact between a superior and inferior is regarded as a deviation in some parts of the continent of Asia. Avoiding eye contact is regarded as a sign of guilt and hide. Ideas of what is normal and abnormal also change over time. At one time, adult boy or a girl living without marriage in India was considered as abnormal, but now, most of the cases of 'Live in relationships' is accepted and legally, homosexuals can marry, which is considered as a normal.

Maladaptive Behavior

Behavior is abnormal if it is Maladaptive, i.e. it has an adverse effect on the well-being of the individual or society. For example, a person who is frightened of crowds that he cannot leave his house or persons who drinks so much alcohol that he cannot live a normal life. Individuals who are violent and aggressive have a bad effect on society. They may vent out their aggression on the roads and cause traffic accidents or indulge in crime.

Personal Distress

In this criteria one would look at the person's subjective (internal) feelings rather than their (external) behavior. They may feel unhappy, depressed and agitated. They maybe unable to concentrate or sleep. They may hide these feelings from others and their behavior may appear normal. There maybe the 'smiling depression' where an individual is very depressed but hides that depression from family and friends. Often the first that his family knows of the depression is when he attempts to kill himself.

Models of Abnormality

The Lay Model

People are labeled as 'looney' when they are confusing, depressing and frightening others. This is often framed as bad nerve or nervousness. It overlaps with ideas of mental illness. The lay model also exaggerates the connection between violence and schizophrenia. It is said that a person who diagnosed with schizophrenia is more likely to commit a violent crime than a normal person.

The Legal Model

Nowadays, experts in legal model team have a psychiatric expert because of two reasons:
- The absence of precise legal definition of mental illness and
- Psychiatric opinion in court is viewed as expert view on the presence or absence of four legal categories: mental illness, mental impairment, severe mental impairment and psychopathic disorder.

The Psychological Model

Buss (1996) outlines three main psychological concepts on normality and abnormality:
- *Statistical concept:* Frequently occurring behaviors in a population are normal and thus infrequently occurring behaviors are not normal.
- *Concept of ideal:* When a person's consciousness dominates the unconsciousness (psychoanalytic) and who can fulfill their human potential (humanistic).
- *Specific Behavior Concept:* Trying to define abnormality explicitly through behavioral view, but still it reflects the value system which has relationship with culture and time.
  - The issues on normality vs abnormality are not going to be over soon because of the overlapping and lacking of definite definitions and criteria.

Medical Model/Biological Model

Abnormal behavior is caused by biological factors, especially involving genetic material and the brain. Changes in anatomical structure and biochemical transmission in the brain causes abnormal behavior. The brain structures most relevant to abnormal behavior include the thalamus, reticular activating system, limbic system and cerebrum. Imbalances in neurotransmitters are highly associated with mental disorders. Genetics also plays an important role in abnormal behavior.

2 Principles and Concepts of Mental Health Nursing

PRINCIPLES OF MENTAL HEALTH NURSING PRACTICE

Conceptual models and nurse

- Existential models
- Psychoanalytical models
- Behavioral models
- Interpersonal models

CLASSIFICATION OF MENTAL DISORDERS

A classification is a way of seeing the world at a point in time. Classification of mental disorders gives a broad description of various types, or categories of abnormal behavior. Mental disorders are broadly classified on the basis of international classification of disease (ICD-10), diagnose and statistical manual classification (DSM-IVR) and research diagnostic criteria (RDC). This classification helps the health worker to classify, plan and diagnose and helps in research.

ICD-10 CLASSIFICATION OF MENTAL AND BEHAVIORAL DISORDERS

World Health Organization in 2006 published ICD-10 here, alpha numeric code, based on a single letter followed by two numbers at the three character level (A00-Z99) has been adopted in ICD-10. ICD-10 as a whole is designed to be a central related classification. The 'family' also includes classification that cover information on important medical or health implication, e.g. 'The classification of impairment, disabilities and handicaps, the classification of procedures in medicine, and the classification of reasons for encounter between clients and health workers'.

LIST OF CATEGORIES

F00-F09 Organic, Including Symptomatic, Mental Disorders

- F00: Dementia in Alzheimer's disease.
- F00: 1 Dementia in Alzheimer's disease with early onset.
- F00: 2 Dementia in Alzheimer's with late onset.
- F00: 3 Dementia in Alzheimer's disease, atypical or mixed type.
- F00: 4 Dementia in Alzheimer's disease, unspecified.
- F01: Vascular dementia: unspecified.

F01: 0 Vascular Dementia of Acute Onset

- F01: 1 Multi infarct dementia.
- F01: 2 Subcortical vascular dementia.
- F01: 3 Mixed cortical and subcortical vascular dementia.
- F01: 8 Other vascular dementia.
- F01: 9 Vascular dementia, unspecified.
- F02: Dementia in other disease classified elsewhere.

F02: 0 Dementia in Pick's Disease

- F02: 1 Dementia in Creutzfeldt-Zakob disease.
- F02: 2 Dementia in Huntigton's disease.
- F02: 3 Demetia in Parkinson's disease.
- F02: 4 Dementia in HIV disease.
- F02: 8 Dementia in other specified disease classified elsewhere.

F03: Unspecified Dementia

A fifth character maybe added to specific dementia in F00-03 as follows:

- X0: Without additional symptoms.
- X1: Other symptoms, predominantly delusional.
- X2: Other symptoms, predominantly hallucinatory.
- X3: Other symptoms, predominantly depressive.
- X4: Other mixed symptoms.

F04: Organic Amnesic Syndrome, not Induced by Alcohol and Other Psychoactive Substances

F05: Delirium, not Induced by Alcohol and Other Psychoactive Substances

- F05: 0 Delirium, not superimposed on dementia, so described.
- F05: 1 Delirium, superimposed on dementia.
- F05: 8 Other delirium.
- F05: 9 Delirium, unspecified.

F06: Other Mental Disorders due to Brain Damage and Dysfunction and due to Physical Disease

- F06: 0 Organic hallucinosis.
- F06: 1 Organic catatonic disorder.
- F06: 2 Organic delusional (Schizophernia-like) disorder.
- F06: 3 Organic mood (affective) disorder.
- F06: 30 Organic manic disorder.
- F06: 31 Organic dipolar affective disorder.
- F06: 32 Organic depressive disorder.
- F06: 33 Organic mixed affective disorder.
- F06: 4 Organic anxiety disorder.
- F06: 5 Organic dissociative disorder.
- F06: 6 Organic emotionally labile (asthenic) disorder.

- F06: 7 Mild cognitive disorder.
- F06: 8 Other specified mental disorder due to brain damage and dysfunction and due to physical diseases.
- F06: 9 Unspecified mental disorder due to brain damage and dysfunction and due to physical diseases.
- F07: Personality and behavioral disorders due to brain disease, damage and dysfunction.
- F07: Organic personality disorder.
- F07: 1 Postencephalitic syndrome.
- F07: 2 Postconcussional syndrome.
- F07: 8 Other organic personality and behavioral disorders due to brain disease, damage and dysfunction.
- F07: 9 Unspecified organic personality and behavioral disorders due to brain disease, damage and dysfunction.
- F09: Unspecified organic or symptomatic mental disorder.

F10–F19: Mental and Behavioral Disorder due to Psychoactive Substance Use

- F10: Mental and behavioral disorders due to use of alcohol.
- F11: Mental and behavioral disorders due to use of opioids.
- F12: Mental and behavioral disorders due to use of cannabinoids.
- F13: Mental and behavioral disorders due to use of sedatives or hypnotics.
- F14: Mental and behavioral disorders due to use of cocaine.
- F15: Mental and behavioral disorders due to use of other stimulants, including caffeine.
- F16: Mental and behavioral disorders due to use of hallucinogens.
- F17: Mental and behavioral disorders due to use of tobacco.
- F18: Mental and behavioral due to use of volatile solvents.
- F19: Mental and behavioral disorder due to multiple drug use and use of other psychoactive substances.

F20–F29: Schizophrenia, Schizotypal and Delusional Disorders F20 Schizophrenia

- F20.0: Paranoid schizophrenia.
- F20.1: Hebephrenic schizophrenia.
- F20.2: Catatonic schizophrenia.
- F20.3: Undifferentiated schizophrenia.
- F20.4: Postschizophrenia depression.
- F20.5: Residual schizophrenia.
- F20.6: Simple schizophrenia.
- F20.8: Other schizophrenia.
- F20.9: Schizophrenia, unspecified.

F21: Schizotypal Disorders

- F22: Persistent delusional disorders.
- F22.0: Delusional disorder.
- F22.8: Other persistent and delusional disorders.
- F22.9: Persistent delusional disorder, unspecified.

F23: Acute and Transient Psychotic Disorder

- F23.0: Acute polymorphic psychotic disorder without symptoms of schizophrenia.
- F23.1: Acute polymorphic psychotic disorder with symptoms of schizophrenia.
- F23.2: Acute schizophrenia like psychotic disorders.
- F23.3: Other acute predominantly delusional psychotic disorder.
- F23.8: Other acute and transient psychotic disorders.
- F23.9: Acute and transient psychotic disorders unspecified.

F24: Induced Delusional Disorder

F25: Schizoaffective Disorders

- F25.0: Schizoaffective disorder, manic type.
- F25.1: Schizoaffective disorder depressive type.
- F25.2: Schizoaffective disorder mixed type.
- F25.8: Other schizoaffective disorder.
- F25.9: Schizoaffective disorder, unspecified.
- F28: Other nonorganic psychotic disorders.
- F29: Unspecified nonorganic psychotic.
- F30–F39: Mood (affective) disorders.

F30: Manic Episode

- F30.0: Mania without psychotic symptoms.
- F30.1: Mania with psychotic symptoms.
- F30.2: Mania with psychotic symptoms.
- F30.8: Other manic episodes.
- F30.9: Manic episode unspecified.

F31: Bipolar Affective Disorder

- F31.0: Bipolar affective disorder, current episode hypomanic.
- F31.1: Bipolar affective disorder, current episode manic without psychotic symptoms.
- F31.2: Bipolar affective disorder, current episode manic with psychotic symptoms.
- F31.3: Bipolar affective disorder, current episode mild or moderate depression.
- F31.30: Without somatic syndrome.
- F31.31: With somatic syndrome.
- F31.4: Bipolar affective disorder, current episode severe depression without psychotic symptoms.
- F31.5: Bipolar affective disorder, current episode severe depression with psychotic symptoms.
- F31.6: Bipolar affective disorder, current episode mixed.
- F31.7: Bipolar affective disorder, currently in remission.
- F31.8: Other bipolar affective disorders.
- F31.9: Bipolar affective disorder, unspecified.

F32: Depression Episode

- F32.0: Mild depressive episode.
- F32.00: Without somatic syndrome.

- F32.01: With somatic syndrome.
- F31.1: Moderate depressive episode.
- F31.10: Without somatic syndrome.
- F31.11: With somatic syndrome.
- F32.2: Severe depressive episode without psychotic symptoms.
- F32.3: Severe depressive episode with psychotic symptoms.
- F32.8: Other depressive episodes.
- F32.9: Depressive episode, unspecified.

F33: Recurrent Depressive Disorder

- F33.0: Recurrent depressive disorder, current episode mild.
- F33.00: Without somatic syndrome.
- F33.01: With somatic syndrome.
- F33.1: Recurrent depressive disorder, current episode moderate.
- F33.10: Without somatic syndrome.
- F33.11: With somatic syndrome.
- F33.2: Recurrent depressive disorder, current episode severe without psychotic symptoms.
- F33.3: Recurrent depressive disorder, current episode severe with psychotic symptoms.
- F33.4: Recurrent depressive disorder, currently in remission.
- F33.8: Other recurrent depressive disorders.
- F33.9: Recurrent depressive disorder, unspecified.

F34: Persistent Mood (Affective) Disorders

- F34.0: Cryclothymia
- F34.1: Dysthymia
- F34.8: Other persistent mood (affective) disorders.
- F34.9: Persistent mood (affective) disorder, unspecified.

F38: Other Mood (Affective) Disorders

- F38.0: Other single mood (affective) disorders.
- F38.00: Mixed affective episode.
- F38.1: Other recurrent mood (affective) disorders.
- F38.10: Recurrent brief depressive disorders.
- F38.8: Other specified mood (affective) disorders.
- F39: Unspecified mood (affective) disorders.

F10–F48: Neurotic, Stress Related and Somatoform Disorders

- F40: Phobic anxiety disorders.
- F40.0: Agoraphobia.
- F40.00: Without panic disorder.
- F40.01: With panic disorder.
- F40.1: Social phobias.
- F40.2: Specific (isolated) phobias.
- F40.8: Other phobic anxiety disorders.
- F40.9: Phobic anxiety disorders, unspecified.

F41: Other Anxiety Disorders

- F41.0: Panic disorders (episodic paroxysmal anxiety).
- F41.1: Generalized anxiety disorder.
- F41.2: Mixed anxiety and depressive disorder.
- F41.3: Other mixed anxiety disorder.
- F41.8: Other specified anxiety disorder.
- F41.9: Anxiety disorders, unspecified.

F44: Dissociative (Conversion) Disorders

- F44.0: Dissociative amnesia.
- F44.1: Dissociative fugue.
- F44.2: Dissociative stupor.
- F44.3: Trance and possession disorders.
- F44.4: Dissociative motor disorder.
- F44.5: Dissociative convulsions.
- F44.6: Dissociative anesthesia and sensory loss.
- F44.7: Mixed dissociative (conversion) disorder.
- F44.8: Other dissociative (conversion) disorder.
- F44.80: Ganser's syndrome.
- F44.81: Multiple personality disorder.
- F44.82: Transient dissociative (conversion) disorders occurring childhood and adolescence.
- F44.88: Other specified dissociative (conversion) unspecified.
- F44.9: Dissociative (conversion) disorders, unspecified.

F45: Somatoform Disorders

- F45.0: Somatization disorders.
- F45.1: Undifferentiated somatoform disorders.
- F45.2: Hypochondriacal disorder.
- F45.3: Somatoform autonomic dysfunction.
- F45.30: Heart and cardiovascular system.
- F45.31: Upper gastrointestinal tract.
- F45.32: Lower gastrointestinal tract.
- F45.33: Respiratory system.
- F45.34: Genitourinary system.
- F45.38: Other organ or system.
- F45.4: Persistent somatoform pain disorders.
- F45.8: Other somatoform disorders.
- F45.9: Somatoform disorder, unspecified.

F48: Other Neurotic Disorders

- F48.0: Neurasthenia.
- F48.1: Depersonalization derealization syndrome.

- F48.8: Other specified neurotic disorders.
- F48.9: Neurotic disorder, unspecified.

F50–F59: Behavioral Syndrome Associated with Physiological Disturbances and Physical Factors

- F50: Eating disorders.
- F50.0: Anorexia nervosa.
- F50.1: Atypical anorexia nervosa.
- F50.2: Bulimia nervosa.
- F50.3: Atypical bulimia nevosa.
- F50.4: Overeating associated with other psychological disturbances.
- F50.5: Vomiting associated with other psychological disturbances.
- F50.8: Other eating disorders.
- F50.9: Eating disorder, unspecified.

F51: Nonorganic Sleep Disorders

- F51.0: Nonorganic insomnia.
- F51.1: Nonorganic hypersomnia.
- F51.2: Nonorganic disorder of the sleep wake schedule.
- F51.3: Sleep walking (somnabulism).
- F51.4: Sleep terrors (night terrors).
- F51.5: Nightmares.
- F51.8: Other nonorganic sleep disorders.
- F51.9: Nonorganic sleep disorders, unspecified.

F52: Sexual Dysfunction, not Caused by Organic Disorder or Disease

- F52.0: Lack or loss of sexual desire.
- F52.1: Sexual aversion and lack of sexual enjoyment.
- F52.10: Sexual aversion.
- F52.11: Lack of sexual enjoyment.
- F52.2: Failure of genital response.
- F52.3: Orgasmic dysfunction.
- F52.4: Premature ejaculation.
- F52.5: Nonorganic veginismus.
- F52.6: Nonorganic dysparenmia.
- F52.7: Excessive sexual drive.
- F52.8: Other sexual dysfunction, not caused by orgnic disorders or disease.
- F52.9: Unspecified sexual dysfunction, not caused by organic disorders or disease.

F53: Mental and Behavioral Disorders Associated with the Puerperium not Elsewhere Classified

- F53.0: Mild mental and behavioral disorders associated with the puerperium, not elsewhere classified.
- F53.1: Severe mental and behavioral disorders associated with the puerperium, not elsewhere classified.

- F53.8: Other mental and behavioral disorders associated with the puerperium, not elsewhere classified.
- F53.9: Puerperal mental disorder unspecified.

F54: Psychological and Behavioral Factors Associated with Disorders or Disease Classified Elsewhere

F55: Abuse of Non-dependence-producing Substances

- F55.0: Antidepressants.
- F55.1: Laxatives.
- F55.2: Analgesics.
- F55.3: Antacids.
- F55.4: Vitamins.
- F55.5: Steroids or hormones.
- F55.6: Specific herbal or folk remedies.
- F55.8: Other substances that do not produce dependence.
- F55.9: Unspecified.
- F59: Unspecified behavioral syndrome associated with physiological disturbances and physical factors.

F60–F69: Disorders of Adult Personality and Behavior

- F60: Specific personality disorder.
- F60.0: Paranoid personality disorder.
- F60.1: Schizoid personality disorder.
- F60.2: Dissocial personality disorder.
- F60.3: Emotionally unstable personality disorder.
- F60.30: Impulsive type.
- F60.31: Borderline type.
- F60.4: Histrionic personality disorder.
- F60.5: Anankastic personality disorder.
- F60.6: Anxious (avoidant) personality disorder.
- F60.7: Dependent personality disorder.
- F60.8: Other specific personality disorder.
- F60.9: Personality disorder, unspecified.

F61: Mixed and Other Personality Disorder

- F61.0: Mixed personality disorder.
- F61.1: Troublesome personality disorder.
- F62: Enduring personality changes, not attributable to brain damage and disease.
- F62.0: Enduring personality changes after catastrophic experience.
- F62.1: Enduring personality changes after physical illness.
- F62.8: Other enduring personality changes.
- F62.9: Enduring personality change, unspecified.

F63: Habit and Impulsive Disorders

- F63.0: Pathological gambling.
- F63.1: Pathological fire setting (pyromania).
- F63.2: Pathological stealing (kleptomania).
- F63.3: Trichotillomania.
- F63.8: Other habit and impulse disorders.
- F63.9: Habit and impulsive disorder, unspecified.

F64: Gender Identify Disorders

- F64.0: Trans-sexualism.
- F64.1: Dual-role transvestism.
- F64.2: Gender identify disorder of childhood.
- F64.8: Other gender identify disorder.
- F64.9: Gender identify disorder, unspecified.

F65: Disorders of Sexual Preference

- F65.0: Fetishism.
- F65.1: Fetishistic transvestism.
- F65.2: Exhibitionism.
- F65.3: Voyeurism.
- F65.4: Pedophilia.
- F65.5: Sadomasohism.
- F65.6: Multiple disorders of sexual preference.
- F65.8: Other disorders of sexual preference
- F65.9: Disorders of sexual preference, unspecified.

F66: Psychological and Behavioral Disorders Associated with Sexual Development and Orientation

- F66.0: Sexual maturation disorder.
- F66.1: Egodystonic sexual orientation.
- F66.2: Sexual relationship disorder.
- F66.8: Other psychosexual development disorders.
- F66.9: Psychosexual development disorder, unspecified.

A Fifth Character maybe used to be Indicated or Associated with:

- X0: Heterosexuality
- X1: Homosexuality
- X2: Bisexuality
- X8: Other, including prepubertal.

F68: Other Disorders of Adult Personality and Behavior

- F68.0: Elaboration of physical symptoms for psychological reasons.
- F68.1: Intentional production or feigning of symptoms or disabilities either physical, or psychological (factitious disorder)

- F68.8: Other specified disorders of adult personality and behavior.
- F69: Unspecified disorder of adult personality and behavior.

F70–F79: Mental Retardation

- F70: Mild mental retardation.
- F71: Moderate mental retardation.
- F72: Severe mental retardation.
- F73: Profound mental retardation.
- F78: Other mental retardation.
- F79: Unspecified mental retardation.

F80–F89: Disorders of Psychological Development

- F80: Specific development disorder of speech and language.
- F80.0: Specific speech articulation disorder.
- F80.1: Expressive language disorder.
- F80.2: Receptive language disorders.
- F80.3: Acquired aphasia with epilepsy (Landon-Kleffner syndrome)
- F80.8: Other development disorders of speech and language.
- F80.9: Development disorder of speech and language, unspecified.

F81: Specific Development Disorders of Scholastic Skills

- F81.0: Specific reading disorders.
- F81.1: Specific spelling disorder.
- F81.2: Specific disorder of arithmetical skills.
- F81.3: Mixed disorder of scholastic skills.
- F81.8: Other development disorder of scholastic skill.
- F81.9: Development disorder of scholastic skill, unspecified.

F82: Specific Development Disorder of Motor Function

F83: Mixed Specific Development Disorder

F84: Pervasive Development Disorder

- F84.0: Childhood autism.
- F84.1: Atypical autism.
- F84.2: Rett's syndrome.
- F84.3: Other childhood disintegrative disorder.
- F84.4: Overactive disorder disintegrative disorder retardation and stereotyped movement.
- F84.5: Asperger's syndrome.
- F84.8: Other pervasive development disorder.
- F84.9: Pervasive development disorder, unspecified.

F88: Other Disorder of Psychological Development

F89: Unspecified Disorder of Psychological Development

F90–F98: Behavioral and Emotional Disorder with Onset Usually Occurring in Childhood and Adolescence

F90: Hyperkinetic Disorder

- F90.0: Disturbance of activity and attention.
- F90.1: Hyperkinetic conduct disorder.
- F90.8: Other hyperkinetic disorders.
- F90.9: Hyperkinetic disorder, unspecified.

F91: Conduct Disorder

- F91.0: Conduct disorder confined to the family context.
- F91.1: Unsocialized conduct disorder.
- F91.2: Socialized conduct disorder.
- F91.3: Oppositional defiant disorder.
- F91.8: Other conduct disorder.
- F91.9: Conduct disorders, unspecified.

F92: Mixed Disorders of Conduct and Emotions

- F92.0: Depressive conduct disorder.
- F92.8: Other mixed disorder of conduct and emotions.
- F92.9: Mixed disorder of conduct and emotions, unspecified.

F93: Emotional Disorders with Onset Specific to Childhood

- F93.0: Separation anxiety disorder of childhood.
- F93.1: Mobic anxiety disorder of childhood.
- F93.2: Social anxiety disorder of childhood.
- F93.3: Sibling rivalry disorder.
- F93.8: Other childhood emotional disorder.
- F93.9: Childhood emotional disorder, unspecified.

F94: Disorders of Social Functioning with Onset Specific to Childhood and Adolescence

- F94.0: Elective mutism.
- F94.1: Reactive attachment disorder of childhood.
- F94.2: Disinhibited attachment disorder of childhood.
- F94.8: Other childhood disorders of social functioning.
- F94.9: Childhood disorder of social functioning, unspecified.

F95: TIC Disorder

- F95.0: Transient tic disorder.
- F95.1: Chronic motor or vocal tic disorder.
- F95.2: Combined vocal and multiple tic disorder.
- F95.8: Other tic disorder.
- F95.9: Tic disorder, unspecified.

F98: Other Behavioral and Emotional Disorder with Onset Usually Occurring in Childhood and Adolescence

- F98.0: Nonorganic enuresis.
- F98.1: Nonorganic encopresis.
- F98.2: Feeding disorder of infancy and childhood.
- F98.3: Pica of infancy and childhood.
- F98.4: Stereotyped movement disorder.
- F98.5: Stuttering (stammeing).
- F98.6: Cluttering.
- F98.8: Other specified behavioral and emotional disorders with onset. Usually occurring in childhood and adolescence.
- F98.9: Unspecified behavioral and emotional disorder with onset usually occurring in childhood and adolescence.

F99: Unspecified Mental Disorder

F99: Mental Disorder, not Otherwise Specified

PERSONALITY DEVELOPMENT AND DEFENSE MECHANISM

Personality is the total of a person's internal and external pattern of adjustment to life, determined in part by genetically and by life experiences. According to Taylor, 'personality is the aggregate of the physical and mental qualities of the individual as these interact and function in characteristic fashion with his environment'. It is expressed as behavior. Behavior is a combination of physical, psychological and affective characteristic of an individual, differential from another person with his unique identify.

Personality is also expressed in the unique pattern of traits which characterize the individual. Traits are the characteristic of an individual like good natured, calm, shy, irritable, talkative; these are few examples of different traits, from the traits one is to sum up as smart.

Named on these traits, to sum up; an individual's personality is an aggregate conglomeration of decision they have made throughout their life and the memory of experiences to which these decision led. These are inherent natured, genetic and environmental factors that contribute to the development of personality according to the process of socialization. 'Personality also colors our values, belief, and expectation. Hereditary factors that contribute to personality development do so as a result of interactions with the particular social environment in which people live'.

FACTORS CONTRIBUTING TO PERSONALITY

According to Mayer, 'knowledge, skill and language are obviously acquired and represent important modification of behaviors'. Learned modifications in behavior are not passed on to children, they must be acquired by them through their own personal experience.

The probable consensus is that heredity and environment jointly affect personality development. The full potential of a person may or may not be achieved due to environment constraints and requirement, but the potential for development, both physically and psychologically is determined by the complex set of genes.

The factors affecting personality development are, heredity, culture, family, environment, social and situational conditions.

Theories of Personality Development

Each theory of personality tries to define the word 'personality' in coherence with the theory. The most common theories are:

- Dynamic theories
- Type and trait theories
- Learning and behavioral theories
- Humanistic theories

DYNAMIC THEORIES OF PERSONALITY

Dynamic theories search for the processes by which needs, motives and impulses often hidden from view interact to produce the individual behavior.

Sigmund Freud's Theory of Psychoanalysis

Sigmund Freud's psychoanalysis is both a theory of personality as well as psychotherapy. Psychoanalytic theory has three major aspects.

- A theory of structure of personality in which the ID, ego and super-ego are the principal parts (Fig. 2.1).
  - *ID:* It is the most primitive part and present in the infant. It is completely unconscious, arousal part of the personality that exist at birth, containing all of the basic biological drives. It operates pleasure principles.
  - *Ego:* The ID is managed by the ego. The ego consists of reality. It has the rules of behaving and thinking. The ego delays the satisfying ID motives and channels behavior into some more socially acceptance outlets by taking into account of what is possible in the real world.
  - *Superego:* It means over the self. It is fully 'conscious'. The superego consists mainly of prohibitions learned from parents and other authorities.

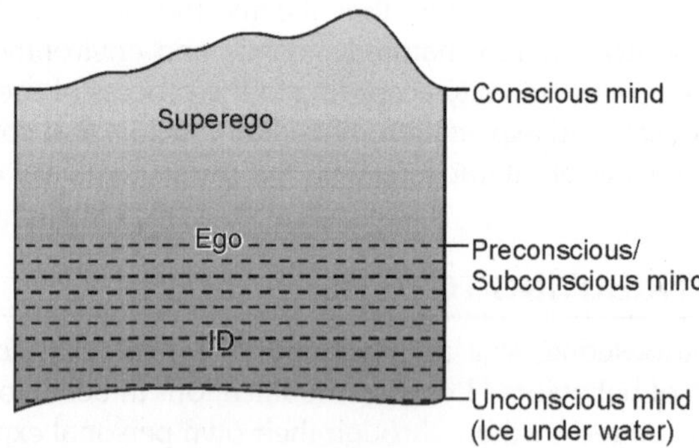

Fig. 2.1: Freud's topographical model

- A theory of personality dynamics in which conscious, preconscious, unconscious, motivation and ego-defense mechanism play a major role.
  - *Conscious level:* At this level, we are aware of certain phenomena around us and of certain thoughts.

   - *Preconscious level:* Here, we find memories and thoughts that are easily available with a moment's reflection. *Example:* what we had in dinner at last night.
   - *Unconscious level:* This level contains memories, thought and motives which cannot easily call up. The entire ID is unconscious, the ego and superego include material at all three levels of conscious.
- *Theory of psychosexual development:* According to Freud, the different motives and body regions influence the different stages of growth child. He believed that if a child's needs at one of psychosexual stages were either over satisfied or unsatisfied, fixation would take place.
   - *Oval stages (Birth–1 year):* In this stage, the infant obtains pleasure first by sucking and later by biting. Fixation at this stage may produce a critical, 'biting' personality.
   - *Anal stage (1–3 years):* Here toilet training takes place, it is the child's first interaction with authority.
   - *Phallic stage (3–5 years):* Genitals are the main organs of focus.
   - *Latency stage (6- puberty):* In this stage, children grow and develop intellectually, physically and socially but not boys, girls play only with girls and each thinks opposite sex is pretty awful.
   - *Genital stage (Adolescence and beyond):* Puberty marks the beginning when mature heterosexual interest appear. Identity and independence are establishment during this phase.

JUNG THEORY OF PERSONALITY

Carl Jung emphasized on people's future-oriented goals, hopes and plans. He credited each individual with collective unconscious and personal unconscious as an important aspect to understand an individual.

Collective unconscious is believed to be part of the unconscious mind that went beyond the personal experiences of the individual. Collective unconscious grows out of the past experiences of the human race which is store house of primitive fundamental images, impression and predispositions. He called these images, impression or predisposition as archetypes. Archetypes are more like subjective recreations that originated in our ancestors in response to certain universal experiences such as rising sun, rain and childbirth.

Personal unconscious: In addition to collective unconscious, each individual is credited with a personal unconscious which develops whenever the individual conscious experience are repressed.

ADLER'S THEORY OF PERSONALITY

Alfred Adler believed that people are forever struggling to overcome their feeling of inferiority people strive continually for superiority and mastery of the world.

- *Inferiority complex:* Adler believed that inferiority complex is the result of repeated failure to overcome weaknesses and inability to master or place excessive emphasis on some particular inferiority. He also stressed on the concepts of 'compensation' and 'over compensation' and pursuit of activities designed to make up for or to overcome inferiority.
- *Styles of life:* According to Adler, each individual has its own personal approach to living. Each of us develops a unique and lasting method of coping with life.

INTERPERSONAL THEORY OF HORNEY

- Karen Horney (1960) proposed that two major components of person is basic anxiety and basic hostility.
- *Basic anxiety:* It is a feeling that arises in childhood when the child feels helpless in a threating world. Loving and reliable parents can create a feeling of security, but erratic, indifferent or rejecting parents may increase the child sense of helplessness and vulnerability, this sets, the stages for basic anxiety.
- *Basic hostility:* It usually accompanies basic anxiety because the hostility (negatively) cannot be expressed directly to parents. It is typically represented, which only enhances for child's anxiety.
- Horney also proposed three different modes of social behavior. Horney believed that normal people use all three modes of social interaction at all times in a relatively balanced and flexible manner, adjusting their approach to situational demands. But disturbed neurotic individual allow one approach to dominate their social interaction and this rigidity gets into trouble.
  - *Moving towards other:* This involves excessive compliance obeying.
  - *Moving against other:* This behavior involves pursuing of satisfaction by dominating others.
  - *Moving away from other:* This is self-protection by withdrawal.

TYPE AND TRAIT THEORIES OF PERSONALITY

The Greek physician Hippocrates proposed his first type theory. The grouping or sets of types are called typologies. He grouped people into four temperament types.

- *Sanauine:* Cheerful, vigorous, confidently optimistic.
- *Melancholic:* Depressed, remorse, gloomy.
- *Choleric:* Hot tempered, angry.
- *Phlegmatic:* Slow moving, calm and unexcitable.

Trait Theory of Allport

Golden Allport described personality in three terms:

- *Cardinal traits:* These traits are dominating and influencing feature on the personality in such a way that it overshadows the influence of other traits in the same individual. These broad, highly influential traits are often called by names drawn from key historical figures.
  - *For example:* If you say someone is the, 'Jhansi lakhsmi bai' or Kittur Chennamma, it describes the cardinal trait of courage.
- *Central traits:* Central traits are those that might be mentioned in a careful letter of recommendation. These traits are not so prominent as cardinal traits.
  - *For example:* Confident, reliable and punctual etc.
- *Secondary traits:* These are the least generalized of the characteristics of the person, these are traits that are influential but only within a narrow range of situation.
  - *For example:* Like ice-cream.

EYSENCK'S CLASSIFICATION OF PERSONALITY

Hans J Eysenck, a German psychologist proposed that personality consist of four dimensions. They are introversion, extroversion, normal and mental deficiency (Fig. 2.2).

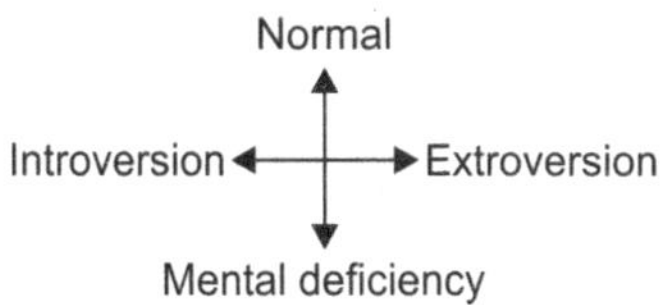

Fig. 2.2: Classification of personality

He observed that the person, who suffer from psychoticism is not fluent in speaking and can not adjust well to a new situation. His intention is not bold and his learning and memory power is not developed well. His level of aspiration is also low. Psychotics suffer from mental disorders. They are quite different from introvert and extrovert persons suffering from mental deficiency and are different from introverts and extroverts. They show different symptoms. In their case, psychological factors are main cause for symptoms. On the other hand, the man suffering from mental deficiency is dominantly influenced by heredity and nerve sensations. After getting three dimension of personality, Eysenck accepted intelligence as the fourth dimension.

LEARNING AND BEHAVIORAL THEORIES OF PERSONALITY

According to learning and behavioral theorist, personality is a learned phenomena. Learning theorists seek to understand people's behavior by studing their learning history, their current environment or both.

Dollard and Miller—Theory of Social Learning

The basic ideas behind these theories is that the behavior can be explained by means of basic learning principles derived from experiments.

Radical Behaviorism of Skinner/Reinforcement Theory

According to BF Skinner, personality is actually a collection of reinforced responses. He placed strong emphasis on behavior that can be observed. The theory deals with the processes by which reinforcement (reward) and punishment influence the likelihood of behavior.

Social Learning Theory

Social learning theory was proposed by Albert Bandura and Richard Walters. They focused on observational learning or imitation. They used concepts of internal cognitive processes to explain imitation and delayed performance. It is used to treat phobias and abnormal personality traits.

HUMANISTIC THEORY OF PERSONALITY

Humanistic theorists emphasized on self-concept of an individual.

Roger's Self Theory

Carl Roger's self theory extracted from client centered approach to psychotherapy and behavior. As children grow, parents and others react to their behavior. Sometimes in a positive manner and sometimes with disapproval. He believed that in mature, adjusted people, there is matching (congruence) between the total person and the self. With this feeling, well adjusted people can accept the full range of their experiences without distorting or avoiding them. They coined the term called 'phenomenal field'. It means the whole of experience. This is the individual subjective frame of reference and it may or may not correspond to external reality out of the phenomenal field, a self-concept gradually develop.

MASLOW'S THEORY OF SELF-ACTUALIZATION

Abraham Maslow (1967) emphasized on the development of the self. According to him, self-actualization is a goal that people are always striving to reach in life. These people live as a fully functioning person and fulfilled their basic potentialities.

ERIK ERIKSON'S PSYCHOSOCIAL DEVELOPMENT THEORY

Erikson believed that personality develops in series of stages. He also believed that the ego exists from birth and that behavior is not totally defensive. Research on Sioux Indians on a reservation, Erikson felt that development is determined by the interaction of the body (Indians genetic biological observation programming), mind (psychological) and cultural (ethos) influences. His developmental stages were based on his philosophy that the world gets bigger as we go along and failure is cumulative. He organized life into eight stages that extend from birth to death.

Infancy: Birth to 18 Months

- **Ego development outcome:** Trust vs mistrust.
- **Basic strength:** Drive and hope.
  - Erikson also referred to infancy as the oral sensory stages where the major emphasis is on the mother's positive and loving care for the child; with a big emphasis on visual contact and touch. If we pass successfully through this period of life, we will learn to trust that life is basically good or okay and have basic confidence in future. If we fail to experience trust and are constantly frustrated because one's needs are not met, we may end up with a deep-seated feeling of worthlessness and mistakes of the world in general.

Early Childhood: 18 Months to 3 Years

- **Ego development outcome:** Autonomy vs shame.
- **Basic strength:** self-control, courage and will.
  - During this stage, we learn to master skills for ourselves not only do we learn to walk, talk and feed ourselves but we are learning fine motor development as well as the much appreciated toilet training. Here, we have the opportunity to build self-esteem and autonomy as we gain role control over one's body and acquire new skills learning right from wrong. It is also during this stage, however, that we can be very vulnerable. If we are shamed in the process of toilet training or in learning other important skills, we may feel great shame and doubt of our capabilities and suffer low esteem as a result. The most significant relationship are with parents.

Play Age: 3 to 5 Years

During this period the child experiences a desire to copy the adults around us and take initiative in creating play situation. The child makes up its own stories with toys, phones and toy cars, playing out roles in a trial universe, experimenting with the blueprint what we believe it means to be an adult. The child also begins to use the word 'why' and in this stage the most significant relationship is with the basic family.

School Age: 6 to 12 Years

- **Ego development outcome:** Industry vs inferiority.
- **Basis strength:** Maturity and competence.
  - During this stage, often called in latency, capable of learning, creating and accomplishing numerous new skills and knowledge, thus developing a sense of industry. This is also a very social stage of development and if we experience unresolved feeling of inadequancy and inferiority among our peers, we can have serious problem in terms of competence and self-esteem.
  - As the world expands a bit, the child's most significant relationship is with the school and neighborhood. Parents are no longer the complete authorities they once were, although they are still important.

Adolescence: 12 to 18 years

- According to Erikson, development mostly depends upon what is done to us. From here onwards development depends primarily upon that what we do. And while adolescence is a stage at which we are neither a child nor an adult, life is definitely getting more complex as we attempt to find our own identity, struggle with social interactions and grapple with moral issues.
- In this stage, the task is to discover who are as individual separate from our family of origin and as member of a many of us go into a period of withdrawing from responsibilities which Erikson called a 'moratorium' and if we are unsuccessful in navigating this stage, we will experience role confusion and upheaval.
- A significant task for us is to establish a philosophy of life and in this process we tend to think in terms of ideal, which are conflict free, rather than reality, which is not, the problem is that we do not have much experience and find it easy to substitute ideals for experience. However, we can also develop strong devotion to friends and causes. It is no surprise that one most significant relationships are with per groups.

Young Adulthood: 18 to 35 Years

- **Ego development outcome:** Latancy and solidarity vs isolation.
- **Basic strength:** Affiliation and love.
  - In the initial stage of being an adult we seek one or more companions and love. As we try to find mutually satisfying relationship, primarily through marriage and friends, we generally also begin to start a family, through this age has been pushed back for many couples who today do not start their families until their late thirties. If negotiating this stage is successful, we can experience intimacy on a deep level if we are not successful, isolation and distance from others may' occur successful, and when we don't find it easy to create satisfying relationships, our world can begin to shrink as, in defense we can feel superior to others. Our significant relationships are with marital partners and friends.

Middle Adulthood: 35 to 55 or 65 Years

- **Ego development outcome:** Generativity vs self-absorption or stagnation.
- **Basic strengths:** Production and care.
  - In middle adulthood period, work is most crucial. Erikson observed that middle age is when we tend to be occupied with creative and meaningful work and with issues surrounding our family. Also, middle adulthood is when we can expect to 'be in change' the role we have longer envied. The significant task is to perpetuate culture and transmit values and philosophy of culture through the family (taming and teaching the children, off springs) and working to establish a stable environment. Strength comes through care of others and production of something that contributes to the betterment of society, which Erikson calls generativity, so when we are in this stage we often fear inactivity and meaning lessness.
  - As our children leave home, or our relationships or goals change, we maybe face major life changes the mid life crisis and struggle with finding new meaning and purposes. If we do not get through this stage successfully we can become self-observed and stagnate. Significant relationships are within the workplace, the community and the family.

Late Adulthood: 55 or 65 to Death

- **Ego development outcome:** Integrity vs despair.
- **Basic strengths:** Wisdom
  - Erikson felt that much of life is preparing for the middle adulthood stage and the last stage is recovering from it perhaps that is because as older adults we can often look back on our lives with happiness and are content, feeling fulfilled with a deep sense that life has meaning and we have made a contribution to life, a feeling Erikson calls 'integrity'. Our strength comes from a wisdom that the world is very large and we now have a detached concern for the whole of life. Accepting death as the completion of life.
  - On the other hand, some adults may reach this stage and despair at their experiences and perceived failure. They may fear death as reach struggle to find a purpose to their lives, wondering 'was the trip worth it'? Alternatively, they may feel they have all the answers (not like going back to adolescence) and end with a strong dogmatism that only their view has been corrected the significant relationship is with all of mankind 'my-kind'.

Strength and Weakness of Erikson Theory

Erik Erikson's psychosocial development theory has its strength; Judith Gardiner notes through the same development stages, he believes in basic psychosocial and biological differences in males and females. Gardiner further states the individual achieving maturity is always male. The male centered nature of Erikson's psychosocial development theories causes critics to question its current applicability to female identity development. One more question arises, whether individuals must really pass through one stage in order to get to the next.

PERSONALITY ASSESSMENT

Personality assessment is the measurement of personal characteristic. Assessment is an end result of gathering information intended to advance psychological theory and research and to increase the probability, wise decisions will be made and applied. Personality assessment is based on the assumption that much of the observable variability in behavior from one person to another results from differences in the extent to which individual possess particular underlying personal characteristic (traits). The assessment seeks to define these traits, to measure objectively and to relate them to socially significant aspects of behavior. A personality test is a questionnaire or other standardized instrument designed to reveal aspects of an individual character or psychological in the early 20th century and were intended to ease the process of personnel selection. Since these early efforts of this test, a wide variety of personality tests have been developed; notably the Myers Briggs Type Indicator (MBTI), the MMPI and a number of tests based on the five factor model of personality. Today, these tests are used in clinical settings, counseling, career planning and employee selection, and development.

Personality tests are objective and subjective in nature.

Objective Personality Tests

The objective methods, assessment is made objectively so that the results should be reliable and valid.

OBSERVATION

In observation, trained people look at the behavior in a controlled way. The proceedings are recorded and analyzed. In this, variables of situation can be manipulated to see the effect of changes on the responses of subject. Recorded behaviors are analyzed and interpreted to know the personality of the subject.

BEHAVIORAL/SITUATIONAL TESTS

- This test involves the presentation of an imaginary or hypothetical situation in front of the subject and he/she is asked to give possible reactions to the given situation, sometime subject's possible reply is blocked with modifications in situation and he is encouraged to give more replies.
- **For example:** Subject is asked to imagine that you are at home alone and some antisocial elements enter your home on that time what will you do? Let us assume that subject replies that he will ring to police for help. It can be blocked my modifying that, suppose the phone is out of order. In this way, every reply can be blocked to see the variety of replies subject can give. Subject's imagination of the mind and the kind of replies do help to assess the personality of the subject.

RATING SCALES

- Rating scales are helpful to measure about the different personality traits of a subject, teachers coworkers, parents, etc. can be asked to rate the subject for a particular personality trait.
- **For example:** Teachers are asked to rate the subject for his/her emotionality.

1	2	3	4	5
Manic	Excitable	Stable	Shy	Depressive

- It is also called descriptive scale.
- **For example:** A teacher can be asked to rate a student for his behavior in classes on the following rating scale.

1	2	3	4	5
Very good	good	average	poor	very poor

Maximum 1 to 5 or 1 to 7 digits can be allotted. Rating scales with numerical digits is called numerical scale.

Sociometry

Sociometry was founded by Moreno. It is mainly used to study the group and its relationship with others.

Projective Method

According to Freud, projection is a defense process in which impulses, wishes and ideas are brought into conscious which were repressed in unconscious for being painful and embarrassing. Projection here is an unconscious process which brings out internal unconscious personality dispositions based in fear desires and impulses. To externalize such unconscious personality tendencies subject is presented as a structured stimulus. When the subject interpret and give meaning to it, his responses reflection is unconscious personality dispositions. These are the true reflection of the personality of a person. A trained psychotherapist interprets the type of personality.

Rorschach Inkblot Technique

Hermann Rorschach 1921 developed this test. There are ten inkblots, five in black ink on a whole background and five in colored inks on a white background, these plates are standardized. These plates are presented to subject one by one and subject has to tell what he observes in these ink plates. He can give many responses as he desires by observing from different angles to it. These responses are interpreted from various perspective. The therapist assesses normal and abnormal personality traits by analyzing the information. Rorschach inkblot test is used to describe personality, diagnose psychological disorders and to predict the type of behavior.

Thematic Appreciation Test (TAT)

- The psychologist Henry Murray and his colleagues in 1935 developed thematic appreciation test. It consists of 20 pictures, all black and white, that are shown to a client then, the client is asked to tell a story about the person or people in the picture, who are all deliberately drawn in ambiguous situations. Again, the story developed by the client is interpreted by the psychologist, who looks for revealing sentiments and projection of the client's own problems onto the people in the pictures.
- Three types of projective tests include the sentence completion tests, the client is given a series of sentence beginnings, such as 'I wish my mother' or almost everyday I feel .... And asked to finish the sentence, whereas in the draw, person and house tree person the client is asked to draw the named items in details.

Word Association Test

Word association test was developed by Jung. It consists of hundred words. For example, Sukhjeet is instructed that he will be presented 100 words one by one and he has to respond immediately. This is noted for response. The response is recorded. During this procedure, verbal and nonverbal responses are noted down. From these response various complexes and sensitive areas of his life are identified and helps to understand the personality of the person.

SUBJECTIVE METHOD

These methods are subjective in nature and involve the subjective reporting of the subject. They are as follow:

Interview

Interview is a technique of assessment where the interviewer asks the questions for interviewee. It maybe structured or unstructured. In structured interview, questions for the interview are framed in advance; but in unstructured interview, the questions are framed on the spot according to the need and demand. It has 3 phases open, mid and close. Open phase includes rapport building. Next mid phase involves the questioning on the topic in focus. Both questions and answers are recorded. In last phase, the interview will be winded up in an appropriate manner.

Interview has many drawbacks. It has less reliability and validity. It needs preparation and expertise.

Case History

In this method, expertise information about the subject is collected from his birth to present day. This helps to answer the personality of the subject.

Autobiography

Some people have the habit of noting down in dairy every event of live and sometimes it maybe given a book form. Through this, we can assess the personality of the person by the writings.

Questionnaire

These are widely used test in psychiatry. Questionnaires are developed and consist of various questions to different traits of personality.

Eysenck Personality Inventory

- Eysenck personality questionnaire (EPQ) is a questionnaire to assess the personality traits of a person. It was devised by the psychologists Hans Jurgen Eysenck and his wife Subil G. Eysenck. Han's theory is based on physiology and genetics. Although he was a behaviorist who considered learned habit of great importance, he considers personality differences as growing out of our genetic inheritance. He is therefore, primarily interested in what is usually called temperament. Temperament is that aspect of our personalities that is genetically based, inborn, there from birth or even before. That does not mean that a temperament theory says we do not also have aspects of our personality that are learned.
- Eysenck initially conceptualize personality as two, biologically based independent dimensions of temperament measured on a continuum.

Extroversion/Introversion Scale

Extroversion is characterized by being outgoing, talkative high on positive affect (feeling good) and in need of external stimulation. Introverts are chronically over and around and jittery and are in need of peace and quiet to bring them up to an optimal level of performance.

Neuroticism/Stability Scale

Neuroticism is characterized by high levels of negative effect such as depression and anxiety. Neuroticism, according to Eysenck's theory, is based on activation thresholds in the sympathetic nervous system or visceral brain. This is the part of the brain that is responsible for the fight or flight response in the face of danger. Activation can be measured by heart rate, blood pressure, cold hands, sweating and muscular tension neurotic people, who have low activation thresholds, and unable to inhibit or control their emotional reactions, experience negative effect (fight or flight) in the face of very minor stressors they are easily nervous or upset. Emotionally stable people, who have high activation thresholds and good emotional control, experience negative effect only in the face of very major stressors they are calm and collected under pressure.

Psychoticism/Socialization

Psychoticism is associated not only with the liability to have a psychotic episode (or break with reality) but also with aggression. Psychotic behavior is rooted in characteristics of tough mindedness, non-conformity, inconsideration, recklessness, hostility, anger and impulsiveness. The physiological basis suggested by Eysenck for psychoticism is testosterone with higher levels psychoticism associated with higher levels of testosterone.

Cattle's 16 PF Test of Personality

The sixteen personality factor questionnaire (16PF) is a multiple choice personality questionnaire developed by Raymond B. Cattle in 1940s. He used factor analysis to discover and measure the fundamental traits of human personality.

According to Cattle, there is a continuum of personality traits. In other words, each person contains all of these 16 traits to a certain degree. But they might be high in some traits and low in others. The following personality trait list describes some of the descriptive terms used for each of trait 16 personality dimensions described by Cattle.

1. *Abstractedness*: Imaginative vs practical.
2. *Apprehension:* Worried vs confident.
3. *Dominance:* Forceful vs submissive.
4. *Emotional stability:* Calm vs high strong.
5. *Liveliness:* Spontaneous vs restrained.
6. *Openness to change:* Flexible vs attached to the familiar.
7. *Perfectionism:* Controlled vs undisciplined.
8. *Privateness:* Discreet vs open.
9. *Reasoning:* Abstract vs concrete.
10. *Rule consciousness:* Conforming vs nonconforming.
11. *Self-reliance:* Self-sufficient vs dependent.
12. *Sensitivity:* Tender hearted vs tough minded.
13. *Social boldness:* Uninhibited vs shy.
14. *Tension:* Impatient vs relaxed.
15. *Vigilance:* Suspicious vs trusting.
16. *Warmth:* Outgoing vs reserved.

Cattell developed an assessment on these 16 personality factors. This test is used in business. For employee testing and selection, career counseling and marital counseling the test is composed of forced choice questions in which the respondent must choose one of three different alternatives personality traits are then represented by a range and the individual scores falls somewhere on the continuum between highest and lowest extremes.

MINNESOTA MULTIPHASIC PERSONALITY INVENTORY (MMPI)

MMPI is the most widely and frequently used to help, identify personal, social and behavioral problem in psychiatric clients. It also helps to provide relevant information with the problem identification, diagnosis and treatment planning for a client and often used in job screening and other nonclinical assessment. The newer version of MMPI-2 contains seven validity scales and ten clinical scales. Validity scale contains (variable response inconsistly) L scale, F scale, K scale, VRIN scale, and TRIN (True response inconsistency) clinical scales are:

Scale 1: Hypochondriasis
Scale 2: Depression
Scale 3: Hysteria
Scale 4: Psychopathic deviate
Scale 5: Masculinity femininity
Scale 6: Paranoia (PA)
Scale 7: Psicastenia
Scale 8: Schizophrenia
Scale 9: Hypomania (MA)
Scale 10: Social introversion

The items on this scale are of two general types. One group of items deals with social participation, while the other group deals with general neurotic maladjustment and self-depreciation. High scores are generally seen as socially introverted; while low score tend to be sociable and extroverted. High scorers are very insecure and uncomfortable in social situation. They tend to be shy, reserved, timid and retiring, whole low scorers tend to be outgoing, gregarious, friendly and talkative.

DEFENSE MECHANISMS

In Freud's psychoanalytic theory, defense mechanisms are unconscious psychological strategics brought into play by various entities to cope with reality and to maintain self-image. Healthy persons normally use different defenses throughout life. An ego defense mechanism becomes pathological only when its persistent use leads to maladaptive behavior such that the physical and/or mental health or the individual is adversely affected. The purpose of ego defense mechanisms is to protect the mind/self/ego from anxiety and/or social sanctions and or/to provide a refuge from a situation with which one cannot currently cope.

Compensation

People, who do not possess certain skills, happen to have some other qualities, or skills that overwhelm this inability. The lack of something is hidden by having a more prominent feature of the personality that compensates or makes up for their inability. For example, People who may not be very good in socializing skills maybe very good in singing or dancing. This will get them enough attention which they would have missed otherwise for their lack of socializing skills.

Denial

In order not to face the unpleasant situation, the individual altogether denies the reality. A person instead of learning to accept the reality as something natural and normal tries to escape them by denial. For example, an alcoholic denies the amount to be consumed.

Displacement

In this defence mechanism, an emotional feeling is transferred to person or objects who are less dangerous than those who initially around the emotion. For example, Father blasts the child for not doing well in test. The child gets angry but cannot shout back at father. So, he starts quarelling with brother or sister. It shows that he is displacing his anger from father to his brother or sister.

Fixation

It refers to the point in an individual's development at which certain aspects of the emotional development are not advance and fixated at that stage. This arrest appears to develop from the inability of the individual to solve problems that occurred during the specific phase of development at which progress ceased or stopped. For example, Alcoholics are believed to be fixated at the oral stage of development.

Repression

Repression represents those memories, feelings and thoughts that are stored in the unconscious because their recall maybe painful or fearful. Much of what is repressed occurs in childhood and therefore may not be readily verbalized. Because repression is usually limited to specific areas or topics. Repression operates wholly on an unconscious level. Unacceptable feelings are unconsciously kept out of awareness. For example, A man is jealous of his good friends success but he is aware of his feelings of jealousy.

Rationalization

It is a commonly practiced defense mechanism that seeks to justify or provide a seemingly reasonable explanation to make undesirable or questionable behaviors appear logical, reasonable or acceptable. It is frequently used to modify guilt feelings because the valid or true explanation for the behavior would produce feelings of guilt or anxiety. A phase 'grapes are sour' is an example of rationalization.

Regression

The return to an earlier form of behavior or stage of development is called regression. This usually occurs when the more mature or appropriate behavior is blocked by feelings of uncertainty, anxiety, fear conflict or lack of reward. In some instances, it will also represent a retreat to earlier responses. Sometimes an adult throws temper tantrums and tears is an example of regression.

Identification

Identification gives one satisfaction or compensation by identifying with others and their achievements. In identification with others an individual may actually acquire new and useful behaviors. For example, After hospitalization for a minor surgery, a girl decides to become a nurse because she developed a desirable attitude found in people whom she respects and admires.

Reaction Formation/Over Compensation

Reaction formation is the display of behaviors and attitudes that represent the opposite of one's repressed feelings. Anxiety and guilt feelings are repressed and their opposites expressed instead. For example, A woman who actually dislikes her mother-in-law hides her feelings by being always nice to her.

Conversion

In this mental mechanism, the strong emotional conflicts are expressed as or converted into physical ailments. It operates wholly on an unconscious level. For example, The boy who hates father and likes to strike at him, if he does so develops a paralyzed arm, the conflict is resolved. He cannot strike his father even if he wishes to, and the situation carries no threat of retaliation.

Substitution

Substitution maybe employed to reduce tension resulting from frustration. To get satisfaction and reduce anxiety, resulting from frustration, the substitute action must contain similarities to the frustrated one. For example, A student who has not got admission to medical, try to institute it with a course of nursing.

Introjection

In introjection, the values and characteristics of significant persons are incorporated in one's personality. For instance, a woman who like to live in a simple way introjects in her the sophisticated way of living like her husband.

Suppression

In suppression, conscious effort is made by the individual to dismiss the impulses, feelings and thought that are unpleasant to the preconscious mind so, unacceptable feelings and thought are consciously kept out of awareness. For example, A student taking an examination is upset about an argument with his friend but puts it out of his mind so that he can finish the test.

Transference

In transference, the image of one person is unconsciously identified with that of another. A patient who finds the nurse of the same age and height as his daughter, transfers his positive emotions to his nurse as his daughter. It is also possible that if he dislikes his daughter, he transfers his negative emotions to the nurse by being more, abusive or aggressive without any cause.

Sublimation

It is a positive mechanism. It consists of a redirection of sexual impulses to socially valued and accepted activities. Unacceptable desires find an acceptable outlet.

Projection

Projection is a psychological defense mechanism where a person subconsciously denies his or her own attribute, thoughts and emotion, which are then ascribed to the outside world, usually to other people. Thus, projection involves imagining or projecting the belief that others originate those feelings. Projection means blaming others as a way of coping with one's unwanted motives by shifting them to someone else. A student who wants to skip classes may project that everyone is skipping classes and house, it is okay, but in reality, others may not be skipping classes. If projection is overused, it may give rise to a behaviors disorder called paronia. People with this disorder may translate their own negative feelings on to other, and feel that others are out thereto get them humiliated or even killed.

Sympathism

The individual in sympathism tends to always seek gratification in the sympathy that others show of their plight or condition. While most people do not like the attention others give when they are facing difficult times or situation, there are others showing people who bask in the glory of sympathism and do not like to make any efforts to change the status of their condition. Example, If a psychiatric patient is illiterate, he will not try to learn and change the status of his illiteracy because he likes the sympathy that others show the help that others are willing to render.

Intellectualization

By using this mechanism, the intensity of the anxiety is reduced by restoring to a detached, unemotional, intelligent yet abstract language. Mostly used by professionals like doctors, nurses and lectures. For example, Providing sex education in a conservative setting. Temporarily separating emotional and cognitive components sometimes helps the individual to deal with parts of an experience when the whole is too much to handle and overuse can lead to boredom.
Here, reasoning is used to block confrontation with an unconscious conflict and its associated emotional stress, by using excessive and abstract ideation to avoid difficult feeling, it involves removing one's self, emotionally, from a stressful event.

Fantasy and Day Dreaming

The motives that cannot be fulfilled in reality are fulfilled by resorting to wishful thinkings. Wishful thinking means, thinking a one wishes to. This is done by fantasizing, which means creating a fantasy, imaginary dream world of one's own, it helps in transporting people so places and events not possible in reality. Manic patients usually use fantasy as a defense to fulfill their grandiose thoughts.

Withdrawal

- Withdrawal involves the removal of oneself from anything and everything that carries reminders of painful or stressful thoughts and emotions. Since normal social life involves many situations that are connected to the painful event, and friends or colleagues may ask.
- Uncomfortable question, the use of withdrawal means the end of one's social life. It provides temporary relief by giving the person sometimes to devise alternate modes of dealing with the problem situation by spending some moments alone. But too much of withdrawal will make the person cut off from reality and out of synchronous with the social world. This mechanism is used by depressive, and by hypomanic clients.

Dissociation

Dissociation usually results from a trauma, intense pain, or a serious identity crisis. It may manifest itself in disorders such as post-traumatic stress disorder, memory loss, multiple personality disorder, dissociative amnesia, as well as flash backs and forgetting. However, in dissociation memories are not just lost in the subconscious but they are splintered and distorted. This is as if under intense stress the ability of the consciousness to include all the thought, emotions and somatic sensation fails and some aspects become separated and inaccessible. Thus, a person may remember what happened but forget how it felt or a person may feel depersonalized, like a robot.

Maladaptive Use

- Defense mechanism are helpful and healthy if used in a proper manner. However, if misused or overused, the same defense mechanism may also be unhealthy and gives rise to psychological problems.
- Maladaptive use of defense mechanism can occur in a variety of cases for example, when they become automatic and prevent individuals from realizing their true feelings and thoughts. Frequent or continuous use of defense mechanism disrupts reality testing denial and paranoid projection are considered to be psychotic in nature as their repeated use can cause people to lose touch with the real world and their surroundings and consequently isolate themselves from reality and dwell in a world created of their own design. Use of few and multiple defense mechanism also lead to personality disorders.

Maladaptive Behavior

- Adaptive behavior is a type of behavior that is used to adjust to another type of behavior or situation this is often characterized by a kind of behavior that allows an individual to change an unconstructive or disruptive behavior to something more constructive. These behaviors are most often social or personal behaviors. For example, a constant repetitive action could be refocused on something that creates or builds something's. In other words the behavior can be adapted to something else.
- Maladaptive behavior is a type of behavior that is often used to reduce one's anxiety; but the result is dysfunctional and nonproductive. For example, avoiding situations because you have unrealistic fears may initially reduce your anxiety, but is nonproductive.
- In alleviation the actual problem is in the long-term. Maladaptivity is frequently used as indicator of abnormality or mental dysfunction or psychiatric disorder. For example, if you experience frequent panic (anxiety) attacks and diagnosed with panic disorder, you may have inadvertently developed maladaptive patterns of behavior to cope with your situation. These are also called 'dysfunctional' because they tend to provide only short-term relief from anxiety. They are nonproductive in alienating the actual problem in the long run and may act as reinforcers of the underlying problem.

Avoidance

For many people, the symptoms of panic disorder often trigger an array of avoidant behaviors. This can result in agoraphobia. Agoraphobia can take a little time to develop or it can come on rather suddenly. Once it takes root, avoidance behavior often multiply quickly.

Substance Abuse

People with anxiety disorders including panic disorder and agoraphobia sometimes use alcohol or other drugs and substances as a means of coping with fear and anxiety. The research findings show that people with anxiety disorders are up to three times more likely to have an alcohol or other drugs to control stress and anxiety. It is classified as a maladaptive behavior because it provides only temporary relief from anxiety and actually may create more long-term problems.

Create more long-term problems. Substance abuse does not fix the underlying problem and long-term alcohol or drug abuse can lead to tolerance, dependence and lastly for addiction.

Withdrawing

Many challenges in life require ongoing action both behaviorally and psychologically. Sometimes we struggle and succeed. Sometimes we struggle and fail. When the latter occurs, we can try again, or we can withdraw when it comes to panic disorder or any other anxiety disorder, withdrawing is incompatible with recover. It is a maladaptive behavior because it means we submit to the illness and become unable to meet the demands of life. In essence, withdrawing in this sense is like giving up. For many people, the recovery process from anxiety disorders is slow and filled with setbacks. Recovery is accomplished with diligence and a strong resolve not to accept the control that panic attacks and other anxiety related symptoms have over our lives.

Converting Anxiety to Anger

Frustration erupts from anxiety. Sometimes this frustration can develop into anger ... anger toward himself/herself, anger at situation or toward others and this type of anger is rooted in anxiety. Anger is a powerful feeling that is a normal part of the human experience. Everyone has felt angry at one time or another. Anger itself is not a bad thing but if it is expressed in unhealthy ways, it can become a problem and anger can intensify anxiety and worsen the panic symptoms. Anger management programs can help to find more adaptive ways to deal with anxiety.

STRESS/CRISIS MANAGEMENT

Modern life is full of hassles, deadlines, frustrations and demands, for may people, stress is so commonplace that it has become a way of life. Stress is not always bad. In small quantities it helps to perform under pressure and motivate to do the best but when it is constantly running in emergency mode the body and mind pay the price.

Stress is a normal physical response to events that make to feel threatened or upset the balance of body and mind. When you sense danger whether it is real or imagined the body's defense kick into higher gear in a rapid, automatic process known as the 'flight or fight' reaction or the stress response.

The stress response is the body's way of protecting the individuals. When working properly, it helps to stay focused, energetic and alert. In emergency situation, stress can save your life giving you extra strength to defend yourself, e.g. jumping from moving vehicle to save accident.

The stress response also helps you rise to meet challengers. Stress is what keeps you on your toes during a presentation at work, sharpens concentration or drives you to study for an exam. But beyond a certain point, stress stops being helpful and starts causing major damage to health, mood, beyond productivity, relationship and the quality of life.

STRESS

Stress is a nonspecific response of the body to a demand made upon. Stress is also defined as a broad class of experiences in which a demanding situation taxes a person's resources or coping capabilities causing a negative effect on body and mind.

Eustress vs Distress

- Eustress is a positive stress which helps people to meet their goals, *e.g.* Getting a new job. Getting a promotion.
- *Distress:* Distress is a negative stress which can cause too much pressure and trauma in one's life, *e.g.* Failing in class. Getting fired from a job. Death of a loved one.

Acute vs Chronic Stress

Stress responses occur at physiological, behavioral and at cognitive level. Psychological stresses can potentiate physiological response. Stress has its potentially most deleterious health effects when it becomes chronic. Although there are severe stressors that persist over a long period of time, weaken the ability to cope and adjust. If coping ability is exhausted, more stress and distress follow.

The present views of the physiology of stress can be traced back to the contributions of Walter Cannon and Hans Selye. They focused primarily on the sympathetic nervous system and the role of the hormones, epinephrine and noradrenaline, labeled the 'fight or flight' response that creates a mobilization of energy (increased heart rate, blood pressure, blood sugar...) which potentiates physical action. Selye expanded the understanding of the stress response by identifying the role of the HPA (hypothalamic-pituitary axis) in stress, which included the end product cortisol. Selye's notion was that the body attempted to maintain homeostasis or internal equilibrium by adjusting its physiological processes and resisting physiological change.

STRESSORS

The sources of stress in each person's life are place, people and things that cause stress in day to day life.

- *Biological stressors, e.g.* disease, death.
- *Environmental stressor, e.g.* natural disaster, excessive hot and cold.
- *Cognitive stressors, e.g.* heavy work pressure, too difficulty to do work, major life changes.
- *Personal behavior, e.g.* values, beliefs, goals in life.
- *Life situations, e.g.* social situation, catastrophic events, divorce.

STRESS RESPONSES

Stress can be physical, such as a cold, noise, cold temperature, and strenuous activities. It can also be psychosocial, such as anxiety, guilt or joy.

Each person's threshold to stress is different, but stress is a part of everyday life for everyone. The hypothalamus receives information from almost all parts of the brain including the limbic system, the emotional brain. The hypothalamus responds to signals of stress by recruiting the sympathetic division of the autonomic nervous system, also called the fight or flight response. The body prepares for the fight or flight response by:

- Shunting blood from the skin and digestive organs to the muscles.

- Providing more fuel through an increase in glucagon action, in other words, releasing glucose from stored glycogen. The hypothalamus stimulates a release of ACTH from the anterior pituitary gland to increase cortisol levels from the adrenal glands. Cortisol helps to supply cells with amino acids and fatty acids for energy supply while diverting glucose from muscles for use by the brain. Cortisol and related compounds are sometimes used to reduce inflammation, but the concentration necessary for inflammation reduction is toxic to the body.
- The general adaptation syndrome: Hans Selye is credited with identifying the body's reaction to stress with a syndrome he called the General Adaptation Syndrome; which has three phases, as evidenced by the level of stress (Fig. 2.3).

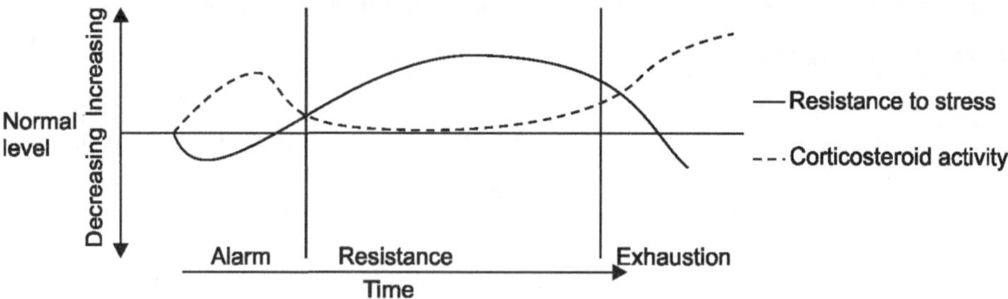

Fig. 2.3: The general adaptation syndrome

a. *Alarm:* The body first organizes physiological responses to threat.
b. *Resistance:* Stress activated responses continue, stabilizing the body's adaptations to stress.
c. *Exhaustion:* The body has depleted its reserves and can no longer maintain response to the stressors.

During the alarm phase, when the body is first aroused, the hypothalamus sends signals to the pituitary glands. This endocrine gland in turn secrets adrenocortic hormone (ACTH), which travels via the bloodstream to the cortex (outer longer) of the adrenal glands, where corticosteroids are released. The hypothalamus also activates the adrenal medulla, the central part of the adrenal gland, which causes adrenaline (epinephrine) to be released and the activation of the sympathetic nervous system. After maintaining high levels of the hormones for a long-time, the body loses its ability to do and exhausts its resources. Selye is credited with identifying the fact that the incidence of certain types of diseases (stress related disorders, such as coronary heart disease) increases. During this stage, exhausted body resources and that a second stressor introduced during the resistance phase or the exhaustion phase further increase the incidence. The research evidence demonstrates that prolonged stress also affect the release of endorphins, chemicals similar in structure to morphine and other opiate drugs used in the modulation of pain.

CRISIS AND DISASTER MANAGEMENT

Crisis

- Most people exist in a state of equilibrium, that is, their everyday lives contain some degree of harmony in their thoughts, wishes, feelings and physical needs. Such an existence generally remains intact unless biological, psychological or social integrity. As undue stress occurs, one's equilibrium can be affected and one may lose control of feelings and thoughts, thus experiencing an extreme state of emotional turmoil. When this occurs, one maybe experiencing a crisis.

- A crisis is defined as 'a state of disequilibrium resulting from the interaction of an event with the individual's or family coping mechanism, which are inadequate to meet the demands of the situation, combined with the individual or family's perception of the situation, combined with the individual or family perception of the meaning of the event (Taylor, 1982).
- According to Roberts (2000), crisis is a period of disequilibrium and decreased functioning as a result of an event or situation that creates a significant problem which cannot be resolved by using familiar coping strategies.
- The event that creates a crisis is significant, only as the individual or family perceives it. The extent of disintegration or disorganization resulting from an event depends on the particular victim's support system including his previous learned experiences, etc.
- A crisis may influence peoples's lives in different ways. As a consequence of a crisis experience, the individual may go down to a lower or less healthy state of function or he may resume the same level of state by repressing the crisis situation. He may function at a healthier level that prior to the crisis because the challenge of a crisis can bring out new strength, skills and coping (Papaport, 1965). Intervention at a crisis state extremely important to prevent psychosocial disorders because long-standing problems that were suppressed can occur at a crisis, making the person totally incapable of handling the situation. If proper guidance and counseling is available at the correct time, the victim will come out of it better equipped to handle further problem in life.

Types of Crisis

Developmental (maturational crisis)

- All human beings go through different stages of life development. The transition between these stages can be emotionally upsetting period, e.g. child's real separation from parents.

Situational Crisis

Situational crisis precipitates by some of the major catastrophes that can happen in life, e.g. sudden death of a loved one, loss of job, etc. The events that precipitate a crisis need not always be strong. Anything that requires a sudden change can be a threat to biopsychosocial equilibrium.

Adventitious Crisis

These crisis occurs very rarely, like natural and national disasters.

Characteristics of a Crisis

A crisis generally occurs suddenly, when a person, family or group of individual is inadequately prepared to handle the event before it arises. Normal and usual coping methods fail, tension rises and feelings of anxiety, fear, guilt, anger, shame and helplessness may occur. Most crisis are generally short in duration, lasting 24 to 36 hours, rarely they last longer than 4 to 6 weeks. They can cause increased biopsychosocial vulnerability, resulting in potentially dangerous, self-destructive or socially unacceptable behavior, or they can provide an opportunity for personal growth. The outcome of a crisis depends on the availability of appropriate helps.

When a crisis occurs, it affects the individual as well as family and society. So, the individual and significant social system have influence on the resolution of the crisis.

Phases of Crisis State

The following phases of a crisis are generally described by theorists.
- Precrisis stage
- Impact phase
- Crisis phase
- Postcrisis phase

The general state of equilibrium in which a person is able to cope with everyday stress is called precrisis phase. When a stressful event occurs, the person is said to be experiencing the impact phase, e.g. a young couple is told by their pediatrician that their toddler has inoperable cancer. Once the shock is over, the young parents become actually aware of their son's critical illness and poor prognosis. This is anxiety to their integrity as a family. They are in the crisis phase and may experience much confusion and disorganization because they feel helpless and are unable to cope with the son's physical condition. When the young parents are able, with or without intervention of others, to regain control of their emotions, handle the situation and work toward a solution concerning their son's illness, they are in the resolution phase of a crisis. If they are able to resume normal activities while living their son's hospitalization and illness, they are in the postcrisis phase. Such an experience may produce permanent emotional injury or may make the young parents feel a stronger bond with each other and their son, depending on their ability to cope.

Paradigm of Balancing Factors

Aguilera (1986) illustrates a paradigm of balancing factors that determine whether a crisis occurs as a result of a stressful event. These factors, which can affect a return to equilibrium, are:
- Realistic perception of an event.
- Adequate situational support.
- Adequate coping mechanisms to help to resolve a problem.

CRISIS INTERVENTION

- Crisis intervention can be defined as an emergency psychological care aimed at assisting individuals in a crisis situation to restore equilibrium to their biopsychosocial functioning and to minimize the potential for psychological trauma.
- Crisis intervention is an active but temporary entry into the life situation of an individual, a family or a group during a period of stress (Mitchell and Resnick, 1981).
- According to Dorland's medical dictionary, crisis intervention is an immediate, short-term, psychotherapeutic approach, the goal of which is to help resolve a personal crisis within the individual's immediate environment. It is an attempt to resolve an immediate crisis when a person's life goals are obstructed and usual problem-solving methods fail. The patient or client is called onto arrive in all steps of the crisis intervention process, including classifying the problem, verbalizing feeling, identifying goals, and options for reaching goals and deciding on a plan.

- Crisis intervention can occur in a variety of settings, e.g. the home, community, casualty, room, industry, classroom, or psychiatric unit. The approach focuses on a particular kind of crisis with direct encouragement of adaptive behavior with general support, environmental manipulation and anticipatory guidance. The individual approach stresses the present, shows little or no concern for the developmental past and places an emphasis on the immediate causes of disequilibrium. It can be used as secondary or tertiary prevention and can be effective in preventing future crisis.

GOALS OF CRISIS INTERVENTION

- To decrease emotional stress and protect the crisis victim from additional stress.
- To assist the victim in organizing and mobilizing resources or support system to meet unique needs and reach a solution for the particular situation, or circumstances that precipitated the crisis. It is hoped that this action will prevent hospitalization, reduce the risk of chronic maladaptation and promote adaptive family dynamics.
- To return the crisis victim to a precrisis or higher level of function.

STEPS IN CRISIS INTERVENTION

Agnikra (1986) mentioned four steps in the process of crisis intervention. These are:

1. Assessment.
2. Planning therapeutic intervention.
3. Implementing techniques of intervention.
4. Resolution of the crisis and anticipatory planning and evaluation.

When working with crisis, the crisis worker should be aware of the following:

- **Most crisis occur suddenly without warning:** Therefore, there is inadequate prior preparation to such a situation.
- The person in crisis prescribes it to be life-threatening.
- There is a decrease or loss of communication with significant other.
- Some displacement from familiar surroundings or significant other occurs.
- All crisis have an aspect of an actual or perceived loss involving a person, object, idea or hope.

Assessment

The first step in the assessment process is to identify the degree of disruption the individual is experiencing. Is the individual anxious, depressed, fearful, confused, disoriented, suicidal or homicidal? The second step is to assess the individual's perception of the event. Is it realistic or distorted? Does he or she perceive the situation as a threat to self-esteem or well-being? Some individuals are unaware of the significance of the event in their lives. Attention is also given to present coping skills and the availability of support system on whom the individual can rely for continued support.

Formulation of nursing diagnoses is the next step. Examples include anxiety, fear, ineffective individual coping, impaired verbal communication, high-risk for injury, altered family processes, etc.

PLANNING THERAPEUTIC INTERVENTION

With information gained throughout the assessment process, and the formulation of one or more nursing diagnosis(es), several specific intervention are proposed. Johnson (1989) states that individuals must learn to ask for help and realize the potential for growth during a crisis.

They should be involved in the choice of alternative coping methods and encouraged to make as many arrangements as possible by themselves. If significant others are involved, their needs and reactions should also be considered. Strength and resources of all person providing support should be identified.

IMPLEMENTING THERAPEUTIC INTERVENTIONS

Therapeutic intervention depends on pre-existing skill, the activity and flexibility of the crisis worker, and the quickness of the person's response. The crisis worker helps the person to establish an intellectual understanding of the crisis by noting the relationship between the precipitating factor and the crisis. He or she also helps the crisis victim to explore coping mechanisms, remember or recreate successful coping devices used in the past, or devise new coping skills. Reducing immobility caused by anxiety and encouraging verbalization of feeling is an immediate goal of the worker. An attempt also is made to establish new supportive and meaningful relationships and experiences, reopening the person's psychosocial world.

The following therapeutic techniques are utilized while performing crisis intervention.

- Display acceptance and concern and attempt to establish a positive relationship.
- Encourage the person to discuss present feelings, such as denial, guilt, grief or anger.
- Help the person to confront the reality of the crisis by gaining an intellectual as well as an emotional understanding of the situation. Do not encourage the person to focus on all the implication of the crisis at once.
- Explain that the person's emotions are a normal reaction to the crisis.
- Avoid giving false reassurance.
- Clarify fantasy, contrasting them with facts.
- Do not encourage the person to place the blame for the crisis on others because such encouragement prevents the person from facing the reality or truth, reduce's the person's motivation to take responsibility for behavior and impedes or discourages adaptation during the crisis.
- Set limit on destructive behavior.
- Emphasize the person's responsibility for behavior and decision.
- Assist the person in seeking help with activities of daily living (ADL) until resolution occurs.
- Evaluate and modify nursing intervention as necessary.

Resolution and Anticipatory Planning

During the resolution phase, reassessment must occur to ascertain that the intervention is reducing tension and anxiety successful rather than producing negative effects. Reinforcement is provided whenever necessary while the crisis work is reviewed and accomplishments of the crisis victim are emphasized. Assistance and guidance is given to formulate realistic plans for the future, and the person is given the opportunity to discuss how present experiences may help in coping with future crisis situation.

Crisis Intervention Model

Crisis intervention maybe provided at individual and family sessions. Crisis group also resolves various issues through use of group process for four to six sessions. They provide support and encouragement to person who depend on others for much of their sense of personal fulfillment and achievement.

Family crisis counseling includes the entire family during sessions lasting approximately six weeks. This type of counseling is considered the preferred method of crisis intervention for children and adolescents.

Telephone hot lines, such as contact and adapt are provided by suicide prevention and crisis intervention counseling centers on a 24 hours basis. They are generally staffed by volunteers who have had intensive training in telephone interviewing and counseling and can give the person in crisis immediate help.

Home crisis visits are available in some situations. For example, if additional information needs to be obtained following a telephone interview; if a caller is assessed as being highly suicidal or if concerned person notify a crisis center of potential patients or clients in crisis.

MODEL OF CRISIS INTERVENTION

- Many crisis intervention models are promulgated over the years. However, Roberts (2005) model represents a practical application.
- It represents a practical example of a stepwise blue print for crisis responding that has applicability across a broad spectrum of crisis situations.

Roberts Seven Stage Crisis Intervention Model

In conceptualizing the process of crisis intervention, Roberts (2005) has identified seven critical stages though which clients typically pass on the road to crisis stabilization, resolution, and mastery (Fig. 2.4). Those stages, listed below, are essential, sequential and sometimes overlapping in the process of crisis intervention.

- Plan and conduct a thorough biopsychosocial and lethality/imminent danger assessment.
- Make psychological contact and rapidly establish the collaborative relationship.
- Identify the major problems, including crisis precipitants.
- Encourage an exploration of feeling and emotions.
- Generate and explore alternatives and new coping strategies.
- Restore functioning through implementation of an action plan.
- Plan follow-up and booster sessions.

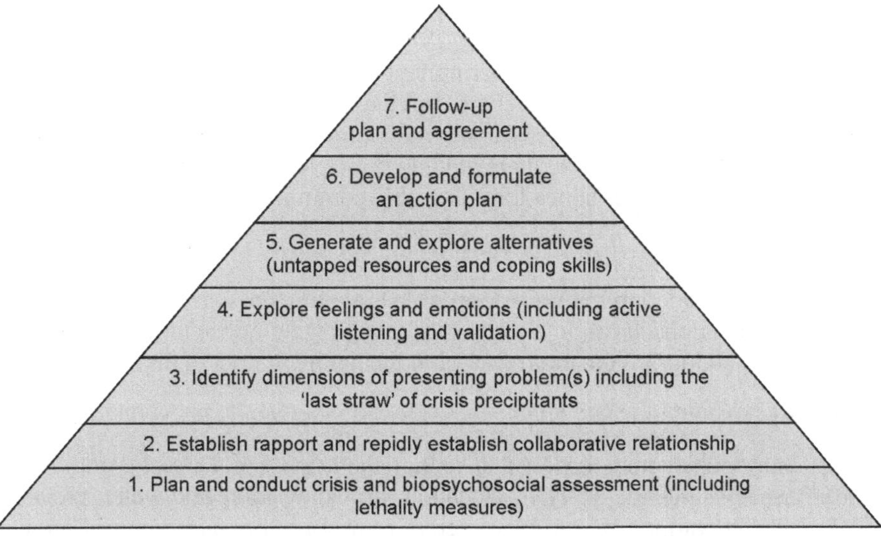

Fig. 2.4: Roberts' seven stage crisis intervention model

DISASTER MANAGEMENT

Disaster management can be defined as the organization and management of resources and responsibilities for dealing with all humanitarian aspects of emergencies in particular preparedness, response and recovery in order to lesson the impact disaster.

Types of disasters: There are four main types of disasters.

- *Natural disaster:* These include floods, hurricanes, earthquakes and volcano exceptions that can have immediate impacts on human health as well as secondary impacts causing further death and suffering from floods causing landslides, earthquakes resulting in fires, tsunamis causing widespread flooding and typhoons, sinking ferries.
- *Environmental emergencies:* These emergencies include technological or industrial accidents, usually involving hazardous material, and occur where these materials are produced, used or transported. Large forest fires are generally included in this definition because they tend to be caused by humans.
- *Complex emergencies:* These emergencies involve a break down of authority, looting and attacks on strategic installations. These include war and conflict situation.
- *Pandemic emergencies:* These emergencies involve a sudden onset of a contagious disease that affects health but also disrupts services and businesses, bringing economic and social costs.
  - Any disaster can interrupt essential services, such as the provision of healthcare, electricity, water, sewage/garbage removal, transportation and communication. The interruption can seriously affect the health, social and economic network of local communities and in large countries. Disaster has a major and long-lasting impact on people long after the immediate effect has been mitigated. Poorly planned relief activities can have significant negative impact not only on the disaster victims but also on donors and relief agencies. Local, regional, national and international organizations are all involved in mounting a humanitarian response to disaster. Each will have a prepared disaster management plan. These plans cover prevention, preparedness, relief and recovery.

Disaster Prevention

These are activities designed to provide permanent protection from disasters. Not all disaster, particularly natural disaster, can be prevented, but the risk of loss of life and injury can be mitigated with good evacuation plans, environmental planning and design standards, the global disaster plan for natural disaster risk offers guiding principles, priorities of action and practical means for achieving disaster resilience for vulnerable communities.

Disaster Preparedness

These activities are designed to minimize loss of life and damage, e.g. by removing people and property from a threatened location and by facilitating timely and effective rescue, relief and rehabilitation. Preparedness is the main way of reducing the impact of disasters.

Disaster Relief

It is a coordinated multiagency response to reduce the impact of a disaster and its long-term results. Relief activities include, rescue, relocation, providing food and water, preventing disease and disability, repairing vital services, such as transportation, telecommunication, providing temporary shelter, food and emergency healthcare facilities.

Disaster Recovery

- Once emergency needs have been met and the initial crisis is over, the people affected and the communities that support them are still vulnerable. Recovery activities include rebuilding infrastructure, healthcare and rehabilitation. These should blend with development activities, such as building human resources for health and developing policies and practices to avoid similar situation in future.
- Disaster management is linked with sustainable development, particularly in relation to vulnerable people, such as those with disabilities, elderly people, children and other marginalized groups.

Levels of Disaster

- *Level III disaster:* Considered a minor disaster. These are having minimal level of damage.
- *Level II disaster:* Considered a moderate disaster. The local and community resources have to be mobilized to manage this situation.
- *Level I disaster:* Considered a massive disaster. This involves a massive level of damage with severe impact.

Phases of Disaster Management

- Prevention phase
- Preparedness phase
- Response phase
- Recovery phase

Prevention Phase

Identify the community risk factors and to develop and implement programs to prevent disaster from occurring.

Preparedness Phase

- Personal preparedness
- Professional preparedness

Community Preparedness:
- The level of community preparedness for a disaster is only as high as the people and organization in the community make it.
- Community must have adequate warning system and a back up evaluation plan to remove people from the area of danger.

Response Phase

The level of disaster varies and the management plans mainly based on the severity or extent of the disaster.

Recovery Phase

- During this phase, actions are taken to repair, rebuild or reallocate damaged homes and businesses and restore health and economic vitality to the community.

- Psychosocial recovery must be addressed. Both victims and relief worker should be offered mental health activities and services.

Disaster Management Cycle

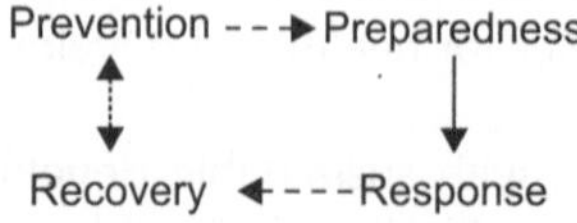

Disaster Nursing

A disaster is a natural or man-made-hazard resulting in an event of substantial extent causing significant physical damage or destruction, loss of life, or drastic change to the environment. A disaster can be defined as any tragic event stemming from events, such as earthquakes, floods, catastrophic, accidents, fires or explosions. It is a phenomenon that can cause damage to life, property and destroy the economic, social and cultural life of people.

Types of Disasters

Disasters are classified as human made, or natural and secondary disaster.

- *According to WHO:* Disaster is any occurrence that causes damage, economic disruption, loss of human life and deterioration in health services on a scale sufficient to warrant an extraordinary response from outside the affected community area. The present century has added a new ecological dimension to the definition of disaster. Chemical and nuclear catastrophes, oil spills, air, water and soil pollution, desertification, the greenhouse effect and environmental effuses.
- *Natural disaster*: For example, earthquakes, floods, hurricane and tsunami.
- *Manmade disaster:* For example, nuclear accident, industrial accident like Bhopal gas tragedy stampede, transport accident, war, airplane crash and terrorist attack.
- *Hybrid disaster*: For example, spread of disease in community and global warming.

Disaster Mitigation

American Red Cross Society defines disaster mitigation refers to actions or measures that can either prevent the occurence of a disaster or reduce the severity of its effects. Disaster mitigation activities include awareness, education and disaster prevention measures.

ORGANIZATIONAL AND PROFESSIONAL ROLE OF DISASTER MANAGEMENT

Healthcare Professional

- Hospitals
- Healthcare professional
- Pharmacies
- Public healthcare facilities

- Rescue personnel
- Trained staff

Nonhealthcare Community

- Fire fighters
- Municipals or government officials
- Media
- Medical supply manufactures
- Police
- Fire
- Volunteers

Disaster Management Plan

Aims of disaster plans

To provide prompt and effective medical care to the maximum possible in order to minimize morbidity and mortality.

Objectives

- To optimally prepare the staff and institutional resources for effective performance in disaster situation.
- To make the community aware of the sequential steps that could be taken at individual and organization levels.

DISASTER MANAGEMENT COMMITTEE

The following members would comprise the disaster management committee under the chairmanship of medical superintendent

- Director/medical superintendent
- Additional medical superintendent
- Chief nursing officer
- Chief medical officer (casualty)
- HODs of surgery, medicine, orthopedics, radiology, anesthesiology and neurosurgery.
- Blood bank in charge
- Security officers
- Transport officers
- Sanitary officers
- Volunteers.

Disaster Control Room

The existing casualty maybe referred as the disaster control room.

Rapid Response Team

- The medical superintendent will identify various specialists, nurses and pharmacological staff to respond within a short notice, depending upon the time and type of disaster.

- The list of members and their phone members should be displayed in the disaster control room.

INFORMATION AND COMMUNICATION

The disaster control team would be responsible for collecting, coordinating and disseminating the information about the situation to all concerned.

Disaster Beds

- Requirement of beds depends upon the magnitude of the disaster.
- Utilization of vacant beds and preoperative beds.
- Convalescing patients, elective surgical cases and patients who can have domiciliary care or OPD basis management should be discharged.
- Utility areas of hospital to be converted into temporary wards such as side rooms, corridors, seminar rooms, etc.
- Creating additional bed capacity by using trolleys, folding beds and floor beds.

Logistic Support System

- Resuscitation equipment
- IV sets/IV fluids
- Disposable needles, syringes and gloves.
- Dressing and suturing material and splints
- Oxygen masks, nasal catheter, suction machine and suction.
- ECG monitors, defibrillators, ventilators.
- Tracheostomy sets and lumbar puncture sets.
- Linen and blankets.
- Key of these cupboards should be readily available at the time of disaster.

Training and Drills

Mock exercise and drill at regular intervals are conducted to ensure that all the staff in the general and those associated with management of casualties are fully prepared and aware of their responsibilities.

Elements of Disaster Plan

A disaster plan should have the following elements:

- Chain of authority
- Lines of communication
- Routes and modes of transport
- Mobilization
- Warning
- Evacuation
- Rescue and recovery
- Triage

- Support of victims and families
- Care of dead bodies

DISASTER AND NURSING PERSPECTIVE

Assessment of the Community at Risk

Assessment: The local climate conducive for disaster occurrence, past history of disaster in the community available community disaster plans and resources personnel available in the community for the disaster plans and management, local agencies and organization involved in the disaster management activities, availability healthcare facilities in the community, etc.

Predisposing Causes

These factors determine an individual's susceptibility to maladaptive and psychotic behavior. They interact with precipitating factors resulting in psychiatric illness.
These are:

- Genetic make up.
- Physical injury to central nervous system.
- Adverse and traumatic psychosocial climate.

PRECIPITATING FACTORS

These are events that occur shortly before the onset of disease and appear to have induced it. They are:

- Stress
- Loss

Perpetuating Cause

These factors are responsible for aggravating or prolonging the diseases already existing in an individual. Psychosocial stress may aggregate the symptoms. Thus, etiological factors of mental illness are amalgamation and interaction of biopsychosocial climate of an individual.

- Biological factors
- Psychological changes
- Physiological factors
- Social/environment factors.

BIOLOGICAL FACTORS

Heredity

Changes in physical and chemical structure of genes give rise to abnormalities in mental and cognitive function.

BIOCHEMICAL FACTORS

Biochemical abnormalities in the brain are the principal factor for psychiatric morbidity. Disturbance in neurotransmitters in the structure, production and discharge level affect the psychomotor function of an individual, e.g. excessive level of non-epinephrine level in brain is seen in mania.

BRAIN DAMAGE

Any damage to the structure and functioning of the brain can give rise to mental illness. Damage to the structure of the brain maybe due to any of the following causes:

- *Infection:* For example, encephalitis, neurosplits, HIV infection, etc.
- *Injury:* Head injury, accident.
- *Vascular:* Intracranial bleeding, hemorrhage, poor blood supply.
- *Intoxication:* Damage to brain tissue due to toxins such as barbiturates, lead, alcohol, etc.
- *Alteration in brain function:* Changes in blood and brain chemistry.
- *Tumors:* Brain tumors.

DIAGNOSE COMMUNITY DISASTER THREATS

Determine the actual and potential disaster threats (e.g. explosion, mass accidents, floods, earthquakes…).

COMMUNITY DISASTER PLANNING

- Develop a disaster plan to prevent or deal with identified disaster threats.
- Identify local community communication system.
- Identify disaster personnel, including private and professional volunteers, local emergency personnel agencies and resources.
- Identify regional back up agencies and personnel.
- Identify specific responsibilities for various personnel involved in the disaster plans.
- Set up an emergency medical system and chain for activation.
- Identify location and accessibility of equipment and supplies.
- Check proper functioning of emergency equipment.
- Identify outdated supplies and replenish for appropriate use.

IMPLEMENTATION OF PLANS

- Focus on primary prevention activities to prevent occurrence of manmade disasters.
- Practice community disaster plan with all personnel carrying out their previously identified responsibilities. (e.g. emergency triage, providing supplies such as food, water, medicine, crisis and grief counseling)
- Practice using equipment: Obtaining and distributing supplies.

EVALUATION OF PLANS

- Critically, evaluate all aspects of disaster plans and practice drills for speed, effectiveness, gaps and revisions.
- Evaluate the response of personnel involved in disaster relief efforts.

ETIOLOGY OF MALADAPTIVE BEHAVIOR

Maladaptive Behavior

- Maladaptive behavior is a set of behaviors the individual might exhibit that are inappropriate or disruptive in nature.
- Maladaptive behavior refers to types of behaviors that inhibit a person's ability to adjust to particular situations. This type of behavior is often used to reduce one's anxiety but the result is dysfunctional and nonproductive.

Etiology

Maladaptive behaviors are caused by multiple factors. These factors may predispose an individual psychiatric morbidity, precipitate or perpetuate the mental illness.

- *Vitamine deficiency and malnutrition:* Vit 'B' complex.
- *Degenerative diseases:* Dementia, Alzheimer's disease.
- *Endocrine disturbances*
- *Physical defects and illnesses:* Chronic illness and physical handicap.

Physiological Changes

Changes in physiological function of an individual in a life span can trigger psychiatric symptoms. The milestones of life like puberty, menstruation, menarche, climacteric, delivery/labour, puerperium. These are marked not only by physiological (endocrine) changes but also by psychosocial and puerperium issues that diminish the adaptive capacity of the individual.

Psychosocial Factors

- Severe psychological trauma suffered as a child, such as emotional, physical or sexual abuse
- An important early loss, such as the loss of a parent
- Neglect
- Poor ability to relate to others
- Death or divorce
- A dysfunctional family life
- Feelings of inadequacy, low self-esteem, anxiety, anger, or loneliness
- Changing jobs or schools.
- Social or cultural expectations (e.g. a society that associates beauty with thinness can be a factor in the development of eating disorders).
- Substance abuse by the person or the person's family members.
- Sexual difficulties arising out of marital life.
- Stress, frustration and seasonal variations also contribute for mental illness (Fig. 2.5).

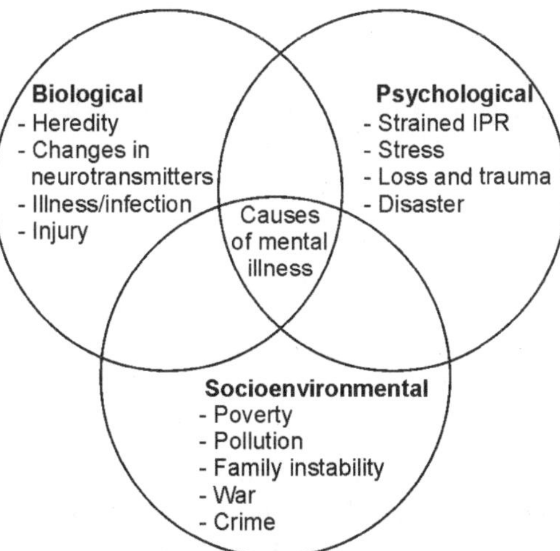

Fig. 2.5: Factors causing mental illness

PSYCHOPATHOLOGY OF MENTAL DISORDERS

- Literally, psychopathology is a term which refers to either the study of mental illness or mental distress or the manifestation of behaviors and experiences which maybe indicative of mental illness or psychological impairment, such as abnormal, maladaptive behavior or mental activity (Atkinson L 2004).
- Actually, psychopathology diverges into two separate routes. It is the study of mental illness or disorders, and is also what emerges as these disorders appear in the individual. For example, a person with certain characteristics like manic and depressed state might have a psychopathology (group of symptoms) indicative of bipolar disorder or other psychopathologies might be suggested with addition of other symptoms.
- The description of psychiatric illness is found in DSM and ICD. With study of these, psychiatric health professionals are able to diagnose disease because of description. This description is part of psychopathology, since intense study of mental health illnesses tends to result in being able to describe the general characteristics of each disease.
- Presence of disease affecting mental processes does not necessarily mean disease originates in the mind. Current and continued research on different forms of disease that manifest 'mental symptoms' suggests the continued work of the psychopathologist. Increasingly, evaluation of different body functions may point to causes of mental illnesses that occur elsewhere anatomically that might need different treatments that in those specifically addressing neurotransmitter. Thus, the study and research in psychopathology is ongoing.
- The other way in which the term is used as descriptive of mental disorders create a common language for mental health practitioners. Yet, no practitioner can make diagnosis unless symptoms manifest. The way in which symptoms manifest can be different with each mental disorder and sometime psychopathologies are immediately evident, while other times they may be hard to observe at first. Having access to diagnostic manuals and possessing significant experiences may make diagnosis better. Wrong diagnosis is not uncommon, since a number of mental conditions share similar psychopathological sign.

REVIEW OF STRUCTURE AND FUNCTION OF BRAIN, NEURAL SYSTEM AND ABNORMAL NEUROTRANSMISSION

Human Nervous System

- As the most complex system, the nervous system serves as the body control center and communications for electrical chemical wiring network. As a key homeostatic regulatory and coordinating system, it detects, interprets and responds to changes in internal and external conditions. The nervous system integrates countless bits of information and generates appropriate reactions by sending electrochemical impulses through neurons to effector organs such as muscles and glands.
- The human nervous system can be divided into two parts: the central nervous system (CNS) and the peripheral nervous system (PNS). The central nervous system consists of the brain and the spinal cord, the peripheral nervous system constitutes of the somatic system and the autonomic system (Fig. 2.6).

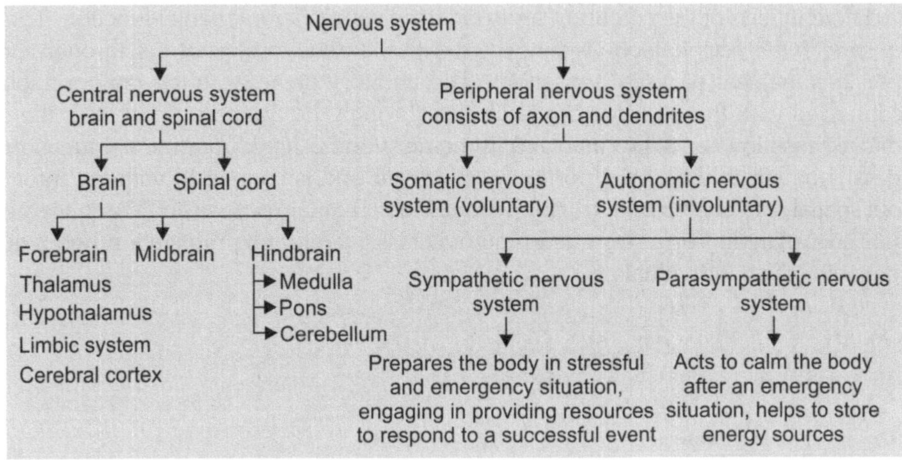

Fig. 2.6: Nervous system

Central Nervous System (CNS)

Central nervous system consists of brain and the spinal cord. Brain is composed of three main divisions: the forebrain, midbrain and the hindbrain (Fig. 2.7).

The Forebrain

- The forebrain consists of thalamus, hypothalamus, limbic system and the cerebrum. All sensory impulses pass through thalamus to the higher center, therefore, it is usually known as relay station. In addition, it controls autonomic nervous system and also plays as a role in the control of sleep and attention.
- Hypothalamus lies below the thalamus. It exerts a key influence on all kinds of emotional as well as motivational behavior, center in the hypothalamus have control over the important body processes like eating, drinking, sleeping, temperature control and sex drive. It also has control over the activities and pituitary gland.
- The limbic system consists of structures in the thalamus, hypothalamus and cerebrum which form a ring around the lower part of the forebrain. Major structures within this system include all the olfactory bulbs, the septal nuclei, and the cingulate gyrus of the cerebral cortex. The limbic system often called the emotional brain. The functions are related to emotional aspects of behavior like so survival, memory, sleep, smell, pleasure and pain, rage, aggression, affection and sexual desire, etc.
- The cerebrum is the most complex and largest part of the brain. The cerebrum is covered by a thick layer of tightly packed nerves called the cerebral cortex. It is divided into two hemispheres; the left and right hemisphere. Different areas of the cerebral cortex are like sensory projection areas, motor for different function like storing sensory information, controlling body movements, coordinating all information that comes to the brain and regulating highly cognitive functions such as thinking, reasoning and problem-solving. Each cerebral hemisphere is divided into four lobes. Frontal, parietal, occipital and temporal lobes.

- The different parts of the cerebrum are connected with different mental function. The visual area lying in the occipital lobe is connected with the visual organs or eye through the optic nerve. It is the seat of visual sensations. The auditory area lies in the temporal lobe and is connected with the auditory organ or ears through the auditory nerve. It is the seat of auditory sensations and also involved in memory and other higher mental functions. The parietal lobe lies in the upper portion of the brain and is connected with the information about spatial relationship and structure. Frontal lobes contain several and are concerned with organizing, planning or actions, learning new tasks, generating motivation and regulation of behavior of an individual.

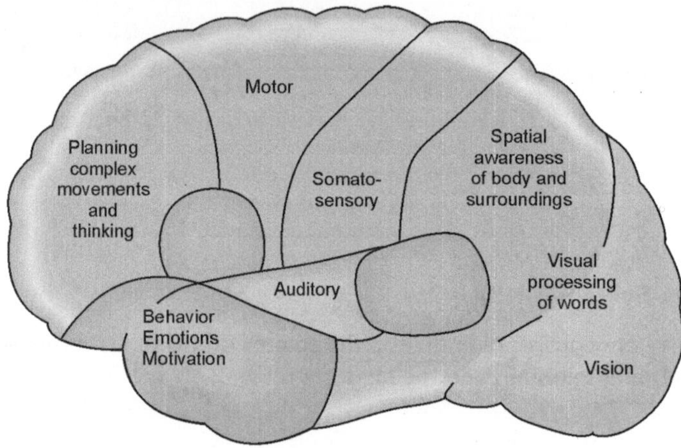

Fig. 2.7: Parts of brain

The Midbrain

It is concerned with the relaying of messages particularly those related to hearing and sight to higher brain center. One of its important structure is known as reticular activating system (RAS). With the help of RAS, an individual is able to decide which impulses should be registered consciously and which should be rejected.

The Hindbrain

It is composed of three structures, the medulla, the pons and the cerebellum (Fig. 2.8). Medulla controls eating and many important reflexes, such as those help us maintain our upright postures. It also regulates the highly complex processes

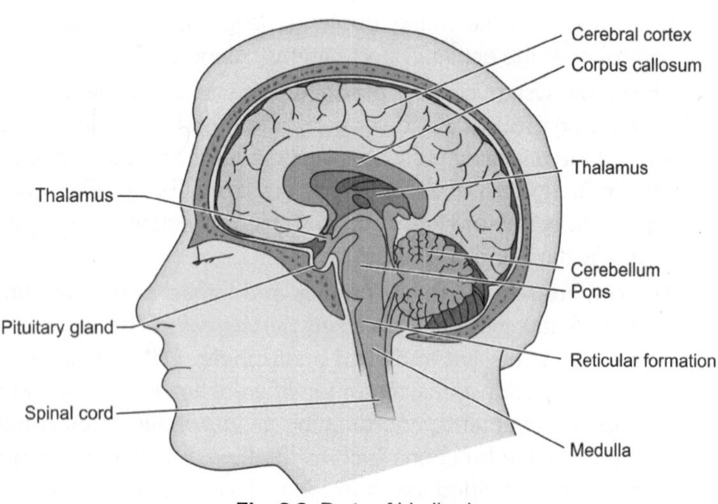

Fig. 2.8: Parts of hindbrain

like digestion, respiration and circulation. The pons assists in breathing, transmitting impulses from the cerebellum of both sides of the brain. Cerebellum is responsible for body balance and the coordination of body movement like dancing, typing, playing, etc.

Spinal Cord

The spinal cord is a continuation of the brainstem. It is long, cylindrical and passes through a channel in the vertebrae called the vertebral canal. The spinal cord has many spinal segments, which are spinal cord regions from which pairs (one per segment) of spinal nerves arise. Like the cerebrum and cerebellum, the spinal cord has gray and white matter; although here the white matter lies outside. The spinal cord carries messages between the CNS and the rest of the body; and mediates numerous spinal reflexes such as knee-jerk reflex.

Peripheral Nervous System (PNS)

- The peripheral nervous system includes sensory receptors, sensory neurons and motor nerve receptors are activated by a stimulus. The stimulus is converted to an electrical signal and transmitted to a sensory neuron. Sensory neurons connect sensory receptors to the CNS. The CNS processes the signal and transmits a message back to an effector organ through a motor neuron.
- *The PNS has two parts:* The somatic nervous system and the automatic nervous system. The somatic nervous system or voluntary nervous system enables human to react consciously to environmental changes. It includes 31 pairs of spinal nerves and 12 pairs of cranial nerves. This system controls movements of elected (voluntary) muscles.
- Thirty one pairs of spinal nerves emerge from various segments of the spinal cord. Each spinal nerve has a dorsal root and ventral root. The dorsal root contains afferent (SENSORY) fibers that transmit information to the spinal cord from the sensory receptors. The ventral root contains efferent (motor) fibers that carry messages from the spinal cord to the effectors. Cell bodies of the efferent fibers reside in the spinal cord gray matter. These roots become nerves that innervate and transmit nerve impulse to muscles and organs throughout the body.
- Twelve pairs of cranial nerves transmit from special sensory receptors information on the senses of balance, smell, sight, task and hearing (Fig. 2.9). Cranial nerves also carry information from general sensory receptors in the body mostly from the head region. This information is processed in the CNS; the resulting orders travel back through the cranial nerves to the skeletal muscles that control movements in the face and throat; such as for smiling and swallowing. In addition, some cranial nerves contain somatic and autonomic motor fibers.
- The involuntary nervous system (autonomic nervous system) maintains homeostasis. As its name implies, this system works automatically and without voluntary input. Its parts include receptors within viscera (internal organ) the afferent nerves that relay the information to the CNS, and the efferent nerves that relay the action back to the effectors. The effectors in this system are smooth muscle, cardiac muscle and glands; all structures that function without conscious control. An example of autonomic control is movement of food through the digestive tract during sleep.
- The efferent portion of the autonomic system is divided into sympathetic and parasympathetic systems. The sympathetic nerves mobiles energy for the 'fight or flight' reaction during stress, causing increased blood pressure, respiratory rate and blood flow to the muscles. Conversely, the parasympathetic nerves have a calming effect; they slow the heartbeat and breathing rate

and promote digestion and elimination. This shows an intimate interaction with the endocrine system which explain why the two systems are called the neuroendocrine system.

- The relationship between sensory and motor neurons can be seen in a reflex. Reflexes are quick because they involve few neurons. Reflexes are either somatic or autonomic. All reflex arcs have five basic elements. A receptor, sensory neuron, integration center, motor neuron and effector. Spinal reflexes are somatic reflexes mediated by the spinal cord. These can involve brain centers. In a spinal reflex the message is simultaneously sent to the spinal cord and brain. The reflex triggers the response without waiting for brain analysis. If a finger touches something hot, the finger jerks away from the spot. The burning sensation becomes an impulse in the sensory neurons. These cause the burned finger to pull away. This spinal reflex is a flex or withdrawal reflex.
- The stretch reflex occurs when a muscle or its tendon is struck. The jolt causes the muscle to contract and inhibits antagonist muscle contraction. For example, the patellar reflex, or knee jerk reflex. This occurs when the patellar tendon is struck. The impulse travels via interpreted neurons to the spinal cord where the message is interpreted. Two messages are sent back, are causing the quadriceps muscles to control and the other inhibiting the antagonist hamstring muscles from contracting. The contraction of the quadriceps and inhibition of hamstrings cause the lower leg to kick or knee jerk.

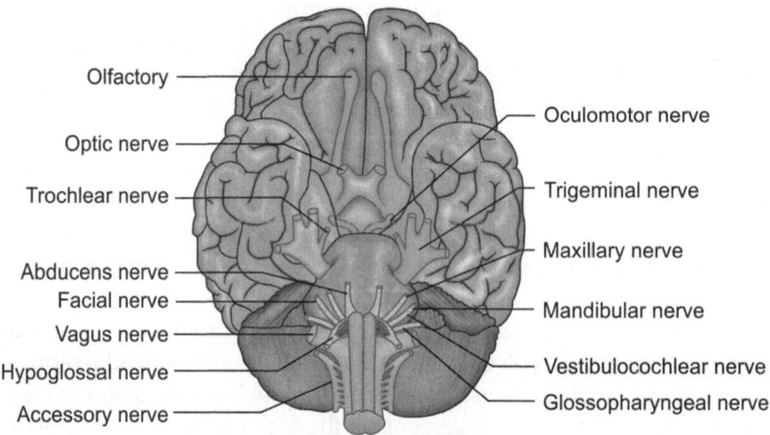

Fig. 2.9: Cranial nerves

BRAIN AND BEHAVIOR

The entire behavior of a person is totally controlled and managed by brain. The new clinical and experimental evidence suggest that the left hemisphere of the brain is specialized for speech activity where the right hemisphere is specialized for many nonlinguistic functions. Researchers believe that complex thinking involves both sides of the brain. The process of learning, emotional control and as well as growth and development is directly and relatively controlled with great extent by the brain. So, any abnormality in physiological and anatomical function can give risk to physio-psychiatric disorder.

NEURON

A neuron is a nerve cell that is the building block of the nervous system. Neurons are specialized to transmit information throughout the body. Humans have about 100 billion neurons in their brain alone. While variable in size and shape, all neurons have three parts, dendrites receive information from another cell and transmit the message to the cell body (Fig. 2.10). The cell body contains nucleus, mitochondria and other organelles. The axon conducts messages away from the cell body.

Three types of neurons occur. Sensory neurons typically have a long dendrite and short axon, and carry message from sensory receptors to the central nervous system. Motor neurons have a long axon and short dendrites and transmit messages from the central nervous system to the nucleus. Interneurons are found only in the central nervous system where they connect neuron to neuron.

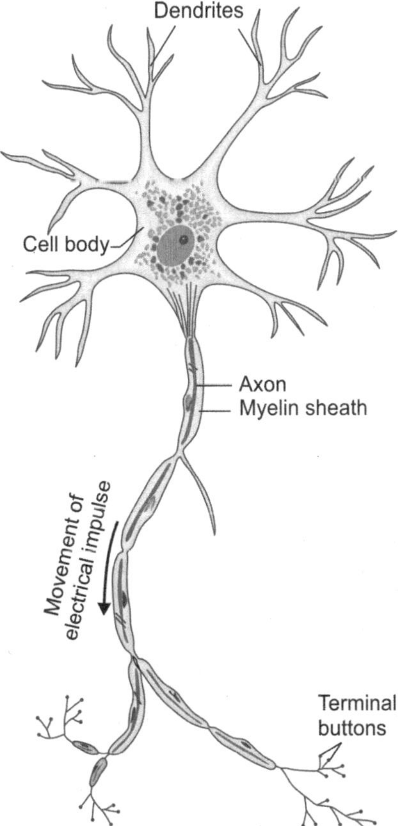

Fig. 2.10: Parts of neuron

Synapses

The junction between a nerve cell and another cell is called a synapse (Fig. 2.11). Message travel within the neuron as an electrical action potential. The space between two cells is known as the synaptic cleft. To cross the synaptic cleft, it requires the actions of neurotransmitters.

Neurotransmitters are stored in small synaptic vesicles clustered at the tip of the axon. Neuron of the action potential causes some of the vesicles to move to the end of the axon and discharge their contents into the synaptic cleft. Released neurotransmitter diffuse across the cleft, and bind to receptors in the other membrane causing ion channels on that cell to open. Some neurotransmitter cause an action potential while others are inhibitory.

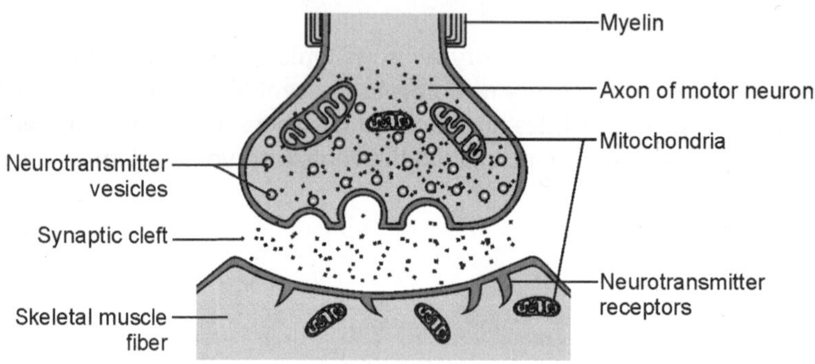

Fig. 2.11: The synapse

- Neurotransmitters tend to be small molecules, some are even hormones. The time for neurotransmitter action is between 0.5 and 1 millisecond. Neurotransmitters are either destroyed by specific anzymes in the synaptic cleft, diffuse out of the cleft, or are reabsorbed by the cell. More than thirty organic molecules are thought to act as neurotransmitters. The neurotransmitters cross the cleft, binding, to receptor molecules on the next cell, prompting transmission of the message along the cell membrane. Acetylcholine and norepinephrine acts each other in different response. Once in the cleft, neurotransmitters are active for only a short time. Enzyme in the cleft inactivates the neurotransmitters. Inactivated neurotransmitter are taken back into the axon and recycled.
- Disease that affects the function of signal transmission can have serious consequences. Parkinson's disease has a deficiency of the neurotransmitter dopamine. Progressive death of brain cells increase this deficit, causing tremors rigidity and unstable posture. Levodopa is a chemical related to dopamine that causes some of the symptoms (acts as substitute neurotransmitter) but cannot reverse the progression of the disease.
- GABA is important in conceptualizing the pathology and treatment of phobia and other anxiety disorders. The bacterium *Clostridium tetani* produces a toxin that prevents the release of GABA. GABA is important in control of skeletal muscles. Without this control, regulation of muscle contraction is lost; it can be fatal when it affects the muscles used in breathing.
- Glutamate is an excitatory neurotransmitter and plays important role in the pathology and treatment of Alzheimer's disease
- Serotonin is also a neurotransmitter which regulates the mood. Abnormality can cause mania and depressive disorders.
- Norepinephrine is important in conceptualizing the pathology and treatment of mania and depression.
- *Clostridium botulinum* produces a toxin found in improperly canned foods. This toxin causes the progressive relaxation of muscles and can be fatal. A wide range of drugs also operate in the synapses. Cocaine, and caffeine and insecticides.

- Biological theories postulate that psychiatric disorders are caused by imbalance in the complex process of brain structure communication with each other through neurotransmission.
- The neuroendocrine theory deals with the interaction between the nervous and endocrine system and the hormones that react to stimulation from the nerve cells.
- *Psychoimmunology:* It studies the interaction between psychological processes and the nervous immune system of the human body. In 1975, *Robert Ader and Nicholoas Cohen* at the university of Rochester coined the term 'psychoimmunology'. Psychoimmunology looks for the exact mechanism by which specific brain immunity effects are retrieved. In this, two major pathways are involved the hypothalamic pituitary adrenal axis (HPA AXIS) and the sympathetic nervous system (SNS). HPA axis responds to physical and mental challenge to maintain homeostasis in part by controlling the body's cortisol level. Dysregulation of the HPA axis is implicated in stress and other mental disorders.

PRINCIPLES OF MENTAL HEALTH NURSING

- Human behavior is the amalgamation of physical, psychosocial, emotional and spiritual components. Illness affects these components in different needs in an unique pattern. These needs will be felt by each client in a different manner at different stages of illness.
- The mental health nursing principles are formulated on the concept that every individual client has an intrinsic worth and dignity, potentialities and capabilities to grow utmost. These following principles help to bring changes in behavior. The principles focus on the specified utilization of client and care with respect and dignity as a human being.
- Accept the client exactly as his acceptance involves the feeling of being loved, cared and harmony. By recognizing nurses acceptance, it will lower the anxiety and non-fearing experience among psychiatric client: it will unlearn the unwanted behavior and relearn the coping behavior among clients. Nurses should consider the client as a 'whole' in holistic way. The psychiatric nursing care activation must focus on emotional needs.

Being Nonjudgmental and Nonpunitive

Psychiatric nurses should provide care by non-judgmental basis, i.e. not considering clients' psychosocial behavior, client should not be punished for his undesirable behavior either directly (e.g. changing) or indirectly (e.g. ignoring). Nurses will not judge the client's behavior on moral or ethical ground. Even if clients behave against the expectation of nurses.

Sincerity and Positive Interest

Nurses has to exhibit sincerity and positive interest towards the client. This is achieved by

- Studying the client's behavior patterns, living style.
- Showing concern and positive interest towards the clients welfare by actively listening and trying to understand the feeling of clients and therapeutic communication.
- Recognizes sincerity for his clients care.
- Accepting clients fears as real to him.
- Explaining the client when his demands were not fulfilled.
- Avoid probing into sensitive matters.

Recognizes and Reflects on Client Feeling, Which He Expresses

Nurses must assess the behavioral pattern, i.e. his inner needs, potentialities, interaction pattern of the client and ability to differentiate between needs and demands. Nurses will give more importance to recognize the clients emotional feelings actually expressed by the client in his conversation and not to the context. Discussion of personal relationships and personal values has to be initiated only by the client, observation of client behavior is directed towards analysis of why the client behaves as he does.

Listening

Always listening is an active process. The nurses must imbibe the act of listening by consuming time and energy to the client. Nurse must be a sympathetic listener and show genuine interest.

Use of Self-Understanding as a Therapeutic Tool

A mental health nurse primarily should have her own self-concept and able to recognize one's feelings attitudes and response. Her limitations and strength makes other to own. Self understanding helps to be assertive in life situation without being aggressive and feeling guilty.

Use of Consistency of Client's Security and Safety

Consistency in care is necessary to develop a feeling in the client that he/she can depend upon the people who are working in the ward. It lowers clients anxiety and provides psychosocial security feeling. It must reflect in their attitudes. Routine care or by defining limitations on the clients behavior; although permitting him to feel free. This is practiced by:

- Providing acceptance constantly and continuously to the client.
- Maintain consistency in the presence of nurse round the clock with prior proper planning and validating.

Reassurance should be given in a Subtle and Acceptable Manner

Reassurance is building psychological strength in clients, confidence. To provide reassurance, the psychiatric nurse needs to understand and analyze the situation as to how it appears to the client false reassurance demonstrates lack of interest and understanding/unwillingness on the part of the nurse to empathize with the client life situation.

Change the Client Behavior by Emotional Experience Rather than by Rational Interpretation

One of the major focus in mental health nursing is on feeling and not much on the intellectual part of client merely adversing or rationalizing with client is not effective in changing behavior. Role play psychodrama and transactional analysis are a few avenues of providing corrective emotional experiences to a client and facilitating insight into his own behavior. These experiences truly charge the undecided behavior.

Unnecessary Increase in Client Anxiety should be Avoided

The following instances may enhance the client anxiety and therefore, be avoided.

- Showing own anxiety and fear to nurses.
- Showing attention to the clients deficits.

- Making the client to face repeated failures.
- Placing demands on client which he/she obviously cannot meet.
- Direct contradiction of clients psychotic ideas.
- Telling sharp comments and showing bias.

Objective Observation of Client to Understand his Behavior

Objectivity is an ability to evaluate exactly what the client wants to say and not mixup one's own feelings, opinion or judgement. To be objective the psychiatric nurse should indulge introspection and make sure that her own emotional needs do not take precedence over clients needs.

Maintain Realistic Nurse-Client Relationship

Professional relationship focuses upon the personal and emotional needs of the client and most on the nurses needs. To maintain and sustain professional relationship the nurse should have a realistic self-concept and should be able to empathize and understand the feelings of the client and the meaning of his behaviors. Always the relationship between nurse and client is therapeutic in nature. Therapeutic nurse patient relationship is an experience of mutual learning for the nurse and the client as well as a corrective emotional experience for the client. The relationship is developed on the basis of the underlying humanity of nurse and client, with both respecting and accepting each others ethnocultural differences.

Avoid Physical and Verbal Force as Much as Possible

Abuse and punishment must be avoided to the greatest extent. If the nurse is an expert in providing care she can predict clients behavior and she can mostly prevent an onset of undesirable behavior.

Nursing Care is Centered on the Client as a Person and not on the Control of Symptoms

The nurse has to look into the client as a person, in a holistic manner. The needs of same symptom clients will be varied. So, nursing care should be centered on individual clients.

- All explanations of procedures and other routines are given according to the clients level of understanding.
- The extent of explanation that can be provided to a client mainly depends on his overall understanding and retention of material, but explanation should never be withheld on the basis that psychiatric client are not having any contract with reality or have no ability to understand.
- Many procedures are modified but basic principles remain unaltered.
- In psychiatric mental health nursing setup, many methods are adapted to individual needs of the clients, but the underlying nursing scientific principles remain the same. Some nursing principles to be kept in mind are: safety, comfort, privacy, maintain therapeutic effectiveness, economy of time, energy, material, etc.

STANDARDS OF MENTAL HEALTH NURSING PRACTICE

The purpose of standards of psychiatric and mental health nursing practice is to fulfill the nursing professions obligation to provide a means of improving the quality of care. The revised 2000 ANA standard are given below.

• **Standard I: Assessment**	The psychiatric mental health nurse collects patients health data.
• **Standard II: Diagnosis**	The psychiatric mental health nurse analyzes the assessment data in determining diagnoses.
• **Standard III: Outcome identification**	The psychiatric mental health nurse identifies expected outcomes individualized to the patients.
• **Standard IV: Planning**	The psychiatric mental health nurse develop a plan of care that is negotiated among the patient, family, and health care team and prescribes evidence of based intervention to attain expected outcomes.
• **Standard V: Implementation**	The psychiatric mental health nurse implements the intervention identified in the plan of the care.
• **Standard V a: Counseling**	The psychiatric mental health nurse uses counseling intervention to assist patients in improving or regaining their previous coping abilities, fostering mental health and preventing mental illness and disability.
• **Standard V b: Milieu therapy**	The psychiatric mental health nurse provides, structures and maintains a therapeutic environment in collaboration with the patient and other health care clinicians.
• **Standard V c: Promotion of self-care activities**	The psychiatric mental health nurse structures intervention around the patient activities of daily living to foster self-care and mental and physical well-being.
• **Standard V d: Psychobiological intervention**	The psychiatric mental health nurse uses knowledge of psychobiological interventions and applies clinical skills to restore the patients health and prevent further disability.
• **Standard V e: Health teaching**	The psychiatric mental health nurse through health teaching, assists patients in achieving satisfying, productive and healthy pattern of living.
• **Standard V f: Case management**	The psychiatric mental health nurse provides case management to coordinate comprehensive health services and ensure continuity of care.
• **Standard V g: Health promotion and health maintenance**	The psychiatric mental health nurse employs strategies and interventions to promote and maintain mental health and prevent mental illness.
• **Standard V h: Psychotherapy**	The advanced practice registered nurse in psychiatric mental health (APRN-PMH) Uses individual, group and family psychotherapy, child psychotherapy and other therapeutic treatments to assist patients in preventing mental illness and disability, treating mental disorders, and improving or regaining previous health status and functional abilities.

Contd...

Contd...

• **Standard V i: Prescriptive authority and treatment**	The APRN–PMH uses prescriptive authority, procedures and treatments in accordane with state and federal laws and regulation to tract symptoms of psychiatric illness and improve functional health status.
• **Standard V j: Consultation**	The APRN-DMH provides consultation to enhance the abilities of other clinicians to provide services for patients and to affect change in the system.
• **Standard V k: Evaluation**	The psychiatric mental health nurse evaluates the patients progress in attaining expected outcomes.

Conceptual Models and Role of Nurse

Behavior is a complex phenomena to explain the scientists put forth their views in the form of theory as well as conceptual models to explain the domains of behavior. A conceptual model is a framework of related concepts. Conceptual model used by mental health practioners address the bases for behavior in order to direct and implement psychotherapeutic interventions. The most important conceptual models are the psychoanalytic, interpersonal, behavioral, cognitive, developmental and neurobiological models.

PSYCHOANALYTIC MODEL (1856–1939)

Sir Sigmund Freud is the founder of psychoanalytic model. Freud was an Austrian physician who began his career as a neurologist. He developed an elaborate theory of human behavior based primarily on his work with persons suffering form disabling anxiety. The treatment approach derived from his theories is known as psychoanalysis. Freud believed that the personality is formed in early childhood and that knowledge of how an individual drives, instincts, psychoenergy or libido and psychosexual attitude are formed during the first 5 to 6 years of life is crucial to an understanding of the personality. Key Freudian concepts include levels of consciousness, structure of the personality and psychosexual development.

Three Levels of Consciousness

Freud believed in three levels of consciousness. The first level of consciousness is the conscious mind, that part of the mind which is aware of the present situation and function only when the person is awake. It represents the smallest part of the mind and directs an individual rational and thoughtful behavior.

The second level of consciousness is the preconscious. The preconscious (subconscious) is the part of the mind in which thought, feelings and sensations are stored. Although material stored in the preconscious mind are outside of awareness, they can be brought to the conscious mind the proper stimulus such as by asking direct question.

The third level of consciousness is the unconscious. The unconscious represents the largest part of the mind and is the storehouse for all of the thoughts, feelings and sensations experienced during the life span of an individual. The individual is rarely aware of the unconscious mind, except when it demonstrates its presence through dreams, jokes, slips of the tongue, unexplained behavior and lapses of memory. These thoughts, feelings and sensations cannot be recalled at will, but nevertheless exert powerful influence on the individual behavior. Belief in the existence of the unconscious is the basis to say 'all behavior has meaning'.

Structure of Personality

The second major concept developed by Freud is the structure of personality. Freud believed that the personality consists of three aspects. The ID, the ego and the super ego.

The ID is part of and derived from the unconscious. It is unlearned, primitive and selfish in nature. The ID does not have a sense of right or wrong and ruthlessly insists on immediate satisfaction of its impulses and desires which are geared toward avoiding pain and experiencing pleasure. The personality of small children consists of mainly ID, a belief that is not difficult to accept when one observes the behavior of infants. They may cry instantly when hungry, regards of the social appropriateness of such behavior. Even mature adults unceasing pressure from the ID to satisfy its demands. The other parts of the personality are responsible for keeping the ID under control.

The ego develops as a result of the child's interaction with her/his surrounding and evironment it establishes an acceptable compromise between the crude, pleasure seeking compromise between the inhibitions of the superego through reality testing. Reality testing is a process the ego employs to ascertain the likely consequences of behavior. The ego is the practical part of the personality. As an individual matures, the ego becomes the rational, reasonable, conscious part of the personality and strives to integrate the total personality into a smoothly functioning coherent whole. In the mature adult the ego represent the self to others and individuals the person from other human beings.

Chronologically, the superego develops at last. The superego acts as the moral judge of the individual based on what the person has learned from significant others, such as parents, teachers and others. It operates mostly at the unconscious level and control the ID. The two aspects of the superego are the conscience, which punishes individuals through guilt and anxiety when their behavior deviates from the standards of the superego; and the ego-ideal, which reward individuals with feelings of well-being when their behavior achieves those standards believed desirable by the superego. Neither the punishing nor the rewarding functions of the superego are based on the reality of the situation. Rather, they are based on the individual internalized standard of right and wrong, good and bad, that were learned at early and are stored primarily in the unconscious.

Freud believed that when ID impulses unacceptable to the superego threaten to emerge, the individual experiences anxiety. Anxiety is a diffuse, vague as a negative emotion. Therefore, the person experiencing anxiety works to get rid of this feeling, often through the use of ego defense mechanism or mental mechanism. These are derived from the ego that are designed to affect a compromise between the demands of the ID and the superego to overcome anxiety ego defense mechanism.

Operate on the unconscious level, although an objective observer maybe able to discern when others are using them. For example, a student who perceives herself as very intelligent but who fails in a test may rationalize, otherwise it produces anxiety in her. To overcome this anxiety she tells herself and others that 'test is not so important.

Table of Details Commonly Used Defense Mechanism

Defense mechanism	Definition	Examples
• **Denial**	Failing to perceive some threatening object or event in the entire world	An alcoholic denies the amart he consumed
• **Compensation**	Exaggerating one trait to make up for feelings of inadequacy or inferiority in another dimension	A physically handicapped man verbally abuses his employees.
• **Displacement**	Attributing feelings to a person or object that are really directed at another person or object	A young woman kicks her cat after arguing with her boss.
• **Fixation**	Remaining 'stuck' in a developmental stage.	A husband depends totally on his wife for most of his activities of daily living.
• **Sublimation**	Redirecting socially unacceptable urges into socially acceptable behavior.	An angry, hostile young man becomes a boxer player.
• **Reaction formation/ over compensation**	Substituting directly opposite wishes for one's true wishes	A woman who actually dislikes her mother in law hides her feelings by being always very nicc to hcr.
• **Identification**	Integrating desired attributes of an admired person to compensate for perceived inadequacy	A shy girl styles her hair similarly that of manner
• **Introjections**	Incorporating another person to avoid the threat posed by the person or by one's own urges	A psychotically depressed women attempts suicide to kill her mother, whom she states that she is in her stomach.
• **Undoing**	Engaging in certain thoughts and actions so as to cancel out or alone for threatening thought or actions that have previously occurred	A business woman studies to become a nursery school teacher after having an abortion
• **Isolation**	Severing the connection between the thought and feeling associated with an event so the event can remain conscious without undue anxiety	A single parent talks unemotionally about her only child's recent diagnosis of brain tumor
• **Rationalization**	Substituting a fictitious, socially acceptable reason for the genuine, unacceptable reason for one's wishes or actions	'I would have helped you if I could, but I have to take my dog to show to veterinary doctor'.
• **Repression**	Forcibly dismission anxiety producing thoughts feelings	A woman is unable to remember being raped by her brother when she was child.
• **Regression**	Returning to patterns of behavior characteristic of a less anxiety producing stage of development	A 6-year-old girl begins to wet the bed at night after her mother's remarriage .
• **Projection**	Attributing to others are objectionable trait or feeling that really emanates from one self.	'My husband is cheating on me'

Contd...

Contd...

Defense mechanism	Definition	Examples
• **Symbolization and condensation**	Using a neutral idea or object to represent an inacceptable idea or objects	A 40 years old man has unconscious feelings of inadequacy as a male and spends all his money on guns and all his time polishing and cleaning them.
• **Conversion**	Expressing unconscious emotional conflicts through a physical symptom with no demonstrable organic basis.	A young woman wakes up paralyzed on the morning of her wedding day.

In contrast to the unconscious nature of defense mechanism, coping mechanism are conscious mental strategies or behavior the individual employs to lower anxiety. Coping mechanism are categorized as short-term or long-term.

Short-term coping mechanisms are designed to address the immediate problem. For example, a person experiencing a great deal of work related stress may drink alcohol a means of coping. Although alcohol may relieve anxiety for time being but it does not address.

The sources of the stress or prevent the anxiety form emerging in contrast, long-term coping mechanism address the cause of the anxiety and are likely to benefit the individual more than short-term coping mechanism. Some examples are relaxation techniques, bio-feedback, exercise, associativeness training, setting goals, classifying communication, visualization and guided imagery, meditation, yoga, seeking out support from peers and self-hypnosis.

PSYCHOSEXUAL THEORY OF PERSONALITY DEVELOPMENT

Fraud stresses that the first five years of life are crucial to the formation of adult personality. The ID must be controlled in order to satisfy social demands. This sets up a conflict between frustrated wishes and social norms. The ego and superego develop in order to exercise this control and direct the need for gratification into socially acceptance channels. Gratification centers of different areas of the body at different stages of growth, making the conflict at each stage psychosexual.

Oral Stage (0–1 Year)

The first stage of personality development is libido. Libido is centered in a body's month. It gets much satisfaction from putting all sorts of things in its month to satisfy libido, and thus its ID demands. Which at this stage in life are oral or mouth oriented, such as sucking, biting and breastfeeding. Freud said that oral stimulation could lead to an oral fixation in later life. We see oral personalities all around us such as smokers, nail biters, finger chewers and thumb suckers. Oral personalities engage in such oral behaviors particularly when under stress.

Anal Stage (1–3 Year)

The libido now becomes focused on the anus and the child derives great pleasure from defecating. The child is now fully aware that they are a person in their own right and that their wishes can bring them into conflict with the demands of the outside world (i.e. Their ego has developed). Freud believed that this type of conflict tends to come to a lead in toilet training, in which adults impose restrictions on when and where the child can defecate. The nature of this first conflict with authority can determine the child's future relationship with all forms of authority.

Phallic Stage (3–6 Year)

Sensitivity now becomes concentrated in the genitals and masturbation (in both genders) become a new source of pleasure. The child becomes aware of anatomical sex differences, which set in motion the conflict between erotic attraction, resentment, rivalry, jealousy and fear which Freud called the Oedipus complex (in boys) and the Electra complex (in girls). This is resolved through the process of identification which involves the child adopting the characteristics of the same sex present.

Latency (5 or 6 to Puberty)

No further psychosexual development takes place during this stage. The libido is dormant. Freud thought that most sexual impulses are repressed during the latent stage and sexual energy can be sublimated towards school/work, hobbies and friendship. Much of the child energies are channeled into developing new skills and acquiring new knowledge and play becomes largely confined to other children of the same gender.

Genital Stage (Puberty to Adult)

Genital stage is the last stage of Freud psychosexual theory of personality development and begins in puberty. It is a time of adolescent sexual experimentation. The successful resolution of which is setting down in a loving one to one relationship with another in the age 20s or so. Sexual instinct is directed to heterosexual pleasure, rather than self-pleasure during the phallic stage. For Freud, the proper antler of the sexual instinct in adults was through heterosexual intercourse. Fixation and conflict may prevent this with the consequence that sexual perversions may develop. For example, Fixation at the oral stage may result in a person gaining sexual pleasure primarily from kissing and oral sex, rather than intercourse.

Application of Freud Theory in Clinical Practice

This theory is based on verbal techniques. Its basic purpose is to solve psychological problems by bringing the unconscious conflict into the conscious mind, where they maybe confronted and resolved. The focus is on underlying ways of experiencing things and thinking about them rather than on behavior. It aims to change the client's personality rather than just certain behaviors. In Freudian's terms, psychoanalysis is designed to strengthen the ego, increase the awareness of the ID, and bring the superego under control. Psychoanalysis is usually involved process that takes years to complete. The role of the psychoanalyst is largely passive like a guide and interpreter than a teacher. One of the major problems the analyst must deal with is the emotion resistance of the client to the painful awareness that an emotional problem exists. Therefore, analysis must uncover the emotional origins of problem; if therapy is to be effective; it must enable the person to acknowledge and confront this problem.

Existential Model (Ellis, Rogers)

The existential model focuses on the person's experience here and now, with much less attention to the person's past.

View of Behavioral Deviations

Existential theorist believes that behavioral deviations result when the individual is out of touch with the self or the environment. This attention is caused by self-imposed restrictions. The individual is not free to choose imposed restrictions. The individual is not free to choose from among all alternative behaviors. Deviant behavior frequently is way of avoiding more socially acceptable or more responsible behavior. The person who is self-alienated feels helpless, sad and lonely. Self-criticism and lack of self-awareness prevent participation in authentic, rewarding relationships with others. Theoretically the person has many choices in terms of behavior. However, existentialists believe that people tend to avoid being real and instead given into the demands of other.

Existential Therapeutic Process

There are several existential therapies, all of which assume that the patient must be able to choose freely from what life has to offer. Although the approaches are somewhat different, the goal is to return the patient to an authentic awareness of being. The existential therapeutic process focuses on the encounter. The encounter is not merely the meeting of two or more people; it also involves their appreciation of the total existence of each other. Through the encounter the patient is helped to accept and understand personal history, to live fully in the present, and to look to the future.

Roles of Patients and Existential Therapist

Existential theorist emphasizes that the therapist and the patient are equal in their common humanity. The therapist acts as a guide to the patient, who has gone astray in the search for authenticity. The therapist is direct in pointing out areas where the patient should be considered charging. However, caring and warmth are also emphasized. The therapist and the patient must be open and honest. The therapeutic experience is a model for the patient; new behavior can be tested before; risks are taken in daily life.

The patient is expected to assume and accept responsibility for behavior. Dependence on the therapist generally is not encouraged. The patient is treated as an adult. Frequently, illness deemphasizes the patient and he is viewed as a person alienated from the self and other; but for whom there is hope if the therapy is trusted and directions are followed. The patient is always active in therapy, working to meet the challenge presented by the therapist.

INTERPERSONAL MODEL (SULLIVAN, PEPLAU)

The Interpersonal model was first developed by American psychiatrist, Harry Stack Sullivan 1892–1949. He considered the healthy person as a social being with the ability to live effectively in relationship with other; mental illness was viewed as any degree of lack of awareness of the processes in interpersonal relationship. In addition, attention is given to the interpersonal nursing theory of Hildergard Peplau. Her theory focuses primarily on the nurse client relationship in which problem-solving skills are developed.

View of Behavioral Deviation

Sullivan's theory states that the person's behavior is based on two drives; the drive for satisfaction and the drive for security. Satisfaction refers to the basic human drives including hunger, sleep, lust and loneliness. Security is related to culturally defined needs such as conformity to the social norms and value system of the individual's ethnic group. Sullivan states that when the nature of a person's self-system interferes with the ability to attend to the need for either satisfaction or security, the person will become mentally ill.

When Peplau defined nursing as an interpersonal process, she also discussed the importance of basic human needs. Needs must be met if a healthy state is to be achieved and maintained for Peplau, the two interacting components of health are psychological demands and interpersonal conditions.

Interpersonal Therapeutic Process

The therapist helps the patient to identify interpersonal problems and then encourages attempts at more successful styles of relating. For example, client often has a fear of intimacy. The therapist allows the patient to become close while clearly showing there is no threat of sexual involvement. It is believed that closeness within the therapeutic relationship builds trust, facilitates apathy, enhances self-esteem, and foster growth toward healthy behavior. Peplau described this process as " psychological emergency" which include the following steps:

- The patient is accepted unconditionally as a participant in a relationship that satisfies the needs.
- Therein the relationship shifts to the patient's readiness for growth as initiated by the patients.
- Power in the relationship shifts to the client, as the patient is able to delay gratification and to invest energy in goal achievement.
- This therapy is completed when the patient can establish satisfying human relationship, thereby meeting basic needs.

Roles of Patient and Interpersonal Therapist

The patient therapist dyad is viewed as a partnership in interpersonal therapy. Sullivan describes the therapist as a 'participant observer' whose role is to engage the client, establish trust, and empathize the therapist interacts as a real person who also has beliefs, values, thoughts and feelings. The patients' role is to share concerns with the therapist and to participate as fully as possible in the relationship. The therapist helps the patient to meet the goals of therapy; needs satisfaction and personal growth.

Behavioral Model

Human behavior is learned, thus all behavior can be unlearned and new behaviors learned in its place. Behaviorism is concerned primarily with the observable and measurable aspects of human behavior. Therefore, when behaviors become unacceptable, they can be unlearned.

Behavior model depends on the theories of Ivan Pavlov and Skinner. This model assumes that all maladaptive behavior is essentially acquired through one's environment. Those practicing this model, believes that this model would be to prioritize changing the behavior over identifying the cause of the dysfunctional behavior. The main solution to psychological illness under this model is aversion therapy, where the stimulus that provokes the dysfunctional behavior is coupled with a second stimulus, which aims to produce a new reaction to the first stimulus based on the experience of the second. Also systematic desensitization can be used, especially where phobias are involved by using the phobia that currently causes the dysfunctional behavior and coupling it with a phobia that produces a more intense reaction. This is meant to make the first phobia seem less fearsome, etc, as it has been put in comparison with the second phobia. This model is helpful to treat phobia and compulsive disorder.

The behavioral model overcomes the ethical issues of 'ill or abnormal'. It concentrates on behavior and whether it is 'adaptive' or 'maladaptive'. The model also allows individual and cultural differences to be taken into account. Provided the behavior is presenting no problems to the individual or to other people, then there is no need to regard the behavior as a mental disorder.

The cognitive behavior model teaches the patient to behave differently, it teaches the patient to think differently. It is hoped that if the patient's feelings and emotions towards something are influenced to change, it will induce external behavioral change. The main model is rational emotive therapy (RET) is based on the priniciple that an 'activating' emotional event will cause a change in thought toward that situation, even if it is an illogical thought. So, with this therapy, it is the therapist's job to question and change the individual thoughts.

MEDICAL MODEL

Medical model is based on the traditional physician-patient relationship. It focuses on the diagnosis of mental illness, and subsequent treatment is based on the diagnosis. Somatic treatments, including pharma therapy and ECT are important component of the treatment process. The interpersonal aspects of the medical model varies widely, from intensive insight oriented intervention to brief session involving medical management of medications.

Most of modern psychiatric care is dominated by the medical model. Other health professionals maybe involved in interagency referrals, family assessment and health teaching but physicians are viewed as the leaders of the team when this model is in effect. Elements of other model of care maybe used in conjunction with the medical model for instance, a client maybe diagnosed with schizophrenia and treated with phenothiazine mediaction. This patient may also be participating in a token economy program to encourage socially acceptable behavior.

A positive contribution of the medical model has been the continuous exploration for causes of mental illness using the scientific process. Recently, great research studies are undertaken in learning about the functioning of the brain and nervous system. Thus progress has led to beginning of understanding of the probable physiological components of many behavioral disorders and increasingly specific and sophisticated approaches to psychiatric care.

View of Behavioral Deviations

The medical model proposes that deviant behavior is a symptom of a central nervous system disorder. Currently, the exact nature of the psychological disruption is not well understood. It is thought that the psychotic disorders such as bipolar disorder, depression and schizophrenia involve an abnormality in the transmission occurred at the synaptic level and involves neurochemicals such as dopamine, serotonin and norepinephrine. Stress and its effects on body and mind are also viewed as a major cause of mental disorders.

Roles of Patient and Medical Therapist

The roles of physician and patient have been well defined by tradition and applied in the psychiatric setting. The physician as the healer, identifies the patient illness and institutes a treatment plan. The patient may have multiple problem, but the physician prescribes the therapy.

The role of the patient involves admitting being ill which can be a problem in psychiatry. Patients sometimes are not aware of their disturb behavior and may actively resist treatment. This is not congruent with the medical model the patient is expected to comply with the treatment program and to try to get well. If observable improvement does not occur, caregivers and significant others often suspect that the patient is not trying hard enough. This can be frustrating to a patient who is trying to get well and is disappointed with the lack of progress. The patient also may have difficulty letting people extend care and at the same time be self-sufficient.

The Nursing Process: Assessment and Evaluation of Psychiatric Clients

The evaluation of psychiatric clients is a multifaceted task, mostly performed by multidisciplinary team of mental health professionals. A comprehensive, holistic psychiatric assessment examines the physical, psychosocial, intellectual, sexual, and spiritual aspects of the client. The physical assessment includes physical examination, a study of the client's biologic life stage and genetic predisposition, laboratory tests and diagnostic tests such as MRI, EEG, etc. The psychological evaluation includes childhood experiences, personality, and current symptoms of psychiatric illness. This information is gathered by multiple skills such as interviewing, observation, carry on the Mental Status Examination. Mental Status Examination and also by administering specific psychosocial tests and rating scales.

Cognitive functioning is best assessed by utilizing a standard measure such as the Mini Mental State Examination. The social assessment consists of an exploration of cultural, environmental and familial influences on the expression and experience of illness, and the spiritual assessment is an exploration of the patient's religious and spiritual dimensions.

The psychiatric nursing evaluation covers the assessment, diagnosis, outcome identification and planning stages of the nursing process. The evaluation is ongoing process and new insights into his or her issues come to light the diagnosis and treatment plan evolve accordingly.

ASSESSMENT

The assessment phase of the nursing process includes the collection of data about a client, family or group by the methods of observation, examination, and interviewing. Two types of data are collected: objective and subjective. Objective data include information obtained verbally from the client, as well as the results of inspection, palpation, precursor, and by auscultation during an examination. Subjective data are obtained as the client, family members or significant others provide information spontaneously during collection of data.

Psychiatric nurses must collect in-depth data about the client. It is the quality and not be quantity of the assessment data that matters (Regan-Kubinski, 1995). The following guidelines for a holistic psychiatric nursing assessment should be tailored to meet the specific needs of the nurse, client and the situation.

PSYCHIATRIC NURSING INTERVIEW

Psychiatric nursing interview is a therapeutic communication between the client and nurse. The purpose of the psychiatric nursing interview is to gather the information necessary to understand, evaluate, and treat the client.

Content of the Psychiatric Nursing Interview: Biopsychosocial History

Biopsychosocial history is a comprehensive assessment of the client's lifetime biological, psychological and social functioning.

Identifying Data

A written biopsychosocial history begins with a comprehensive summary of the client's demographic profile; name, age, gender, marital status, address, residence, religion, nationality, education, occupation and current socioeconomic living situation.

Chief Complaint

The client's chief complaint is the reason for current admission to the hospital. It should be obtained in the client's own words. Mention the duration of complaints is necessary. The chief complaints provides valuable data concerning the client's illness.

History of Presenting Complaint

Describing the period or leading up to admission assess the presenting complaint as any history. It must include the following points.

- Nature of problem
- Onset
- Triggers
- Exuberating/relieving factors
- Progression (improving, worsening or staying the same, intermittent or continuos)
- Associated symptoms
- Disability (effect on life)

  The nature of the presenting complaint is the form the problem takes, e.g. worry, mood, delusion, hallucination, physical complaint, social problem.

  Before finishing, summarize the client's problem and ask 'is there anything you think I should know'.

PAST PSYCHIATRIC HISTORY

Ask about previous contact with psychiatrists, general practitioners and times of severe stress or depression which the patient handled alone.

- Has anything like this ever happened before?
- Have you had any stress related or mental health problems before?

  Find out past episodes occurred, how long they lasted and whether they required admission to hospital. Note past diagnosis and treatment. Always check for previous risky behavior while unwell (self-harm, suicide attempts or violence).

PAST MEDICAL HISTORY

List out past and present physical problems, not only can physical problems relate to the presentation (e.g. multiple sclerosis can cause depression) but awareness of them is vital in treatment.

DRUG HISTORY

List the client's current medications; both prescribed and over the counter. Always note drug allergies and side effects.

FAMILY HISTORY

Drawing a genogram with the client is the clearest way to present their family. For each relative, include:

- Name, age, occupation.
- Any history of mental illness.
- Physical illness.
- Age and cause of death, of applicable.
- Consanguinity of the marriage, etc.

  Obtaining a family history of mental illness is important; because many of these disorders are hereditary. Bipolar and unipolar mood disorders, schizophrenia and attention deficit disorder (ADD) have significant genetic components. The client's response to specific interventions maybe inherited as well and should be included in the family history.

PERSONAL HISTORY

This is patient's life story.

Birth and Early Development

Unless you are assessing a child or someone with a learning disability or neurological problem, it is usually enough to ask two questions.

- Do you know if there were any problems with your mother's pregnancy and your birth?
- As far as you know, did you walk and talk at the normal ages?

As a general rule of thumb, if someone does not know much about these things, they were probably 'normal (i.e. a full term spontaneous vaginal delivery with normal mile stones) if there were any problems, find out details including:

- Prematurity.
- Labor complications/birth trauma/interventions, e.g. cesarean section.
- Time in special care/being unable to go home immediately.
- Need for pediatric follow-up.

Family Background and Early Childhood History

Record periods of serious or lengthy illness, separation from parents, and neglect or abuse.

- What was it like growing up in your family?
- What were your parents and siblings like? How did you get on with them?
- Was early childhood a happy or a difficult time?

Education

This section explores and provides a lot of information about personality and social abilities; and some data about intelligence. Note age and level of achievement on leaving education.

- What was school like for you?
- Did you have any problems at school?

- What were your friendships like?
- Were you shy or outgoing?
- Were you bullied or did anything traumatic happen?
- Were you ever in trouble for things like bullying or taunting?
- Did you get on with teachers?
- Were you near the top, middle or bottom of the class?

Occupation

Chronologically list out client's job pattern, including duration and reasons for leaving job (e.g. Promotional resignation/dismissal). Did they enjoy working? Look for trends, e.g. numerous brief job, that ended due to arguments with employers. This may say something important about their interpersonal relationships or response to authority.

PSYCHOSEXUAL HISTORY

List out relationships chronologically. Note the longest and shorter relationship with reasons. What were the characteristics and can your client see any recurring patterns?

- Age of first intercourse and number of sexual partners.
- Long-term/brief.
- Current employment/training.
- Activities or interest.
- Carrier's duties.
- Social network.

COLLATERAL HISTORY

A history from someone who knows the client well is useful especially if the patient is uncooperative or would not talk to you. Other people maybe better placed than the patient to say whether behavior or personality have changed. Take consent from significant relatives of the client. If a relative approaches you (e.g. while on the ward); there is no breach of confidentiality in listening to them, although you must explain the procedure.

Coping Skills

Coping skills are mechanisms people use to manage internal and external stressors. Coping behaviors can enable an individual to alter a stressful situation by controlling or at least minimizing the stress resulting from the situation. Clients with chronic psychiatric illness maybe unable to alter their condition, but can attempt to control the stress and minimize their stress on their lives.

A client in this situation may reveal several behavioral signs. They may seek more information about their illness and treatment options to care providers and may attend to support groups and express their feelings about self-concept, body image, and physical functions. They may practice yoga and relaxation techniques.

Conversely, maladaptive coping mechanisms are behaviors that ultimately interfere with the clients' ability to confront the stressor, maybe harmful and usually produce additional stress. Such behavior include smoking, drug abuse, alcohol intake, overeating, inappropriate anger and social withdrawal.

Discerning the client's characteristic pattern of coping whether it is adaptive or maladaptive—helps the nurse to predict how the client may react during a current stressor. Assessment of coping helps the nurse to teach positive coping measures.

MENTAL STATUS EXAMINATION

The biopsychosocial history is a record of the client's entire lifetime, the mental status examination is an evaluation of the client's present state. Behavior and general appearance, mood and affect, speech, thought process and content, perceptual disturbances, impulse control, cognition, knowledge, judgment and insight are assessed.

The acronym BEST PICK can be used to recall the main elements of mental status examination. Behavior and general appearance, emotions, mood and affect, speech, thought content and process, perceptual disturbances, impulse control, cognition and sensorium and knowledge of insight, and Judgment.

Behavior and General Appearance

Note the client's body frame, posture, dress, grooming and age appropriateness of appearance. Some common adjectives used to describe the client's general appearance include disheveled, well-groomed, heavily made-up, younger or older looking than biologic age, tensely prostured, under- or overweight and casually dressed.

In terms of behavior, assess the client's gait, activity level, gestures, mannerisms and psychomotor activity. Observe for rare symptoms such as echopraxia, catatonia, and waxy flexibility; akathisia or dyskinesia.

The psychiatric nurse should always evaluate how the client relates to the interviewer and to the interviewing process. Is the client cooperative or uncooperative, bored or angry will be noted.

Emotions: Mood and Affect

The client's mood is the pervasive subjective emotional state, and the visible expression of this state is termed as the affect. Observe the depth, range and fluctuation of emotional expression during the interview. Ask the client directly about his or her mood if the information is not offered spontaneously. Both mood and affect can be described as erythemic (normal), labile (rapidly charging from one mood state to another), depressed, irritable, anxious, euphoric (excessive happiness), frightened or empty. Variability in the client's affect should be noted; ranging from flat (no variability) to labile (rapid changes in affect). Note congruity or incongruity of mood and affect. For example, some depressed clients look depressed, where as others who are depressed appear euthymic.

Speech

Observe for the rate, amount, style, and tone of speech of the client. Speech may range from pressured to hesitant, loud to inaudible, spontaneous to nonspontaneous, slurred to clear and monotonous to dramatic. The client maybe described as talkative or taciturn, depending upon the quantity of speech. Observe for evidence of dysarthria (physical difficulty in vocalizing), echolalia (the repetition of interviewer's words), preservation (repetition of same words of themes), aphasia (difficulties in understanding or producing speech) and other disorders of speech.

Thought Content

The interviewer should note any abnormalities in the client's thought content. Obsessions are intrusive thoughts or ideas that the client recognizes as 'crazy' but acts in accordance with anyway (e.g. compulsive handwashing from an obsessive fear of infection. Hypochondriasis is an obsession with physical concerns that do not exist in reality.

Delusions are convictions that have no basis in reality. Delusions may be paranoid, grandiose, somatic, guilty, bizarre or referential. Note for the degree of congruence between the client's mood and the type of delusion.

Assess for suicidal and homicidal thoughts. Suicidal thoughts are the client's desires to kill or harm him or herself and homicidal thoughts are the client's desires to kill or harm others. The presence of active suicidal thoughts or homicidal thoughts constitutes a psychiatric emergency, and immediate action is necessary to correct it.

Thought Process

The thought process is the way in which the client thinks. It is assessed by client's speech. Assess for loose associations, tangentiality, word salad and neologisms. These symptoms are often seen in schizophrenic disorders.

Circumstantial thought is demonstrated by clients who get lost in details but eventually return to the relevant topic. Thought blocking occurs when the thinking process stops altogether and mind goes 'blank'. Flight of ideas as usually seen in mania, involves pressured speech with rapid topic changes the topic maybe associated, but in a strange way. For example 'I can see! The sea is washing away the shells'. Confabulation, often observed in dementia, is a filling up of information to fill in for memory gaps. For example, a client may given an elaborate but untrue story about how he or she spent the last holiday.

A client with a concrete thought process as opposed to an abstract thought process is only able to understand conversations literally. For example, a client who is asked what brought him or her to the hospital and responds, 'an ambulance' is manifesting concrete thinking. A client's ability to think abstractly maybe ascertained by assessing the client's interpretation of a proverb such as 'all that glitters is not gold' or the client's ability to describe similarities between objects such as chair and table. Concrete thinking is commonly seen in schizophrenia.

Perceptual Disturbances

Main perceptual disturbances are illusions and hallucinations. Theses are misinterpretations of true stimuli, seen in delirium. For example, illusion—a curtain in a dark room is mistaken for a person.

Hallucinations are defined as sensations experienced by the client without real external stimuli. A patient may not have intact reality testing, the ability to accept evidence that these perceptions nor to real. Clients who appear to be talking to imaginary others or pointing at nonexistent objects during the assessment are probably experiencing hallucinations or illusions. Direct questioning regarding perceptual disturbances is usually required to elicit the specific symptoms. Hallucinations maybe auditory, visual, gustatory, olfactory or tactile, client may hear, see, smell, or feel things that in reality do not exist.

Hypnagogic and hypnopompic hallucinations are false sensory perceptions that occur while falling asleep and while awakening from sleep, respectively. Depersonalization is a perceptual difficulty in which the client feels unreal, dead or mechanical; derealization is the sensation that the outside world is unreal.

Impulse Control

Impulse control is the ability to delay, modulate or inhibit the expression of behaviors and feelings. Clues to the client's ability to control his or her impulses are found in the content and process of the interview. For example, a client who describes a recent story of binge drinking and indiscriminate sexual contacts has poor impulse control. A person who storms out of an interview when difficult topics are asked also shows poor impulse control. Assessing the client's ability to control impulses is an integral part of determining potential for acting on suicidal or violent thoughts.

Cognition and Sensorium

Assess for level of consciousness, orientation, concentration and memory. During the interview, clients provide many clues to their sensorium. A client with an altered level of consciousness during the interview demonstrates a fluctuating ability to maintain awareness of the environment.

Orientation is assessed by asking the client regarding his full name, location, address, date and time.

A client's memory and concentration are determined by the ability to answer questions regarding psychiatric history. Concentration can be assessed by asking the client to count backward from 100 by 7s (100,93,86....) and memory is tested by asking the client to remember three objects immediately and to recall them after few minutes. Note for impairments in memory, remote, recent, past, recent, and immediate memory. The client's intellectual functioning (below average, average, superior) maybe estimated from interview considering his/her academic ground.

Knowledge, Insight, and Judgment

Knowledge, insight, and judgment are related concepts usually ascertained while taking history, observation and discussion. Judgment is the capacity to identify possible courses of action, anticipate their consequences and choose the appropriate behavior. Insight refers to the extent of client's awareness of illness and maladaptive behaviors. A client who tells the interviewer of reuniting with his abusive spouse because she feels that the spouse will change demonstrates poor judgment and little insight. A client who is admitted to the hospital for a third time because of noncompliance with antipsychotic medication and who states that he stopped taking the medication because he is not really mentally ill, lacks knowledge and insight into his illness and demonstrates poor judgment in regard to treatment. It may also be assessed by evaluating the answer to a hypothetical question such as: 'what would you do if you found a stamped, addressed envelope in the street?' or 'what would you do at night if your room got the fire?'

The Process of the Psychiatric Nursing Interview

The interview between client and nurse is a therapeutic communication which has beginning, middle and termination phase. Initially the nurse should begin to develop a rapport with the client and to engage the client in the meeting. Establishing a good rapport with a client is necessary and more over empathetic, listen compassionately, become the client's partner and instil trust. The nurse must clarify the purpose of the meeting, which is to gain an understanding of the client's problems and to determine the best way to care. The client should be informed about the health care setting and the interviewer's credentials; and the rules of confidentiality should be discussed; these are requisite to making the client feel comfortable enough to share information.

During the middle phase of the interview, data are collected and processed. The nurse obtains information from and gives information to the client. For example, the nurse may assist the client in the identifying ways to cope with symptoms.

The last stage, i.e. termination phase of the interview summarises what has been accomplished during the meeting. A tentative diagnosis and nursing care plan are planned. This phase is used to help the client relax from the often emotional interaction. If the nurse fails to elicit significant information during these phases, she can go for process recording to elicit most needed information from the client. Lastly, she can conclude the elicited symptoms with ICD-10 criteria and can be evaluated further.

MINI MENTAL STATUS EXAMINATION (MMSE)

Mini Mental State Examination (MMSE) is also known as Folstein test. It was introduced by Folstein et al, in 1975. It is a brief 30-point questionnaire test that is used to screen for cognitive impairment. The MMSE test includes simple questions and problems in a number of areas: the time and place of the test, repeating list of words, arithmetic such as the serial seven, language use and comprehension and basic motor skills. For example, one question asks to copy a drawing of two pentagons (Fig 3.1).

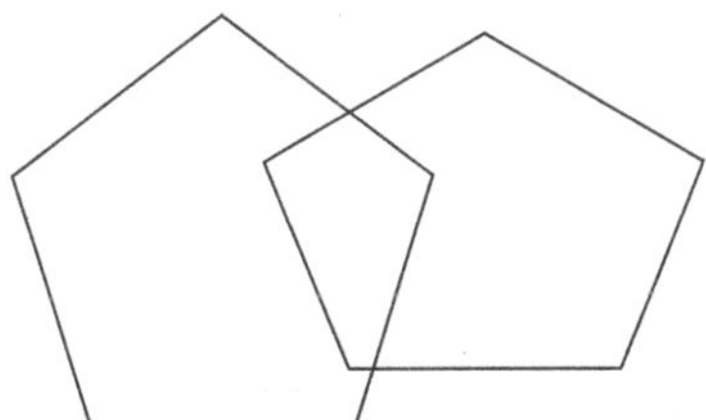

Fig. 3.1: Pentagons

Category	Point	Description
• **Question to time**	5	From broadest to most narrow: Orientation to time has been correlated with future decline.
• **Orientation to place**	5	From broadest to most narrow. Ask about place, name of the street, postbox number, etc.
• **Registration**	3	Repeating named prompts
• **Attention by calculation**	5	Serial seven or spelling 'world' backwards
• **Recall**	3	Registration recall
• **Language**	2	Naming a pencil and a watch
• **Repetition**	1	Speaking back a phrase
• **Complex commands**	6	Varies. Can involve drawing a figure.

INTERPRETATION OF MMSE

Any score greater than or equal to 25 points (out of 30) indicates a normal cognition. Below this, score indicate severe (≤ 9 points), moderate (10–20 points) or mind (21–24 points) cognitive impairment. The raw score may also to be corrected for educational attainment and age. That is, a maximal score of 30 points can never rule out dementia. Low to very low-correlate closely with the presence of dementia; although other mental disorders can also lead to abnormal finding on MMSE testing. The presence of purely physical problems can also interfere with interpretation if not properly noted. For example, a patient maybe physically unable to hear or read instructions probably, or may have a motor deficit that affects writing and drawing skills.

Neurological Examination

Neurological examination is an evaluation of a person's nervous system. It includes the assessment of motor and sensory skills, balance and coordination, mental status, reflexes, and functioning of the nerves.

The complete neurological examination maybe performed:

- During a routine physical examination.
- Following any type of trauma.
- To follow the progression of a disease.
- If the person has any of the following complaints
  - Headaches
  - Blurry vision
  - Change in behavior
  - Fatigue
  - Change in balance or coordination.
  - Numbness or tingling in the arms of legs
  - Decrease in movement of the arms or legs
  - Injury to the head, neck or back
  - Fever
  - Seizures
  - Slurred speech
  - Weakness
  - Tremor

Process of Neurological Examination

During a neurological examination, the psychiatric nurse will 'test' the functioning of the nervous system. Psychiatric nurse will test functioning the nervous system is very complex and controls many parts of the body. It consists of brain, spinal cord and 12 nerves that come from the brain; and that nerves that comes from the spinal cord. The circulation to the brain, arising from the arteries in the neck is, also examined. In infants and younger children, a neurological examination includes the measurement of the head circumference.

The following is a format for assessment during neurological examination.

Mental Status

Mental status (the patient's level of awareness and interaction with the environment) maybe assessed by conversing with the client and establishing their awareness of person, place and time. The person will also be observed for clear speech can making sense while talking. This is usually assessed by observation and keeping rapport.

Motor Function and Balance

This is tested by having the patient's push and pull against the nurses hands with his/her arms and legs. Balance maybe checked by having the patient's stand with his/her eyes closed while being gently pushed to one side or the other. The patient's joints may also be checked by passive and active movement.

Sensory Examination

Sensory examination tests his/her ability to feel. This may tested by tools like dull needles, tuning forks, tuning forks alcohol swabs or other objects. The nurse may touch the patient's legs, arms or other parts of the body and have him/her identify the sensation (i.e. Hot/cold/sharp/dull).

Newborn and Infant Reflexes

There are different types of reflexes that maybe tested in newborns and infants, reflexes are evaluated. Each of these reflexes disappears at a certain age as the infant grows. These reflexes include:

- *Blinking:* An infant will close her/his eyes in responses to bright lights.
- *Babinski reflex:* As the infant's foot is stroked, the toes will extend upward.
- *Crawling:* If the infant is placed on his/her abdomen crawling motions will be made.
- *Moro's reflex:* A quick change in the infant's position will cause the infant throw the arms outward, open the hands and throw back the head.
- *Palmer and plantar grasp:* The infant fingers or toes will curl around a finger placed in the area.
- *Startle reflex:* A loud noise will cause the infant to extend and flex the arms while the hands remains in a fist.
- *Reflexes in the older child/adult:* These are usually examined with the use of a reflex hammer. The reflex hammer is used at different points on the body to test numerous reflexes, which are noted by the movement that the hammer causes.

Evaluation of the Nerves of the Brain

There are 12 main nerves of the brain called the cranial nerves. During a complete neurological examination, most of these nerves are evaluated to help determine the functioning of the brain.

Cranial Nerve I (Olfactory nerve)

This is the nerve of smell. The patient maybe asked to identify the different smells with his/her eyes closed.

Cranial Nerve II (Optic nerve)

This is one of the nerves of the eye that helps control vision. A visual test maybe given and the patient's eye maybe examined with a special light.

Cranial Nerve III (Oculomotor)

This is another nerve that controls part of the eye. This nerve is responsible for the pupil size and the movement of the eye. The nurse may examine the pupil (black part of eye) with a light and have the patient follow the light in various directions.

Cranial Nerve IV (Trochlear nerve)

This nerve also helps with the movement of the eyes.

Cranial Nerve V (Trigeminal nerve)

This nerve allows for many functions, including the ability to feel the face, inside the mouth, and move the muscles involved with chewing. The nurse may touch the face at different areas and watch the patient as he/she bites down.

Cranial Nerve VI (Abducens nerve)

This nerve helps with the movement of the eyes. The patient maybe asked to follow a light or finger to move the eyes.

Cranial Nerve VII (Facial nerve)

This nerve is responsible for various functions, including the movements of the face muscle and taste. The patient maybe asked to identify different tastes (sweet, bitter, sour) asked to smile, move the cheeks or show the teeth.

Cranial Nerve VIII (Acoustic nerve)

This nerve is involved with hearing. A hearing test maybe performed on the patient.

Cranial Nerve IX (Glossopharyngeal nerve)

This nerve is involved with taste. Once again, the client maybe asked to identify different tastes on the back of the tongue.

Cranial Nerve X (Vagus nerve)

This nerve is mainly responsible for the ability to swallow, the gag reflex, some tastes and part of speech. The patient maybe asked to swallow and a tongue blade maybe used to elicit the gag response.

Cranial Nerve XI (Accessory nerve)

This nerve is involved in the movement of the shoulders and neck. The patient maybe asked to turn his/her head from side to side against mild resistance or to shrug the shoulders.

Cranial Nerve XII (Hypoglossal nerve)

This nerve is mainly responsible for movement of the tongue. The patient maybe instructed to stick out her/his tongue and speak.

Investigations

Investigations exclude physical causes of the problem (e.g. hypothyroidism in depression); check general physical health and provide baseline measures before administering medications.

- Biological, e.g. Blood test, CT scans, EEG, MRI
- Psychological, e.g. Symptom rating scales, IQ testing
- Social, e.g. Collateral history.

Psychological Tests

- Many personality tests are used in clinical setting. But mainly Myers-Briggs test and the Big Five tests are common. Almost all of the other personality tests are variations on these two types of tests. The core purpose of these tests is to determine and quantify personality characteristics. The Myers-Briggs test sorts the population into distinct categories on various different topics, while the Big Five tests rate each person as a percentage of each category.

IQ Tests: (Intelligent Quotient)

- IQ originally coined by William Stern. The most common IQ tests are of the William Stern. This is calculated by $IQ = MA/CA \times 100$. MA refers to mental age and CA refers to chronological age.

Process Recording

Process recording is a tool to analyze nurse-patient interactions to find out the real cause of disease of problem. It focuses on verbal and nonverbal communication. The following format has been used to note it.

- *Client's initials:*
- *Age:*
- *Diagnosis:*
- *Goal/aim of interaction:* State your goal—Be very specific.
- Time taken: 10–20 minutes.
- *Venue/description of environment:* Provide a visual description of the setting in which the conversation took place, including disturbing factors, as well as the patient's physical appearance. Verbal communication, state the communication verbatim, including what the client states and your responses. List in sequential order and identify therapeutic and nontherapeutic techniques used during the conversation. Identify any defense mechanisms used by the client.
- *Nonverbal communication:* Include your thoughts and feelings, as well as any facial expressions, gestures, position change or changes in eye contact, voice quality, and voice tone by the client or yourself.
- *Evaluation of interaction:* Discuss whether the goal was met. What changes would you make, if any, after evaluating this interaction?

Psychiatric Nursing Care Management

The nursing diagnosis is a statement of an existing actual problem or of a potential health problem that a nurse is licensed and competent to care. In 1990, the North American Nursing Diagnosis Association (NANDA) defined nursing diagnosis as 'a clinical judgment about individual, family or community responses to actual or potential health problems/life processes'. Nursing diagnosis provides the basis for selection of nursing intervention to achieve outcome for which the nurse is accountable.

Carpenito (1991) classifies nursing diagnosis as actual high risk or possible. An actual nursing diagnosis is based on validated data, high risk nursing diagnosis is based on psychiatric client's degree of vulnerability to develop a specific problem; and possible nursing diagnosis describes a suspected problem requiring additional data to confirm or rule out its presence.

Examples

Type	Diagnosis
• **Actual**	Ineffective individual coping related to forced relocation as evidence by clinical symptoms of depression (e.g. Insomnia, lack of appetite, apathy and low self-esteem).
• **High risk**	High risk for violence (self harm) as evidenced by presence of suicidal ideation.
• **Possible (potential for)**	Noncompliance related to inability to follow directions (e.g. How to take medication secondary to impaired hearing and poor memory).

Nursing Diagnoses in Psychiatric Mental Health Nursing

- Aggression (mild, moderate, severe/extreme/violent)
- Agitation
- Anger
- Anxiety (mild, moderate, severe/extreme/panic)
- Bizarre behavior
- Boredom
- Communication, impaired verbal
- Coping, family, potential for growth
- Coping, ineffective individual
- Crisis, maturational or situation
- Decisional conflict (specify)
- Defensive coping
- Depression
- Diversional activity
- Emotional lability
- Fear
- Grieving, anticipatory or dysfunctional
- Growth and development, altered
- Guilt
- Health maintenance, altered
- Injury, high risk for
- Knowledge deficit

- Loneliness
- Manipulation
- Noncompliance (specify)
- *Nutrition altered:* Less than body requirements
- Parenting, altered (actual, high risk for)
- Perception/cognition altered
- Postoverdose syndrome
- Post-trauma response
- Powerlessness
- Rape trauma syndrome
- Regressed behavior
- Resources management, impaired (specify)
- Ritualistic behavior
- Self-care deficit
- Self-concept disturbance (identify self-esteem, body image or role performance)
- Sexual dysfunction
- Sleep pattern disturbance
- Social interaction impaired
- Somatization
- Spiritual distress
- Substance abuse (alcohol)
- Suicide, high risk for
- Substance abuse (drugs)
- Suspiciousness
- Wellness-seeking behavior.

FORMULATION OF PLAN OF NURSING CARE

This phase includes setting priorities, goals and planning interventions. Priority setting considers the urgency or seriousness of the problem or need and its impact on the person. Is there a threat to the person's life, dignity or integrity? Are there problems or needs that negatively affect the patient? Do problems exist that affect normal growth and development? Consider Maslow's hierarchy needs generally is used as a guide for problem-solving during the formulation of a plan of care. These needs include physical needs, safety, love and belonging, self-esteem and self-actualization.

Ideally, goal setting occurs as the psychiatric nurse and client mutually discuss and state expected outcomes. If the client is actively psychotic and unable to participate in the development of the care plan, the mental health team will formulate a plan of care for the patient. Goals should be sort-term as well as long-term in order to evaluate the patient's progress. Short-term goals are individualized and derived from the diagnosis and can be met in a short amount of time. They should be realistic and achievable, measurable, observable and behavioral, patient centered and time designated. Long-term goals (LTGs) are future oriented and considered the desired result of nursing interventions.

According to Carpenito (1992), care plans have two professional purposes—administrative and clinical. Administrative purposes include defining the nursing focus, differentiating the accountability of each professional of the multidisciplinary treatment team, providing criteria for review of quality care and providing criteria for client classification and financial reimbursement.

Clinical purposes include providing a blue print for charting; communicating information and appropriate interventions about client care to all caregivers; providing individualized, comprehensive care focusing on both short-term and long-term goals; providing continuity of care around the clock and facilitating an ongoing, accurate evaluation of care.

General principles to be considered in writing care plans include the following:

- Individualize or personalize the plan of care according to the nursing diagnoses or problems of client.
- 'Use simple understandable language to communicate information about the client's care.
- Be very specific when stating nursing interventions.
- Prioritize nursing care (e.g. list nursing actions for effective airway clearance before those for impaired physical mobility or sexual dysfunction).
- State short- and long-term goals.
- Indicate the responsible nurse or team member for each nursing intervention.

IMPLEMENTATION OF NURSING ACTIONS/INTERVENTIONS

During implementation phase, nurse utilizes various skills to perform or assist the patient in performing specific activities; promote independence and self-care whenever possible; engage in client psychoeducation, counsel new client as the need arises and implement nursing orders (e.g. measure abdominal growth, monitor intake output, etc.)

Evaluation

The evaluation phase of the nursing process focuses on the psychiatric client's status. Progress towards goal achievement and ongoing reevaluation of the care plan.

Four possible outcomes may occur:

- The client may respond favorably or as expected to nursing interventions.
- Short-term goals maybe met but long-term goals may remain unmet.
- The client maybe unable to meet or achieve any goals and,
- New problems or needs maybe identified.

  All members of the multidisciplinary and interdisciplinary treatment team, as well as the client, should be encouraged to provide continuous feedback regarding the effectiveness of the plan of care. As a result of the evaluation process, the care plan is maintained, modified or totally revised. A brief sample care plan for the client with the ICD-10 diagnosis of depression is shown in display-1.
- *Display-1:* Example of nursing diagnosis and goal-related nursing interventions.

The Patient with Depression/Depressive Disorder

- *Nursing diagnosis:* Ineffective individual coping related to depression in response to/reaction to death of spouse.
- *Goal:* Before to discharge the client will demonstrate a beginning coping to the loss.

Nursing intervention	Outcome criteria
Within 48 to 72 hours, the client will try to do the following:	
• Encourage verbalization of feelings	• Begin to verbalize feelings to staff and others
• Identify prior coping skills	• Identify one or two effective coping skills
• Explore current support systems	• Identify one or two available support systems
• Educate about grief process	• Identify present stage of grief process
• Administer antidepressant medication, instruct patient about medication and its common side effects.	• Demonstrate an understanding of the purpose of the specific antidepressant medication and its common side effects.

Summary: This unit focused on psychiatric client assessment and evaluation. It also includes psychiatric nursing process and care plan. A definition of nursing diagnosis was cited. Psychiatric nursing diagnoses, denoting those approved by NANDA were listed. Principles to be considered in writing a care plan were given. The rationale for the evaluation process, including four possible outcomes or responses to care was discussed. A brief sample care plan for a client with the nursing diagnoses of ineffective individual coping related to depressive disorders was noted.

Self-test

- Name the five steps of the psychiatric nursing process.
- List out the components of mental status examination.
- Briefly explain about neurological examination.
- Enumerate the principles of writing a care plan.
- State several and different activities that occur during the implementation of nursing interventions.
- Describe the evaluation step of the nursing process.
- State nursing diagnosis related to common psychiatric problems according to NANDA.

Therapeutic Communication

INTRODUCTION

According to Webster, an interaction is a mutual or reciprocal action that can occur between or among people. Interaction that facilitates growth, development, maturity, improved functioning and improved coping is considered therapeutic (Rogers, 1961).

Therapeutic communication, relationship, interventions, environment and milieu all are terms that refer to nurse patient interaction. The focus of this unit is to discuss in detail about a therapeutic relationship through communication and interaction.

Communication

In simple way, communication is imparting or interchange of thoughts, opinions or information by speech, writings or signs. The process of communication includes three elements. The sender, the message and the receiver. Communication is the giving and receiving of information. The sender prepares or creates a message when need occurs and sends the message to a receiver or listener, who then decodes it. The receiver may then return a message or feedback to the sender of the message. Communication is a learned concept process influenced by one's attitudes, sociocultural or ethnic background, past experiences, knowledge of subject matter and ability to relate to others. Interpersonal perceptions also affect one's ability to communicate because they influence the initiation and response of communication. Such perception occurs through the senses of sight, sound, touch and smell. Environmental factors that influence communication include time, place/context and the presence of one or more person.

The factors influencing communication are listed below:

- *Attitude:* Attitudes are developed in various ways and maybe the result of interaction with the environment, assimilation of other's attitudes, life experiences, intellectual processes or a traumatic experience. The terms like accepting, caring, judgmental, open or closed minded and prejudiced are used.
- *Sociocultural background:* Communication is vastly influenced by sociocultural philosophy and fabric of the society.

  Past experiences: Previous positive or negative experiences influence one's ability to communicate.

  For example, children who have been told continually to be quiet, or to speak only when spoken to, may become withdrawn and more communicative. Teenagers who have been put down by their parents or teachers whenever attempting to express any feelings may develop a poor self-image and feel their opinions are not worthy. As a result they avoid interacting with others.

- *Knowledge of subject matter:* A person who is well educated or knowledgeable about certain topics may feel more secure when discussing topics with others.
- *Ability to relate to others:* Expressing relevant information to others is an art. This ability is an learned process, the result of practicing communicative skills over a period of time.
- *Interpersonal perceptions:* Interpersonal perceptions like feeling, moving, speaking, etc. all influence the communication process.
- Environmental factors such as time, place and the presence of people. Timing is quite important factor during a conversation. Place and presence of strange people also influences communication.

Types of Communication

Communication takes place at two levels:

a. **Verbal communication:** It occurs through words, spoken or written.
b. **Nonverbal communication:** It occurs through gestures or behavior that do not involve the spoken or written words. This occurs through vocal, gestures, physical appearance, space, gesture, posture, touch and facial expression.

- *Position or posture*: The position one assumes can designate authority, cowardice, boredom or indifference. For example, a nurse standing at the foot of a client's bed with arms folded across chest gives the impression that the nurse is in charge of any interaction that may occur.
- *Gesture:* Pointing out, finger tapping, winking, and clapping, eyebrow raising, palm rubbing, hand wringing and beard stroking are examples of nonverbal gestures that communicate various thoughts and feelings. Reflect on these gestures and your reactions to them. What gestures are common in your nonverbal therapeutic communication. Do they betray feelings of insecurity, anxiety, eagerness or genuine interest?
- *Touch:* Touch conveys many messages. Handshaking, hugging, holding hands and patting all denote positive feelings for another person. Reactions to touch depend on one's age, gender, sociocultural background, interpretation of the gesture and appropriateness of the touch. The nurse should exercise caution when touching people. Before touching any psychiatric client, nurse should take consent. The depressed or grieving client may respond to touch as a gesture of concern; whereas the sexually promiscuous person may consider touching an invitation to sexual advances. An abused child may recoil from the nurse's attempt to comfort, whereas the dying patient maybe comforted by the presence of a nurse sitting by the bedside silently holding the client's hand.
- *Physical appearance:* People who are depressed may pay little attention to their appearance. They may appear unkempt and unconsciously wear dark-colored clothing; reflecting their depressed feelings, confused or disoriented persons may forget to put on items of clothing, put them on inside out, or dress inappropriately. Weight gain or weight loss also maybe form of nonverbal communication. People who exhibit either maybe experiencing a low self a concept or feelings of anxiety, depression or loneliness. The manic client may dress in brightly colored clothes and with many items of jewelry and excessive make-up. People with a positive self-concept may communicate such feelings by appearing neat, clean and well dressed appropriately.
- *Facial expressions:* A blank stare, startled expression, sneer, grimace and broad smile are examples of facial expression denoting one's innermost feelings.

- *Vocal cues:* Pausing or hesitating while speaking, talking in a tense or flat tone, or speaking tremously are vocal cues that can agree with or contradict one's verbalization. Speaking softly may be the result of feelings of anger or hostility. For example, a person who is admitted to the hospital for emergency surgery may speak softly but tremulously, stating 'I' am okay. I just want to get better and go home as soon as possible. The nonverbal cues should indicate to the nurse that the client is not feeling well and the client's feelings should be explored.
- *Distance or spatial territory:* Hall (1966) describes four zones of distance awareness in people. They include the intimate, personal, social and public zones. Actions that involve touching to another body, such as love-making and wrestling, occur in the intimate distance zone. The personal zone refers to an arm's length distance of approximately 1.5 to 4 feet. Physical contact, such as hand holding, still can occur. The social zone, in which formal business and social discourse occurs, occupies a space of 4 to 12 feet. The public zone, in which no physical contact and little eye contact occurs; ranges from 12 to 25 feet. People who maintain communication in this zone remain strangers.

Communication Skills

The following are the effective points to consider and to develop good communication skills for effective therapeutic interactions:

- *Know yourself:* What motivates your interest in helping other. Identify your emotional needs to that they do not interfere with the ability to relate to others. Be aware of any mood swings that you may show. Clients are very sensitive to the emotions of helping individuals.
- *Be honest with your feelings:* The nurses body language, gestures and tone of voice can reveal true feelings or reactions to client behavior. Honesty is the key factor for communication. Your nonverbal communication may contradict your spoken word if you are not honest with the client. For nurses who work with cancer clients often find it hard to relate to terminally ill person. They may avoid contact as much as possible, so that their emotions are not revealed to the clients when they are asked questions such as will I be getting better?, Is it cancer? or Am I going to die?, etc.
- *Be secure in your ability to relate to people:* Do not allow the behavior of others to threaten or intimidate you. Remember that all behavior has meaning. Ask yourself 'what is the client trying to communicate'?
- *Be sensitive to the needs of other:* Listen attentively by using eye to eye contact; focusing your attention on the speaker and assuming a personal distance of 1.5 to 4 feet. Use tact and diplomacy while conversing with others.
- *Be consistent:* Consistency in what you speak and do encourages the development of trust.
- *Recognize symptoms of anxiety:* Knowing anxiety when it appears in yourself and those you relate to it is important. Anxiety impairs communication if the person is unable to concentrate or express feelings.
- *Watch your nonverbal reactions:* Be aware of your body language because it punctuate and modifies verbal messages. Use gestures cautiously to emphasize meanings, reactions or emotions.
- *Use words carefully:* When relating to others, these words should be used continuously. Example, I, you, but, if, then, always, should and ought. Satir (1976) refers to these words as 'powerful words' that may be used thoughtlessly, appear to be accusations, be easily misunderstood, or cause confusion and ambivalence.

- *Recognize differences:* While communication, note the fact of age differences or may have conflicting loyalties can impair communication.
- *Recognize and evaluate your own actions and responses:* Evaluate your own mind, i.e. open or closed-minded, cooperative or incooperative, supportive, or nonsupportive when you converse with someone. Are you available when needed or do you tend to put someone on hold if you are busy? Never cut short a conversation short in the middle of a self-disclosing interaction. Refer the person to someone whom you feel can be supportive regarding the issues at hand.

Ineffective Communication

Disturbances can occur during the process of communication. The nurse needs to be aware of the various reasons for ineffective communication.

These reasons include:

- Ineffective communication skills used by the helping person. The psychiatric nurse may not send the message what is intended.
- Failure to listen on the part of the helping person. Some individuals are doer rather than listeners. They focus on task oriented nursing instead of therapeutic communication. The client also may not hear the message sent because of many reasons, such as stress, anxiety, fear, denial or anger.
- *Conflicting verbal and nonverbal messages:* Ambivalence on the part of the sender may confuse the receiver, who senses conflicting signals and doubts the helping person's interest in him or her.
- *A judgmental attitude:* Anyone who displays prejudice or a judgmental attitude when relating to others may never really get to know the person. A sensitive person may pick-up on judgmental attitudes and refuse to relate to others, thinking that all people are judgmental.
- Misunderstanding because of multiple meaning of language words. Consider the word 'cup'. It may mean a drinking vessel, a hole in a golf green, or a winner's trophy. The sender should select words that are not confusing in meaning.
- *False reassurance:* Sayings such as 'Everything will be okay' or 'Don't worry, the doctor will make you well' are considered examples of false reassurance. No one can always predict or guarantee the outcome of a situation. There are too many variables, such as persons who desires to maintain a sick role, nonsupportive families or an illness that is irreversible (e.g. cancer or multiple sclerosis) clients who receive false reassurance quickly learn not to trust people if they do not respond to treatment as predicted.
- Providing advice rather than encouraging the person to make decision, however small they maybe. Giving advice may facilitate dependency and may also cause the client to feel inadequate because he or she is not given the opportunity to make choices pertaining to personal care. The client will accept advice when wanted. Feelings of dependency and inadequacy may occur and impair therapeutic communication; if the client fails to receive positive feedback during nurse-client interactions. It is much more constructive to encourage problem-solving by the client.
- Disagreeing with or criticizing a person who is seeking support. Belitting a person may result in the development of low self-concept and inability to cope with different stressors. Consider both thoughts and feelings during conversation.
- The inability to receive information because of a preoccupied or impaired thought process. The receiver maybe prepared to hear a different message from the one sent. Someone who is

preoccupied with thoughts is not as receptive to message as a person with a clear mind. Impaired thought process, such as delusions or hallucinations also interfere with communication. A client who hears voices saying he or she is being poisoned by others is not receptive to a nurse's, request to take medication.
- Changing the subject if one becomes uncomfortable with the topic being discussed.

Nurse Client Interactions

We find two types of interactions—social and therapeutic may occur when the nurse is working with clients or families who seek help for physical or emotional needs. Social interactions occur daily as the nurse greets the client and passes the time of day; so to speak, with what is referred as short or small talk. Saying 'Good morning', It's a beautiful day and have you heard any jokes are examples of socializing.

During a therapeutic interaction the nurse helps or encourages the patient to ventilate feelings of perceptions, the nurse helps or encourage the patient to ventilate feeling of perceptions, fears, anxieties, frustrations, expectations and increased dependency needs. For example, you look upset, would you like to share your feelings with someone.

Therapeutic Communication

Therapeutic communication is an interpersonal interaction between the nurse and the client during which the nurse focuses on the clients' specific need to promote an effective exchange of information.

A comparison of social interactions and therapeutic interaction is given below (Purtilo 1978). He also recommends the following approaches when communicating in a therapeutic ways.

Social vs Therapeutic Interaction

Social interaction	Therapeutic interaction
• Social interaction maybe referred as doing a help or favor for another person such as giving someone money, etc.	• Therapeutic interaction promotes the functional use of one's latent inner resources. Encouraging verbalization of feelings following the death ones child or exploring ways to cope with excessive stress are examples of therapeutic help.
• A personal or intimate relationship occurs.	• A personal, but not intimate relationship occurs.
• Not necessarily concerned with the identification of needs.	• Needs are identified by the person with the help of the nurse.
• Personal goals may or may not be discussed.	• Personal goals are set by the client.
• May create constructive or destructive dependency.	• Promotes constructive dependency, interdependency and independency.
• May use a variety of resources during socialization.	• Uses specialized professional skills while employing nursing interventions.

Approaches to Therapeutic Communication (Purtilo, 1978)

- Translate any technical information into simple terms.
- Clarify and restate any instructions or information given. Clients usually do not ask doctors or nurses to repeat themselves.
- Display a caring attitude.

- Exercise effective listening.
- Do not overload the listener with information.

Roger's (1961) lists eight conditions essential for a therapeutic relationship to occur. They include:

- *Empathy:* The helper is able to understand and feel on the feeling of another person. He/she has to 'walk in another's shoes' shows empathetic understanding because such actions enables one to experience the feelings of another and respond to them. A person seeking help feels understood and accepted. The person is able to relate to another, to explore feelings and to try new behaviors.
- *Respect:* The helper considers the person to be deserving of high regard and cares deeply for the person as a human being. Consistency on the part of the helper conveys respect.
- *Genuineness:* The helper is sincere, honest, and authentic in responses. The helper becomes a role model as he/she meets the patient's needs rather than wants.
- *Self-disclosure:* Exposing a view of one's attitudes, feelings and belief is self-disclosure. It can occur on the part of the helper as well as the client. Appropriate self-disclosure by the helper provides a role for the other person to model, allowing the person to become more open, reveal more about self and feel more secure.
- *Concreteness and specificity:* The ability to identify feelings by skillful listening requires the helper to be realistic, not theoretical; while assisting the person in expressing specific feelings.
- *Confrontation:* Discussing misunderstandings in the person's thought and behavior must be done in an acceptable manner after good establishment of rapport. Those with emotional problems may perceive themselves differently than they think others regard them. Such feelings may result in anxiety and inappropriate behavior in an attempt to reconcile these perceived misunderstandings.
- *Immediacy of relationship:* Recognizing one's own feelings and sharing with the client is essential to a therapeutic relationship. The helper needs to be able to share spontaneous feelings but not necessarily all of them. The sharing of too many negative expressions can be detrimental during the beginning of a relationship. Once a relationship exists, the helper shares immediate feelings when the helper feels the patient will benefit from communication.
- *Self exploration:* If the client is to make progress, he or she needs to engage in self-exploration. Feelings of discomfort or fear may initially emerge; however; the more the client investigates feelings, the more the client learns to adapt and cope with the problem.

Confidentiality

Confidentiality is very important during a nurse client interaction. The client has a right to privacy. All information concerning the client is considered personal property and is not to be discussed with other clients or outside the hospital setting. When discussing any information with a client, as in nursing conference, the client's name and identity should be kept secret. It may be necessary for a student nurse to reassure a client that confidentiality will be maintained except when:

- The information maybe harmful to the client or others.
- The client does not intend to comply with the treatment plan.
- The patient threatens self-harm. One way to convey this is simply to state 'only information that will be helpful in management to others on the staff'. Family members should be informed to get permission from clients 18 years old and older before seeking any health team member.

THERAPEUTIC RELATIONSHIPS: ESTABLISHING AND MANAGEMENT OF ROLES

Peplau (1952) describes six subroles of the psychiatric nurse during a therapeutic relationship. They are teacher, mother, surrogate, technical nurse expert, manager, socializing agent and counselor or nurse therapist. For example, the nurse-manager is accountable for creating a therapeutic environment in which the clients feel safe and accepted. The subrole of teacher enables the nurse to educate client about specific illnesses and medication prescribed to promote early recovery. Social skills such as participating in groups are promoted by the nurse who acts as a socializing agent. The nurturing needs of clients who are unable to carry-out simple tasks are met by mother surrogate. Recording vital signs, medical or surgical procedures, administration of medication and physical assessment are generally carried out by the technical nurse. Lastly, the nurse therapist or nurse counselor employs therapeutic skills to help patients identify and deal with various stressors or problems that have resulted in dysfunctional coping. Each of these roles can be effective during the various phases of the therapeutic relationship.

During the therapeutic relationship, clients try to distort their perceptions of others. Therefore, they may relate to the nurse not on the basis of the nurse's realistic attributes but wholly or chiefly on the basis of interpersonal relationships existing in their environment. This is termed as transference or paratoxic distortion (Yalom 1985). Countertransference occurs when the nurse responds unrealistically to the client's behavior of interaction. Negative transference can interfere with the development of a therapeutic relationship.

THE ONE-TO-ONE NURSE CLIENT RELATIONSHIP

Peplau (1952) discusses the phases of one-to-one nurse client relationships established in psychiatric mental health nursing. Such relationships can be divided into three phases. Initiating or orientation phase, working and terminating phases. These phases are important and effective in both inpatient and outpatient setting. Following is a description of each of the phases, including therapeutic tasks or goals to be fulfilled.

Orientation Phase/Initiating Phase

This is the first step in therapeutic relationship. During this phase the nurses set the stage for a one-to-one relationship by becoming acquainted with the client. Both the nurse and the client may experience anxiety when they met first time. Very little it exists. Assessment of the client occurs as the nurse and client agree on the time, place and duration of each setting of the meeting. Communication styles of the nurse and the client are explored to facilitate rapport and open communication as the client begins to share innermost feelings, anxieties and conflicts. Client must feel accepted as he or she develops a feeling of trust toward the nurse. Allow the client to set the pace of the relationship. The client is a unique person who is ill and maybe experiencing feelings of loneliness, fear, anger, disgust, despair, frustration and rejection. As a client, the person seeks comfort and help in handling various stressors. In doing so the client accepts another assistance in problem-solving or goal setting.

The following tasks to be accomplished during the first phase

- Building trust and rapport by acceptance.
- Establishing a therapeutic environment.
- Establishing a mode of communication acceptable to both the client and nurse.

- Initiating a therapeutic contract by establishing a time, place and duration of each meeting as well as the length of time the relationship will be in effect.
- Assessing the client's strengths and weaknesses.

Working Phase/Middle Phase

The second phase of therapeutic relationship is known as the working or middle phase. In this phase, the client begins to relax, starts to trust the nurse, and is able to discuss mutually agreed upon goals with the nurse as the assessment process continues and a plan of care action develops. Perceptions of reality, coping mechanisms and support systems are identified at this time. Alternative behaviors and techniques are identified at this time. The nurse are explored to replace those that maladaptive. The nurse and the client, both discuss the meaning behind behavior the working as well as any reactions by the nurse such as fear, embarrassment, anger or intimidation. During the working phase, the client is able to focus on unpleasant, painful aspects of life with the nurse's support and help.

Therapeutic tasks accomplished during the working phase include:

- Exploring perception of reality
- Developing positive coping behaviors
- Identifying available support systems
- Promoting a positive self-concept
- Encouraging verbalization of feelings
- Developing a realistic plan of action
- Implementing the plan of action
- Evaluating the results of the plan of action
- Promoting independence.

Terminating Phase

The last step of the therapeutic relationship is the termination phase. The nurse terminates the relationship when the mutually agreed-upon goals are reached, the patient is transferred or discharged. As separation occurs, the client may exhibit symptoms like regressive behavior, hostility or experience sadness. The client may attempt to prolong the relationship as clinical symptoms of separation anxiety are experienced.

Termination needs to occur if a therapeutic relationship is to be a complete process. Preparation for last step begins during the initiating phase.

There are some mutually accepted goals resulting in the termination of a therapeutic relationship include the ability to:

- Provide self-care and maintain one's environment
- Demonstrate independence and work independently with others
- Recognize signs of increased stress or anxiety
- Cope positively when experiencing feelings of anxiety, anger or hostility
- Demonstrate emotional stability and equality.

Therapeutic Communication Techniques

Therapeutic communication is used to encourage the expression of feelings and ideas.

- *Active listening:* It is being attentive to what the client is saying; verbally as well as nonverbally. Sit facing the client, open posture, lean toward the client, keeping eye contact and relax.

It is an active process of receiving information responses on and other forms of receptive nonverbal communication convey to the client he/she is being listened to understand.
Therapeutic value: Nonverbally communicates to the client the nurse's interest and acceptance.

- *Making observations:* It is done by commenting on how the other person looks, sounds or acts. For example, 'You look tired' or 'I have not you eating anything today'.
- *Broad opening:* Encouraging the client to select topics for discussions. For example, 'what are you thinking about'?
- *Restating:* Repeating the main thought expressed by the client. For example, 'you say that your mother left you when you were five years old'.
  Therapeutic value: It indicates that the nurse is listening and validates, reinforce or calls attention to something important that has been said'.
- *Using touch:* This is most potent form of communication. Comfort touch such as holding a hand, is especially important for vulnerable clients who are experiencing severe illnesses.
- *Clarifying:* To check whether understanding is accurate, or to better understand, the nurse restates an unclear or ambiguous message to classify the sender's meaning 'I' am not sure what you mean. Could you tell me about that again?
  Therapeutic value: It helps to clarify feelings, ideas and perception of the client and provides an explicit correlation between them and the client's action.
- *Reflection:* It is directing back the client's ideas, feelings, questions and content. For example, you are feeling tense and anxious and it is related to a conversation you had with your husband at night.
  Therapeutic value: It validates the nurse's understanding of what the client is saying and signifies empathy, interest and respect for the client.
- *Sharing Humor:* Sharing humor contributes to feelings, of togetherness, closeness and friendliness. It promotes positive communication in prevention, and perception. Here the discharge of energy through comic enjoyment of the imperfect. For example, that gives a whole new meaning to the word 'nervous' said with shared kidding between the psychiatric nurse and the client.
  Therapeutic value: Care promote insight by making repressed material conscious, resolving paradoxes, tempering aggression and revealing new options and is socially acceptable form of sublimation.
- *Informing:* The skill of information-giving. For example, I think you need to know about your medications.
  Therapeutic value: Helpful in health teaching or client education about relevant aspects of client's well-being and self-care.
- *Focusing:* Taking note of a single idea expressed or even a single word. An example is: On a scale of 0 to 10, tell me the level of the pain you are experiencing in your great to right now. Questions or statements that help the client expand on a topic of importance. For example, I think that we should discuss more about your relationships with your father.
  Therapeutic value: It allows the client to discuss central issues and keeps the communication process goal directed.
- *Sharing perceptions:* Asking the client to verify the nurses understanding of what the client is thinking or feeling. For examples, You are smiling but I sense that you are really very angry with me.

Therapeutic value: Conveys the nurse understands to the client and has the potential for clearing up confusing communication.

- *Theme Identification:* This involves identification of underlying issues or problems experienced by the client that emerge repeatedly during the course of the nurse client relationship. For example, I noticed that you said, you have been hurt or rejected by the man. Do you think this is an underlying issue?
  Therapeutic value: It allows the nurse to promote the client's exploration and understanding of important problems silence.
- Time for the nurse and client observe one another, sort out feelings, think of how to say thing and consider what has been verbally communicated. The nurse should allow the client to break the silence. Lack of verbal communication for therapeutic reasons. For example, sitting with the patient and nonverbally communicating shows interest and involvement.
  Therapeutic value: Allows the client, time to think and gain insight, slow pace of the interaction and encourages the client to initiate conversation while enjoying the nurse's support, understanding and acceptance.
- *Suggestions:* Presentations of alternative ideas for the client's consideration relative to problem-solving. For example, have you thought about responding to your boss in a specific problem has occurred.
  Therapeutic value: It increases the client's perceived notions and or choices.
- *Providing information:* Relevant information is important to make decision experience less anxiety and feel safe and secure. For example, Raman is getting an echocardiogram right now which is a test that uses painless soundwaves to create a moving picture of her heart structures and values and should tell us what is causing her murmur.
- *Sharing empathy:* The ability to understand and accept person's reality, to accurately perceive feelings and to communicate understanding. For example, 'It must be very frustrating to know what you want and not be able to do it'.
- *Sharing Hope:* Communicating a 'sense of possibility' to others. Encouragement when appropriate and positive feedback. For example, 'I believe you will find a way to face your situation because I have seen your courage in the past'.
- *Sharing feelings:* Nurses can help clients to express emotions by making observations, acknowledging feelings and encouraging communication, providing permission to express 'negative' feelings and modeling healthy anger.
- *Paraphrasing:* Restating another's message more briefly using one's own words. It consists of repeating in fewer words the essential ideas of the client. For example, the client says, ' I cannot, focus': my mind keeps wandering. The student nurse says' you are having difficulty in concentrating'.
- *Asking relevant questions:* To seek information needed for decision-making. Asking only one question at a time and fully exploring one topic before moving to another area. Open-ended questions allows for taking the conversational lead and introducing pertinent information about a topic. For example, 'what is your biggest problem at the moment or How has your pain affected your life at home'.
- *Summarizing:* It is pulling together information for documentation. It gives a client a sense of closure. For example, it is my understanding that your arm pain is you understand. It is a concise review of key aspects of an interaction. Summarizing brings your arm pain to level 1 since you have taken a vovoran one hour ago. Taking your pain medication before physical therapy seems to help you complete the activities which the doctor wants you to for

your psychosocial rehabilitation. Is this correct? Client responds 'yes', it really helps to take the medicine before I do my physical therapy, because it helps reduce the pain in my arm.

- *Self-disclosure:* Subjectively true personal experiences about the self, are intentionally revealed to another person for the purpose of emphasizing both the similarities and the differences of experiences. These exchanges are offered as an expression of genuineness and honestly by the nurse and disclosures should be relevant and appropriate. They are used sparingly so the client is the focus to the interaction; 'that happened to me once, too. It was devastating and I had to face about myself that I did not like. I went to counseling and it really helped. What are your thoughts about meeting a counselor?
- *Confrontation:* It is helping the client become more aware of inconsistencies in his or her feelings, attitudes, beliefs and behaviors. Only to be used after trust has been established and should be done gently with sensitivity. For example, 'you say, you have already decided what to do, yet you are still talking a lot about your options.
- *Encouraging formulation of a plan of action:* Encourage the client for therapeutic decision-making, e.g. if this situation occurs again, what options would you have?
- *Asking direct questions:* Ask direct questions to ventilate his/her inner feelings and thoughts, e.g. how does your wife feel about your hospitalization?

NONTHERAPEUTIC TECHNIQUES OF COMMUNICATION

- Nontherapeutic communication 'blocks' to communication of feelings and ideas.
- *Reassuring:* The nurse implies that anxious client has no cause for worry or concern, *e.g. nurse with child:* Do not cry, mummy will come back.
  Nurse with adult: you have nothing to worry about anything.
  Someone will come along who will love you and make you very happy.
- *Promoting:* The nurse mechanically repeats the client's words without thinking, without evaluating what has been said and without helping the client to think things through. It indicates a lack of interest, respects and relatedness on the part of the nurse, *e.g.* adolescent: I hate you.
  Nurse: You hate me.
- *Giving approval:* The nurse provides positive sanction for client's thinking or behavior, thereby setting and maintaining standards of good and bad. The client may work to earn the nurses praise rather than to make progress, *e.g. nurse with child:* You are a good boy.
  Nurse with adult: Your's choice was only the correct one.
- *Rejecting:* The nurse refuse to consider or shows contempt for the client's thinking. Rejection closes the topic of exploration, *e.g. nurse with adult:* Do not let me hear my more about ……
- *Probing:* The nurse digs for information or persistently questions the client even after the client indicates unwillingness to discuss the issues, *e.g. nurse with adult:* Tell me about your history of alcohol abuse.
- *Challenging:* The nurse insists the client provides a rational basis for irrational thinking, the client then becomes defensive, *e.g. Nurse with adult:* If you really have no legs, how can you walk up here to the nurse's station?
- *Requesting an explanation:* The nurse asks 'why' to the client, thereby asking for the reason for feelings and behaviors when the client may not know the reason, *e.g. nurse with client:* Why did you do that?

- *Using denial:* The nurse refuses to acknowledge that a problem exists, there by cutting of exploration of the problem with the client and denying the validity of the client's perception. *e.g. nurse with adult:* I am not going to be able to stop drinking. *Nurses:* Of course, you will.
- *Blaming:* The nurse inappropriately expresses feelings or anger or impatience with the client as a means of faulting the client because the nurse-patient relationship is not progressing well. This the therapeutic dead end that negates that nurse's role as a client advocate; destroy trust and takes away clients motivation to work with the nurse to identify and explore sensitive topics, *e.g. nurse with adult:* I know the pain is bad when I have to try to turn you, but it was you who climbed up on the ladder and risked breaking a hip, not me.
- *Disapproving:* The nurse makes a negative value judgment about the client's behavior and thinking. *Nurse with the child:* That was bad to do, *e.g. nurse with adult:* I am afraid, I cannot approve of such behavior.
- *Advising:* The nurse literally tells the client what to do. This implies that nurse knows best and the client is incapable of independent problem-solving, *e.g. nurse:* You should use acne medication and stop drinking soft drinks.
- *Interrogating:* The nurse bombards the client with multiple questions that do not allow the client time for a thoughtful response. The question interrupts therapeutic communication, e.g. *Nurse:* How did you feel after the surgery? When they took out the bandage off were you nervous?

  Did you dread looking in the mirror who was with you at that time?
- *Introduction of unrelated topic:* The nurse changes the subject when the clients bring up material the nurse prefers not to discuss, *e.g. adult:* I wish I could die. *Nurse:* What dress you are wearing today?
- *Using jargon:* The nurse excludes the client and makes the interaction incomprehensible by using nursing jargon, e.g. *nurse with adult:* Ingestion of a cholecystocholangiographic medium (gallbladder pill) is necessary.
- *Asking personal questions:* Asking personal questions that are not relevant to the situation is not professional or appropriate. Do not ask question just to satisfy your curiosity, why are not you married to Kamal? It is not appropriate. Instead it can be asked like how would you describe your relationship with Kamal.
- *Giving personal opinions:* Giving personal opinions, takes away decision-making for the client. Remember the problem and solution belongs to the patient not to the nurse. 'If I were you' I would put your father in a nursing home 'can be reframed to say Let us talk about what options are available to your father'.
- *Changing the Subject:* 'Let us not talk about your insurance problems, its time for your walk'. Changing the subject when someone is trying to communicate with you is made and shows a lack of empathy. It tends to block further communication and seems to say that you do not really care about what they are sharing. 'After your walk, let's talk some more about what is going on with your insurance company.
- *Automatic responses:* Saying—Administration does not care about the staff or older adults are always confused. These are generalizations and stereotypes that reflect poor nursing judgment and threaten nurse-client or team relationships.
- *False reassurance:* Do not worry, everything will be all right. When a client is seriously ill or distressed, the nurse may be tempted to offer hope to the client with statements such as 'you will be fine' or 'there's nothing to worry about'. When a patient is reaching for understanding these phrases that are not based on fact or based on reality can do more harm than good.

The nurse maybe trying to be kind and think he/she is helping, but these comments tend to block conversation and discourage further expressions of feelings. A better response would be It must be difficult not to know what the surgeon will find. What can I do to help?

- *Sympathy:* Sympathy focuses on the nurses feelings rather than the client's saying, 'I' am so sorry about your amputation, it must be terrible to lose a leg'. This shows concern but more sorrow and pity than trying to understand how the client feels. Sympathy is a subjective look at another person's world that prevent a clear perspective of the issues confronting that person. A more empathetic approach would be 'the loss of your leg is a major change, how do you think this will affect your life'?
- *Asking for explanations:* Why are you so upset ? A nurse maybe tempered to ask the other person to explain why the person believes, feels or is acting in a certain way. Clients frequently interpret why question as acquisition. Why question can cause resentment, insecurity and mistrust? It is better to phrase a question to avoid using the word 'why, 'you seem upset, what is in your mind'?
- *Approval or disapproval:* You should not even think about assisted suicide. It is just not right. Nurses must not impose their own attitudes, values, beliefs and moral standards on others, while in the professional helping role. Judgmental responses by the nurse often contain terms such as should, ought, good, right or wrong. Agreeing or disagreeing sends the subtle message that nurses have the right to make value judgments about the client's decisions. Approving implies that the behavior being praised is the only acceptance one.
  Disapproving implies that the client must meet the nurse's expectations or standards. Instead the nurse should help clients explore their won beliefs and decision. The nursing response 'I am surprised you are consider assisted suicide. Tell me more about it.......' gives the client a chance to express ideas or feelings without fear of being judged.
- *Defensive responses:* 'No one here would intentionally lie to you'. When clients express criticism, nurses should listen to what they are saying. Listening does not imply agreement. To discover reasons for the client's anger or dissatisfaction, the nurse must listen uncritically. By avoiding defensiveness the nurse can defuse anger and uncover deeper concerns. 'You believe have been dishonest with you. It must be hard to trust anyone'.
- *Passive or aggressive responses:* Things are bad and there is nothing you can do about it or 'being sick is bad and its all your fault'. Passive responses serve to avoid conflict or side step issues. They reflect feelings of sadness, depression, anxiety, powerlessness and hopelessness. Aggressive responds provoke confrontation at the other person's expense. They reflect feelings of anger, frustration, resentment and stress. Assertive communication is a far more professional approach for the nurse to take.
- *Arguing:* 'How can you say you did not sleep a wink when I heard you snoring all night long !!' Challenging or arguing again perceptions denies that they are real and valid to the other person. They imply that the other person is lying, misinformed or uneducated. The skillful nurse can provide information or present reality in a way that avoids argument 'you feel like you did not get any rest at all last night, even though I thought you slept well since I heard you snoring'.

TECHNIQUES THAT ENHANCE THERAPEUTIC COMMUNICATION

Maximizing therapeutic communication requires the use of techniques that encourage clients to open up and speak more freely and frankly. There are number of such therapeutic techniques of communication that are generally considered helpful for nurse to use.

Some guidelines are:

- Individualize each technique to your client level of understanding.
- Vary the therapeutic techniques used. Particularly avoid using any one type of techniques repeatedly.
- Use language appropriately.
- As you enter the clinical area to take with a client for the first time, relax and realize that most clients want very much to talk to you.
- Any specific techniques of communication might be used at anytime, according to the client and situation.

INEFFECTIVE THERAPEUTIC COMMUNICATION

These include:

- Failure to listen
- Conflicting verbal and nonverbal messages
- A judgmental attitude
- False reassurance
- Giving of advice
- The ability to receive information because of preoccupation of impaired thought process and changing of the subjects.

THERAPEUTIC IMPASSES

Therapeutic impasses are block in the process of the nurse-client relationship. Impasses provoke frustration feelings in both the nurse and the client, which may range from anxiety and apprehension to frustration, love or intense anger.

ELEMENTS OF THERAPEUTIC IMPASSES

- *Resistance:* It is the client's attempt to remain unaware of anxiety producing aspects within the self.
- *Transference:* It is an unconscious response in which the client experiences feelings and attitude towards the nurse that were originally associated with significant figures in the client's early life. For example, a client perceives the nurse as acting the way that his mother did, regardless of how the nurse is truly acting. Transference can be positive if client view the nurse as helpful difficult because of unpleasant emotions that interfere with treatment such as anger and fear.
- *Counter transference:* It refers to a specific emotional response by the nurse towards the client that is inappropriate to the content and the context of the therapeutic relationship or inappropriate in its emotional intensity.

Counter transference are usually of three types:

1. Reaction of intense love or caring.
2. Reaction of intensive hostility or hatred.
3. Reaction of intense anxiety often in response to a patient's resistance.

Forms of counter transference displayed by the nurse:

- Difficulty in empathizing with client in certain problem areas.
- Recurrent anxiety, unease or guilt related to the client.

- Personal and social relationship with the client.
- Encouraging patient's dependency, praise or affection.
- Sexual or aggressive fantasies towards client.
- Arguing with client or tendency to push client 'before' he is ready.
- Feeling angry or impatient because of patient's unwillingness to change.
- *Boundary Violation:* It occurs when a nurse goes outside the boundaries of the therapeutic relationship and establishes a social economic or personal relationship with a psychiatric client, *e.g.* possible boundary violation.
  Nurse accepts free gifts from client.
  Having personal or social relationship with client.
  Nurse attends a social function of client.
  Nurse regularly reveals personal information to the client.
  Nurse routinely hugs or has the personal contact with client.
  Nurse does business with or purchases services from client.

INTERVENTIONS TO OVERCOME THERAPEUTIC IMPASSES

- Nurse must have knowledge of the impasses and recognize behaviors that indicate their existence.
- Nurse must reflect on feelings, explore reasons behind such behavior.
- Coworkers are more likely than others to recognize the phenomenon initially and provide feedback to the nurse about it.
- Nurses must examine their strength, weaknesses, prejudices and values before they can interact more appropriately with client.
- The transference reactions of client must also be examined, gently but directly.
- Nurses must be open and clear about their genuine reactions when clients misperceive behavior.
- Nurses should also state actions that they can and cannot take to meet the client's needs.
- Limit settings is useful when clients act appropriately towards the nurse.
- Maintain open communication with her supervisor, who can then guide her in making adequate progress in handling, such resistant reactions.

Treatment Modalities and Therapies in Mental Disorders

PSYCHOPHARMACOLOGY

Treatment modalities of psychiatric client's are multimodal in practice. Primarily, the psychiatric client is treated by drugs. These drugs in psychiatric care are known as psychiatric drugs. The study of these drugs are known as psychopharmacology.

Psychotropic or psychoactive drugs are chemicals that affect the brain and nervous system; alter feelings, emotions and conscious in various ways; and frequently are used therapeutically in psychiatry to treat a broad range of mental and emotional illnesses.

The different categories of psychiatric drugs include:

- Antipsychotic agents
- Antianxiety/anxiolytics
- Antidepressants
- Mood stabilizers.
- Anticonvulsants
- Hypnotics and other related drugs.

Anticholinergic or anti-Parkinson's drugs are utilized to alleviate extra pyramidal symptoms (EPS) or side effects. Each category of these drugs which focus on principles or rationale and therapy contraindication, side effects, implications for nursing actions and client and family psycho education are discussed in this chapter.

ANTIPSYCHOTIC DRUGS

A psychoactive drug, psychopharmaceutical or psychotropic is a chemical substance that crosses the blood-brain barrier and acts primarily upon the central nervous system where it alters brain function resulting in changes in perception, mood, consciousness, cognition and behavior.

An antipsychotic (neuroleptics) is a tranquilizing psychiatric medication primarily used to manage psychosis. It was first discovered in 1950s. Chlorpromazine was first antipsychotic used as a surgical anesthetic. It was used to calm the patient. The discovery of chlorpromazine as psychoactive effect in 1952 led to great reduce in use of restrints, seclusion and sedation in the management of agitated client.

Antipsychotics are the psychotropic drugs which are used in the treatment of major psychotic disorders and psychotic symptoms. These are also called as major tranquilizers, neuroleptics as well as antischizophrenic drugs and dopamine receptors blockers.

Types of Antipsychotic Drugs

First generation antipsychotics/typical antipsychotics:

- *Butyrophenones:* Haloperidol (haldol, serenace)
  Droperidol (droleptan)
- *Phenothiazines:* Chlorpromazine (thorazine, largactil)
  Fluphenazine (prolixin)
  Perphenazine (trilafon)
  Thioridazine (mellaril)
  Trifluoperazine (stelazine)
  Triflupromazine (vesprin)
  Levomepromazine (nozinan)
  Promethazine (phenergan)
  Pimozide (Orap)
  Cyamemazine (Tercian)
- *Chlorprothixene:* Chlorprothixene(Cloxan, taractan.)
  Clopixol (Sordinol)
  Flupenthixol (depixol)
  Thiothixene (navane)
  Zuclopenthixol (cisordinol)

Second generation antipsychotic/atypical antipsychotics:

- Clozapine (clozaril)
- Olanzapine (zyprexa)
- Risperidone (Risperdal)
- Quetiapine (secoquel)
- Ziprasidone (geodon)
- Amisulpride (solian)
- Paliperidone (invega)
- Iloperidone (fanapt)
- Sertindole (serdolect)
- Lurasidone (latuda)

Third Generation Antipsychotics:

- Aripirazole (ability)
- Partial agonists of dopamine.

First Generation Antipsychotic/Typical Antipsychotics

- These are classic, typical antipsychotics and are usually called 'phenothiazines'.
- These are primarily dopamine receptor blockers, preventing the stimulation of the postsynaptic neurons by dopamine. It causes several adverse effects associated with dopamine blockade, including hypotension, anticholinergic effects and extrapyramidal side effects.

Second Generation Antipsychotics/Atypical Antipsychotics

These are newer generation, atypical antipsychotics, block both dopamine receptors and serotonin receptors. This dual neurological effects and depression are associated with the typical antipsychotics.

MECHANISM OF ACTION

The exact mechanism of antipsychotics in not well known. One of the major mechanisms appears to be antidopaminergic activity. These drugs block dopamine receptors in the brain. Dopamine receptors is blocked with the blockage of postsynaptic dopamine receptor in the basal ganglia, hypothalamus, limbic system, brainstem and at medulla. The medication exerts antipsychotic properties by blocking actions on receptors specific to dopamine, serotonin and other neurotransmitters.

PHARMACOKINETICS

- The orally administered antipsychotics are absorbed erratically and variability from gastro-intestinal tract.
- IM/IV administration provides much more reliable blood level.
- The oral liquid dose produces a peak level at 1.5 hours and IM peaks at 30 minutes.

Indications

It is indicated in various psychiatric disorders.

- *Organic psychiatric disorder*
  - Delirium.
  - Dementia.
  - Delirium tremens (psychoses occurring in drug and withdrawal states. (Ex., haloperidol, risperidone).
  - Drug induced psychoses.
  - Other organic mental disorder: organic hallucination and delusional disorders.
- *Nonorganic psychotic disorders*
  - Schizophrenia.
  - Schizoaffective disorder.
  - Acute psychoses.
  - Mania maintenance treatment of bipolar disorder.
  - Major depression.
  - Delusional disorder.
- *Neurotic and other psychiatric disorders*
  - Severe intractable and disabling anxiety.
  - Obsessive compulsive disorder.
  - Anorexia nervosa (rarely used).
- *Medical disorders*
  - Huntington's chorea.
  - Intractable hiccups (low dose of chlorpromazine).
  - Nausea and vomiting (e.g. an ondansetron is an antiemetic drug and is a weak antipsychotric).
  - Tic disorder.

CONTRAINDICATIONS/PRECAUTIONS

These drugs are contraindicated in clients with known

- Hypersensitivity.
- Evidence of CNS depression.
- Blood dyscrasias
- Parkinson's disease.
- Liver, renal and cardiac insufficiency.

Cautiously used in:

- Elderly clients
- Severally ill/ depilated client
- Diabetic client
- Respiratory insufficiency
- Prosthetic hypertrophy
- Intestinal obstruction
- Individual should avoid exposure to extremes in temperature while taking antipsychotic drugs.

SIDE EFFECTS OF ANTIPSYCHOTICS

Sl. No.	System Involvement	Side Effects	Possible Cause
A.	Autonomic side effects	Dry mouth Constipation Cyclopedia Mydriasis Urinary retention Orthostatic hypertension Impotence Impaired ejaculation	Muscarinic cholinergic blockade
B.	Extrapyramidal side effects (EPS)	Parkinson's syndrome, akathisia, acute dystonia rabbit syndrome, tardive dyskinesia, neuroleptic effects.	Dopaminergic receptor blockade
C.	Other CNS effects	Seizures, sedation, depression or pseudodepression.	Decreased seizures threshold
D.	Metabolic and endocrine side effects	Weight gain, diabetes, galactorrhea with or without amenorrhea.	Dopaminergic blockade in hypothalamus
E.	Allergic side effects	Jaundice	Hypersensitivity reaction
F.	Cardiac side effects	ECG changes sudden death (rare cases)	Anticholinergic reaction
G.	Ocular side effect	Retinopathy	Not known
H.	Dermatological side effect	Contact dermatitis	Allergic reaction

DRUG INTERACTIONS

- *Methyldopa:* Increased risk of EPS.
- *Levodopa:* Decreased action of levodopa.
- *Tricyclic antidepressants:* Increased toxicity.

- *Carbamazepine, phenobarbital, rifampicin:* Plasma level of haloperidol decreases.
- *Lithium:* Antihypertensive action antagonized.

BASELINE CLINICAL OPINION

It is important to monitor physical health before prescribing antipsychotics and following are the minimum suggestions and investigations based on the clinical opinion.

- Obtain detailed personal and family history, weight BMI, BP, WBC and neutrophils, and FBC.
- *After one month:* Weight, BMI, BP and FBS.
- *After three months:* Weight, BMI, BP and FBS.
- *After six months:* Weight BMI, BP and FBS serum lipids and liver function test.
- *After twelve months:* Weight BMI, BP and FBS and serum lipids.

General principles regarding routine clinical use.

Some general principles regarding routine clinical use of antipsychotics include:

- Atypical antipsychotics are usually preferred.
- Whenever possible, the lowest effective dose should be used.
- Routinely only one antipsychotic should be used at one time.
- High dose of antipsychotic should be avoided.
- It is really important to monitor physical health.
- An oral atypical antipsychotic drug should be considered as first line of treatment for individuals with newly diagnosed schizophrenia.
- Routine blood and clinical monitoring should be recommended.

DEPOT ANTIPSYCHOTICS

The use of a depot or long acting injectable (LAI) formulation of antipsychotic drug is a therapeutic option for clients demonstrating significant adverse consequences resulting from significant noncompliance with oral antipsychotic treatment. To improve compliance, liquid doses are available.

Practice Guidelines

- For client who have never taken oral risperidone, administer a test dose of 1–2 mg/day for two consecutive days to rule out idiosyncratic hypersensitivity to risperidone.
- The starting dose of LAI risperidone is determined by a client's prior antipsychotic history.

Guidelines for switching from oral risperidone to IM/IV RISPERIDONE

Dose of oral risperidone mg/day	Dose of 1 ml. IM/ IV. risperidone mg/fortnight.
• < 2 mg–25 mg	• Between 2 and 4 mg
• > 4 mg 37.5–50 mg	• 25–37.5 mg

At present, two depot antipsychotics are marketed:

- *Fluphenazine decanoate:* Injection dose 12.5–25mg 1M/sk.
- *Haloperidol decanoate:* Injection dose should not exceed 100 mg. It is administered every 4 week or monthly once.

Administration of Depot Antipsychotic Injection

- Parental product should be inspected visually for particulate matter and discoloration.
- A dry syringe and 21-gauze needle should be used. Use of wet syringe will cloud the solution.
- Maximum volume per site per injection should not exceed 3 ml.
- Before administration a depot injection, it is always advisable to start with a short acting dosage. So that client can be assessed with potential side effects.

Nursing Implications

- *Closed observation:* The nurse has to monitor the client for adverse effects, specially when the antipsychotics are just started. The expected results are reduction in the aggressive hyperactive behavior and disorganized thoughts.
- *Extrapyramidal reaction:* Observe for Parkinson's disease, akinesia, akathisia, dystonia and tardive dyskinesia.
- *Observe for drowsiness:* Medicines should be administered at bed time. Report if the drowsiness persists for a very long time. The client should be advised not to drive and handle machinery while taking antipsychotic drugs.
- *Record blood pressure:* B.P. should be recorded every half an hour. If it develops by 20 to 30 mm/hg in the client, immediate reporting and interventions should be done.
- *Accurate route of medication:* Antipsychotics are not given subcutaneously unless specially prescribed as they cause tissue irritation. These drugs should be given deep intramuscularly in a 'Z' track manner.
- *Dry mouth:* It may be reduced by encouraging the client to rinse his/her mouth frequently. Give a piece of lemon or chewing gum. Good oral hygiene should be maintained.
- *Blurred/impaired vision:* Blurred vision or night blindness can be permanent due to pigmentary retinopathy.
- *Weight gain:* The client on antipsychotic drugs may have weight gain. Weight record should be maintained. The client may be encouraged on a low salt and planned caloric daily.
  - An intake output chart should be maintained specially for male client's who are confined to bed and have an enlarged prostate gland. Encourage to take at least 2500 ml of liquid intake.
  - The client should be advised to protect his skin, by not going in the sun and to wear protective clothing and sunglasses.
  - The client should be explained not to increase or decrease or stop taking drugs without consulting doctor. The drug should be withdrawn slowly to avoid nausea and seizures.

Reassurance to Relatives

The client and his relatives should be explained that desired effects will be achieved after weeks of mediation, so the relatives need to wait for the effects of the drugs.

NURSING MANAGEMENT

The following nursing diagnoses are may be considered for client receiving antipsychotic therapy:
- Risk for other directed violence related to panic anxiety and mistrust of other.
- Risk for injury related to medication side effects of sedation. Photosensitivity, reduction of seizure threshold, extrapyramidal symptoms.

- Risk for activity intolerance related to medication side effects of sedation, blurred vision and weakness.
- Noncompliance with medication regimen related to suspiciousness and mistrust of others.

NURSING PLANNING AND IMPLEMENTATION

Anticholinergic Effects

- *Dry mouth*
  - Provide the client with sugarless candy or gum, ice and frequent sip of water.
  - Ensure that the client practice strict oral hygiene.
- *Blurred vision*
  - Explain that these symptoms will most likely subside after a few weeks.
  - Advise the client not to drive a car/vehicle until vision clears.
  - Clear small items from the pathway to prevent falls.
- *Constipation*
  - Order foods high in fiber.
  - Encourage increase in physical activity and fluid intake.
- *Urinary retention*
  - Instruct the client to report any difficulty with food to minimize GI upsets.

Sedation

- Discuss with the physician the possibility of administering the drug at bedtime.
- Discuss with the doctor, the possible decrease in dosage or order for less sedating medication.
- Instruct the client not to drive /swim or to operate dangerous equipments while experiencing sedation.

Orthostatic Hypertension

- Instruct the client to rise slowly from a lying or sitting position.
- Monitor blood pressure and vital signs.
- Document and report significant changes.

Photosensitivity

- Ensure that the client wears protective sunscreens, clothing and sunglasses while spending time at outdoors.

Hormonal Effects

- Decreased libido, retrograde amnesia, ejaculation, gynecomastia (men).
- Amenorrhea (women).
- Weight gain.

Salivation: (with clozapine)

- A significant number of clients receiving clozapine therapy experience extreme salivation. Offer psychosocial support to the client.

Extrapyramidal Symptoms (EPS)

- Observe for symptoms and report immediately to doctor.
- Symptoms may appear 1 to 5 days following initiation of antipsychotic medication occurs most often in women, the elderly and dehydrated client.

Neuroleptic Malignant Syndrome (NMS)

- It is a rare but potentially fatal complication of treatment with narcoleptic drugs.
- Onset can occur within hours or even years after drug initiation and progression is rapid over the flowing 24–72 hours.
- NMS symptoms include severe parkinsonian muscle rigidity, hyperpyrexia up to 107 °F, tachycardia, tachypnea, fluctuations in BP, diaphoresis, rapid deterioration of mental status stupor or coma.

Tardive Dyskinesia (TD)

- Symptoms of TD are marked by bizarre facial and tongue movements, stiff neck and difficulty in swallowing.
- Client's receiving long term (month/year) antipsychotics therapy are at risk.
- The symptoms are potentially irreversible.
- The drugs should be withdrawn at the first sign, which is usually vermiform movements of the tongue, prompt actions may prevent irreversibility.

Dystonia

- Marked by involuntary muscular movements, spasm of face, arms, legs and neck.
- This occurs most often in men and in client younger than 25 years.
- Psycho education:
  - Use caution when driving or operating dangerous machinery, drowsiness and dizziness can occur.
  - Do not abruptly stop the drug, slowly taper the dosage.
  - Strict follow up.
  - Rise slowly from a sitting/lying position to prevent sudden drop in blood pressure.
  - Be aware of possible risks of taking neuroleptics during pregnancy. Safe use during pregnancy and lactation has not been established. Neuroleptics thought to cross the placental barrier to fetus could experience adverse effects of the drugs.
  - Continue to take medication, even if he is feeling well and as thought it is not needed. Symptoms may return if medication is discontinued.

Outcome Criteria/Evaluation

The following criteria may be used for evaluation to know the effectiveness of therapy with antipsychotic medication of the client:

- Has not harmed others.
- Has not experienced injury caused by side effects.
- Maintain WBC within normal limits.

- Exhibits no symptoms of EPS, TD or NMS.
- Maintains weight within normal limits.
- Takes drugs willingly. Verbalizes understanding of medication regimen and the importance of regular administration.

ANTIANXIETY DRUGS/HYPNOTICS

Antianxiety agents (i.e. Sedatives) and hypnotics are referred as hypnosedatives. Antianxiety agents are primarily used to treat daytime tension and hypnotics to relieve insomnia.

Antianxiety drugs also known as minor tranquilizers. These are medication that relieve anxiety by slowing down the central nervous system. Their relaxing and calming effects have made them very popular. They are also prescribed sleeping pills and muscle relaxants.

Indications

- Generalized anxiety disorder; adjustment disorder with anxious mood.
- Panic disorder, agoraphobia and school phobia.
- Agitative depression.
- Insomnia.
- Stage-IV NREM sleep disorder like enuresis, somnambulism.
- Nightmares.
- Premedication anesthesia.
- Anticonvulsant use.
- As a skeletal muscle relaxant.
- Treatment in alcohol and other drug withdrawal syndromes.
- For minor surgical, endoscopic or obstetric procedures.
- Acute mania.
- Antipsychotic induced akathisia.
- Emergency management of acute psychoses.
- Narcoanalysis or abreaction therapy.
- Acute alcohol withdrawal.

Classification of Anxiolytics

Antianxiety drugs are classified into 6 types:

- Benzodiazepines (BDZ).
- Buspirone.
- 5 HT reuptake inhibitors (5 HTRI).
- Antidepressants.
- Beta adrenergic blockers.
- MAO inhibitors.

Benzodiazepines (BDZ)

- **Short-acting benzodiazepines (3–5 hours)**
  - Triazolam 0 25 mg
  - Midazolam 0.25–0.5 mg
- **Intermediate benzodiazepines (6–24 hours)**
  - Alprazolam (1–4 mg)
  - Lorazepam (1–6 mg)
  - Oxazepam (15–120 mg)

- **Long-acting benzodiazepines (24–72 hours)**
  - Clonazepam (0.5–10 mg)
  - Chlordiazepoxide (10–40 mg)
  - Diazepam (2–40 mg)
  - Flurazepam (15–30 mg)

Mechanism of Action

Antianxiety drugs depress subcortical level of the CNS, particularly the limbic system and reticular formation. They may potentiate the effect of the powerful inhibitory neurotransmitter gamma amino butyric acid (GABA) in the brain, these produces calmative effect. All level of CNS depression can be affected from mild sedation to hypnosis to coma.

Use

Benzodiazepines are used to relieve short-term anxiety, generalized anxiety disorder, OCD, panic disorder, sleep disorders, epilepsy and as preanesthetic agent.

Buspirone

- *Dose:* 15–60 mg: Half life – 2.5 mg.

Mechanism of action: Partial agonist to 5 HT receptors thought to balance serotonin level by lowering them in anxious persons.

- *Uses:* As anxiolytic in mild anxiety.
  - Generalized anxiety disorders.
  - Not much effective in severe and chronic anxiety/panic anxiety.

Selective Serotonin Reuptake Inhibitors (SSRIs)

- *Example:* Fluoxetine (20–60 mg)
- *Mechanism of action:* acts by blocking uptake of 5HT
- *Uses:*
  - Panic disorders
  - OCD depression
  - Generalized anxiety disorders
  - Phobias.

Tricyclic Antidepressants

- Doxepin (150–300 mg)
- Imipramine (150–300 mg)

- *Mechanism of action:* TCA'S act by reducing uptake of 5HT and norepinephrine.
- *Uses:* Anxiety associated with depression
  - Panic anxiety states.

Beta Adrenergic Blockers

- *Example:* Propranolol (120–160 mg)
  - Atenolol (50–100 mg)

Mechanism of action: It acts by blocking peripheral sympathetic system and reduces physical or somatic symptoms of anxiety. It decreases BP and slows heart rate.

- *Uses:* Social phobia.
  - Less effective for other forms of anxiety.

Monoamine Oxidase Inhibitors (MAOI)

- *Example:* Phenelzine (45–90 mg).
- *Mechanism of action:* Acts by blocking the action of MAO enzymes.
- *Uses:* Panic attacks of anxiety and phobia.

SIDE EFFECTS OF ANTIANXIETY DRUGS

- Nausea
- Vomiting
- Weakness
- Epigastric pain
- Diarrhea
- Vertigo
- Blurring of eyes.
- Body aches
- Urinary incontinence

Impotence
Ataxia
Dry mouth
Retrograde amnesia
Sedation
Lassitude
Increased reaction time
Dry mouth

RISK FACTORS

Anyone who takes antianxiety drugs can experience unpleasant or dangerous side effects but certain individuals are at a higher risk.

- *People over sixty five years:* Older adults are more sensitive to the sedating effects of anti-anxiety mediation; even small dose can cause confusion, amnesia, loss of hips to dementia. Antianxiety drug use in the elderly is associated with an increased of falls, broken hips and legs, road traffic accidents.
- *Pregnancy:* Expectant mother should avoid antianxiety drug. Since these anxiety medications cross the placenta, their use during pregnancy can lead to dependence in the baby. Then following birth, the baby will then go through withdrawal, with symptoms such as muscle weakness, irritability sleep and breathing problems and trembling. These drugs are excreted in breast milk, so they should be avoided while breastfeeding the baby.
- *People with a history of substance abuse:* Anyone with a current or former problem with alcohol or drugs should avoid antianxiety drugs or use them only with extreme caution. The greatest benefit of benzodiazepines is, an that they work quickly, but makes individual to be addictive. This can quickly lead to their abuse, often very dangerous in combination with alcohol or other illicit drug consumption.

INTERACTIONS

Increased effects of antianxiety agents can occur when taken with alcohol, narcotic, antipsychotic, antidepressant, antihistamine, neuromuscular, blocking agents, cimetidine or disulfiram. Increased effects also occur with consumption of cigarette and caffeine.

ANTIANXIETY DRUG DEPENDENCE AND WITHDRAWAL

Antianxiety medications including popular benzodiazepines are meant for short term use. However, many people take regularly and lead to physical dependence. Drug tolerance also acts as anxiety relief as before. According to American Academy of Family Physician, benzodiazepines lose their therapeutic antianxiety effect after 4 to 6 months of regular use.

Most people become addicted to their antianxiety drugs within a couple of months but problem may arise soon. For some clients, drug dependency develops after a few shorts of week. Once physical dependency occurs, stopping will be very difficult. The body is used to the medication, so withdrawal symptoms occur if the dose is decreased or discontinued. Psychological dependence may be an issue too. If you' have been relying on drug to keep your anxiety in check, you may lose confidence in your own abilities to deal with life's difficulties and start to think you 'need' the medication to survive.

NURSING THERAPEUTICS

- Assessment of the client, prior to the use of antianxiety, sedative, and hypnotic agents. If the client complains of sleep disturbance, the causative factor should be identified.
- Teach the client regarding the proper use of prescribed medications and explain their adverse effects.
- Caution-not to use in combination with other CNS depressants.
- While administering the drugs, delayed dose should be given at bed time to promote the normal sleep pattern, so that daily activities are not affected.
- Look for side effects, record and report immediately.
- If the client complains of drowsiness, tell him to avoid using knife and instruct not to drive.
- Instruct the client not to take any stimulants like coffee, alcohol as they alter the effect of drugs.
- Avoid excessive use of drug to prevent the onset of substance abuse.
- Drug should be reduced gradually; sudden stoppage of the drug may cause REM, insomnia, dreams or nightmares, mare convulsion, agitation.
- Assess for oversedation especially in old people.

MOOD STABILIZERS

Mood stabilizers or antimanic agents are psychopharmacological agents used for stabilizing mood wings, particularly those of manic in bipolar disorders. These include anticonvulsants, calcium channel blocker, adrenergic blocking agents and atypical antipsychotics.

Classification

- *Class A:* The primary acute and prophylactic effect by treating the depressed phase, preventing or delaying manic episodes without destabilizing the overall course of the illness by exacerbation of depression. Example Lithium.
- *Class B:* The primary acute and prophylactic effect by treating the manic phase, preventing or delaying depressive episodes without destabilizing the overall course of the illness by exacerbation of manic episode. Example, Lamotrigine.
  - Bauer (2004) defines mood stabilizers are a group of medication which can treat both mania and depression or at minimum, they treat one of the two and rarely cause the other people to become worse in the process.

Mood stabilizers are classified on the basis of action as follows:

Classification	Generic name	Daily recommended dosage (mg)
• **Antimania**	Lithium carbonate (ESKALITH, Lithane, lithobid)	**Acute mania:** 1800–2400 **Maintenance:** 900–1200
• **Anticonvulsant**	Clona ceptam (klonopin)	0.75–1.6
	Carbamazepine (tegretol)	200–1200
	Valproic acid (depakene; depakote)	500–1500
	Lamotrigine (lamictal)	100–200
	Gabapentin (neurontin)	900–1800
	Topiramate (topamax)	50–400
	Oxcarbazepine (trileptal)	600–2400
• **Calcium channel blockers**	Verapamil (calan isoptin) Nifedipine, Adalat, Procardia	80–320 60–180
• **Benzodiazepines**	Alprazolam (xanax)	1–4
	Chloradiazepoxide (librium)	10–40
	Diazepam (valium)	2–40
	Lorazepam (ativan)	1–6
• **Atypical antipsychotic**	Olanzapine (zyprexa)	5–20
	Aripiprazole (abilify)	10–30
	Chlorpromazine (thorazine)	75–400
	Quetiapine (seroquel)	400–800
	Risperidone (risperdal)	1–6
	Ziprasidone (geodon)	40–160

- *Lithium:* Lithium, a naturally occurring salt, is a first line treatment for client with acute mania and for the long-term prevention of recurrent episodes. It has been postulated that lithium may correct an ion exchange abnormality in the neuron, normalize synaptic neurotransmitter of norepinephrine, serotonin, dopamine and acetylcholine. It likely regulated by second-messenger systems during neurotransmission.
- *Anticonvulsants:* A variety of anticonvulsant drugs have beneficial effects in the treatment of bipolar disorder. It is postulated that the anticonvulsant/mood stabilizing agents work in bipolar disorder by enhancing the effects of the inhibitory neurotransmitter (GABA) and by desensitizing the 'kindling' effect in bipolar illness.
  - Kindling occurs when the brain becomes neurochemically sensitized to events such as stress, trauma or the effects of street drugs and eventually seems to cause the brain to spontaneously respond in a dysfunctional manner even in the absence of these events. Kindling is a model used to explain the causes of cyclical.
  - Illnesses, such as bipolar illness and intermittent symptoms of other illness, such as panic attacks.

- *Calcium channel blockers:* Dysregulation of intracellular calcium may be involved in some affective disorders and this can lead to the investigation of a class of drugs primarily used to treat hypertension and angina. Calcium channel in the postsynaptic neuron, affecting the nonadrenergic neurotransmitter system and are used primarily when other mood stabilizers have failed.
- *Benzodiazepines:* Used in acute mania. Benzodiazepines allows for rapid induction of sleep with earlier resolution of mania without necessitating high dosage of antipsychotic medication in the acute phase.
- *Atypical antipsychotics:* These are used to treat acute mania in bipolar disorder and are becoming more first line treatment because of the side effects, profile and tolerability compared with other mood stabilities.

MOOD STABILIZING AGENTS

Classification	Mode of action	Indications	Contraindications
• Antimanic • Lithium	Enhance reuptake of norepinephrine and serotonin, decreasing the level in the blood, resulting in decreased hyperactivity	• Prevention and treatment of bipolar disorder, also used for bipolar depression • Major depression • Neutropenia • Alcohol dependence	• Hypersensitivity • Sodium depletion • Brain damage • Pregnancy and lactation • Caution with thyroid disorder, diabetes, urinary retention, seizure disorders
• Anticonvulsants • Clonazepam	Action in the treatment of bipolar disorders is unclear.	• Abscess, kinetic and myoclonic seizures • Bipolar manic	• Hypersensitivity • Glucoma, liver disease lactation • Pregnancy • Elderly
Carbamazepine	Action in the treatment of bipolar disorder is unclear.	• Grand mal and psychomotor seizures • Bipolar mania	• Hypersensitivity • Lactation • Caution in elderly • Liver/renal/cardiac disease Pregnancy
Valproic acid	Action in the treatment of bipolar disorders is unclear	Absence seizures	• Hypersensitivity • Lactation • Elderly
Lamotrigine	Action in the unclear bipolar disorder	• Generalized tonic-clonic seizure, absence or myoclonic seizures • Bipolar disorder	• Hypersensitivity • Liver disease • Caution in renal and hepatic insufficiency • Pregnancy, lactation and children <16 years
Gabapentin	Action in the treatment of bipolar disorders is unclear	Partial seizures with or without generalization, in adults with epilepsy Bipolar disorders	• Hypersensitivity • Liver disease • Caution in renal and hepatic insufficiency, pregnancy, lactation children and elderly
Topiramate	Action in the treatment of bipolar disorders is unclear	Partial onset of seizures	Hypersensitivity
Calcium channel blockers	Action in the treatment of bipolar not well known	Angina, arrhythmias, hypertension	• Hypersensitivity • Heart block, shock, pregnancy lactation

Contd...

Contd...

Classification	Mode of action	Indications	Contraindications
Verapamil			
Antipsychotics	Action in the treatment of bipolar disorders is unclear	Schizophrenia, Bipolar mania	• Hypersensitivity • Children and lactation • Caution with hepatic or cardiovascular disease comatose oracle depression, pregnancy elderly

Lithium Toxicity

The margin between the therapeutic and toxic level of lithium carbonate is very narrow. Because lithium is excreted by the kidney, can adversely affects the thyroid and has a narrow therapeutic index and can quickly become fatal, initial and on going health assessment and laboratory monitoring is essential. Lithium toxicity is a medical emergency requiring rapid assessment and treatment.

The usual range of therapeutic serum concentrations are:

For acute mania: 1.0 to 1.5 mEq-/L

For maintenance: 0.6 to 1.2 mEq-/L

Serum lithium levels should be monitored once or twice a week after initial treatment until dosage and serum levels are stable, the monthly during maintenance therapy. Blood sample should be drawn 12 hours after the last dose.

Lithium levels should be monitored prior to medication administration. The dosage should be withheld and the physician to be notified if the level reaches 1.5 mEq-/L or at the earliest observation and report by the client of even mildest symptom. If left untreated, lithium toxicity can be life threatening.

Symptoms of Lithium Toxicity

- Symptoms of lithium begin to appear at blood levels greater than 1.5 mEq-/L; blurred vision, ataxia, tinnitus, persistent nausea and vomiting, severe diarrhea, fine tremors.
- *At serum level of 2.0 to 3.5 mEq-/L:* Excessive put of dilute urine, increasing tremor, muscular irritability, psychomotor retardation, mental confusion, giddiness.
- *At serum level above 3.5 mEq-/L:* Impaired consciousness, nystagmus, seizures, coma, oliguria/anuria, arrhythmias, psyhomotor retardation, mental confusion, cardiovascular collapse, disorientation, death.
- Lithium is similar in chemical structure to sodium. Behaving in the body in much the same manner and competing with sodium at various sites in the body. If sodium intake is reduced or body is depleted of its normal sodium, lithium is reabsorbed by the kidneys, increasing the possibility of toxicity. Therefore the client must consume or diet adequate in sodium as well as 2500 to 3000 ml of fluid intake per day. Accurate record of vital signs, intake- output and client's weight should be monitored on a daily basis.

STABILIZING LITHIUM LEVELS

Common causes for an increase in lithium levels:

- Decreased sodium intakes.
- Diuretic therapy.

- Decreased renal functioning.
- Fluid and electrolyte loss, sweating diarrhea. Dehydration, fever, vomiting.
- Overdose.
- Nonsteroidal anti-inflammatory drugs

Ways to Maintain or Stable Lithium Level

Stabilize dosing schedule by dividing doses or use of sustained release capsules:
- Ensure adequate dietary sodium and fluid intake (2–3 L/day).
- Replace fluid and electrolytes lost during exercises or gastroillnesses.
- Monitor signs and symptoms of lithium, side effects and toxicity.
- If client forget a dose, a dose may be taken if less than 2 hours have elapsed; if longer than 2 hours, the dose should be stopped and the next dose taken as scheduled. Never double upon doses.

Management of Lithium Toxicity

- *Assess quickly:* Obtain rapid history of incident, especially during night and offer support and explanation to patients.
- Hold up all lithium doses.
- Record BP, pulse, temperature, respirations and level of consciousness. Be prepared to initiate stabilization procedures, protect airway and provide supplemental oxygen.
- *Obtain lithium blood level immediately:* Obtain electrolytes BUM, creatinine, urine analysis, CBC when possible.
- Electrocardiogram, monitor cardiac status.
- *Limit lithium absorption:* If acute overdose provide emetic and nasogastric suctioning.
- *Vigorously hydrate:* 5–6 L/day balance electrolytes IV line, indwelling urinary catheter.
- Client will be bedridden, provide range of motion exercises and frequent turning.
- Ascertain reasons for lithium toxicity, increase health teaching efforts, arrange for more frequent clinical visits and blood checks, assess for depression and suicidal intention.

CENTRAL NERVOUS SYSTEM STIMULANTS

The CNS stimulants are a diverse group of pharmacological drug whose first action is stimulation of CNS.

Mechanism of Action

There is a fine balance between excitation and inhibition in the CNS. Information is transmitted along neurons by action potentials. Depolarizing post synaptic potential in an excitatory post synaptic potential. If the degree of this action potential is of magnitude an action potential will be produced in an all or nothing manner through this second neuron. The purpose of the inhibitory postsynaptic potential (1 PSP) is to decrease the number of nerve impulses generated per unit of time. If this did not occur the client would be in a constant state of stimulation.

Classification of CNS Stimulants

- Analeptic stimulants
- Psychomotor stimulants
- Methylxanthines.

ANALEPTIC STIMULANTS

The agent in this group are very different in chemical composition, which makes it difficult to classify each one reference to absorption, distribution and metabolism. Doxapram and nikethamide were historically used as CNS and respiratory stimulants. They still have limited clinical use.

Mechanism of Action

Most of the agents in this group possess the ability to interact with amino acid neurotransmitter. Recent interact studies have explored that GABA receptor chloride ionophore interaction. These clinical trials have postulated that the analeptic stimulants have the ability to change the way chloride ions travel across the neuronal membrane. The inhibitory action of some amino acid neurotransmitters involves an increase in conduction.

Adverse Reactions

- Produce adverse reactions that are exaggerations of their therapeutic effects.
- Produce life-threatening clonic tonic seizures than can lead to death.
- Prior to these seizures, there may be tachypnea, tachycardia and severe hypertension.
- Extreme atmospheres and increased sensitivity to sensory stimuli induced seizures.

PSYCHOMOTOR STIMULANTS

Amphetamines, methamphetamine, methylphenidate psychomotor stimulant mostly have activities similar to amphetamines. Methylphenidate and pemoline have different chemical structures. All these agents are absorbed following oral administration, and most are distributed in the tissues, with concentrations in the brain and CSF. They are metabolized in the liver and excreted in urine. Alkaline urine promotes reabsorption and lengthens the duration of action. All psychomotor stimulants have same action, contraindication/precautions and interaction.

Mechanism of Action

Amphetamines release catecholamines. In PNS, there is a release of norepinephrine from adrenergic nerve terminal and a direct stimulating action on alpha and beta receptor sites. The central mechanism has yet been determined. The central sites are cerebral cortex and reticular activation system. They also produce an anorexigenic effect, leading to weight loss. They may cause a loss of smell and taste, which may height the anorexigenic effects. The overall effects are CNS and respiratory stimulation, mydriasis, bronchodilatation, anorexigenic effects and contraction of urinary bladder sphincter.

Uses/Indications

Therapeutic uses are very limited. Used in management of ADHD, neurolepsy, and obesity. Obesity is usually managed with amphetamines like compounds.

Contraindications and Precautions

- Contraindicated in client's with hypertension, advanced arteriosclerosis, agitated states, cardiovascular disorders, drug abuse, glaucoma, MAO inhibitors and hypersensitivity.

- Not given under 12 years of age.
- May aggravate motor and vocal tics.

Adverse Reactions

Nervousness, irritability, talkativeness, insomnia, dizziness, headache, increased motor activity, mydriasis, depression, hypertension, vomiting, anorexia, cardiac arrhythmia, constipation, dry mouth, metallic taste and increase libido.

DRUG INTERACTIONS

Drug-Drug Interaction:

- Avoid with guanethidine.
- Avoid with sodium bicarbonate and acetazolamide (may cause activation of urine, decrease, urinal excretion of amphetamines and results in an increasing effects of amphetamines).
- With phenothiazines and lithium carbonate.
- Oral dextroamphetamine nicotine induces a dose related increase in cigarette smoking in 'normal' smokers. It is a behavioral stimulant that increase the rate of a variety of learned and stereotyped behaviors.

Drug Laboratory

Elevated level of growth hormone, change in cortisol level and fecal discoloration.

METHYLXANTHINES

These are also called xanthenes or xanthine derivatives. They occur naturally in plants and are consumed in beverages. Coffee and cola contains caffeine, tea contain caffeine and theophylline.

Uses

- As a CNS depressant over dosages.
- Reducing fatigue.
- Headaches.
- Causes vasoconstriction of cerebral arteries, reducing compression of pain sensitive structures.
- Theophylline relieves paroxysmal dyspnea associated with left heart failure.
- Aminophylline (bronchodilator) used for treatment of asthma, bronchospasm and paroxysmal dyspnea.

ADVERSE REACTIONS

- These are very similar of CNS stimulants.
- The CNS and CVS are major system effected.
- Toxicity results in nervousness, insomnia,tachycardia, extrasystole, increased respiration and diuresis.

CAFFEINE

It is absorbed from gut and distributed in tissues. It is metabolized in liver and excreted in urine. The half life is 3–4 hours in adults.

EFFECT ON SYSTEM

- Low to moderate intake produce stimulation of cerebral cortex, causing increased alertness and decreased fatigue. As one approaches 250 mg or more (2–3 cups coffee/tea), the chances of developing more signs of CNS stimulation like nervousness, restlessness, insomnia and tremors.
- Exerts positive inotropic effects on myocardium and positive inotropic effects at the SA node, causing transient increase in heart rate, force of contraction and cardiac output. It may cause increased sinus rates, extrasystole, or ventricular dysrhythmias.
- Stimulates gastric acid and pepsin secretion.
- Weak diuretic (increases renal blood flow and GFR and decrease proximal tubular reabsorption of sodium and water.)
- Increase BMR (intake of 3–9 mg/kg body weight, i.e. 225–675 mg caffeine or 2–6 cups of coffee, can increase BMR by 10%).

Contraindications and Precautions

- Myocardial infarction, dysrhythmias.
- Palpitations, heart failure.
- Hypersensitivity.
- Pregnancy.
- Use cautiously in peptic ulcers.

PSYCHOLOGICAL THERAPIES

Therapeutic Community

Therapeutic community also called as Milieu therapy, and therapeutic milieu are term used interchangeably to describe, explain an environment that utilizes various adaptive psychosocial skills in coping with self, others and the environment. The main focus is on social interpersonal relationship as well as occupational and recreational activities. The concept of deinstitutionalization, the use of psychotropic agents, respect for client's rights, creation of multidisciplinary treatment team and use of therapeutic groups are changes that have contributed for the development of a therapeutic community.

Criteria of Therapeutic Community

Therapeutic milieu can exist in a variety of settings such as the hospital, community center, home or at private nursing home/clinic. Regardless of the setting, certain criteria must be met to help clients to develop a sense of self esteem and personal growth to feel secure to establish trust, to improve their ability to relate to others and to return to the community.

The milieu should

- Be specific and purposeful and planned to provide safety from physical danger and emotional trauma. It should be well furnished to facilitate a home like atmosphere with privacy and provisions for physical needs as well as promote opportunities for interaction and communication among clients and personnel.
- Provide a testing ground for new patterns of behaviors while client's taken responsibility for their actions. Behavioral expectation should be explained to client, including the existing rules, regulations and policies.

- Be consistent when setting limits. This criterion reflects aspects of a democratic society. All clients are treated as equally as possible with respect to restrictions, rules and policies.
- Encourage participation in group activities and free flowing communication in which clients have the freedom to express themselves in a socially acceptable manner.
- Provide respect and dignity to client. Adult-adult interaction should prevail, when appropriate promoting equal status of interaction and exchange of interpersonal information and avoiding any power plays. Client should be encouraged to use personal resources to resolve conflicts.
- Covey an attitude of overall acceptance and optimism. Conflict between staff members must be handled and resolved in same manner to maintain a therapeutic environment. Clients are perceptive of such reaction and may feel these are the cause of conflicts among personal.
- Continually assess and evaluate patient's progress modifying treatment and nursing interventions as needed.
  - The Ward Atmosphere Scale (WAS) is an instrument used to evaluate the effectiveness of a therapeutic milieu. Ten subscales are rated by staff and clients to provide information regarding what actually exists and what should exist.

Subscale items focus on

- Staff control of rules, schedules, and client's behavior.
- Progress, clarity of day-to-day routine.
- Measurement of client's involvement in social functioning, attitudes and general enthusiasm.
- Practical preparation of the client for discharge and transition into the community.
- Supportive atmosphere of staff, doctors and peers towards client.
- Degree of spontaneity the environment allows the client to freely express feelings.
- Promotion of responsibility, self direction and independence as well as staff response to client suggestion or criticisms.
- Order and organization of the unit including staff and client's responses.
- Encouragement of verbalization of feelings such as anger and the channeling of feelings into appropriate behavior.
  - This scale/ instrument is appropriate to evaluate inpatient setting. Partial hospitalization programs, day care treatment centers and community-based mental health programs.
  - From the above discussion, therapeutic community is defined as a scientific structuring of the environment to effect behavioral changes and to improve the psychological health and functioning of the individual.

BASIC ASSUMPTIONS

- The health of each individual is to be realized and restored, encouraged to grow at maximum limit.
- Every interaction is an opportunity for therapeutic intervention.
- The client owns his or her own environment.
- Each client owns his or her own behavior.
- Peer pressure is a useful and powerful tool.
- Inappropriate behaviors are dealt with as they occur.
- Restrictions and punishment are to be avoided.
- A treatment plan is directed by an interdisciplinary team.

- The plan is formulated by collective measures.
- Team members of all disciplines sign the plan and meet weekly to update the plan as needed.
- Disciplines may include psychiatry, psychiatric nursing, social work, occupational, recreational therapy, art therapy, music therapy, diet therapy and Chaplain service.

Role of Nurse

- Through use of the psychiatric nursing process, nurses manage the therapeutic environment on a 24 hours basis.
- Nurses have the responsibility for ensuring that the client's physiological and psychological needs are met.
- Nurses are also responsible for
  - Medication administration.
  - Development of a one-to-one relationship.
  - Setting limits on unacceptable behavior.
  - Client education.

PSYCHOTHERAPY

- Psychotherapy has been referred to as a process in which a person attempts to relieve symptoms, resolve problem or seek personal growth by entering into an implicit or explicit contract with a psychotherapist.
- According to Quentin Crisp "psychotherapy is a friendship and expensive way of tempering with the lives of clients weak enough or foolish enough to seek outside help with personal problem for which infact, only will power is any solution.
- In the words of Jerome Frank (1991) despite their diversity, all psychotherapies attempt to relieve suffering and psychological disability by inducing changes in patient's attitudes and behavior.
- The goals of psychotherapy relieving patient's discomfort/pain, improving the client social functioning and improving the client to perform or act appropriately.

These goals are achieved by:

- Establishing a therapeutic therapist-client relationship.
- Providing an opportunity for the client to release tension as problems are discussed.
- Assisting the client in gaining insight about the problem.
- Providing the opportunity to practice new skills.
- Reinforcing appropriate behavior as it occurs.
- Providing consistent emotional support.
  - Types of individual psychotherapy include psychoanalysis, uncovering therapy, hypnotherapy, reality therapy, supportive therapy and behavior therapy.

PSYCHOANALYTIC PSYCHOTHERAPY

The term psychoanalysis was introduced by Sigmund Freud. It is used to describe a lengthy method of psychotherapy in which the client talks in an uncontrolled, spontaneous manner termed as free association. Here, the psychoanalysis therapist tries to bring into conscious awareness the repressed childhood experiences with associated feelings. The therapist assists the client in exploring repressed anxieties, fears and images of childhood by interpreting dreams, emotions and behavior. A relieving experience is encouraged by the therapist to enable the client to deal with harmful emotions. Only trained analyst is capable of doing it very effectively. The analyst should be aware of his own unconscious conflicts and feelings so that he/she will be aware when those conflicts and feelings interfere with the analysis of client's feelings. Psychoanalysis sessions last approximately 45 minutes, 4 to 5 days a week for approximately 3 to 5 years. It is a long and expensive procedure.

UNCOVERING THERAPY

Uncovering therapy also referred as intensive explorative psychotherapy which assists the person in gaining insight by uncovering conflicts, mainly unconscious, so that they can be treated openly and effectively. The client then works through the conflict and repeated exploration of the newly gained insight.

HYPNOTHERAPY

The word hypnosis is derived from the Greek literature. Hypnos means sleep. Hypnosis was discovered by James Braid in 1841. It is an adjunct to inotropic used to help to learn to relax, effect behavioral changes, control attitudes and uncover repressed feelings and thoughts. The therapist places the person in a trance mood and encourages discussion of emotional conflicts. A person who undergoes hypnosis, generally is submissive, abandons control and responds with a high degree of mental and physical suggestibility. It is effective in the treatment of overeating, smoking and other addictive disorders. The hypothesized persons cannot be forced to perform action that conflict with the person's values and beliefs.

REALITY THERAPY (RT)

Reality therapy is an approach to psychotherapy and counseling. It is developed by William Glasser in 1960s. It is considered as a form of cognitive behavior therapy. It focuses on 3Rs realism, responsibility and right and wrong; rather than symptoms of psychiatric illness.

Reality therapy maintains that the individual is suffering from a socially universal human condition rather than a mental illness. It is in the unsuccessful attainment of basic needs that a person's behavior moves away from the norm; since fulfilling essential needs is part of a person's present life. Reality therapy does not concern on client's past or unconscious mental processes.

Reality therapy mainly focuses on the here-and-now action of the client and the ability to create and choose a better future. Usually client seek to discover what they really want and how they are currently choosing, to behave in order to achieve the goals.

Reality therapy is based on the premise that persons who are mentally unhealthy are irresponsible. They cannot meet all of their basic needs and they refuse to face reality. Responsibility either was never learned or was abandoned at some point in life. The therapist helps the person to overcome denial of the real world and meet needs by assuming responsibility for action. This is done as the therapist becomes involved in an active relationship with the client, rejects unrealistic behavior displayed by the client, and teaches the client better ways to meet needs in the real world. It stresses on present state because the past cannot be changed. It also forces the client to make value judgments by facing issues of right and wrong, and by assuming responsibility for action.

SUPPORTIVE PSYCHOTHERAPY

Supportive psychotherapy is used primarily to reinforce a patient's ability to cope with stressor through a number of key activities, including attentively listening and encouraging expression of thought and feelings; assisting the individual to gain a greater understanding of their situation and alternatives. Helping to boost the individual's self esteem and resilience; and working to instill a sense of hope. It may be provided short term as well as long term depending on the individual and the specific set of circumstances.

Supportive psychotherapy is best suited for people who are trying to cope with an acute crisis or for those where attempting to promote fundamental changes may be more disruptive than useful to the person.

It is also used to handle conscious conflicts or current problems. The therapist utilizes techniques such as reassurance, unburdening, environmental modification, persuasion and classification. Reassurance helps the patients to regain self-confidence and decrease feelings of fear and anxiety. Psychological reassurance occurs, for example when parents are told it is normal to experience occasional feelings of hostility and aggression towards one's children.

Through supportive psychotherapy, clinicians help client learn how to move forward and make decision or changes that may be necessary to adapt either to an acute change such as the loss of a loved one or severe disappointment or to a chronic situation, such as an ongoing illness, for example recurrent depressive episodes. Before this it can be accomplished that client needs to be given the opportunity to express their feelings and thought about the issues, and this is an important part of supportive psychotherapy.

In this form of therapy, a trusting relationship between the client and the therapist is an integral to the client's healing or progress. It is important that the individual has confidence that the therapist can understand their feeling of despair or anger yet still maintain a belief in their ability to recover.

The therapist must also help the patient to understand the difference between recovering and gaining back what has been lost. In many cases, re-establishing the past or prior pattern of life if not possible, and the client will need to come to terms with the changes that need to be made.

The main techniques used are reassurance, unburdening, environmental modification, persuasion and classification. Reassurance helps the client to regain self confidence and decrease feelings of fear and anxiety.

Another technique involves ventilation. Ventilating one's feelings through conscious free expression is referred to as unburdening. Two purposes are served by unburdening, intense and revealing oneself, resulting in a form of self punishment.

Environmental modification or manipulation is done to relieve a client's symptoms and distress. Advising a young mother to hire a babysitter, so that she can have time to herself, planning a child in a hostel because of a poor interpersonal relationship with the parents, who are undergoing a divorce or suggesting that a middle aged man take a vacation to overcome feeling of prolonged or unresolved grief are examples of environmental modification or manipulation.

Persuasion is used to give direct suggestions to influence behavior and may include an elements of environment modification. For example, A teenager who smokes and drink excessively when feeling stressed is told to try jogging, swimming or other physical exercise to release tension, anxiety or frustration.

Clarification is a process by which the therapist helps the client to gain a clearer picture of reality by understanding feelings and behavior. Explaining to a man with alcoholism that his illness is a result of a poor self image or to a woman that she needs to be hospitalized because of self destructive behavior are both examples of clarification of reality.

For some people, supportive psychotherapy can lead to improvements in adaptation, interpersonal functioning, emotional stability, resilence, coping and self esteem. It, this form of therapy, is often most useful in supporting patients through a period of crisis but can also be effective in achieving gains over the long term with regard to chronic situation.

BEHAVIOR THERAPY

Behaviorism looks psychological disorders as the result of maladaptive learning as people are born with tabula rasa (a blank state). They do not assume that sets of behaviorism assumes that all behavior is learnt from the environment and symptoms are acquired through classical conditioning and operant conditioning.

According to American Psychiatric Association (1980), behavior therapy is a mode of treatment that focuses on modifying observable and at least in principle, quantifiable behavior by means of systematic manipulation of the environment and behavioral variables thought to be functionally related to the behavior. It aims to eliminate symptoms such as behavior tantrums or bedwetting or to develop desirable behavior. Behaviorirst believe that problem behaviors are learned and therefore can be eliminated or replaced by desirable behaviors through new learning experiences.

Rowe (1989) lists the following general principles of behavior therapy.

- Faulty learning can result in psychiatric disorders.
- Behavior is modified through the application of principles of learning.
- Maladaptive behavior is considered to be excessive or deficient; thus, behavior therapy seeks to promote appropriate behavior and decrease or eliminate the frequency, duration or place of occurrence of inappropriate behavior.
- One's social environment is a source of stimuli that support symptoms. Therefore, it also can support changes in behavior through appropriate treatment measures.
  - Behavior techniques include behavior modification systematic desensitization, aversion therapy, cognitive behavior therapy, assertiveness impulsive therapy and limit setting.

Behavior Modification and Systematic Desensitization

Classically two theories of learning used in behavior modification. Pavlov's theory of conditioning, which states that a stimulus elicits a response (seeing apple stimulates salivary glands) and Skinner's operant conditioning theory which states that the result of a person's behavior determine whether the behavior will recur in the future (a child is given a slap when he breaks a dish). In operant conditioning, good behavior is rewarded with physical reinforcers (food) or social reinforcers (approval, appreciation, token of exchange) and these reinforcers are withheld if maladaptive behavior positive or good behavior, bringing about a change in attitudes and feelings. Operant conditioning has been successful in teaching language to autistic children, teaching ADL and social skills to cognitively disabled children and adults and teaching social skills to regressed psychotic clients.

Systematic densensitization is a type of behavioral therapy works on the principle of classical conditioning. This therapy aims to remove the fear, anxiety or a phobia and substitute a relaxation response to the conditional stimulus gradually using counter conditioning.

This is done by forming a hierarchy of fear, involving the conditional stimulus (e.g. A spider, /dog) that are ranked from least fearful to most fearful. The client works with the their way up starting at the least unpleasant and practicing their relaxation techniques as they go. When they feel comfortable with this, they move on to the next stage in the hierarchy.

Thus, for example, a spider phobic might regard one small stationary spider 5 meter away as only modestly threatening but a large, rapidly moving spider 1 meter away as highly threatening. The client reaches a state of deep relaxation and is then asked to imagine (or is confronted by) this situation until it fails to evoke any anxiety at all indicating that the therapy has been successful. This process is repeated while working through all of the situation in the anxiety hierarchy until the most anxiety provoking event occurs. The client is also given training in relaxation techniques, e.g. Control over breathing muscle, detensioning.

The number of sessions required depends on the severity of the phobia. Usually 4–6 session up to 12 for a severe phobia. The therapy is complete once the agreed therapeutic goals are met.

AVERSION THERAPY

Aversion therapy is a form of treatment that utilizes behavioral principles to eliminate unwanted behavior. In this therapeutic method, the unwanted stimulus is repeatedly paired with discomfort. The goal of the conditioning process is to make the individual associate the stimulus with unpleasant or uncomfortable sensation.

During aversion therapy, the client may be asked to think of or engage in the behavior they enjoy while at the same time being exposed to something unpleasant such as a bad task, a foul smell or even mild electric shocks. Once the unpleasant feelings become associated with the behavior, the hope is that the unwanted behavior or action will begin to decrease in frequency or stop entirely.

Uses of Aversion Therapy

- Bad habit
- Addictions
- Alcoholism
- Smoking
- Gambling
- Violence or anger issues
  - The overall effectiveness of aversion therapy can depend upon a number of factors including the methods used and whether or nor the client continues to practice relapse prevention after treatment is concluded. In some instance, the client may return to previous pattern of behavior once they are out of treatment and no longer exposed to the deterrent. Consider ethical parameters while using this method.

COGNITIVE BEHAVIOR THERAPY

Cognitive behavior therapy (CBT) is a form of treatment that focuses on examining the relationships between thought feeling and behavior. By exploring patterns of thinking that lead to self destructive action and the belief that direct those thoughts. People with mental illness can modify their thoughts and the client will actively work together to help the patient recover from their mental illness. People who seek CBT can expert their therapist to be problem focused, and goal directed in addressing the challenging symptoms of mental illness. Because CBT is an active intervention, one can also expert to do homework or practice outside of sessions.

Uses of CBT

CBT is used to treat a range of psychological problems including:
- Anxiety
- Anxiety disorders such as social phobia, OCD, PTSD.
- Depressive disorder
- Uncontrollable anger
- Irrational fears
- Hypochondriasis
- Substance abuse like smoking/alcohol and other drug abuse
- Gambling
- Eating disorders
- Insomnia
- Marital problems
- Emotional or behavioral problems in children.
- Sexual disorders.

The Interaction of Thought, Feeling and Behavior

- The main focus is that thought, feelings and behavior combine to influence a person's quality of life. For example, severe shyness in social circle. Phobia may come from the person thinking that other people will always find them boring or stupid. This belief causes the person to feel extremely anxious in social situation. This behavior may include stammering, sweating and other uncomfortable symptoms. The person then feels overwhelmed with negative emotions (such as shame) and negative self talk (I am such a idiot), their fear of social situation may become work with every bad experience.
- CBT aims to teach people that it is possible to have control over their thoughts, feelings and behavior. CBT helps the person to challenge and overcome automatic belief and use practical strategies to change or modify their behavior. The result is more positive feelings, which in turn lead to more positive thoughts and behavior.

Assertiveness Training

Assertiveness is a particular mode of communication. Joseph Wolpe in 1958 coined the term behavior therapy. Wolpe's belief was that a person could not be both assertive and anxious at the same time and thus being assertive would inhibit anxiety.

Goals of Assertive Training

- Increase awareness of personal rights.
- Differentiation between nonassertiveness and assertiveness.
- Differentiation between passive aggressiveness and aggressiveness.
- Learning both verbal and nonverbal assertiveness skills.
  - During assertiveness training, clients are taught how to relate appropriately to others using open, frank, honest and direct expressions whether these are positive or negative in nature. In other words, one voices opinions openly and honestly without feeling guilty. One is encouraged not to be afraid to show an appropriate response, negative or positive,

to an idea or suggestion. Many people are unable to say how they feel and hold back their feelings. They may show inconsiderate aggression and disrespect for the rights of others. Assertive training teaches one to ask for what is wanted, take a position on various issues, and initiate specific action to obtain what one wants while respecting the rights of other. This training is beneficial to mentally healthy and unhealthy or for both persons.

IMPLOSIVE/FLOODING

The nongradual extinction approach flooding consists of rapidly exposing the client to the conditioned stimulus, while minimizing the client to escape from the conditioned stimulus. It is also called as response prevention. In practice, it is almost opposite of systemic desensitization. Persons are exposed to intense forms of anxiety producers either an imagination or real life. Such flooding is continued until the stimulant no longer produce disabling anxiety. It is used in the treatment of phobia, obsessive compulsive neurosis, and problems causing maladaptive anxiety as well as to other therapies.

IMPLOSIVE THERAPY

A variation of flooding was developed by Stample and Levis in 1967. It is impulsive therapy or implosion. Implosive therapy is flooding with these characteristics.

- All presentation of anxiety situations are done by hearing or client to imagine the scene.
- The imagined scenes are often ones of exaggerated or impossible situation designed to elicit as much anxiety as possible.
- The scenes are often based on hypothesized sources of anxiety, some of which are psychodynamic in nature. These hypothesized sources of anxiety center around such things as hostility toward parental figures, rejection sex, and dynamic concepts where oedipal complex and death wishes.
  - This treatment usually consists of first having the client to imagine an anxiety producing scene and realize that although unpleasant, the anxiety is not unbearable. Then the client is given a sequence of high anxiety scenes to imagine, often in order of increasing anxiety, hence a hierarchy to some extent. This treatment, generally accompanied by strong emotional reactions of the client, is continued over a few treatment sessions until the anxiety is assessed to have extinguished.

Limit Setting

Limit setting is an important aspect of the therapeutic milieu. Limits reduce anxiety, minimize manipulation, provide a framework for the client to function and enable the client to learn to make request. Naturally the client learns to control his or her own behavior. The first step in limit setting is to give advance warning of the limit and the consequences that will follow if the client does not adhere to the limits. Choices should be given whenever possible. This allows the client a chance to participle in the limit setting. For example, a 18 year old substance abuse client is informed that he is to keep his room orderly practice good personal keep like this hygiene and attend therapy sessions twice in a week. If he does not follow these regulations he is to loose one or more of his privileges. He will be allowed to state his feelings about the limits and to decide which of his privileges will be discontinued temporarily.

The consequence of limit setting should neither provide a secondary gain (e.g. Individual attention) nor lower self esteem. The consequences should occur immediately after the client has exceeded the limit. Consistency must occur with all personnel on all shifts acting to contribute to a person's security and to convey to the client that someone cares.

MANAGEMENT THERAPY

Other therapies like occupational, educational, art, music and recreational activities all have psychotherapeutic values and are called management therapy.

Occupational therapy uses purposeful activities as a way of meeting a person's needs and provides for personal change and growth. Creative media such as clay moulding, wood burning, painting, gardening or housekeeping are used to express creative needs or feelings and conflicts that a person is unable to express verbally. Activities such as bakery items preparation, wearing or standing, candle making provide outlets for the release of anger and negative emotions as well as thought, hostility and frustration. The occupational therapist also may focus on activities that improve living life style skills, such as grocery shopping, cooking and self-care activities.

FAMILY THERAPY

Family therapy focuses on relationships within the family unit and takes place with other family members present. It is used as the main treatment modality or it could be used as a supplement to other therapies.

Virginia Satir, Salvadoe Minuchin, Murray Bowen and Milton Erickson are few theorists who have contributed to family therapy.

Family therapy is a technique that employs a psychotherapeutic approach in helping family members to gain insight into their problems and change behavior and emotions from dysfunctional to healthy relationship. Using this method, the family can perform the basic functions necessary for the well being of all its members. Therapy is indicated when the family does not perform its basic functions adequately. The therapist views the family as the client and looks at the family members in relationship to the individual client therapist also encourage family involvement in the treatment of family members.

Family therapy differs from individual therapy. However, in the former it is assumed that outside or external influences play a major role in personality development and the regulation of members lives. Individual therapy, however, is believed that internal or intrapsychic thoughts, feelings and conflicts are the major components of personality developments.

In family therapy the family is seen as a whole system rather than just the sum of its individual members. As with individual and group therapy, family therapy is used to approach a wide variety of therapeutic goals. Rather than viewing problems as owned and caused by a particular family member. It helps to identify the ways that relationship and individual problems are caused and maintained by the family dynamics. For example, if a child is having academic and social problems the focus will be on identifying the family pattern that have contributed to the child acting out, rather than on wording intrapsychically with the child none.

Changes in families occur during family therapy because of the individual's desire to confirm to the groups or family, as problems are worded through by the family the individual member's become aware of their mutual problems of specific areas that are deviated and of the family member needs each individual member role should become clear. Thus, it helps to maintain healthy relation mutually with each other.

DIFFERENT APPROACHES TO FAMILY THERAPY

Jones (1980) describes seven approaches to family therapy.
These are briefed as follows:

Integrative Approach

- Nathan Ackerman considered to be the grandfather of family therapy, uses an integrative approach. To varying degrees, he rejected the view of the family as a system, his focus was on family values. Ackerman believed in interlocking pathology, which occurs when an individuals are locked into a neurotic interaction.
- Therapists using the integrative approach consider the interactions between the person and her or his social environment. The family needs to share concern for each member welfare. A problem arises if there is too much fluidity or rigidity of family role relationship. These relationships are analyzed so that therapy focuses on the family dynamics of illness.

Psychoanalytic Approach

- Therapists using the psychoanalytic approach base many of their views on Sigmund Freud's theory, believing that family members are affected by each member's psychological make up. Individual behaviors are regulated by the family's feedback system. Problems arise from this feedback system when there is an internalization process or introjections of prenatal figures. This occurs from an unconscious incorporation of another's personality into one's own.
- Psychoanalytic therapy is intensive in nature over a long period of time and focuses on cognitive, affective and behavioral components of family interaction. The goal is to guide the family member to exhibit pathology into a restructuring change in their personality.

Bowen Approach

- Murray Bowen's approach to family therapy viewed the family as consisting of emotional and relationship system. He believed an individual's behavior is a response to the behavior of another person. The intellect is not autonomous but is responsive to others feelings and logical reasoning is impaired. Bowen states that pathology develops if a family member is dominated by the feelings of those around him or her, and boundaries of self are not clearly differentiated from the family system. Thus, relationship with other can cause emotional disturbance in the individuals.
- Therapy is based on therapeutic techniques that are teachable and is graded toward helping the person to differentiate between feelings and thinking. Bowen believed that appropriate responses could be taught. The goal is to help each member not to be dominated by the feelings of others but to active a better differentiation of self.

Structural Approach

- According to Salvador Minuchin, view the family as a system of individuals. The family develops a set of invisible rules and laws that evolve over a period of time and are understood by all family members.
- A hierarchical system or structure develops within the family. The problems arise if family boundaries become enmeshed or disengaged. Problems in families also arise due to poor coping towards changes.

- The structural therapist observes the activities and function of family member. Therapy is short term and action oriented. It is geared toward changing the family organization and its social context. A holistic view of the family is developed focusing upon influence that family members have on one another. Guidance is given towards developing clear boundaries for individual members and towards changing the families structural pattern.

Interactional or Strategic Approach

- The interactional or strategic approach uses communication theory and was pioneered by Virginia Satir and Jay Haley. The therapist studies the interactions between and among family members, recognizing that engage in one family member occurs in relation to change in another family member. Family members develop a calibration and feedback system so that homeostasis or equilibrium may be maintained. Interactionists agree with structuralism that a set of invisible laws emerge in the family relationship and problem arises if these rules are very vague and ambiguous. When power struggles develop within a family, strategies employed to control the situation may provide symptoms. These symptoms are interpersonal with at least one family member contributing to the dysfunction of another.
- This therapy is based on the concept of homeostasis. According to this concept, as one member gains insight and becomes better, another family member may become worse. Communication is considered the basis for all behaviors. Therapy deals with the interpersonal relationship among all family members and focuses on why the family is in therapy and what changes each member expects. The family thus helps to set goals for the treatment approach.

Social Network or Systemic Approach

- Many modern therapists believe that the family operates as a social network. They believe that healing comes from social relationship, problem ensured from family illness or change a system approach is utilized but is not clearly defined. The growth model is used to understand emotional difficulties that arise during different stages of developments.
- This therapy emphasizes the natural healing powers of the family. It involves bringing several people together as a social network. For the first few meetings, this may encompass people who are outside of the family but have similar ideals and goals. Family members are helped to set goals for optimal outcomes or solving of problem.

Behaviorist Approach

- The behaviorist believe that the family is a system of interlocking behavior, that one type of behavior will cause another. They deny internal motivation forces but believe individual react to external factors and influences. The individual's certain response to other individual. Behavior is learned and reinforced by family members, who respond either positively or negatively and sometimes a peculiar behavior is exhibited to gain attention.
- Therapy includes interpreting family member's behavior but not necessarily changing it, although change may be brought about by restricting and reframing the interpersonal environments. Thus, therapy is based on an awareness process as well as on behavioral change. Therapeutic approaches using principles of learning theory are taught. This is an

effort to bring about change, positive reinforcement is given for desired behavior. Approaches are direct and clearly stated. The full family is involved in goal setting for desired outcomes, and a contract may be established for this cause.

GOALS OF FAMILY THERAPY

- When meeting with a family or identified client in a family, it is important for the therapist to assess the family problems and goals may need to be modified according to the family values system. The therapist needs to have insight into his/her own value system so as not to influence the direction of treatment. What the family identifies as problems may not be what the therapist identifies as problems owing to differences in values, culture and socio-economic class. The therapist needs to remember to work on the problems the family identifies, or to explain to the dysfunctional family why, the therapist sees the problems differently change the family not the therapist, should provide the information for and determine the direction of charge when goals are being set. Each family member should state his or her goals and the outcomes expected from the therapy if the therapist and family are from similar backgrounds. The problem identification and the methods of resolving them tend to be more similar.
- A major goal of family therapy is to facilitate positive changes in the family. The other goals include fostering open communication of thoughts and feelings and promoting optimal functioning in interdependent roles. The therapist needs to assess the various roles each family member fulfills and determine if these roles are rigid or inflexible. In addition to these, the therapist needs to function as a role model and demonstrate how to deal with conflict. Developing contracts for the family members may be useful in goal setting (e.g. Keeping a room clean, having fewer fights, paying more attention to others needs.
- Initially, the therapist determines which family members need to participate or continue in family therapy and how the problems of the identified interlock with the relationships of other family members. His interlocking relationship may need to be modified finally, the therapist helps family member with a realistic view of their relationship with one another and the overall effect of their behavior on each other.

STAGES OF FAMILY THERAPY

There are three main stages of family therapy. These are the initial interview, working phase/ intervention phase and the termination phase.

The Initial Interview

- Initial phase, usually a family therapist is contacted by the identified patient or by another or significant family member. He /she express concern to setup an appointment for an initial interview with the family. Most therapist's ask all family members to be present at the family sessions. The information collected earlier period can be useful in forthcoming sessions. During initial period, therapist gather information about family in general, dynamics family history and present functioning.
- If a certain family member is reluctant to come to for the initial interview, it may be helpful if the therapist states the rationale for seeing all family member at that time. For example, the

therapist could state that the problem affects all member of the family and that is important to attend. The therapist can explain that therapy will not be effective without that member's attendance and active participation.

The Intervention/Working Phase

The goal of the working phase is to help the family accept and adjust to change. During this phase the therapist needs to identify the strengths and problems of the family. According to Otto, he identified 12 family strengths. The therapist should determine which of these strengths are present in the family seeking help.

- The ability to provide for the physical, emotional and spiritual needs of each family member.
- The ability to be sensitive to the needs of family members.
- The ability to communicate feelings, emotions, beliefs and values effectively.
- The ability to provide support, security and encouragement to enhance creativity and independence.
- The ability to initiate and maintain growth producing relationship within or without the family system.
- The capacity to maintain and create constructive and responsible community relationship in the neighborhood, school, town, local and state governments.
- The ability to grow with and through children.
- The ability for self help and the ability to accept help when appropriate.
- The ability to perform family roles flexibly.
- The ability to show mutual respect for the individual and independence of each family member.
- The ability to use a crisis as a unearn of growth.
- The ability to have a concern for family unity and laxity and for cooperation among family members.

During this second phase, families do a lot of working and the therapist participates in the therapeutic process. Usually family sessions occur once a week for one hour. Some family member may be motivated to participate in order to help the identified client. Other member may be reluctant to participate owing to fears of having family secrets revealed. It would be unusual if all family member were willing and eager to participate in family therapy sessions. The therapist can ask all members, their view of the problem; what they would like to see changed and their thought and feelings about other members of the family. Through this technique the therapist can learn a great deal about the problems and conflicts that are occurring in the family system.

Soon the family members will be able to recognize that the therapist's role is to offer suggestions and guidance. The therapist will not assume the role of a parent, child or arbitrator. The therapist will facilitate open, honest communication among family members. Learning appropriate methods of expressing themselves if there has been anger out burt's, hostility or very little communication. Also, some secssions particularly pose dealing with conflicts and altercations may make family members feel uncomfortable. As therapy continues, family members will begin to realize that relationships can change. They will recognize that roles do not have to be fixed and rigid; they may change as personal growth occurs within the family member will become more autonomous. If the sessions are helpful and changes occur in the family, understanding and insight may be the cause. Increased understanding occurs after a long sessions.

Termination Phase

If the family has achieved the goals and the identified specific problems have been resolved, then it is time to initiate the termination phase. However, the therapist should remember that no family terminates therapy without some reason or problem. Also, some family members may be somewhat reluctant terminate the sessions, nevertheless, termination should take place. By the time, the family has learned how to solve its own problems in a healthy manner, has developed its own internal support system and has learned to communicate in an open, honest and direct manner. Power has been appropriately assigned and redistributed; and family members are able to work out and resole problems at home without the therapist's interventions.

NURSES ROLE IN FAMILY THERAPY

Higher educated psychiatric nurse practitioner can serve as a family therapist. Involving the full family when one is ill is mandatory to solve the problem during the initial assessment, whether for medical or emotional illnesses, nurses obtain information about the client's family members, including grandparents, aunts and uncles. Nurses include family members in health education and teaching family assessment, participating in family teaching and education and also providing family therapy are the main roles of psychiatric nurse.

One assessment tool that nurse can utilize in determining the family constellation of members is a genogram, a diagram of family members usually over three generations. The genogram is simple to use and can convey a great deal of information about the family.

In a genogram the names of family members are placed on horizontal lines to indicate separate generations. Any children are denoted by vertical lines. The children are ranked from oldest to youngest, going from left to right. The symbols used to depict each individual family members are usually squares for males and circles for females. Inside the square or circle is the family member name and age. Outside of the symbols pertinent information can be written, such as depressed, alcoholic, cancer, hypertension and so on. Other symbols can be used to denote marriage, death, adoption, divorce, separation, miscarriage, abortion or twins. A basic genogram is shown is Figure 5.1.

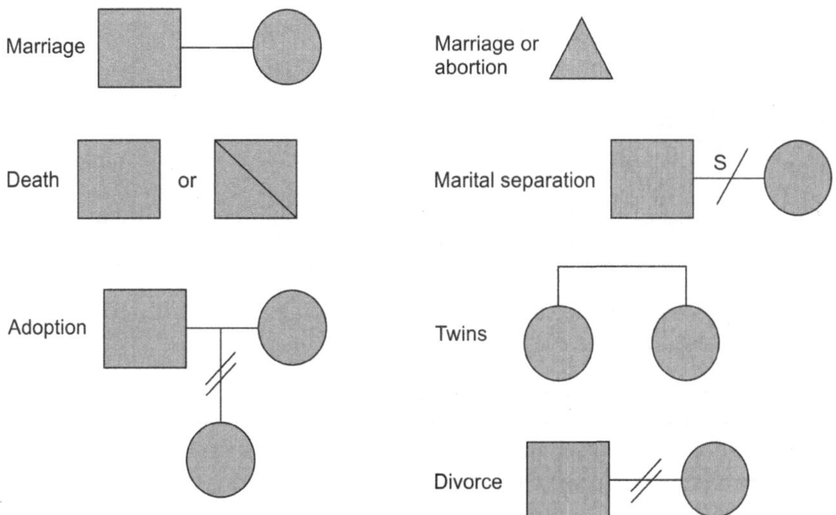

Fig. 5.1: Basic genogram

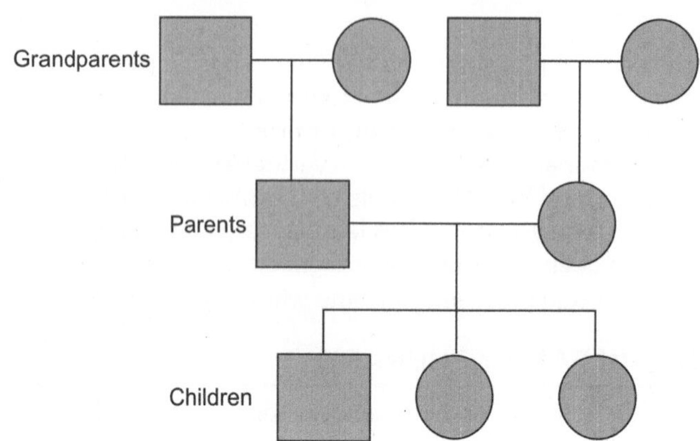

Fig. 5.2: Genogram

From the Figure 5.2 a lot of information can be gathered. A family is often interested in doing a genogram because it gives them a diagram of family relationship including significant information. The genogram is useful in teaching the family members about family system. It is important for family members to begin to understand the role(s) they fill and how their roles influence the family system. Once they realize that roles are learned and that they have the choice of altering their roles, change can occur. At that point, the family can begin to work on its own. The common nursing diagnoses include the following.

Nursing diagnoses are utilized to identify functional characteristics of facilities.

According to Carenito (1992), three nursing diagnoses are specific to families:

- Ineffective compromised family coping refers to inadequate comfort, assistance or encouragement provided by the primary support person to an individual experiencing a need or health challenge.
- Ineffective disabling family coping. It describes a family with a history of overt or covert destructive behavior.
- Altered family processes describes change within the family due to a stressor that has altered individual responses.

GROUP THERAPY

Introduction

Group therapy is a type of psychotherapy that involves one or more therapist working with several people at the same time. This type of therapy is widely available at a variety of location, including private therapeutic practices, nursing homes, clinics, community health center. Group therapy is sometimes used alone, but it is also commonly integrated into a comprehensive treatment plan that also includes individual therapy and medication.

DEFINITION OF GROUP THERAPY

Nudelman (1986) defines group therapy as 'an identifiable system comprised of at least three people who share a common goal'. Nudelman explains that group therapy helps members be knowledgeable about their goals and work toward their achievement. Psychological forces are cooperative in group therapy, and each member is affected by the unique behaviors, personality traits and emotional energy of the others in the group. Sadock (1985) suggests that in group therapy, member gain personal insights, improve there and make necessary alterations, in their personality. Gardner and Lasalle (1987) define group therapy as the treatment of emotional stress and disorder through the means of group method and process. Within their proposed framework, group processes are planned, goal oriented, systematic, and based on sound theoretical theories. Yalom (1985) considered to be one of the leading practitioner in the field of group therapy, believes that therapy group is composed of many forms, with the major emphasis on the importance of the 'here-and-now' experience.

Therapeutic group focuses on the stress and emotional problems that can arise in relation to a physical illness, a developmental crisis or a lack of social complex task of attempting to prevent further emotional control and disturbance. Therapeutic groups usually center on a specific theme and are educational in nature. The leaders of these groups hope to teach members to better cope with the emotional stress that they are experiencing and, if possible, to eliminate the sources of stress.

Gardner and Lasalk (1987) identify the following goals:

- Decreased sense of isolation.
- Promote readjustment to former community involvement and relationship.
- Enhance the skills of problem solving.
  - Some examples therapeutic groups are groups of person with a terminal illness like cancer, groups with birth defects, etc.
  - Adjunctive groups make use of specialized activities such as sensory and perceptual stimulation, socialization, a daily orientation for chronically psychotic client on a short-term hospital inpatient department.

PRINCIPLES/CHARACTERISTICS OF GROUP THERAPY

Group therapy differs most significantly from individual therapy in that it is more effective in treating problems of with interpersonal relationship. It creates a greater opportunity for reality testing and experiencing mutual concern and support. On the other hand, members of groups may feel more vulnerable, frightened and at risk and the transference process may be diluted. Yalon (1985) has identified eleven important characteristics of group therapy.

These are:

- *Instillation of hope:* It is of primary concern. According to White (1987), people participating in the group experience was initially feeling demoralized and helpless and points out that providing them with hope is therefore a most worthwhile achievement. Clients should be encouraged to believe that they can find help and support within the group and that it is realistic to expect that problem will be solved.
- *Universality:* It is the sense of realizing that one is not completely alone in any situation. Group members often identify this factor as a major reason for their seeking group therapy. During the therapy sessions, members are encouraged to express complex and often very negative feelings in the hope that they will experience understanding and support from others with similar thoughts and feelings.
- *The imparting of information:* Includes both indirect and direct advice and refers to the imparting of specific educational information plus the sharing of advice and guidance among members. The transmission of this information also indicated to each member and the others concern and trust.

- *Altruism:* It is the act of giving and taking. Clients have the experience of learning to help others and in the process, they begin to feel better about themselves. Both the group therapist and the member can offer invaluable support, insight and reassurance while allowing themselves to gain self knowledge and growth.
- The corrective recapitulation for the primary family group allows members within the group to correct some of the perceptions and feelings associated with unsatisfactory experiences they have had with their family. The participants receive feedback as they discuss and retrieve early familial conflicts and experience corrective response. Family roles are explored, and members are encouraged to resolve unfinished family business.
- The development of socializing techniques is essential within the group as members are given the opportunity to learn and test new social skills. Persons also receive information about maladaptive social behaviors.
- Imitative behavior refers to the process in which member observe and model their behavior after one another. Imitation is an acknowledged therapeutic force: a healthy by interactive group environment provides valuable opportunities for experimenting with desired changes and behavior.
- *Interpersonal learning:* Includes the gaining of insight, the development of the transference relationship, the experience of correcting emotional thoughts and behavior and the importance of learning about oneself in relation to other.
- Group cohesiveness is the development of a strong sense of group membership and alliance. Ideally each member should feel acceptance and approval from all others within the group. The concept of cohesiveness refers to the degree to which a group function as a supportive problem solving unit. This factors plays an important in ensuring optimal individual and group growth.
- Catharsis, is similar to group cohesiveness, involves members relating to one another through the verbal expression of positive and negative thoughts and feelings.
- Existential factors that are constantly operating within the group make up Yalom's final factor. These intangible issues encourage each group member to accept the motivating idea that he or she is ultimately responsible for his or her own life choices and actions.
  - In 1982, Taylor expands Yalom's theory and states that members of group therapy reflect person in the larger society and that group conditions replicate reality. Within this structure, group participants present their concerns and problem and in turn receive direct feedback and solutions.
  - Sadock (1985) views that the key elements of group includes therapy for various types of member's participation and the skill and expertise of the group leader.

TYPES OF GROUP THERAPY

There are a wide variety of therapy groups that make use of the major theoretical frame works. Lego (1982) classifies all group therapy as either open or closed. Open group do not have specific boundaries; members may join and leave the group at different times. Group cohesion and leadership stability are identified as major elements. Closed groups may have either a set of membership, a specific time frame or both of characteristics. Specific membership may address the needs of a particular kind of client such as a group of female college students who are bulimic or a rehabilitative group. Most closed groups require members to start the group at the same time and then terminate the group after a predetermined length of time. Both open and closed therapy groups are used extensively inpatient and outpatient treatment settings.

According to Marrom, mostly five types of groups for therapy are seen. The five groups are as follows.

- Support groups focus on increasing the member's adaptation, self esteem, and sense of emotional well-being.
- Reeducation and remotivation group often very beneficial for psychiatric clients who are withdrawn or socially isolated. The attempt to increase communication and interaction among members to foster more acceptable and appropriate behaviors.
- Problem solving therapy groups focus on the resolution of specific problems that patients have identified.
- Insight without reconstruction groups have group leader who place their major emphasis on interpersonal communication and work on effecting change by increasing the member's cognitive and emotional understanding of their problem.
- Personality reconstruction groups make use of psychoanalytical theory and encourage the member to explore former relationship and problems and their impact on the present.

Construction and Establishing a Group

- Therapist's personal treatment choice and his or her own philosophies, as well as client needs, determine the selection of group therapy participants. Consideration is given to the desired size of the group (nearly 10 members) diagnosis of member, age, gender, intellectual level, verbal or communication skills, motivation and social skills, during the selection process, a decision to make as to whether the group will be homogeneous or heterogeneous in nature. For example, a group focusing on women's issues such as single parenting may not be therapeutic for teenagers, women in their 70s or male client. On the other hand, a group focusing on loss and grief could be suitable for various age groups either gender and person's married, widowed, single or divorced participants.
- Attention is also laid to the environmental setting, room temperature, lighting, sound, furnishing, privacy, location and seating arrangement are important factors that contribute to an atmosphere conducive to therapeutic group process.

Stages of Group Development

All therapy groups have three major phases:

- A beginning or orientation phase.
- A middle or working phase.
- An ending or termination phase.

During each of three stages, significant issues concerning group growth and development arise and are dealt by the group. The key issues involve dependency and interdependency. In the view of Inckman, the primarily focus is on the completion of a specific task, viewing all interactions among members as related to that task.

According to him, phases of group development are:

- *Forming:* Orientation of members.
- *Storming:* Members are resistant to task and group influence.
- *Norming:* Overcoming of resistance
- *Performing:* Problem-solving stage.

Initially, forming a group is a major task. It involves anxiety and stress among group members. Each member is concerned norm and acceptable behavior are identified. During this stage, there may be frequent testing, minimal disclosure and periods of strange, ackwardness and uncomfortable silence. The major task is for the group to resolve these initial feelings and to achieve a sense of group identification and definition of purpose. The tasks of the leader are to create a supportive and accepting environment to promote unification and to encourage verbalization of feelings.

During the middle phase, the working phase, the group becomes more cohesive and members explore relationship and conflicts. The group begins to express all kinds of feelings, thoughts both positive and negative; and unhealthy behaviors are openly criticized. Throughout this stage, there may still be evidence of continued resistances as increased pressure is placed on members to participate in risk taking. The major tasks for members during the working phase are to develop a sense of reliance on each other, promote trust, to assume a highest sense of responsibility for the group direction and to maintain trust and openness within the group relationships.

The therapist role is to encourage actively the members to explore their conflicts and goals to identify repetitive behaviors and to continually classify the group goals and tasks. During the final stage of group therapy, termination may occur in several different ways, depending upon whether the group is open or closed. As the members prepare to leave, they reflect on the insights and growth that they have made within the group. They share feedback with one another as they experience ambivalence about leaving the group. Most members feel both sadness and optimism as they anticipate the future. They may feel a sense of loss and rejection by the group. Therapist assumes a less active role during the termination phase as he or she helps the members to integrate the changes and to say goodbye. In this time, it is better to conduct exit interview for evaluation of group experience.

The Effectiveness of Group Therapy

Group therapy can be very effective, especially in certain situations. Research studies have shown that group therapy can be an effective treatment choice for depression and traumatic stress.

ADVANTAGES OF GROUP THERAPY

The key advantages of group include:

- Group therapy allows people to receive the support and encouragement of the other members of the group. People participating in the group are able to see that there are others going through the same kind of problem; which can help them feel less alone.
- Group members can serve as role models to others members of the group. By seeing some one who is successfully coping with a problem, other members of the group can view that there is hope and recovery is possible. As each person processes, they can in turn serve as a role model and support figure for others. This can help to foster feelings of success and accomplishment.
- Group therapy is very cost effective. Instead of focusing on just one client at a time, the therapist can devote his or her time to a much larger group of people.
- Group therapy offers a safe heaven. The setting allows people to practice behavior and action within the safety and security of the groups.

- By working in a group, the therapist can see first hand, how each person responds to other people and behavior in social situation. Using this information, the therapist can provide valuable feedback to each client.

ROLE OF THE NURSE

Working with groups nurses are having many multiple opportunities to assume the role of group leader, group therapist or co-therapist, apart from these roles, nurse has the function of task manager and maintenance role. Group task functions are concerned with the more practical issues of leading a group while group maintenance functions focus on less tangible group process.

PLAY THERAPY

Introduction

To understand play therapy, it is necessary to consider how children learn. A child plays his work, the old saying goes, infants first learn about object and people in their environment by touching and exploring. Later in creative play, children reveal their understanding of the world and their relationship to it. Children are unable to verbalize many of their thoughts, feelings, wishes and fears in play therapy, toys become medium of communication between child and therapist. It was first introduced by Virginia Axline in 1947.

Definition

According to Charles Schaefer, in his writing 'the therapeutic power of play' – 'play is a universal in nature'. Children's play has the power not only to facilitate normal child development but also to alleviate abnormal behavior. Play therapy can be defined as an interpersonal process where a trained therapist systematically applies the curative power of play to help clients to resolve their psychological difficulties.

Garry Landreth a play therapist, wrote in his book entitled play therapy : the art of the relationship, 'play is the singular control activity of childhood occurring at all times and in all places'.

Many experts say that play is a child's form of work; others say is the opposite of work. Regardless of how play relates to work, it is the way a child learns to make sense of his or her world, by trying out roles, reenacting important events, practicing nurturing skills, exploring different themes, and pretending to have various experiences all within a safe, nonthreatening environment, the child can build confidence, resolve emotional conflicts and develop one-on-one social skills.

To know the power of play therapy, Charles Schaefer provided the following of therapeutic factors:

- *Overcoming resistance:* Play is the best way to build rapport with a child and establish a therapeutic relationship.
- *Communication:* Play is to the child what verbalization is to the adult. The most natural medium for self expression. Play gives children the chance to enact the thoughts, and feelings which they cannot express in words. It also provides insight into the inner world of the child.
- *Mastery:* A child develops self efficiency by mastering his environment and learning that what he/she does, makes a difference in the world.

- *Creative thinking:* The use of creativity and flexibility helps the child to develop problem solving skills especially pretend play.
- *Catharsis:* Strong emotions can safely be played out without harm to others within the safe environment of the play therapy room.
- *Abreaction:* Children can recreate past events, release appropriate affect and gain mastery over the situation by producing a different outcome.
- *Role play:* Children can try out different behaviors and identities. They can experience what it is like to be a hero one day and a villain the next.
- *Fantasy:* Play facilitates the child's imaginative and creative abilities. Pretending given a child power over the world even when he/she does not have much control in real life.
- *Metaphoric teaching:* This involves myth-making which communicates with the right side of the brain. It provides a means to changing unrealistic expectations.
- *Attachment formation:* Play that involves touch and smiling helps from the natural attachment with a child. It involves shared sensor motor activities and appropriate forms of touch which evoke feelings of intense pleasure and fun in the child.
- *Relationship enhancement:* The therapist should be warm caring and accepting. This is best accomplished when the goal of play is fun rather than achievement.
- *Enjoyment:* The experience of positive affect is uplifting and decrease anxiety, play is free from external demands obligation and serious intent.
- *Mastering developmental fears:* Play incorporates a form of systematic sensitization. The child can be exposed to a fearful situation, and the fearful or anxious feelings that would otherwise accompany that experience are reduced while relaxing and experimenting the pleasure of fun in play.
- *Game play:* Therapeutic broad games provide children with opportunities to practice cooperative play, practice problem solving skills and not have to be concerned with winning or losing.

GOALS OF PLAY THERAPY

The important goals of play therapy includes the following:

- To boost self-acceptance, self-confidence and self-reliance.
- Facilitate learning about self and others.
- Explore and express feelings and thoughts.
- Encourage ability to make good decision.
- Arrange opportunities to practice control and responsibility.
- Explore alternative views of problems and relationship.
- Learn and practice problem solving and relationship skills.
- Increase feelings, vocabulary and emotional concepts.

These goals can be achieved in either a directive or non directive approach to play therapy.

A non-directive approach focuses on letting the child to determine what activities he or she likes to engage, and works with the assumption that the child will eventually breach the subject of his trauma and work enough in his therapy.

Virgina Axline (1947) outlined some important elements of non-directive play therapy.

- To provide a warm, friendly environment.
- Accepting, permissive relationship.
- Responsive with reflection of feelings.

- Structured time boundaries.
- Safe physical and eye contact allowed.
- Emphasize child as independent and responsible for action.

A directive approach encompasses the above elements while simply giving more direction, setting goals with the child and actively promoting exposure to the trauma. Some techniques may involve asking the child to take on different roles in the play of his trauma, asking directive question about what the different figures mean, asking 'what would happen if........', asking child to differentiate between past and present, videotaping the play, observing it together and discussing on it.

STAGES IN PLAY THERAPY

There are three identifiable stages in play therapy which will guide the therapist for interventions.

- *Safety stage:* In this stages, child is learning to trust and feel safe with the therapist and in the therapy environment using active intervention. During this phase will it not only be effective at exposure but may serve to retraumatize the child. Simply focus on therapeutic relationship at this point. This stage may last from a few weeks to a few months.
- *Trauma processing:* The child begins to express some of the elements of his trauma through play. This marks that the child is using his play to work through the trauma.
- *Reconnection:* The child has worked on mattering his past experiences and is now faced with the future and how he/she will react to individual in the environment.

Categories of Play

Categories of play are not mutually exclusive; different forms or categories of play may overlap. Having choices is important since an action that appears to one child may be of no interest to another, and the child's interest is likely to change through the play period. An understanding of play in many forms can help parents to understand its importance for children of all ages. Some specific categories of play are as follows:

- *Physical play:* When children run, jump and play games such as chase, hide and seek, tag and engage in physical play. This play has a social nature because it involves other children. It also provides exercise, which is essential for normal growth and development.
- *Expressive play:* Certain forms of play gives children, opportunities to express feelings by engaging with material. Material used in expressive play include temporary paints, fingerprints, water color, crayons, colored pencils and markers, drawing paper, clay, water, sponges, beanbags, pounding benches, punching bags, rhythm instruments, sharing cream, pudding and gelatin.
- *Manipulative play:* Children control or master their environment through manipulative play. They manipulate the environment and other people as much as possible. Manipulative play starts during infancy. Infants play with their parents, for example, they drop a toy, wait for the parent to pick it up, clean and return it, and then they drop it again. This interaction brings the infant and parent/therapist together in a game that children move objects such as puzzle piece and gadget to better understand how they work.
- *Symbolic play:* Certain games can symbolically express a child's problems. Because there are no rules in symbolic play, the child can use this play to reinforce, learn about and imaginatively alter painful experiences. The child who is from abusive family may pretend

to be a mother who loves and cradles her child rather than one who verbally or physically abuse her child, or in this play this same child might act out abusive experience by letting or screaming at a doll that symbolizes the child. Parents can be surprised by their child's perception of family issues. Children mimic their parent in certain ways; in other games they may pretend that they are the heroes as they read about in books or see television. At certain development, symbolic play may be used by children to cope with fear of separation when they go to school or hospital.

- *Dramatic play:* Children act out situation as they suspect what used to happen to thereon, that are useful to them or that they have witnessed. Dramatic play can be either spontaneous or guided and may be therapeutic for children in the hospital.
- *Familiarization play:* Children handle material and explore experiences in reassuring, enjoyable ways. It prepares children for potentially fearful and painful experiences such as surgery or parental separation.
- *Games:* Some video and computer card games, are played by one child alone, games with rules are rarely played by children younger than four years of age. Board games, card games and sports once enjoyed typically by school age children. In these games children learn to play by the rules and to take turns. Older children enjoy games with specific rules. However younger children tend to like games that allow them to change the rules.
- *Surrogate play:* For children who are too ill or incapacitated to play, another child or a parent may serve as surrogate. Watching the surrogate who plays on behalf of the sick child is stimulating to the sick child. When parents engage in expressive art by painting or redecorating a room while the physically challenged child watching which this stimulates the child.

FUNCTIONS OF PLAY

Play reinforces the child's growth and development. Some of the more common function of play are to facilitate physical, emotional, cognitive, social and moral development.

PHYSICAL DEVELOPMENT

Play aides in developing both fine and gross motor skills. Children repeat certain body movements purely for pleasure and these movements develop body control, e.g. an infant will first hit at a toy, then will try to grasp it and eventually will be able to pick it up. Next, the infant will shake the rattle or perhaps bring it to the mouth. In these ways, the infant moves from simple to more complex gestures.

EMOTIONAL DEVELOPMENT

Children who are anxious may be helped by role playing. Role playing is a way of coping with emotional conflicts. Children may escape through play into a fantasy world in order to make sense out of the real one. Also, a child's self awareness deepens as he/she explores an event through role playing or symbolic play.

When a parent or sibling plays a board game with a child, shares a bike ride, plays baseball or reads a story, the child learns self-importance. The child's self esteem gets a boost. Parents send positive message to their child when they communicate pleasure in providing him or her with daily care. From these early interactions, children develop a vision of the world and gain a sense of their place in it.

COGNITIVE DEVELOPMENT

- Children gain knowledge through their play. They exercise their abilities to think, remember and solve problems. They develop cognitively as they have a chance to test their belief about the world.
- Children increase their problem solving abilities through games and puzzles. Children involved in make-believe play can stimulate several types of learning. Language is strengthened as the children model, others and organize their thoughts to communicate. Children playing house create elaborate narratives concerning their roles and the nature of daily living.
- Children also increase their understanding of size, shape and texture through play. They begin to understand relationships as they try out to put a sequence-object in a round opening or a large object in a small space. Books, videos and educational toys that show pictures and matching words also increase a child's vocabulary while increasing the child's concept of the world.

PHASES OF PLAY THERAPY

- *Introductory phase:* The first task of the therapist is to gain child's trust. This may happen in 5 minutes to 5 months, depending on the personality and prior experience of the child. Until trust has been firmly established and the child is able to reveal inner thoughts and feelings, it is difficult to accomplish other goals.
- *Honeymoon phase:* Children, like adults in therapy, usually go though a honeymoon period. When the relief from finally being able to express some of their anxieties is so great that their demeanor at home and school improves dramatically.
- *Rebellious phase:* At this point, the child often voices strong anger about having to attend therapy sessions. Usually the child is voicing strong anger about almost everything else as well, and parents begin to wonder whether therapy is constructive or destructive endeavor. This sudden rebellion, the constant venting of anger is actually a positive sign. It indicates that a repressed feeling that has resulted in much anxiety or depression is beginning to surface. In the therapy, the child is encouraged to express feelings and temper tantrums are mostly seen by children.
- *Working phase:* Becoming aware of what one is feeling, learning more productive method of expressing feelings, and developing healthier defense are some of the tasks achieved in this phase. Occasionally the behavior may actually deteriorate or symptoms may intensify. Such period is relatively shot lived. Such regressive episode may indicate that old defense is weakening.
  - The old defense that served to ward off feeling of insecurity is no longer operative. While this may increase the child's distress, it provides an opportunity for an examination of the underlying feelings of worthlessness, the child has harbored all along, so the heathier defense against threats to his self confidence can be developed.
- *Termination phase:* The longer and more intense the sessions, the more difficult to terminate the therapy. Many of the child's original symptoms do reappear. This is due to stress caused by the termination, it may be the child way of convincing everyone that the therapy is still needed. If proper time is not allowed to work through the emotions generated by separation, therapeutic gains may not be maintained.

- The therapist must help the parents to be as realistic as possible in setting goals for the child. At the end, the therapy is like an education, the conditions for learning are provided but it is up to the child to accept or reject the available possibilities for growth and change.

Advantages of Play Therapy

The play therapy, specially non-directive play therapy offers the child an opportunity to experience growth under the most favorable conditions. Because play is the child's natural medium for self expression. He/she uses the therapy time to play out her/his accumulated feelings of fear, tension, frustration and aggression.

When the child plays out his feelings he/she allows them to surface, faces them and learns to control, accepts and abandon them. Through this process, the child gradually relates that he/she is an individual in his/her right and is capable of thinking and making decision for him or her.

MUSIC THERAPY

Music is a moral law. It gives soul to the universe, wings to the mind, flight to the imagination, a charm to sadness gaiety and life to everything. It is the essence of order and leads to all that is good and beautiful.

History of Music Therapy

Music has been used as a healing force for centuries. Music therapy goes back to Biblical times, when David played the harp to rid King Saul of a bad spirit. As early as 400 BC, Hippocrates, Greek-father of medicine, played music for his mental patients. Aristotle described music as a force that purified the emotions. In the 19th century, Arab hospital contained music rooms for the benefit of the patients. In USA, American medicine men often employed chants and dances as a method of healing for patients. Music therapy, knows to begin in the after math of World War I and II. Musicians would travel to hospitals, particularly in the UK and play music for soldiers suffering from war related emotional and physical trauma patient. Indian musical treatment approaches, the Vedic Hindu chants were used for healing the souls. The newer practice involve the use of archika, gathika and samika to enhance attention and to improve concentration and to help get into meditative and relaxed states. These recitals called proto raga-s one used in mental retardation and in behavioral disorders. Earlier, Indian physicians used nadopasana, raga chikitsa, as treatment modalities in practice.

Definition

The American music therapy association (1981) defines music therapy as an established health care profession that uses music to address physical, emotional, cognitive and social needs of individual of all ages. Music therapy improves the quality of life for person who are well and meets the needs of children and adult with disabilities or illness.

The National Association of Music Therapy has defined music therapy as the therapeutic tool for the restoration, maintenance and improvement of mental and physical health. It is the systemic application of music, as directed by the music therapist in a therapeutic environment to bring about desirable changes in behavior. Such changes enable the individual underlying therapy to experience a greater understanding of himself and the concepts about him, thereby achieving a more appropriate adjustment to the society. Neurologic music therapy is defined as the therapeutic application of music to cognitive, sensory and motor dysfunction due to neurologic diseases of the nervous system. It is based on a neuroscience model of music perception and production and the influence of music on functional changes in nonmusical brain and behavior function.

Goals of Music Therapy

Music therapists work with people of all ages to address limitation in non-musical areas.

- *Communication skills:*
  - To improve expressive language (ability to communicate thoughts/feelings).
  - To improve receptive language (ability to understand).
  - To improve speech and verbal communication.
  - To promote effective use of nonverbal communication.
- *Academic/behavior skills:*
  - To encourage ability to imitate.
  - To improve ability to comprehend written language.
  - To improve ability to count associate numbers with concepts.
  - To improve ability to discriminate colors.
  - To promote reality orientation.
  - To improve memory skills.
  - To increase the task behavior
  - To improve ability to follow direction.
  - To increase participation.
  - To decrease interfering behavior.
  - To promote ability to complete activities of daily living.
- *Motor skills:*
  - To maintain/improve fine motor functioning.
  - To maintain/improve gross motor functioning.
  - To promote identification of body parts.
  - To maintain/reach/grasp/release skills.
  - To improve eye hand coordination.
  - To improve auditory and visual perception.
- *Emotional skills:*
  - To increase verbal/nonverbal expression of feelings.
  - To improve self esteem.
  - To improve impulse control.
  - To increase attention span.
  - To develop coping skills.
  - To decrease stress and anxiety.
  - To facilitate the grieving process.
  - To teach relaxation techniques.
  - To facilitate and exploration of spiritual concern.

- *Social skills:*
  - To improve social interaction with others.
  - To improve appropriate eye contact.
  - To increase ability to touch others appropriately.
  - To increase willingness to be touched by others.
  - To increase ability to share material and equipment with others.
  - To improve ability to make choices and initiate responses.
  - To improve ability to accept praise and give praise to others.
  - To decrease isolation.
  - To improve ability to participate in appropriate play activities.
  - To improve interpersonal skills.
  - To build relationship.
- *Leisure skills:*
- To develop skills to participate in appropriate leisure activities.
- To develop knowledge of available leisure time activities.
- *Other skills:*
  - To decrease pain.
  - To teach pain management skills.
  - To promote independence.
  - To facilitate reminiscence and life review.
  - To develop creativity and sense of identity.

Therapeutic uses of Music

Music stimulates and utilizes many parts of the brain. It captivates and maintain attention.

- Music is an effective motivator.
- Music provides a safe, structured setting for verbal and nonverbal communication.
- Music uses sounds and silence to structure time in an understandable way.
- Music provides both structure and freedom through the use of form and improvisation.
- It provides a meaningful, enjoyable context for repetition.
- Music activities encourage social interaction.
- Music is an effective memory aid.
- Music supports and encourages movement.
- Music taps into memories and emotions.
- Music provides nonverbal immediate feedback.
- Music activities are easily adapted to each person abilities.
- Music interventions can be designed to be success oriented.
- Music uses concrete concepts that are easily demonstrated and understood fast, slow, up and down loud and soft, long and short, etc.
- Many activities utilize many senses at the same time to enhance the learning experience, hearing seeing by feeling.
- Overall, music therapy can be designed to promote wellness, manage stress, alleviate pain, express feeling, enhance memory, improve communication and promote physical rehabilitation. Research in music therapy support its effectiveness in a wide variety of health care setting and in educational setting.

MECHANISM

The exact mechanism of music therapy is under research. But it is assumed to be an effective therapy because it stimulates peptides, endomorphins and natural opiates secreted by the hypothalamus that produces pleasurable feelings and reduces the unwanted stimuli.

The music therapy has the potential to synchronize body rhythms with rhythm of music. The synchronization and entertainment is thought to decrease, the symptoms of pain. The sympathetic nervous system activity leads to relaxation response. The pitch also affects the autonomic nervous system, increasing tension when high and relaxing it when low; therefore, music with slow, steady relaxing rhythm and low pitch orchestral effects would be appropriate for the client.

CLINICAL EFFECTS OF MUSIC THERAPY

- Music has distinct effects on the human organism. Soothing music can be used to achieve an alpha wave brain state which initiates a state of relaxed awareness.
- Soothing music with a flowing, lyrical, melodious, single, harmony and soft tone helps to stimulate the relaxation response.
- It can stimulate the release of endorphins from the brain and reduce the level of ADH, increase phenylethylamine can trigger autonomic nervous system and produce relaxation in muscle tone, brain wave frequency, galvanic skin response and papillary reflexes. Music also facilitates emotional homeostasis.
- According to Dr. Barbara Crowel (1992), the former President of Association of Music Therapy, said that music makes the difference between isolation and interaction, between chronic pain and comfort between demoralization and dignity.
- Music therapy influence the physiological variables like blood pressure, heart rate, respiration, EEG measurement, body temperature and galvanic skin response.
- It alleviates pain, anxiety, nausea, fatigue and depression.
- Lowers apical heart rate and raises peripheral temperature.
- It reduces stress and anxiety, decrease blood pressure and heart rate during music therapy.
- Music therapy creates a difference in elderly.
- Music stimulates all the senses and involves the elderly at many levels. The multimodal approach facilities many skills related to activities of daily living.
- Quality relearning and maximum participation occurs when the elderly is permitted to experience the joy of activity with music. The medium of music therapy allows his/her activity to occur naturally and frequently.
- Music is highly motivating catalyst, it can also have relaxing effect. Enjoyable music activities are designed to be success oriented and elderly to feel better about them.
- Music can encourage socialization, social expression, communication and motor development. Because the brain processes music, in both hemispheres, music can stimulate cognitive functioning and maybe used for recommendation in some speech and language skills enhancement.
- To conclude, music is esthetically appealing and can be justified as use as therapy in psychiatric setting.

PSYCHODRAMA

Introduction

For thousand of years drama has been used in healing methods. In the new millennium, drama is used as a therapy to express not only feelings but also the inner thoughts through talking. Each night we enter the strange theatre of our dreams where we experience images and dramas that have meaning in our lives. In psychodrama, images are explored and its meaning is discovered.

Psychodrama is a method of psychotherapy in which client use spontaneous dramatization, role playing and drama tie self-presentation to investigate and gain insight into their lives. It was developed by Dr. Jacob L. Moreno (1889–1974). It maybe used in a variety of clinical and community based setting and is most often utilized in a group scenario, in which each person in the group can become therapeutic agents for one another scenes. Psychodrama encourages the spontaneity and creativity of client for therapeutic purposes.

Definitions

- Psychodrama is an experiential form of therapy that allows for correction through the re-experiencing and then dynamic improvement through expression and role rehearsal. (Serge Lebovici 2011).
- According to Auckland Training Center for Psychodrama, defines psychodrama is an experiential group approach to creating life that can incorporate any aspect of human experience, real or imagined. It can be defined as the science which explores the truth by dramatic methods.
- It is therapeutic, invigorating, cosmic and earthy at the same time. It is the theatre of truth. It is about getting clearer with people looking at relationship in the past, present and future.
- Psychodrama is a specialized type of group therapy that employs a dramatic approach in which patient becomes actors in life situation scenarios with the goal to resolve interpersonal conflict in a less threatening atmosphere than the real life situation would present.

History of Psychodrama

Dr. J.L. Moreno (1889–1974) was the founder of psychodrama and sociometry and one of the forerunners of the group psychotherapy movement. Around 1910, he developed the theatre of spontaneity, which is based on the acting out of improvisational impulses. The focus of this exercise was not originally on the therapeutic effects of psychodrama. These were seen by Moreno, to simply be positive side effects.

Another important practitioner in the field of psychodrama is Carl Hollander. Hollander was the 37th Director certified by Moreno in Psychodrama. Although psychodrama is not widely practiced, the work done by practitioner of psychodrama has opened to research possibilities for other psychological concepts such as group therapy and expansion of the work of Sigmund Freud. The method of psychodrama are also used by group therapy organization such as alcoholic anonymous and also find place in other types of therapy, such as post divorce counseling for children.

Concept of Psychodrama

The inventor of the psychodramatic method, JR Moreno said psychodrama incorporated the whole of the universe in your being. The method recognizes the roles we live out of their history and connection to act spontaneously and create life a new, moment by moment. It is a lot of fun. It is an opportunity to become who you were originally meant to be.

It is a rehearsal for life. It is about expansiveness and role development. It also includes developing flexibility, i.e. the movement between fantasy, reality, play and healing. It uses a stage or action space to explore reality, express truth and develop roles that contribute to rewarding creative ways of being in the world.

Methods of Psychodrama

- In psychodrama, participants explore internal conflicts by acting out their emotions and interpersonal interactions on stage. A psychodrama session (typically involves 1–2 hours) focuses principally on a single participant known as protagonist. Protagonists examine their relationships by interacting with the other actors and the leader, known as the director. This is done using specific technique, including mirroring–doubling (psychodrama), soliloquy and role reversal.
- The session is often broken up into three phases: The warm-up—the action and the post-discussion session. During a typical psychodrama session, a number of clients gather together. One of these clients is chosen as the protagonist.
- During the warm-up stage, the actors are encouraged to enter into a state of mind where they can be present in and aware of the current moment and are free to be creative. This is done through the use of different games. One such game is called the 'life boat warm-up' in this warm-up. In that the client are told that they are in a life boat with a limited amount of space. In order to survive, an actor must convince the client that he or she deserves a seat on the lifeboat.
- The action section of the psychodrama session is the time in which the actual scenes themselves take place. Finally, in the postdiscussion phase, the different actors are able to comment on the action and share their empathy and experiences with the protagonist of the scene.
- Mirroring is an important technique in psychodrama. In mirroring, the protagonist is first asked to act out experience. After this, the client steps out of the scene and watches as another actor steps into their role and portrays the clients.
- Doubling is another psychodramatic technique in which the client is joined by another actor in his or her portrayal of him or herself. The second actor assumes the role of an 'auxillary ego' which reveals hidden parts of the protagonists behavior, by acting as him or her. Role playing is another method in which the client portrays a person or objects that is problematic to him or her.
- In soliloquy, another technique, the client speaks his or her thoughts aloud in order to build self-knowledge.
- Finally, role reversal is a technique in which a client is asked to portray another person while a second actor portrays the client in the particular scene.

DANCE THERAPY

Dance therapy is also known as movement therapy. Dance therapy is the therapeutic use of movement to improve the mental and physiosocial well-being of a person. It focuses on the connection between the mind and body to promote health and healing. Dance therapy can be considered as expressive therapy.

Definitions

- Dance therapy is a type of psychotherapy that uses movement to further the social, cognitive, emotional and physical development of the individual.
- According to American Dance Therapy Association the psychotherapeutic use of movement is a process that furthers the emotional, cognitive, social and physical integration of the individual.
- Dance therapy/movement therapy, a creative art therapy, is rooted in the expressive nature of dance itself. Dance is the most fundamental of the arts, involving a direct expression and experience of oneself through the body. It is a basic form of authentic communication, and as such it is an especially effective medium for therapy. It is based on the concept and the body, mind and the spirit are interconnected.

Brief History of Dance Therapy

The roots of dance/movement therapy can be traced to the early 20th century and the work of pioneer Marian Chance. She was a modern dancer of US.
- In soliloquy, another technique, the client speaks his or her thoughts aloud in order to build self-knowledge
- Finally, role reversal is a technique in which a client is asked to portray another person while a second actor portrays the client in the particular scene.

PSYCHOLOGICAL APPLICATIONS

- Psychodrama can be used in both clinical and non clinical areas. For example, used in business, education and professional training.
- One specific application in clinical situation is for people suffering from dysfunctional attachment, and PTSD. For this reason, it is often utilized in the treatment of children who have suffered emotional trauma, PTSD, depression and abuse.
- Using role play and story telling, children maybe able to express themselves emotionally and reveal truth about their experience. They are not able to openly discuss with their therapist and rehearse new ways of behavior.
- Moreno's theory of child development is divided into three stages. Finding personal identify, recognizing oneself (the mirror stage) and recognizing the other person (the role reversal stage). Mirroring, role playing and other psychodynamic techniques are based on these stages. Moreno believed that psychodrama could be used to help individuals continue their emotional development through the use of these techniques. Who began teaching dance in 1930. She noticed that some of her students were much more interested in the emotions they expressed in dancing than in the mechanics and technique of dance, and so she began to encourage this form of self-expression. Word spread of the dance student reported feelings of well-being after they mentally unburdened themselves through dance and doctors become intrigued. They began to send their patient to change many of whom were people with psychiatric illness.

Therapeutic Uses of Dance Therapy

- It helps to develop communication skills, a positive self-image and emotional stability.
- Used to relieve stress, treatment in PTSD.

- Relaxation therapy.
- Used as a adjunct therapy with palliative care in cancer and pain disorder.

TECHNIQUES OF DANCE THERAPY

- Dance therapist uses many techniques to cure illnesses. Some of the major 'school of thought in dance' therapy include the Freudian approach, Jungian technique, and object-relations orientation.
- The authentic movement technique is derived from the Jungian method of analysis in which people work with recurring images in their thoughts or dreams to drive meaning in their life. Instead of asking the patient to dance out certain emotions, the therapist instructs the patient to move when he or she feels 'the inner impulse'. The moves are directed by the patient and the therapist is a noncritical witness to the movement. The moves are supported to emerge from a deep level within the patient.
- In Freudian technique, dance therapist work with patients to uncover feelings which are hidden deep in the subconscious by expressing those feelings through dance.
- In object relations technique, the therapist often helps the patient to examine problems in his or her life by considering the primary initial relationship with the parents. Emotions are expressed in a concrete, physical way. For instance, a client would work out his or her fears of abandonment by repeatedly coming close to and dancing at a distance from the therapist.
- Dance therapist sometimes use other types of therapy along with the dance, such as art or drama. Therapists also discuss what happens during a dancing sessions by spending time in 'talk therapy'. For example. The therapist might instruct patient to imagine they are on a beautiful peaceful beach as they dance.
- The one frequently used technique is the therapist mirrors the movement of the patient as he or she expresses important emotions. This is especially powerful in patient one-on-one therapy. It is thought that this device provides a sense of safety and validates the patient emotions.
- The underlying premise of dance therapy is that when people dance, they are expressing highly significant or a head bent in shame has deep significance to a dance therapist. Through dance therapy, the theory goes, patients are able to move easily express painful, frightening emotion and can progress from there after experiencing dance therapy. They can talk about their feelings more freely and tear down the barriers they have erected between themselves and other people. The hope is that eventually they can go on to live more psychologically healthy lives.

Research and General Acceptance

Dance therapy was earlier considered as simply a 'feel good' treatment, but it is now more respected and used therapeutically. The current research on dance therapy have proven that dance therapy can be effective tool to help people overcome psychological problems.

INDIVIDUAL THERAPY

Introduction

Individual therapy is a confidential relationship between the client and therapist, that may occur in different settings like therapist office, chappel or in hospital. It is a method of bringing about changes in a person by exploring his or her feelings, attitude, thinking and behavior.

Definitions

Individual therapy is a form of therapy in which the client is treated one-on-one with a therapist. The most popular form of therapy, individual therapy may encompass many different treatment styles including psychoanalysis and cognitive behavior therapy.

Individual psychotherapy involves meeting with a therapist one-on-one for the purpose of reducing internal suffering which may occur in the form of problematic behavior, beliefs, feelings, and somatic response.

Aim

- To modify the maladaptive behavior.
- To improve interpersonal relationship.
- To get relief from stress or unhappiness.
- To make personal changes.

Goals

- Establishing a healthy relationship with the client.
- Providing opportunity for the client to release tension as problems are discussed.
- Assisting the client in gaining insight about the problem.
- Providing opportunity to practice new skills.
- Reinforcing appropriate behavior as it occurs.
- Providing consistent emotional support.

PROVIDER OF INDIVIDUAL THERAPY

- Client seeking therapy may see a psychiatric, a psychologist, a nurse, a social worker or a therapist/counselor.
- Registered psychiatric nurse may provide counseling and client education related to crisis, stress, mental health and may also provide referral to community source for both therapy and counseling.

Indications

- Anxiety disorders and personality disorder.
- Mood disorders
- OCD
- Eating disorders.
- Substance abuse
- Schizophrenia
- Sexual dysfunction
- Suicidal client/homicidal clients.

Contraindications

- Dangerous behavior, i.e. violent, restless, resistive and noncooperative.
- Too much disorganized, i.e. confused, disoriented.
- Uncommunicative, i.e. mute.
- Patient's who are receiving ECT and physical illness.

Phases of Individual Therapy

- Introductory phase.
- Working phase.
- Termination phase.

INTRODUCTORY PHASE

In this phase, the therapist and client establish boundary of relationship. The client's problem is noted, present coping skills are identified, strength and attributions are explored and communication established. During the introductory phase, the therapist forms some preliminary ideas about the client needs. Together, client and therapist discuss issues such as the length of time therapy will require, meeting dates, location, fees and so forth. The goal of this first stage of therapy is to establish a degree of trust that will allow clients to give up their defenses so they can enter into the second or working stage of treatment.

WORKING PHASE

This phase occurs when the therapist and client focus on client's problem and reach on understanding of why the problem has occurred. In the past, this exploration may have taken months or years to complete. Today, the whole process may be completed in 20 sessions. Increased trust allows the client to experience greater recall and insight and to express previously repressed feelings.

TERMINATION PHASE

This phase occurs when the client achieves maximum benefits of therapy. It occurs at any time during the session of the client and is resistance to treatment. In this stage, the client achieves a higher level of understanding or the self and relationships with others and begins to try out new ways of perceiving, thinking, feeling and behaving. As the client interact with others and sees newly acquired coping skills, changes are reflected in external behavior and in interaction with others.

TECHNIQUES OF INDIVIDUAL THERAPY

- When the client comes to OPD, the therapist observes the behavior and assess whether the client is indicated for psychotherapy, if indicated then, the therapist's schedule, value and time must be allocated.
- The therapist provides conducive environment with comfortable seating arrangement to enhance relaxation to the client.
- Physician assesses the physical condition of the client and exclude if any physical illness is present.
- Alter gaining confidence, the therapist explain the theoretical information about the principle of treatment, structure of mind-body-relationship, role of conscious mind in determining behavior of normal person, influence of emotions and the body functions.
- Encourage the client to ventilate his/her idea, feeling and painful experience without any inhibition.
- The therapist plays as an active listener and notes the health and records the essential information and makes an occasional remarks.

- During interaction, the therapist analysis the situation and gives valuable suggestion whenever necessary.
- The client is encouraged to discover the reason for his odd behavior, there by therapist allows the client for in depth understanding of himself and help him to find a solution to a problematic situation.
- The process is continued till there is satisfactory improvement of the client condition and extent of the nature of handling the psychological conflict by the client himself.
- The therapeutic procedure and ways of handling the problem are modified according to client's needs.
- The frequency of therapeutic session, decided upon client's needs.

INDIVIDUAL THERAPY WITH CHILDREN AND ADOLESCENTS

The need for psychotherapy for a child or adolescent is based upon such factors as the client's current problem, life history, level of development, ability to cooperate in treatment and what interventions are most likely to help with present concerns. Psychotherapy is often used in combination with other intervention such as administration of medicine, use of behavior management, cooperative work with school. They must have an understanding of normal adjustment at child or adolescent at any given age as well as understanding of individual life history. Individual psychotherapy focuses on improving child's adaptive skills.

Skill and outside the family coping. The relationship that develops between the therapist and client is very important. Most pediatric and adolescent client do not voluntarily seek treatment, they are referred to treatment because of a disturbance noted by a family member, teacher or pediatrician. If client feels comfortable, safe and understood, it is much easier to express his/her thoughts and feelings.

Psychotherapy provides emotional support, helps the client to resolve conflict with people, helps the client to understand problem and feelings and assist the client in trying out new solution to a new problem. Parents may be involved in varying degree. The therapist acts as an advocate and may called to make recommendation that affects various aspects of client's life. Individual psychotherapy for children and adolescent, including techniques utilized to help a child to express emotions, fear and concern.

ROLE OF NURSE IN INDIVIDUAL THERAPY

When a nurse provides individual psychotherapy, the nurse is functioning as a therapist such as that all professional actions are grounded in the theory or approach of the therapy. While the therapist does the nursing process requires assessment and analysis of data that results in nursing diagnosis. The nurse's role in individual therapy is a teacher, counselor, an advocate and researcher.

LIGHT THERAPY

Introduction

Light therapy is an alternative or complementary approach includes such techniques as the use of colored light or colored gemstones directed at or applied to various parts of the body. In some alternative forms of light therapy, the person visualizes being surrounded by and breathing in light of a particular color. It is also called as phototherapy.

Definition

Light therapy is a way of alternative treatment modality, where light is used to treat psychological disorders especially seasonal affective disorder.

HISTORY OF LIGHT THERAPY

Light therapy for seasonal affective disorder (SAD) was first introduced in 1980s. It has become the recommended treatment of choice for seasonal depression by American Psychiatric Association in 1980, Dr A J Lewy and coworkers at National Institute of Mental Health Demonstrated that high intensity light affects the neural release of melatonin by the pineal gland in the brain of people.

DESCRIPTION OF LIGHT THERAPY

- Light therapy uses specialized artificial light to treat mood disorder, shift one's biological clock, or synchronize one's sleep wake cycle with the day/light cycle.
- It may also be useful in normalizing sleep and behavior in people with dementias, although more research is needed in this field to show its efficiency.
- The artificial light consists of either a light box which emits up to 10000 lux of light, much brighter than lamp or a lower intensity of specific wavelengths of light from the blue (470 nm) to the green (525 nm) areas of the visible spectrum.
- Light therapy refers to two different categories of treatment one used in mainstream medical practice and the other in alternative/complementary medicine.
- Mainstream light therapy/photo therapy includes the use of ultraviolet light to treat psoriasis and other skin disorders and the use of full spectrum or bright light to treat seasonal affective disorder (SAD).

PURPOSE

Mainstream Light Therapy

- The purpose of light therapy in mainstream psychiatric treatment is the relief of seasonal affective disorder, a form of depression mostly associated with shortened daylight hours in northern latitudes from the late full to the early spring.
- It is occasionally employed to treat such sleep related disorder as insomnia and jet lag. Recently, light therapy has also been found effective in the treatment of nonseasonal forms of depression as bipolar disorders.
- Light therapy for SAD and nonseasonal forms of depression is thought to work by triggering the brain's production of serotonin. Other researchers postulated that light therapy may relieve depression or jet lag by resetting the body's circadian rhythm or inner biological clock.
- In dermatology, ultraviolet (UV) light therapy is used to treat rashes, psoriasis, other skin disorders and jaundice. OPD treatment for psoriasis usually requires three treatment sessions per week until the skin clears which takes about seven weeks.

Alternative Light Therapies

Alternative light therapies are generally used to treat energy imbalances in the seven major Chakras. Chakras are defined by eastern system of traditional medicine as energy centers in the human body located at different points along the spinal column. Each Chakra is thought to absorb a certain vibration of light in the form of one of the seven colors of the rainbow and to distribute this color energy throughout the body.

The seven major Chakras in the body and their associated colors are:

- *Red*: The root chakra, located at the base of the spine.
- *Orange*: The sacral/chakra, located at back.
- *Yellow*: The solar plexus area.
- *Blue*: The throat or thyroid chakra.
- *Indigo*: The so called 'third eye' located in the head at the level of the pineal gland.
- *Violet/white*: The crown chakra, located at the level of the pituitary gland.

Precautions

- Patients with eye disorders should consult an ophthalmologist before being treated with any form of phototherapy.
- Clients who are taking medication that make their skin sensitive to UV rays or bright light should also consult their health care provider. Although there are no reports of permanent eye damage from either light box therapy or UV treatment for skin disorders, client's sometimes experience headaches, dry eye, mild sunburn or fatigue. These problems can usually be relieved by adjusting the length of time for light treatment and by using a sunscreen and nose/eye drops.

Indication

Light therapy is useful in the treatment of depression (SAD), bulimia nervosa and premenstrual syndrome.

PROCEDURE OF ADMINISTRATION OF LIGHT THERAPY

Mainstream Light Therapy

Mainstream phototherapy for skin disorders, the exposure of the affected areas of skin to UV light. It is most often administered in an out-patient clinic or doctor's office. Light therapy for seasonal affective disorder and other forms of depression can be self-administered at home or in a private room in the work place. The client sits in front of a light box mounted on or near a desk or table for a period of time, each day ranging from 15 minutes to several hours, depending on the severity of the SAD symptoms. Some SAD clients may have two or three session of light therapy each day. Treatment typically begins in the fall, when the days grow noticeably shorter and end in the spring.

Light Box

- The right box itself maybe equipped with full spectrum bulbs, which do emit UV rays as well as visible light or it may use bulbs that filter out the UV rays and emit bright light only.
- Most light boxes emit light ranging from 2500–10000 lux, being a unit of light measurement equivalent to 1 lumen per square meter. For purposes of comparison, average in-door lighting in 300–500 lux, and the sunlight outdoors on a sunny day in summer is about 100000 lux.

- Clients are instructed to sit facing the light box but to avoid staring directly at it. They can read or work at their desk while sitting infront of the light box.
- Newer forms of light therapy for SAD include the light visor, which resembles a base ball cap with a light source attached underneath the front of the device, above the wearer's eyes. The light visitor allows the patient to walk more while receiving light treatment.
- Another new treatment is dawn simulation, which appears to be especially helpful for SAD clients who have difficulty in getting up in the morning. In down simulation, the lighting fixture is programmed to turn gradually from dim to brighter light to simulate the sunrise. Dawn simulation is started around 4:30 or 5'o clock on the morning, while the patient is still asleep.

Alternatives of Light Therapies

- Chromotherapy may be administered in several different ways.
- The first step is determining the source or location of patient's energy imbalance. Some color therapists or chromopaths are sensitive to the colors in the aura or energy field surrounding a person's physical body that is invisible to most people.
- Another technique involves suspending a quartz crystal on a pendulum over each chakra while the client lies on a table or on the floor. The crystal swings freely if the chakra is open and energy is moving normally, but stops or moves irregularly if the chakra is blocked.
- In the second stage of treatment, colored light is directed at specific areas of the body. The cromopath may use either colored light bulbs.
- The red, orange and yellow rays are thought to enter the body more effectively through the soles of the feet; patient receiving these colors of light may be asked to sit on the floor with their base feet 12–14 inches from the light source.
- Blue light can be used to irradiate the whole body for the relief of physical pain, and violet light can similarly used to relieve nervous strain and mental disorders.

BIOLOGICAL CLOCK

- Biological clock keeps out body rhythms and sleep wake cycles in synchro with the light day cycle of the earth.
- It is located in the suprachiasmatic nucleus in the hormone control center of the brain, the hypothalamus.
- When light enters the eye, it activates this part of the brain and reduces production of the sleep hormone (melatonin) produced in the pineal gland of the brain. The light also acts to the release of a variety of other hormones and affect body temperature.
- We are programmed to cycle every 24 hours but our exposure to light on a regular basis keeps us linked closely to the earth's rhythms.
- Four neruotransmitters (dopamine, norepinephrine, glutamate, GABA) have roles in controlling the biological clock. If you have sleeping problem in addition to noting the amount of light you get each day, have your thyroid hormone levels checked.
- Generally, the more bright light one gets during the day (especially earlier in the day) the more likely one is to make more melatonin during the night and the less sensitive one is to minor light exposure in the evening or night time.

Application and Timing of Light Therapy

If one wants to delay sleep onset, it is best to give light therapy in the hours before bedtime, when core body temperature is beginning to go down. On the other hand, if one wants to move earlier in the day/night cycle, it is best to administer light therapy in the second half of the night.

For Mood Disorder

- Seasonal affective disorder (SAD) is strictly defined as present when a person has a mood disorder which occurs during a particular time/season of the year, then clear completely at other times of the year.
- If one is treating mood disorder, light therapy is best for duration of 30 minutes for every hour, one sleeps 8 hours, they would require one hour of light therapy given one hour before they would normally sleep.
- Light therapy for mood disorder should usually begin about one week before depressive symptoms tend to begin or as soon as they begin. It should be tapered as the day lengthens. The transition dates are around the spring and fall equinox (March 20 or 21th and September 22 or 23 each year).

For dementia

It is possible that bright light between 7–9 pm may help people with dementia to sleep better, have fewer night time awaking, reduce the decrease of cognitive symptoms at night.

Mechanism of Light Therapy

- The therapeutic level of illumination has several known physiological effects, though its mechanism of effect is still not fully known, blood levels of the hormone melatonin, which may be abnormally high at certain times of day, are rapidly reduced by light exposure.
- Depending on when bright light is presented, the body's clock which control daily rhythm of body's temperature, hormones, secretions and sleep patterns shifts ahead or is delayed when stimulated by light. These physiological time shifts maybe the basis of the therapeutic response.
- On the other hand, the antidepressant effect may not involve rhythm shift, but rather overall changes in neurotransmitter activity such as serotonin and dopamine.

Preparation of client

- Client should consult their health care provider before mainstream phototherapy in order to determine possible sensitivity to bright light and adjust medication dosages if necessary.
- Holistic and alternative practitioners usually ask client to bathe or shower before phototherapy and to wear loosely fitting while on neutral colored clothing.
- Washing is considered necessary to remove any negative energy that the patient has picked up from other people or from the environment.
- Wearing light colored loose clothing is thought to minimize interference with the vibrations form the colored light.
- The final step in preparation is a brief of meditation or creative visualization for the practitioners as well as the client. This step helps to create an atmosphere of calm and relaxation for the client.

Aftercare

- No aftercare is necessary for mainstream light treatments.
- Practitioners of alternative light therapies recommend that clients sit or rest quietly for a few minutes after the treatment rather than returning abruptly to their daily routines. This brief rest is thought to maximize the benefits of the treatment.

Risks of Light Therapy

- Mainstream light therapies may produce minor side effects (headache, insomnia, mild sunburn or skin irritation, dry eyes) in some patients.
- In addition some clients receiving phototherapy for SAD may experience hypomania, which is a feeling of euphoria or upbeat mood.
- As with the physical side effects, hypomania can usually be managed by adjusting the frequency or length of light therapy sessions.
- There are no known risks associated with alternative light therapies.

Normal Result

Normal result for mainstream light treatments are clearing of the skin disorder or a lifting of depressed mood. Normal results for alternative light therapies include a sense of heightened energy and relief from negative thoughts or preoccupations. Some chromopaths also consider relief of physical or symptoms to be normal results for chromotherapy.

AROMATHERAPY

Introduction

Aromatherapy is the practice of using volatile plant oils, including essential oils for psychological and physical well-being. The essential oil profiles are details of over 90 essential oils, absolutes, carbon dioxides, and hydrosols that are also commonly utilized in Aromatherapy. Although essential oils, carbon dioxide, extracts and absolutes are distilled by different methods. The term essential oil is sometimes used as a blanket term to include all natural, aromatic, volatile, plant oils including carbon dioxides and absolutes.

Definition

- Aromatherapy is a form of alternative medicine that uses volatile plant materials, known as essential oils and other aromatic compounds for the purpose of alternating a person's mood, cognitive function or health.
- A complementary therapy based on the healing properties of essential plant oils. The oils are usually massaged into the body; but they can be inhaled; used on a bath or in a cold compress placed next to the skin.

History of Aromatherapy

Aromatherapy is the word coined by Heri Maurice Cattefosse in France in 1928. He was beginning to explore, that of using the aromatic components of plants to facilitate healing. These aromatic oils had been used for healing. These are recorded in Chinese and Ayurveda, from 2000 BC, as well as passages of the Bible that speak of their healing properties. These are liquids extracted from plants, which evaporate at room temperature with characteristic aromas. They are also called 'volatile oils' because of their ability to evaporate easily. Most of these oils have a protective function, killing microorganisms.

THE BENEFIT OF AN AROMA WITH ESSENTIAL OILS

- *Benefits of inhaling essential oil:* Essential oils that are inhaled into the lungs offer both psychological and physical benefits. It stimulates the brain to trigger a reaction, but when inhaled into the lungs, the natural constituents (naturally occurring) chemical can supply therapeutic benefit.
- *The benefits of physical application:* Essential oils that are applied to the skin can be absorbed into the bloodstream. The constituents of essential oils can aid in health, beauty and hygiene conditions. Since essential oils are so powerful and concentrated, they should never be applied to the skin in their undiluted form. To apply essential oils to the skin, essential oils are typically diluted into a carrier such as a cold pressed vegetable oil, also known as a carrier oil. Common carrier oils include sweet almond oil, apricot kernel oil and grape seed oil.
- *Other benefits:* In additions to therapeutic benefit at the emotional and physical level, essential oils are helpful in other application. Essential oils can be used in household and laundry cleaner. Some oils acts as a natural insect repellent and pesticide. You may recall using citronella candles during the summer to keep mosquitoes away. Citronella essential oil is the ingredient in the candles that is responsible for repelling the mosquitoes.

Modes of Application

The modes of application of aromatherapy include:
- *Aerial diffusion:* For environment fragnancing or aerial disinfection.
- *Direct inhalation:* For respiratory disinfection, decongestion, expectorant as well as psychological effects.
- *Topical application:* For general massage, bath, compresses, and therapeutic skin care.

Indications

- Alopecia areata (hair loss)
- Agitation, possibly including agitation related to dementia
- Anxiety
- Constipation
- Insomnia
- Pain
- Itching and psoriasis
- Depression.

Contraindications

- Pregnant women, people with severe asthma and people with a history of seizures should avoid hyssop oil.
- People with history of allergies should only use essential oils, such as rosemary and spike lavender.

- People with estrogen dependent tumors (breast cancer/ovarian cancer) should not use oils with estrogen like compounds, such as fennel, anise, sage and clary sage.
- People receiving chemotherapy should consult to their doctor before trying aromatherapy.

MATERIALS USED IN AROMATHERAPY

Some of the material employed include:

- *Absolutes:* Fragrant oils extract primarily from flowers or delicate plant tissues through solvent or supercritical fluid extraction (e.g. rose absolute). The term is also used to describe oil extracted from fragrant butters, concretes and enfleurage pomades using ethanol.
- *Carrier oils:* Typically, oily plant base triacylglycerides that dilute essential oils for use on the skin (e.g. sweet almond oil).
- *Essential oils:* Fragrant oils extracted from plants chiefly through steam distillation (e.g. eucalyptus oil) or expression (grapefruit oil). However, the term is also occasionally used to describe fragrant oils extracted from plant material by any solvent extraction.
- *Herbal distillates or hydrosols:* The aqueous by-product of the distillation process (e.g. rosewater). There are many herbs that make herbal distillates and they have culinary uses, medical uses and skin care use. Common herbal distillated are chamomile, rose and lemon balm.
- *Infusion:* Aqueous extracts of various plant material (e.g. Infusion of chamomile).
- *Phytoncides:* Various volatile organic compounds from plants that kill. Many turpentine based fragrant oils and sulfuric compounds from plants in the genus 'allium' are phytoncides though the latter are likely less commonly used in aromatherapy due to their disagreeable odors.
- *Vaporizer (volatized) raw herbs:* Typically higher oil content plant based material dried, crushed and heated to extract and inhale the aromatic oil vapors in a direct inhalation modality.

THERAPEUTIC EFFECTS OF AROMATHERAPY

- Aromatherapy is the treatment or prevention of disease by use of essential oils.
- It includes pain and anxiety reduction, enhancement of energy and short-term memory, relaxation, hair loss prevention and reduction of eczema induced itching.
- Aromatherapy does not use conditions, but helps the body to find a natural way to cure itself and improve immune response.
- Practitioners tend to emphasize the use of oils in massage.

USING NATURAL REMEDIES IN THE TREATMENT OF EMOTIONAL AND MENTAL STATES

- Natural healing is an ancient practice, documented in care painting at least 80000 years old. Through the ages more than three fourths of the world's population have relied on remedies from nature.
- Most people associate this approach with physical health needs. The healers of the past knew better; they treated the mind, the spirit and emotions with the same remedies given to heal the body.
- The holistic way of thinking is returning, accompanied by a revival of herbal, homeopathic, nutritional, orthomolecular and other treatments in matter of the mind.

EXAMPLES OF OILS

Antidepressant	Ylang-ylang, geranium, jasmine, sandalwood, lemon, mandarin
Anxiety	Petigreen, neroli, bergamot, cypress, lavender, lime marjoram rose, violet.
Innervating	Basil peppermint, rosemary
Sedative	Neroli, pet grain, cedar wood, chamomile, melisa, valerina

Research studies since 1920's shows the following benefits of oils.

Lavender	Relaxing, circulation, meditative
Pine	Strengthening, stabilizing
Angelica	Anorexia, relieving hopelessness
Basil	Fatigue, general nerve tonic, antidepressant soporific, confusion, melancholy, mental well being, classify and concentration, reduces anxiety
Bay	Antihysteric, sedative, hypotensive
Bergamot	Sedative for anxiety and antidepressant, stimulates appetite
Chamomile	Calming, hyperactivity, good for use with children
Clary sage	Sedative and nervine for insomnia, paranoia, panic and hysteria
Cypress	Anxiety, confusion
Everlasting	Grounding, increases dream activity
Juniper	Apathy, paranoia, confusion, anxiety, nervous trembling and paralysis, diuretic
Marjoram	Grief, insomnia
Spikenard	Grounding

Usage

- Baths : 8–10 drops
- Massage : 10–20 drops in 1 ounce of oil
- Inhalation : 2–5 drops on a tissue of cotton ball
- Diffusers : Use pure oiles only
- Body lotion : 15–20 drops in 1 ounce of lotion
- Spritzer : 4 ounces of distilled water with 40–60 drops of pure essential oil, shake before using.

Other Therapeutic Uses

- Pure essential oil of rosemary is very effective for Alzheimer's disease.
- Aromatherapy is excellent for almost everything under sun.

Nervous Tension

The following blend will relax the nervous system. Ease tension and brief emotional equilibrium.

- 10 drops lavender
- 10 drops petitgrain
- 4 drops roman chamomile.

Nervousness/anxiety/insomnia

The following blend will profound and relax the individual, induce sleep, bring calm to an active mind that is controlling the correct emotional balance and total relaxation.

- 10 drops lavender
- 10 drops basil
- 3 drops neroli.

Role of Nurse in Aromatherapy

The use of Aromatherapy in nursing care continues to be popular in many settings. Most of the nursing literature relates to the use of essential oils in low doses for massage and use of the oils as environmental fragrances. Since the 1990s nurses have considered that the increased technology of health care threatens their ability to practice holistic care, which is positively entrenched in the philosophy of nursing.

- Florence Nightingale's lasting legacy on the profession of nursing is widely known. She was known for the use of Aromatherapy in the nursing profession.
- The nurse should assess the patient before the application of Aromatherapy.
- Knowledge about oils and its effects should be discussed with the client before the application.
- The patient should be made relaxed with loose clothing.
- Client should be advised to take bathe before the therapy.

RELAXATION THERAPIES

Introduction

Constant stress is one of the defining features of modern life, and it is the source of many health ill-health conditions, specially psychological problems. Stress plays an obvious role in nervousness, anxiety and insomnia. The newer research findings shown that it contributes to a vast number of illness. There are many several ways to mitigate the damage caused by stress. Increased physical exercise, taking relaxation breaks and vacations, and therapeutic use of relaxation techniques.

Relaxation Techniques

There are many types of relaxation therapies and use a variety of techniques. For example, a simple lying down or assuming a relaxed, seated posture in a quiet place and closing the eyes. The next step differs depending on the method. The techniques like autogenic training, guided-imagery, progressive muscle relaxation and meditation, are some of the examples.

Therapeutic Benefits of Relaxation Therapy

Numerous research findings have evaluated relaxation therapies that are useful in the following conditions.

- Insomnia
- Asthma
- Anxiety
- Hypertension
- Angina

- Back pain
- Bulimia nervosa
- Treatment of cancer
- Depression
- Congestive heart failure
- Fibromyalgia
- Stroke and ulcers
- Arthritis and headaches
- Irritable bowel syndrome and OCD, PMS.

Over all, relaxation therapy encourages a more relaxed state, long after the session and facilitates better coping skills.

Function

During stressful situation, the sympathetic nervous system increases activity that leads to the 'fight or flight' response. During this response, heart rate and blood pressure increase and breathing becomes irregular and increased. When experiencing physical reaction to stress, people often have difficulty in calming themselves down. Thus, the body's natural relaxation response is a powerful antidote to stress.

Types of Relaxation Techniques

The major types of relaxation techniques are as follows:

1. *Autogenic training:* This technique uses both visual imagery and body awareness to move a person into a deep state of relaxation. The person imagines a peaceful place and then focuses on different physical sensations, moving from the feet to the head, e.g. one might focus on warmth and heaviness in the limbs, easy, natural breathing or a calm heartbeat.
2. *Breathing:* In breathing techniques, you place one hand on your chest and the other on your abdomen. Take a slow, deep breath, sucking in as much air as you can inhale. As you are doing this, your belly should push against your hand. Hold your breath and then slowly exhale. Deep breathing exercises helps a lot.
3. *Progressive muscle relaxation:* This technique involves slowly tensing and then releasing each muscle group individually starting with the muscle in the toes and finishing with those in the head.
4. *Medication:* The most two popular forms of medication useful clinically are, transcendental and meditation (repeating a mantra... a single word or phase) and mind fullness meditation (focusing on thoughts and sensation.)

USES

- Research suggests that meditation can help improve a peron's quality of life and reduce stress hormones.
- Clinical trial studies also show that relaxation techniques reduce the perception of pain.
- Meditation is used as a treatment in PTSD.

YOGA

Definition

Yoga is a philosophy and practice that connects the body, breath and mind to energize and balance the whole person. This mind-body therapy involves physical postures, breathing exercises and meditation to improve overall well-being.

HISTORY

The word 'Yoga' is derived from a Sanskrit, which means 'union'. It appeared more than 2000 years ago and was practiced thousands of years before that. It is both a spiritual practice as well as exercise to reduce stress. In its traditional form, yoga is considered a complete lifestyle that provides a path to spiritual enlightenment.

The dimensions of yoga are:
- Pranayama (breathing)
- Asan (postures)
- Yama (restraint)
- Niyama (healthy observances)
- Pratyahara (sensory withdrawal)
- Dharana (meditation)
- Samadhi (higher consciousness)

Type of Yoga

The following are the different branches of yoga:
- *Bhakti yoga:* This form of yoga aims to take all of the love in one's heart and direct it towards the divine. By seeing God in all of concern, the person who practices regularly has respect for all life and is encouraged to treat others generously.
- *Hatha yoga:* Hatha yoga emphasizes physical postures or exercise, known as asanas, with the goal of balancing the opposites in one's life. During the exercise, flexion is followed by extension; a rounded back is followed by an arched back and physical exercise are followed by meditation.
- *Jnana yoga:* This form of yoga emphasizes deep contemplation. Practitioners seek jnana or 'wisdom' through meditation and the goal is to be one with god.
- *Karma yoga:* Karma yoga is based on the philosophy that yesterday action determine today's circumstances perform selfless acts of kindness. By making today's action positive, they hope they can improve tomorrow's circumstances for both themselves and other, and overall for the world.
- *Raja yoga:* This paves way to reintegration. Raja yoga blends the four layers of self: the body : the individual consciousness, the individual sub consciousness and the universal and infinite consciousness. Raja yoga, being most concerned with the mind and, spirit. It gives more importance to meditation.
- *Tantra yoga:* Like hatha yoga, practitioners of tantra yoga seek to balance the opposites in their lives. They also try to break free of the 'six enemies' (physical longing, anger, greed, variety, obsession, jealousy) and the eight fetter (hatred, apprehension, fear, shyness, hypocrisy, pride of ancestry, variety of culture, egoism) by using discipline, training and rituals.

- *Function of yoga:* Health scientists postulated that yoga reduces stress. They also believe that yoga promotes the release of endorphins, natural painkillers and mood elevators from the brain. Study findings shown that yoga can lower heart rate and blood pressure, increase muscle relaxation and increase breathing capacity.

All branches of yoga have three major techniques breathing, exercise (asana or postures) and meditation.

- *Breathing exercise:* In yoga, breath work is lesson as pranayama. Pranayama increases blood circulation and reduces oxygen consumption. That brings more oxygen to the brain and improves the way our body uses oxygen. It also increases how much air you can draw into your lungs. Getting much air into the lungs help to feel alert and focused.
- *Asanas (postures):* It provides a gentle to intense workout that enhances strength, flexibility and balance.
- *Meditation:* Meditation practice quiets the mind and brings on both physical and emotional relaxation, which helps to reduce blood pressure, chronic pain, anxiety and cholesterol levels.
- *Therapeutic benefits of yoga:* (yoga therapy)
- Yoga therapy derived from yoga tradition of Patanjali and the ayurvedic system of health care refers to the adaptation and application of yoga techniques and practices to help individual facing health challenges at any level to manage their condition, reduce symptoms, restore balance, increase vitality and improve attitude. (Gary draftsow. USA 2011)
- It is also defined as, yoga therapy is that facet of the ancient science of yoga that focuses on health and wellness at all levels of the person physical, psychological and spiritual. Yoga therapy focuses on the path of yoga as a healing journey that brings balance to the body and mind through an experiential understanding of the primary intention of yoga, awakening of spirit, our essential nature. (Joseph le Page. intergative yoga therapist 2011)
- Yoga improves fitness, lowers blood pressure, promotes relaxation and self confidence and reduces stress and anxiety people who practice yoga tend to have good coordination, posture, flexibility, range of motion, concentration, sleep habits and digestion. Studies show that yoga may help in the following conditions.
- Anxiety and stress
- Arthritis
- Asthma
- Cancer
- Chronic back pain
- Depression
- Diabetes
- Epilepsy
- Hypertension
- Irritable bowel syndrome
- Lung disease
- Pregnancy
- Migraine headaches.

In addition to the above, yoga postures that stretch and strengthen the points in the body may improve grip strength and reduce pain among people with carpel tunnel syndrome.

Biofeedback

Biofeedback is a treatment technique in which people are trained to improve their health by using signals from their own bodies. Physical therapist uses biofeedback to help stroke victims regain movement in paralyzed muscles, psychologists used it to help tense and anxious client learn to relax. Clinical specialists in many different fields use biofeedback to help their client to cope with pain.

Biofeedback is a technique that trains people to improve their health by controlling certain bodily processes that normally happen involuntarily, such as heart rate, BP, muscle tension, and skin temperature. Electrodes are attached to skin to measure the processes and display them on a monitor. With the help from a biofeedback therapist, one can learn to change your heart rate, BP, e.g. at first you use the monitor to see your progress, but eventually you will be able to achieve success without the monitor or electrodes. Biofeedback is an effective therapy for many condition but it is primarily used to treat high blood pressure, tension headache, migraine headache, chronic pain and urinary incontinence.

Types

The three most commonly used forms of biofeedback therapy are:
- Electromyography (EMG), which measures muscle tension.
- Thermal biofeedback, which measures skin temperature, neurofeedback or electroencephography (EEG), which measures brain wave activity.
- *Functioning of biofeedback:* Usually in a normal session, electrodes are attached to the skin. They send information to monitor by the translates the measurements into a tone which varies in pitch, a visual meter that varies in brightness or a computer screen that show lines moving across a grid. The therapist then leads him/her in mental exercises. Through trial and error, the client can learn to identify the mental activities that will bring about the physical changes that client want.

Therapeutic uses of Biofeedback

Biofeedback in the following health problems:
- Anorexia nervosa
- Anxiety
- Asthma
- Autism
- Back pain/chronic pain
- Bedwetting
- Depression
- Diabetes
- Seizure and migraine
- Head injuries
- Hypertension, motion sickness
- Sexual disorders including pain while intercourse
- Spinal cord injuries.

Each session generally lasts less than one hour. The number of sessions required depends on the condition being treated. Many clients start to see results within 8–10 sessions. Treatment of headache, incontinence and Raynold's disease requires at least 10 weekly session and some follow up session as health condition improves. Conditions like high BP, usually requires more than 20 weekly biofeedback session. It is considered a safe treatment, modality.

ALTERNATIVE SYSTEM OF MEDICINE

Alternative medicine is also called as complementary medicine is a term used to describe a wide range of healing systems that are not considered part of mainstream or conventional western medicine. The goal of conventional medicine is to find the physical source of a particular disease and then cure it, e.g. if a person has an infection, a conventional doctor may prescribe an antibiotic to kill the invading bacteria. Alternative medicine practitioner on the other hand, take more 'holistic' approach to health care. They believe that health and disease involve a complex interaction of physical, spiritual, mental, emotional, genetic, environmental and social factors in order to treat a disease or promote good health. Alternative practitioner treats the whole person.

Principles of Alternative Therapy

The basic principles of alternative therapies include the following:

- The focus is on the whole person physical, emotional, social and spiritual.
- Preventing of illness is a primary concern.
- Treatments are highly individualized.
- Treatments are aimed at the causes of illness rather than at its symptoms.
- Treatments are designed to support the natural healing process of the body.

Types of alternative therapies

The National Center for Alternative Medicine classifies alternative therapies into five major groups.

Alternative medical systems

These are built upon complete system of theory and practice, e.g. homeopathy, naturopathy, ayurveda and traditional chinese medicine.

Biological medicine

It is the use of substance found in nature, such as herbs, food and vitamins to promote health.

Energy medicine

- It involves the use of energy field to promote health. These aim to influence energy field believed to surround and penetrate the human body.
- For example reiki, therapeutic touch, Yi Yong, and electroacupuncture.

Manual Medicine

It is based on manipulation and movement of one or more parts of the body, e.g. osteopathy, physical therapy, massage, chiropractic and reflexology.

Mind/body medicine

It uses a range of techniques that help to boost the mind's ability to influence bodily functions, e.g. biofeedback, deep relaxation, guided imagery, hypnotherapy, meditation, prayer, yoga and support groups.

AYURVEDA

Ayurveda is considered to be the oldest healing science. It is a holistic approach to health, that is designed to help people live long, healthy and well-balanced lives. The term 'ayurveda' is derived from Sanskrit literature. Ayur meaning 'life' or 'life span' and 'veda' meaning 'knowledge. It has been practiced in India for at least 5000 years. The basic principle of ayurveda, is to prevent and treat illness by maintaining balance in the body, mind and consciousness through proper drinking, diet, lifestyle as well as with herbal remedies.

There are two main types of ayurveda traditional and maharishi. Maharishi is a version of traditional ayruveda based on translations from the classical texts by Maharishi Mahesh yogi. Both types of ayurvedic practitioners prescribe herbs, believe that disease results from an imbalance in the doshas and use many of the same remedies for treating illness. Maharishi ayurveda emphasizes the role of supreme consciousness in maintaining good health and promotes transcendental meditation (TM), as a way to experience the pure conscious of the universe. It also highlights the expression of positive emotions and the needs to attune the life to the natural rhythms of the body.

CONCEPT OF AYURVEDA

According to ayurvedic belief, each person has a distinct pattern of energy. A specific combination of physical, mental and emotional characteristics. It is also believed that there basic energy types called doshas, present in every person.

- *Vata:* The energy that controls bodily functions associated with motion, including blood circulation, breathing, blinking and heartbeat. When vata energy is balanced, there is creativity and vitality. Out of balance, vata produces fear and anxiety.
- *Pitta:* The energy that controls the body's metabolic systems, including digestion, absorption, nutrition and intelligence. In balance, pitta leads to contentment and intelligence. Out of balance, pitta can cause ulcers and arouse anger.
- *Kapha:* The energy that controls growth in the body. It supplies water to all body parts, moisturizes the skin, and maintains the immune system. In balance, kapha is expressed as love and forgiveness. Out of balance kapha leads to insecurity and envy.
- Everyone has vata, pitta and kapha, but usually one or two are dominant in a particular person. Many things can disturb the energy balance, such as stress, an unhealthy diet, the weather and strained family relationship. The disturbance shows up as disease. Ayurvedic practitioners prescribe treatment to bring the doshas back into balance.

Treatment Modalities in Ayurveda

Ayurvedic practitioners practice more than 20 types of treatment, but most commonly prescribed include:

- *Pranayama:* It is a breathing exercise. Practicising pranayama helps to feel calm and quiet.
- *Abhyanga:* It is rubbing the skin with herbal oil to increase blood circulation and draw toxins out of the body through the skin.

- *Rasayana:* It is using mantras (repeating words or phrases) during meditation combined with certain herbs to rejuvenate a person.
- *Yoga:* Combining pranayama, movement and meditation it improves circulation and digestion and to reduce blood pressure, cholesterol level, anxiety and chronic pain.
- *Panchakarma:* Cleansing the body to purify it and reduce cholesterol. Practitioners use methods that cause sweat, bowel movement and even vomit to cleans the body of toxins.
- *Herbal medicines:* Prescribing herbs to restore dosha balance.

Ayurveda and Psychiatry

Ayurveda has differentiated human organs into dyanendriya (organs of perceptions) and karmendriye (organs of action). It has given the special status of ubha dynedriyas (organs of both, perception as well as action) to man or manas (mind). Ayurveda also says that in one body-mind apparatus, our mind, control our body and is more important for perception, thinking, understand, taking the right decisions at the right time, etc.

If the mind is sick, then the body-mind apparatus is in danger. When the mind is in a status of health, it contains positive feelings like those of love, affection, sharing, caring, etc. Due to improper diet and action, the natural state of mind is disturbed and these positive feelings are driven out. They then give place to negative feelings like those of anger, jealousy, cruelty, laziness, etc... which further leads to mental disorder.

Ayurveda also says that these negative feelings are emotional toxins. If they are not driven out of body in a stipulated time, they give rise to chronic mental disorders like anxiety neurosis, depression, etc. If this is further, it turns into permanent mental disorder like unmad (unreasonable and irrational state of mind, like hysteria). Ayurveda has also included apasmara (epilepsy) in the category of mental disorders.

As for the causes, ayurveda mentions improper diet, actions committed in this birth, bad deeds done in the last birth, physical and overindulgence in sex. It also includes severe mental or physical stress and unfavourable personal, familial and social environment in the causes of mental disorders. All these hamper the natural vitality of a person and lead to disturbed health.

A person suffering from mental disorder becomes incapable of conducting himself/herself in according to hallucinations, instead of coherent thoughts, social withdrawal, antisocial behavior or extreme violence on the personal, family or social level is seen. A few physical symptoms like tremors, irregular eye ball movement oblivion of one's own body, excessive perspiration and salivation may accompany these behavioral aberrations. Seeking attention is also a symptom, pendulum. All the in between stages like diverting attention, distracting attention, etc. are seen in various mental or psychosomatic disorders purpose sellers movements or compulsive obsessive movements can also be observed at times.

For the treatment of these disorders, prescribes herbs and shrubs. Cooling medicines prepared from rose, brahmi, kevada (pandanus odoratissimus) as well as mixtures such as gulkand (rose petals treated with crystal sugar and sunlight), chyavan prash or morawala (a mixture of made from amla, i.e. Emblica officinalis, sugar, etc.) are recommended to keep the mind balance, fresh and active. Almonds are also effective to keep the mind in balanced fresh and active.

Ayurveda also strongly recommends avoiding alcohol, tobacco, marijuna, and other intoxicating substances. Very hot, spicy food and too much of non-vegetarian items should be avoided. Use of cow milk, homemade ghee, apples, pineapples, grapes, etc. are recommended to enhance mental strength and vitality.

General hygiene maintained by taking a daily bath and changing one's clothes regularly is recommended. Social interaction is advisable and the client is encouraged to keep himself/herself busy in some productive activity. Negative feelings should be kept away by involving the client in religious or social thoughts and activities. Positive thinking, support from family members and a moderate response to the patient's mental tempers and tantrums from the illness. To regain one's social position and lead a normal life again is a difficult task but not impossible. It can be achieved by collective measures.

HOMEOPATHY

Introduction/History

- The main idea behind homeopathy is the law of similar, which is explained as 'like cures like' in the late 18th century, a German physician named Samuel Hahnemann found that quinine containing Peruvian bark (chinchona) cured malaria. Hahnemann swallowed a dose of Peruvian bark and began to feel feverish, drowsy, extremely thirsty and agitated all symptoms of malaria. Hahnemann started to experiment more and formed his theory that like cures like, or the law of similar; that when a substance in large doses causes certain symptoms, in small doses it can cure these same symptoms.
- Herbs and other plants, minerals, venom from snakes and other substances can be used to make homeopathic remedies. They are diluted again and again and successes or shaken vigorously between each dilution. The process of sequential dilution and succession is called potentization.

Functioning of Homeopathy

- Homeopathic remedies start with substances such as herbs, mineral or animal products. These substances are first crushed mechanically shaken, then stored. This is called as 'mother tincture'. Homeopaths then dilute tinctures more with alcohol or lactose, either 1 part to 10 (written as 'x') or 1 part to 100 (written as "c"). These tinctures dilute these tinctures 2 times (2 x or 2c), 3 times (3x or 3c) and so forth. Many times, practitioners will use much higher dilutions, because the more diluted the substance, the more potent its healing powers are thought to be.
- Homeopathic remedies aim to stimulate the body's healing mechanisms. Homeopaths believe that any physical disease has a mental and emotional component. So a homepopathic diagnosis includes physical symptoms (such as feverishness), current emotional and pshychological state (such as anxiety and restlessness) and the person's constitutions. A person's constitution includes qualities related to creativity, initiative, persistence, concentration, physical sensitivities and stamina. The right remedy for a condition will take all of these aspects into account, so each diagnosis and remedy is individualized. That means 3 people with fever could need 3 very different prescriptions. These remedies are usually taken for no more than 2–3 days, although some people may used only 1-2 doses before they start feeling better. In some cases daily dosing may be prescribed.

HOMEOPATHY AND MENTAL HEALTH

- In the area of mental health, Hahnemann was a pioneer. In 1793, he started humanistic treatment for mentally ill patient. In regard to mental disorders, he writes 'almost all so called mental and emotional are nothing but physical disease in which the symptoms of mental health and emotional disorder characteristic of each are increased more or less rapidly as the physical symptoms, diminish, almost like a local disease transferred into the invisible subtle mental or emotional organ
- Hahnemann was a precursor in the field of psychosomatics. He saw the human being having an integrated mind and body, in contrast to the prevailing dualism of his time. According to him in all disease being treated, the psychic condition of the patient should be written down among the totality of symptoms as one of the most important if one desires to have a faithful picture of the disease to make a successful homeopathic cure.
- Hahnemann made a distinction between organic and psychological disease. He prescribed psychotherapeutic techniques. The first homeopathic hospital for the mentally ill was founded in Middletown, New York in may 1974.
- Homeopathic use various remedies with apparently different biological action. Some have acute symptomatology in its picture like belladonna, hyoscyamus, stramonium and veratrum album. In these, the symptoms appear soon after the remedy is ingested.
- The other class of drugs or remedies, like natrum muriaticum (sodium chloride), silica, phosphorus or sepia (cuttlefish tincture) take longer time and repeated doses in order to manifest their particular symptomatology and sphere of action. The selection of remedies is always based on the totality of symptoms of the patient, and in the consideration of the peculiar, or characteristics, qualities of the organism.

Siddha Medicine

Siddha medicine (Tamil traditional) is one of the oldest system of medicine. Plants, animals, metals and some chemicals are used to prepare the Siddha medicines. Various forms of medicines are used for therapeutic purpose. It defines physical disease as 'pini and psychological disease as 'noi...the', kniekai no 64 of agasthiar' is the note worthy book of siddha medicine. Kinekai no. 1 describes about 18 psychiatric diseases. The Siddhars totally denies the concept of demonology and accepts abnormal behavior in terms of pathology.

Symptoms of Abnormal Behavior

- According to Kirusa Nithanam 50 the symptoms for the psychological disorder as follows; standing with upper limbs, restlessness, singing meaninglessly, dancing, laughing, changing postures, sleeplessness.

  Embracing others, loose talking, murmuring , spitting on others, wandering, sexual aggression, rolling on the floors. Standing naked and removal of clothes. They have described abnormal behavior into 18 types including several sexual disorders like male impotency, female frigidity and sexual dysfunction. Siddhars describes the evils of alcoholism and drug abuse.

REASONS FOR ABNORMAL BEHAVIOR ACCORDING TO SIDDHA

The Agasthiar in this book kinekai no 0164 completely describes the demonology.
Siddhars believed that the root cause of the abnormal behaviors are evil desire, disordered thought, passions, morbid imagination, excessive fear, envy, anger and immoral activities. The karma or off shoots or chronic disease are mainly caused by the man's previous action. The law of karma describes that man's sin action. Sin actions of man are the root cause of the present life. Present life is guided by our karma. Siddhars believed that the mental abnormalities are caused by the evil karmas of the man or his/her ancestor's. Another important reasons are their dosham. If the dosham increases, the mental abnormalities occur. Siddhars also believed that the abnormalities may occurred due to sleeplessness and breaking of varma points, for example due to the damages of uchikala varmam, suliyadivarmam due to the damages of uchikala varmam, suliyadivarmam and thudi narambu, traumatic disorder may occur.

REMEDIES RECOMMENDED BY THE SIDDHARS FOR ABNORMALITIES

Siddhars recommended several medications for mental abnormalities. They prescribed aviztham (medicines) as well as manthiram (psychotherapy), e.g. Thuvalai, Vedhu (steam bath), Ullukku Kokuthal, Nasium, Kallikam, etc.

Psychotherapy (Manthiram)

Providing spiritual healing enhancing the speed of recovery. Using manthiram (spiritual words) may cure the disease, particularly for kama disease.

Herbal Medicine

Herbal medicine also called botanical medicine or phytomedicine ... refers to using a plant's seeds, berries roots, leaves, bark or flower for medicinal purposes.

History of Herbal Medicine

- Plants had been used for medicinal purposes long before recorded history. Ancient Chinese and Egyptian papyrus writing describe medical uses of plants, as early as 3000 B C. Indigeneous cultures (such as African and nature American) used herbs in their healing rituals, while others developed traditional medical systems (ayurveda and Traditional Chinese medicine) in which herbal therapies were used. Researchers found that people in different parts of the world tended to use the same or similar plants for the same purposes.
- In the early 19th century, where chemical analysis first became available, scientists began to extract and modify the active ingredients from plants. Later, chemists began making their own version of plant extracts, declined in over time, the use of herbal medicines declined in favor of drugs. Almost one-fourth of pharmaceutical drugs are derived from botanicals.
- Recently the World Health Organization (WHO) estimated that 80% people worldwide rely on herbal medicines for some part of their primary health care.

Functioning of Herbs

In many cases, scientists are not sure what specific ingredient in a particular herb works to treat a condition or illness. Whole herbs contain many ingredients, and they may work together to produce a beneficial effects. Many factors determine how effective a herb will be, e.g. the type of environment (climate, bugs, soil quality) in which a plant grew will affect it, as well how and when it was harvested and processed.

Therapeutic use of Herbal Medicine

- Herbal medicine is used to treat many conditions, such as asthma, eczema, premenstrual syndrome, rheumatoid arthritis, migraine, menopausal symptoms, chronic fatigue, irritable bowel syndrome, and cancer. Some common herbs and their used are discussed below.
  - *Ginkgo (ginkgo biloba):* Used to treat circulatory disorders and to enhance memory.
  - *Kava kava (piper methysticum):* It is believed to elevate mood, enhance well being and contentment and produce a feeling of relaxation. Used to treat anxiety, insomnia and related nervous disorders.
  - *Saw palmetto (serenoa repens)* is used for the treatment of benign prostatic hyperplasia (BPH), a non concerous enlargement of the prostate gland.
- *St. John's wort (hypericum perforatum):* It acts as antidepressant. Used in mild to moderate depression.
- *Valerian (valeriana officinalis):* Used to treat sleep disorder.
- *Echinacea preparation:* (From Echinacea purpurea and other Echinacea species) may improve the body's natural immunity.

Adverse reactions of herbs

- St. John's wort can cause skin to be more sensitive to the sun's ultraviolet rays and may cause an allergic reaction, stomach upset, fatigue and restlessness. It also interferes with the effectiveness of many drugs, including the blood thinner warfarin, protease inhibitors for HIV, birth control pills, certain asthma drugs and many other medication.
- Kava–kava has been linked to liver toxicity.
- Valevian may cause sleeplessness and in some people it may even have the unexpected effect of overstimulating instead of sedating.
- Garlic, ginkgo, fever few and ginger, among, other herbs may increase the risk of bleeding.
- Evening primrose (oenothera binnis) may increase the risk of seizures in people who have seizure disorders and bleeding in people with bleeding disorder or who take blood thinning medications, such as warfarin.
- The herbs are available in the market in different forms. Teas, syrups, oil, liquid extracts, tinctures and dry extract (pills or capsules).

NATUROPATHY

Naturopathy or naturopathic medicine is a system of medicine based on the healing power of nature. Naturopathy is a holistic system, means that, it strives to find the cause of disease by understanding the body, mind and spirit of the person.

Philosophy and Premise of Naturopathy

- Naturopathy deals with the healing power of nature, since it believes that all healing powers are within the body. This means that within every human organism there is a healing energy, which includes the immune system in the fuller sense of both the physical and the psyche, which is responsible for wellness and for maintenance of health.

- Falling ill is when we go against nature; the cause of disease (toxins) is expelled from the body to cure it. Fasting has been described as nature's way to recover. A thorough rest is which includes fasting the most favorable condition in which an ailing body can purify and recover itself.
- Following first premise is the second, that the therapies used to support and stimulate. This healing power of nature must be in 'the gentlest, least invasive, most efficient manner possible'.
- The third naturopathic premise is 'to diagnose and treat the cause'. Naturopaths do not simply treat the manifestation of the disease but rather search for the cause and treat it. To accomplish these goals, naturopathic medicine incorporates many therapeutic modalities; herbal medicine, homeopathy, nutrition, hydrotherapy, food, exercise therapy, physical therapy, manipulation of the bony and soft tissues, life style and counseling.
- *There are two areas of focus in naturopathy:* One is supporting the body's own healing abilities and the other is empowering people to make lifestyle changes necessary for the best possible health.
- Naturopaths consider client to be participant in their health care, so changes in life style, may be considered.

TRADITIONAL CHINESE MEDICINE

Traditional Chinese medicine (TCM) is a complete medial system that has been used to diagnose, treat and prevent illnesses for more than 2000 years. It is based on a belief in Yin and Yang, define as opposing energies, such as earth and heaven, winter and summer and, happiness and sadness. When Yin and Yang are in balance, the person feels relaxed and energized. Out of balance, however Yin and Yang negatively affect the health.

The practitioners also believe that there is a life force or energy, known as Qi (pronounce 'chee') in everybody. For Yin and Yang to be balance and for the body to be healthy Qi must be balance and flowing freely. When there is little or too much Qi in one of the body's energy pathways, called meridians or when the flow of Qi in blocked, it causes illness.

The ultimate aim of TCM treatment is to balance the Yin and Yang in our lives by promoting the natural flow of Qi.

Functioning of TCM

Disease alterations in the normal flow of Qi such that Yin and Yang are imbalanced. It thought to have three major causes. External or environmental factors, internal emotions and lifestyle factors, such as diet. Though the use of its therapeutic modification, TCM stimulates the body's own healing mechanisms.

Practices used in TCM include:

- Acupuncture and acupressure.
- Moxibustion, burning a herb near the skin.
- Herbal medicine
- Nutrition
- Chinese massage, called Tui na.
- Exercise, such as Tai Chi and Qi gong which combine movement with medication.

In TCM, the body's internal organs are thought of not only as individual structures but also as complex network. According to TCM, Qi flows through organ system, kidney, heart, spleen, liver, lung, gallbladder, small intestine and large intestine... by way of meridians. Despite their specific names, these five systems correspond to more than individual body parts. The kidney, for example, represents the entire urinary system along with the adrenal glands, located on top of the kidneys. The heart, unreasonable, represent both the heart and the brain.

Therapeutic use of TCM

TCM is known to be helpful in the following conditions

- Obesity
- Diabetes and its complications
- High cholesterol
- Depression
- Arthritis
- Body pain
- Infertility
- Alzheimer's disease
- Parkinson's disease
- Digestive disorders such as irritable bowel syndrome
- Recurrent cystitis, inflammation of the bladder
- Nausea and vomiting and allergies
- Asthma, cancer, stroke
- Addictions, epilepsy, sleep problems
- Infections of menopausal symptoms
- Epilepsy, stress.

Tai Chi

- Tai Chi is a gentle exercise program that is a part of Traditional Chinese Medicine. It is derived from the martial arts, Tai Chi is composed of slow, deliberate movements, meditation and deep breathing, which enhance physical health and emotional well-being.
- Tai Chi is based on spiritual and philosophical ideas that advocate a need for balance in the body, mind and spirit. Central to Tai Chi is the idea that Qi or life energy, flows throughout the body. Qi must be able to move freely for good health. The principle for Yin/Yang forces in the universe, in the same way as light and dark. Tai Chi is meant to harmonize, these pairs of opposites. Finally, Tai Chi imitates motion found in nature, such as movement of animals, therapy uniting human beings with the natural world.

History

Zhang Sanfeng, a martial artist who lived in China in the late 16th century, created the practice of Tai Chi. According to legend, Sanfeng had a dream about a snake and a crane engaged in battle. Their graceful movements inspired his noncombative style of martial arts. This ancient form of movement has been practiced in China for centuries and is still a daily routine for tens of thousand of people there, especially the elderly.

Functioning of Tai Chi

There are various perspectives on how Tai Chi works. Eastern philosophy holds that Tai Chi unblocks the flow of Qi. When Qi flows properly, the body, mind and spirit are in balance and health is maintained. Others believe that Tai Chi works in the same way as other mind-body therapies and there is sample evidence that paying attention to the connection between the mind and the body can relieve stress, combat disease and enhance physical well being. Tai Chi has 3 major components... movement, meditation and deep breathing.

- *Movement:* All the major muscle groups and joints are needed for the slow, gentle movement in Tai Chi. It improves balance, agility, strength, flexibility, stamina, muscle tone and coordination. This low impact, weight bearing exercise strengthens bones and can slow bone loss, thus preventing the development of osteoporosis.
- *Meditation:* The newer research shows that meditation soothes the mind, enhance concentration, reduces anxiety and lowers blood pressure and heart rate.
- *Deep breathing:* Exhaling air and toxins from the lungs while inhaling a plentitude of fresh air increases lung capacity, stretches the muscles involved in breathing and releases tension. It also enhances blood circulation to the brain, which boots mental alertness. At the same time, the practice supplies the entire body with fresh oxygen and nutrients.

Tai Chi Session

Tai Chi practiced in a group. The session lasts for a hour. Each session begins with a warm-up exercise then the instructor guides the class through a series of 20-100 Tai Chi movements that together comprise a 'Form'. A form can take up to 20 minutes to complete. Each form has a nature-based name that describes its overall action... such as 'wave hands like cloud' or 'grasp the birds tail'. At the same time, participants are asked to focus on the point just below their navels, believed to be the center from which Gi flows. The instructor encourages the client to perform all movements in a slow, meditative manner and to focus on deep breathing. At the end of session, there is usually a wind down exercise, relaxation and meditation.

Therapeutic Benefits of Tai Chi

- Tai Chi improves overall fitness, coordination and agility. People who practice Tai Chi on a regular basis tend to have good posture, flexibility and range of motion, are more mentally alert and sleep more soundly at night.
- Tai Chi is both a preventive and complementary therapy for a wide range of conditions. Specifically, it is beneficial for chronic pain, gout, heart disease, high blood pressure, arthritis, osteoporosis, diabetes, headaches, fibromyalgia, rheumatoid arthritis, osteoarthritis, and sleep disorders. Tai Chi is also beneficial for the immune system and the central nervous system, which makes it especially good for people with a chronic illness, anxiety , viral virtual infections, depression, or any stress related disorder. The deep breathing of Tai Chi regulates the respiratory system, helping to treat respiratory ailments, such as asthma, bronchitis and emphysema. It also stimulates the abdomen, which aids in digestion and helps to relieve constipation and gastrointestinal conditions. Many clinical studies indicate that elderly people who practice Tai Chi has better hand-eye coordination and are much less prone to falls, both serious health risks to people in that age groups. Tai Chi is safe for example, regardless of age or athletic ability and can be modified for most health problems. People with limited mobility... even those in wheelchairs... can learn and successfully use Tai Chi.

UNANI MEDICINE

Unani medicine is based on the Greece philosophy. According to basic elements, i.e. earth, air, water, fire which have different temperaments, i.e. cold, hot, wet and dry. After mixing and interaction of four elements a new compound having new temperament comes into existence.

The simple and compound organs which got their nourishment through four humors, i.e. blood, phlegm, yellow bile, black bile. The humour also assigned temperament as blood is hot and wet, phlegm is cold and hot, yellow bile is hot and wet, phlegm is cold and dry. These principles and doctrines of this system. Both fundamental and applied, have a close similarity to Ayurveda with specialization in Iatro-chemistry. According to this system, the human body is the replica of the universe and so are the food and drugs irrespective of their origins.

HYPNOTHERAPY

The term 'hypnosis' derived from the Greek word 'hypnos' meaning 'sleep'. Hypno therapists be practice exercise that bring about deep relaxation and an altered state of consciousness, also known as trance. It helps to master his/her own awareness. By doing this, it affects bodily functions and psychological responses.

HISTORY

Throughout history, trance states have been used by Shamans and ancient peoples in rituals and religious ceremonies. The use of it was associated with the work of an Austrian physician named Franz Anton Mesmer. In 1700s, Mesmer believed that illnesses were caused by magnetic fields in the body getting out of balance. He used magnets and other hypnotic techniques to treat people.

FUNCTIONING OF HYPNOSIS

When something happens to us, we remember it and learn a particular behavior in response to what happened, each time something similar happens, our physical and emotional reactions attached to the memory are repeated. In some cases, these reactions are unhealthy. In some forms of hypotherapy, a trained therapist guides the client to remember the event that led to the first reaction, separate the memory from the learned behavior and replace unhealthy behavior with new, healthier one's.

During hypnosis, the body relaxes and thoughts become more focused. It lowers blood pressure and heart rate, and changes certain types of brain wave activity. In this relaxed state, the client feels at ease physically yet fully awake mentally and highly responsive to suggestions. In this time, the conscious mind becomes less alert and the subconscious mind becomes more focused.

Stages of Hypnosis

- Reframing the problem
- Becoming relaxed, then absorbed
- Dissociating (letting go of critical thoughts)
- Responding (compiling with a therapist suggestions)
- Returning to usual awareness
- Reflecting on the experience.

Therapeutic Benefits of Hypnosis

- Hypnosis is used in many variety of setting... from emergency rooms to dental treatment to OPD clinics. The clinical trial study suggests that hypnosis may improve immune function, increase relaxation, decrease stress and ease pain and feelings of anxiety.

- Clinical studies on children in emergency department show that it reduces fear, anxiety and discomfort.
- Other problems or conditions that may respond to hypnotherapy include:
  - Irritable bowel syndrome
  - Tension headaches/phobias/addictions
  - Bedwetting
  - Asthma/phobias
  - Labor and delivery
  - Skin disorder/stress
  - Tinnitus/wart
  - Eating disorder
  - Cancer related pain
- Indigestion (dyspepsia)

Risks Associated with Hypnotherapy

Before undergoing session, treat the treatable cause. If the condition is psychological in origin, treat it by medications and have a correct diagnosis. Without an accurate diagnosis, it could make your symptoms worse. Very rarely it leads to the development of 'false memories' made up by the unconscious mind; known as confabulations.

Massage Therapy

- Massage is a 'hands on' treatment in which a therapist manipulates the muscles and other soft tissues of the body to improve health and well being. Varieties of massages ranges from gentle stroking and kneading of muscles of other soft tissues to deeper techniques.
- Massage helps to relieve muscle tension, reduce stress and evoke feelings of calmness. It affects the whole body, it particularly influences the activity of the musculoskeletal, circulatory, lymphatic and nervous system.

Types of Massage

There are nearly 100 different massages and body work techniques. Each technique is uniquely designed to achieve a special goal. *These are:*

- *Aromatherapy massage:* Essential oils from plants are massaged into the skin to enhance the healing and relaxing effects of massage. Essential oils are believed to have powerful effects on mood by stimulating the deep structures in the brain known to store emotions and memory.
- *Craniosacral massage:* Gentle pressure applied to the head and spine to correct imbalance and restore the flow of cerebrospinal fluid in this areas.
- *Lymphatic massage:* Light rhythmic strokes are used to improve the flow of lymph throughout the body.
- *Myofascial massage:* Gentle pressure and body positioning are used to relax and stretch the muscle, fascia and related structures.
- *Onsite/chair massage:* On site massage therapists use a portable chair to deliver brief, upper body massage to fully clothed people in offices and other public places.
- *Polarity therapy:* A form of energy healing, polarity therapy stimulates and balances the flow of energy within in the body to enhance health and well being.

- *Reflexology:* Specialized thumb and finger techniques are applied to the hands and feet. Reflexologists believe that there are certain 'reflex points' or direct connection to specific organs and structures, throughout the body.
- *Rolfing:* Pressure is applied to the fascia (connective tissue) to stretch it, lengthen it and make more flexible. The goal of this technique is to realign the body, so that it conserves energy, releases tension and functions better.
- *Shiatsu:* Gentle finger and hand pressure are applied to specific points on the body to relieve pain and enhance the flow of energy (known as Qi) through the body's energy pathways (called meridians).
- *Sports massage:* It is often used on professional athletes and other active individuals. Sports massage can enhance performance and prevent and treat sports related injuries.
- *Swedish massage:* Here, a variety of strokes and pressure techniques are used to enhance the flow of blood to the heart, remove waste products from the tissue, stretch ligaments and tendons and ease physical and emotional tension.
- *Trigger point massage:* Pressure is applied to 'trigger point' (tender areas where the muscles have been damaged) to alleviate muscle spasms and pain.
- *Integrative touch:* A gentle form of massage therapy that uses gentle, noncirculatory techniques. It is designed to meet the needs of client who are hospitalized or in hospice care.
- *Compassionate touch:* It combines one-on-one focussed attention, intentional touch and sensitive massage with communication to enhance the quality of life for elderly ill or dying clients.

Functioning of Massage

For many centuries, human touch has been shown to be emotionally and physically beneficial. The particular massage technique may either stimulate or calm the body's muscles and tissues to create a desired effect. When a practitioner massage soft tissue, electrical signals are transmitted both to the local area and throughout the body, these signals, in combination with the healing properties of touch, help to heal damaged muscle, stimulate circulation, clear waste products via the lymphatic system, boost the activity of the immune system, reduce pain and tension and induce a calming effect. Massage may also enhance well being by stimulating the release of endorphins (natural painkillers and mood elevators) and reducing levels of certain stress hormones.

Therapeutic use of Massage

- In general, massage is believed to support healing, boost energy, reduce recovery time after an injury, ease pain and enhance relaxation, mood and well being. It is useful for many musculoskeletal problems, such as low back pain, osteoarthritis, fibromyalgia, sprains and strains. Massage may also relieve depression in people with chronic fatigue syndrome, ease chronic constipation, decrease swelling, alleviate sleep disorders and improve self image. In the work place, massage has been shown to melt away stress and enhance mental alertness.
- Clinical trial studies also show that massage may be an effective treatment for young children and adolescents with a wide range of health problems, including:
  - *Autism:* Autistic children, who usually do not like being touched, show less autistic behavior and are more social and attentive often receiving massage therapy.

- *Atopic dermatitis/eczema:* Children with this scaly, itchy skin problems seem to experience less rednes, scaling and other symptoms if receiving massage between flares. Massage should not be used when this skin conditions is activity inflamed.
- *Attention deficit hyperactivity disorder (ADHD):* Massage may improve mood in children with ADHD and help feel less fidgety and hyperactive.
- *Bulimia:* Research findings show that adolescents with bulimic feel less depressed and anxious after receiving massage therapy.
- *Cystic fibrosis:* Massage may reduce anxiety and improve respiration in children with this lung condition.
- *Diabetes:* Massage may help to regulate blood sugar levels and reduce anxiety and depression in children with diabetes.
- *Rheumatoid arthritis:* Children with juvenile rheumatoid arthritis (JRA) have been shown to experience less pain, morning stiffness and anxiety as a result of massage therapy.

Precautions

People with the following conditions should avoid massage:

- Heart failure
- Kidney failure
- Infection of the superficial veins
- Blood clots in the legs
- Bleeding disorders
- Contagious skin conditions.

OCCUPATIONAL THERAPY

Introduction

In its simplest terms, occupational therapist and occupational therapy assistants help people across the lifespan to participate in the things they want and need to do through therapeutic use of every day activities (occupation). Common interventions include helping children with disabilities to participate fully in school and social situations, helping people recovering from injury to regain skills and providing support for older adults experiencing physical and cognitive changes.

SERVICES OF OCCUPATIONAL THERAPY

- An individualized evaluation, during which the client, family and occupational therapist determine the person's goals.
- Customized interventions to improve the person's ability to perform daily activities and reach the goals.
- An outcome evaluation to ensure that the goals are being met and/or make changes to the intervention plan.
- Occupational therapy services may include comprehensive evaluations of the client's home and other environments (e.g. workplace, school), recommendations for adaptive equipment and training in its use and guidance and education for family members and caregivers. The practitioners have a holistic perspective, in which the focus is on adapting the environment to fit the person, and the person is an integral part of the therapy team.

Basic Principles of Occupational Therapy (OT)

- Occupational therapy treatment focuses on helping people to achieve independence in all areas of their lives. It can help kids with various needs to improve their cognitive, physical, motor skills and enhance their self esteem and sense of accomplishment.
- OT can evaluate children's skills for playing, school performance and daily activities and compare them with what is developmentally appropriate for that group.
- According to American Occupational Therapy Association (AOTA), in addition to dealing with an someone's physical well being, OT addresses psychological, social and environment factors that can affect functioning in different ways.

Indications

- Birth injuries or birth defects
- Sensory processing disorders
- Traumatic injuries (brain or spinal cord)
- Learning problems
- Autism/ pervasive developmental disorders
- Juvenile rheumatoid arthritis
- Mental health or behavioral problems
- Orthopedic injuries
- Depression
- Fear/panic
- Anger
- Apathy
- Suicidal behavior
- Denial
- Dependency
- Withdrawal.

When to Refer a Client to Psychiatric Occupational Therapy

Psychiatric clients should be referred whose daily living skills are impaired due to:

- Treatment/non compliance or resistance.
- Severe lack of motivation.
- Depressive symptoms, anhedonia, isolation, social withdrawal evidence, indifference, vegetative state, crying.
- **Adjustment reaction:** Depression, ruminating, reaction out of characters of patient, or out of proportion to physical insult, anger, hostility, blaming and treatment refusal.
- Overall, occupational therapy uses purposeful activities as a way of meeting a person's needs and provides for personal changes and growth. Creative media, such as clay, wood burning or painting are used to express creative needs or feelings and conflicts that a person is unable to express verbally. Activities, such as rug weaving or sanding provide outlets for the release of anger, hostility and frustration. The therapist also may focus on activities that improve living skills, such as grocery, shopping, cooking and self care.

ELECTROCONVULSIVE THERAPY

Introduction

Electroconvulsive therapy (ECT) is a form of shock therapy used to interrupt a client's current maladaptive pattern of thinking, feeling and behaving. It is an adjunctive somatic treatment that is most commonly utilized for agitation or for those who are actively suicidal. In essence, the procedure is undertaken to produce emotional regression of the client in time, thereby bringing about modification of the client's affective response and behavior. This effect is produced when an electrical current is applied to the brain through electrodes placed on the temporal areas of the skill which produce an artificially induced grand mal seizure. Its exact mechanism is uncertain but it is postulated that the electrical change includes a biochemical response.

The treatment is considered effective if the client begins to evidence a feeling of well being, ceases to be preoccupied with morbid ideation or is free from agitation. The outcome of this form of treatment permits the individual to be more accessible to others. This assessibility is observed when the client demonstrates a readiness to socialize and to engage in intensive psychotherapy.

Definitions

- Electroconvulsive therapy (ECT) is a procedure in which electric currents are passed through the brain, deliberately triggering a brief seizure.
- A procedure in which an electric current is passed through the brain to produce controlled convulsions (seizures) to treat patients with depression, particularly for those who cannot take or are not responding to antidepressants, have severe depression or are at high for suicide.
- ECT is a physical/somatic therapy in which with the help of electrodes, current is passed through the temporal region in between the two hemispheres of the brain to produce an artificial grand mal type of seizures.

History of ECT

- In 1500s, the Swiss physician Paracelsus induced seizures by administering camphor by mouth to treat psychiatric illness.
- **1785:** Used seizure to treat mania using camphor.
- **1934:** The Hungarian neuropathologist Ladislas Joseph non marijuna used convulsive therapy by using IM injection of camphor to treat catatonic schizophrenia.
- **1938:** Italian psychiatrist Lucino Bini and
- **1940:** Curatte used muscle relaxant in ECT
- **1950-51:** Succinylcholine was introduced during ECT
- **1978:** ECT ethics are introduced
- **1988:** ECT is used in mania
- **2000:** Sarah Lisanby and colleagues from Columbia university induced convulsive treatment with magnetic stimulation.

Indications

ECT is indicated in patients with major depressive disorder, bipolar disorder, schizophrenia and other disorders.

Major Depressive Disorder

ECT should be considered for client in the acute phase of major depressive disorder who have a high degree of symptoms, severity and functional impairment or who have psychotic symptoms or catatonia.

ECT may be treatment of choice for clients in whom treatment response is urgently needed such as client who are suicidal or those refusing food and nutritionally compromised.

Bipolar Disorder

- ECT may be considered for client with severe or treatment resistant manic or mixed episodes of bipolar disorder.
- In severe mania or depression during pregnancy. Depression/mania with suicidal thought/ attempts.
- Clients who are resistant to antidepressants.

Schizophrenia

- Acute schizophrenia, severe psychosis that has not responded for clients whose acute episode of depression responds to treatment with antipsychotic medication. The greatest therapeutic benefit appears to occur when ECT is administered concurrently with antipsychotic medication. It may also be considered for clients with prominent catatonic features that have not responded to lorazepam.
- ECT is choice for comorbid depression.

Other Psychotic Disorders

- Schizophreniform disorder.
- Schizoaffective disorder.

Comorbid Disorder

- Obsessive compulsive disorder (OCD)
- Mania
- Schizophrenia in client with OCD
- Catatonia
- Neurological malignant syndrome
- Parkinson syndrome
- Pain in delirium.

Contraindications

- ECT has no absolute contraindications. Many medical conditions place clients at an increased risk for complications and warrant closer monitoring.
- Recent MI/coronary ischemia/CHF.
- Cerebral tumor or aneurysm/cerebral infraction/hemorrhage/seizure disorder/severe respiratory failure.

Relative Contraindications

Pregnancy
Thyrotoxiosis
Cardiac dysrhythmias
Glaucoma
Retinal detachment.

Mechanism of Action

ECT induces many physiopsychological changes. ECT affects catecholamine pathways between diencephalon and limbic system causing generalized seizures by increasing the threshold. Thus, causing down regulation of beta receptors in the cortex and hypothalamus.

Technique of ECT

The technique used for ECT administration are of two types.

a. *Direct ECT:*
  - Direct ECT is administered in the absence of muscle relaxant and general anesthesia. Here only injection atropine 0.6 mg (IV/1m/s c) administered half an hour before ECT.
  - Grand mal seizures are induced by passing electric current through the temporal lobe.

b. *Modified ECT:*
  - Modified ECT includes the use of anesthesia, muscle relaxant and oxygenation.
  - Anesthetic medications include methohexital (barbiturate), thiopental (barbiturate) and etomidate propranolol (non-barbiturate) are used commonly. The cognitive outcome after ECT may be affected by the choice of the anesthetic medication. The use of anesthesia is to decrease anxiety and to achieve maximum effects. It is used to modify force of convulsion and to avoid complications like bone fracture.

Common Drugs used in ECT

- *Atropine:* (0.5–0.6 mg) is given IV before the treatment or given S/C or 1M 30 minutes, before treatment. It is administered to decrease oral secretions and to prevent vagal stimulation during ECT which may cause cardiac arrests.
- *Anesthetic agents:* Propofol (0.75 mg/kg) and thiopentone (1.5–2.5 mg/kg) are an anti convulsant, thus it decreases the duration of seizures.
- *Muscle relaxants:* Succinylcholine (0.75–1.5 mg/kg) is a depolarizing blocking agent. Its administration is followed by muscle relaxation which starts from above to downwards, when the fine twitching movement disappear, it is a time of muscle relaxation. It reduces intense muscle contraction associated with ECT.

PLACEMENT OF ELECTRODES

- *Bilateral ECT:* Most commonly used ECT. It involves the placement of electrodes on bitemporal region. An imaginary line is drawn from outer canthus of eye to the targus of ear. Midpoint of imaginary line is located and electrode placed at one inch above the mid point.
- *Unilateral ECT:* In unilateral ECT, electrodes are placed on one side of the head usually on the non dominating side. It is better with lesser side effects particularly those of memory impairment.
- *Amount of current used in ECT:* The usual dose of electricity is 70–150 volts for 0.1–1 second average is 0.5–0.6 seconds. The usual amount of current passed is 200–1600 millivolts.

PHASES

- *Tonic phase:* In this phase, muscles in body that have not been paralyzed contract for a period of 5–15 seconds.
- *Clonic phase:* It is characterized by movement or convulsion and last for 25–30 seconds. There is slow planter and fine movement of toes during clonic phase.

Reflexes

- *In tonic phase:* Blapharospasm a tonic spasm of eye lid muscles is observed when current is applied; and mild grimace.
- *In clonic phase:* Babinski reflex – slow planter flexion during tonic phase and fine movement of toes in clonic phase and planter flexion.

Number and frequency

- *Depression:* Client shows response after few ECT and peak response after 10–12 ECT.
- In bipolar disorder (manic type) schizo-affective or catatonic schizophrenia, peak response is shown after 5–10 ECT.
- In chronically ill schizophrenia peak response is shown after 20–25 treatment.
- Usually, ECT is administered 3 times a week; however the frequency of treatment can be reduced if client shows a severe confusional state, in case of suicidal, it can be on daily basis.

Complications

- *Amnesia:* Retrograde and antergrade.
- Memory loss and confusion.
- Fractures and dislocations.
  - Compression, fracture of dorsal area between 2nd and 8th usually of 3rd, 4th and 5th is very common.
  - Fracture of femur and humerus.
  - Dislocation of jaw and rarely fracture of acetabulum.
- *Apnea:* Apnea is a physiological phenomena. It can be prevented keeping clean, prevent collection of secreations and turning head to outside and if it prolongs, artificial respiration is applied.
- *Other complications:*
  - Headache.
  - Fear due to unpleasant procedure.
  - Backache.
  - Injury to mouth and tongue.

Stuns or Subshocks

Subshocks occur due to insufficient current applied which does not result in full convulsive stage. These stuns sometimes produce cardiac irregularities, respiratory distress and collapse, confusion due to subshock is more marked than after ECT fit. It 3 subshock given on same day, then treatment must be stopped and next day ECT is given with increased intensity. If current is given with more intensity then it leads to intracranial damage.

Pretreatment Evaluation

- Informed consent.
- Detailed medical and psychiatric history.
- General and systematic physical examination.

- Routine laboratory investigations (HB, ESR, DLC, urine routine, ECG, chest X-rays)
- Others like EEG and plasma proteins, cholinesterase.
- Examination of fundus oculi to rule out papilledema.

Role of Nurse

- It is important that client should not hear or see anything before or after treatment.
- In hospital setting where ECT is given nurse should do set up which includes:
  - Waiting room.
  - Treatment room.
  - Recovery room and after care room.

Waiting Room

- Room should be calm with dim lights and light color of walls.
- Decorate/put some flowers to give pleasant feeling to client.
- There should be magazine so that client can divert his mind and reduce anxiety.
- Lavatory should be attached, because client needs to empty his bowel and bladder before treatment.
- Nurse should be available to clear the doubts regarding.

Treatment Room/ECT Room

- It should have low level bed with railings for comfort of client, railing should be well padded to avoid injury to client during convulsions.
- Articles required for ECT are:
  - ECT machine: Check all the plugs are in working conditions.
  - Normal saline to clear temporal region and also to dip electrodes.
  - Endotracheal tube.
  - Sterile suction catheters.
  - Mouth wipes and cotton balls.
  - Emergency drugs.
  - Sterile syringes 2cc, 5cc, 10cc.
  - Ambu bag, BP apparatus. Tongue depressor.
  - Kidney tray and paper bag.
  - Mouth gag.

Recovery Room

- Once client responds to painful stimuli, he/she is transferred to recovery room.
- A floor bed with 1 to 1 padding should be kept ready.
- Observation and monitoring of vital signs.
- Mouth wipe to clear secretions.
- Extra clothes.

Nursing Interventions before Administering ECT

- Check all the investigations–routine and lab.
- Take written consent–explain the procedure.

- Client should be kept NPO (at least 2 to 3 hours before ECT).
- Remove all metallic articles (watch, bangles, jewellery).
- Remove artificial dentures/lipstick/nail polish or any make up.
- Loosen the tight clothes.
- Encourage client to empty his/her bowel and bladder.
- Administer pre-medications as prescribed.
- Transfer the client to waiting room.

Nursing Interventions During ECT

- The client is transferred on a trolley from a waiting room to ECT room and placed in a wheel padded comfortable dorsal position or supine position, small pillow can be kept under lumbar curve.
- Administer anesthetic agent, thiopentone 2.5 mg/kg and succinylcholine 0.75–1.5mg/kg.
- Well padded mouth gag or tongue depressor is placed between the teeth.
- Support the shoulder and arms tightly, restrain the thigh with the help of sheet.
- Hyper extension of head with support to chin by nurse.
- Provide electrodes dipped in saline water or jelly for placing on temporal region.
- Make an observation of granular seizures. The initial tonic stage which lasts for 10–5 seconds followed by convulsions casting for 25 to 30 seconds.
- Do suction immediately.
- Restore respiration by giving oxygen by mask.

Nursing Interventions After ECT

- Observe and record vital signs.
- Put on the railings and place client on a side lying position, wipe the secretions.
- Transfer client to recovery room only when the client answers to simple question like 'open your mouth'.
- Record vital signs every 15 minutes, once client is stable record every half an hour till full recovery.
- Allow the client to sleep for a hour.
- Reassure the client.
- Reorient the client to ward and other settings.
- Make a note of any injuries or complications of pain by client such as body pain and headache.
- Encourage client to go for shower bath and change clothes.
- Allow the client to drink tea followed by breakfast to carry out daily activities.

Schizophrenia and Psychotic Disorders

Psychotic disorders are a group of major serious illnesses that affect the mind and body. These illnesses alter a person's biopsychosocial setup. When psychotic symptoms are severe, claim loose touch with reality and unable to sustain the demands of daily life. However, these are treated by multiple modalities.

SCHIZOPHRENIA

Schizophrenia is considered as main iconic disease of mind. It is a chronic, severe and disabling brain disorder that has affected people throughout the ages. Schizophrenia is a brain disorder that affects a person's ability to perceive the world and to process information. Although schizophrenia is a serious and chronic illness, it can be well treated and rehabilitated to live independently, work and lead normal lives. The advancement in psychiatry has contributed for attainment of meaningful recovery. It is always associated with multiple, complex symptoms, can be termed as a group of disorders.

Schizophrenia affects thinking and psychomotor functions. The client exhibits altered perception of reality, often a significant code of contact with real world. They may hear or see things that do not exist, speak in strange or confusing ways, believes that others are trying to harm them; or fell like they are being constantly watched and monitored. With such a blurred line between the real and the imaginary, schizophrenia makes it difficult ever frightening, to negotiate the activities of daily life. In response, they withdraw themselves from the external world and act out in confirm and fear.

Historical Background

- The word schizophrenia is derived from two Greek words 'schizo'-means to split and 'phren'-means 'mind'. It was found in Ayurveda as long as 1400 BC in the 1st century 4D.
- A French psychiatrist Benedict Moral (1856–1976) formed the term 'demence precoce' to describe deteriorated client whose illness began in adolescence.
- Email Krapeline (1856-1976) as of the founders of modern psychiatry, described 'dementia a praecox', a term that emphasized the change in cognition (dementia) and early onset (precox as a distinct illness were categorized as 'madness'.
- Eugen Bleuler (1857–1939) a Swiss psychiatrist, coined the term 'schizophrenia' and described the symptoms of schizophrenia as positive or negative. He emphasized that schizophrenia consisted of a group of disorders rather than being a distinct entity. Bleuler identified fundamental symptoms of schizophrenia, popularly known as 4As as essential things.

- Association defects or loosening in the logical relationship among thought.
- Affective disturbances like inadequate (blunted or flat) or in appreciate.
- Autism a form of thinking and behavior that is abnormally idiosyncratic and narcissistic.
- Ambivalence-coexistence of two contradictory thought.
- In 1959, Kurt Schneider described certain symptoms of schizophrenia.
- Henri Laborit (1914–1995), a Parisian surgeon, used chlorpromazine (thorazine) in the treatment of schizophrenia.
- In 1970's–Assertive community treatment act was passed to deliver quantity based psychiatric care.
- 1979: The National alliance on mental illness was developed as an advocacy group for people with mental illness and their families. It lobbied for the rights of mentally ill and made great contribution for reducing the stigma of illness.
- The decade of the brain (2000 onwards) put more emphasis on brain research. Use of new research tools (FMRI) helped in know the processes of emotion and experience.
- During 1990's–Atypical antipsychotics like alanzapine, respiridone and quetiapine were developed, when posed less nasal for extrapyramidal side effects than first generation antipsychotics.

Definitions

- WHO defines schizophrenia as 'a severe mental disorder that affects thinking, language, perception and sense of self and often includes hearing voice or delusions.
- ICD- 10 defines' schizophrenia is characterized in general by fundamental and characteristic distortion of thinking, perception and inappropriate or blunted affect. Delusion are bizarre in nature. Auditory hallucinations are common. Thinking is vague and speech sometimes – incomprehensive. Mood is characteristically shallow and incongruous, ambivalence, negativism, stupor or catatonia maybe present. The onset maybe acute or insidious with a seriously disturbed behavior.
- Elizabeth Drew (2010) defines schizophrenia is a psychosis disorder characterized by loss of contact with the environment, by noticeable deterioration in the level of functioning in everyday life, and by disintegration of personality expressed as disorder of feelings thought (as delusion), perception (as hallucinations) and behavior.

EPIDEMIOLOGY OF SCHIZOPHRENIA

Schizophrenia is a chronic, severe and disabling brain disorder that has affected people globally throughout history. Approximately, 1% of the population develops during their lifetime. It affects men and women with equal frequency, the disorder often appears earlier in man, usually in late teens or early twenties, than in women.

The current epidemiological statistic show that

- *Incidence:* 10–20 per lakh population per year.
- *Prevalence:* 1–1.2%
- *Age of onset:* Adolescence or early adulthood.
- *Gender ratio:* Equal
- *Others:* Enhanced in winter births, low birth and low socioeconomic status.

Other Facts

According to WHO report (2009) schizophrenia affecting about 7 per thousand of adult population, mostly in the age group 15 to 35 years, though the incidence is low (3–10,000), the prevalence is high due to chronicity.

Facts

- It affects about 24 million people worldwide.
- Schizophrenia is a treatable disorder, treatment being more effective in its initial stages.
- More than 50% of person with schizophrenia are not receiving appropriate care.
- Ninety percent of people with untreated schizophrenia are in developing countries.
- Care of persons with schizophrenia can be provided at community level, with active family and community involvement.

Common Misconceptions about Schizophrenia

- *Myth:* Schizophrenia refers to a "split personality" or multiple personalities.
  Fact: Multiple personality disorder is a different and much less common disorder than schizophrenia. People with schizophrenia do not have split personalities. Rather they are 'split off' from reality.
- *Myth:* Schizophrenia is a rear condition.
- *Fact:* Schizophrenia is not rare; the life time rise of developing schizophrenia is widely accounted to be around 1 to 100.
- *Myth:* People with schizophrenia are dangerous.
- *Fact:* Although the delusional thoughts and hallucinations of schizophrenia sometimes lead to violent behavior, most people with schizophrenia are able to enjoy life and function with their families.

RISK FACTORS

Schizophrenia is the most common psychotic condition

- *Age:* Schizophrenia can occur at any age, but it tends to first develop (or at list become evident) between adolescence and young adulthood. Schizophrenia in children is likely to be severe. It declines with age, its incidence has been tend to be peak in those who are about 45 years old, and again in people who are in their mid-60s (mostly older). Late onset schizophrenia that devolves in the 40s is most likely to be the paranoid with fewer negative symptoms or learning impairment.

Gender

Schizophrenia affects both men and women, there are some differences:

- Men tend to develop schizophrenia between the ages of 15–24, paranoid schizophrenia is very common in men and symptoms tend to be more severe.
- The onset in women is usually slightly later, between ages 25–34, and the symptoms tend to be less severe. The earlier a girl starts menstruations the longer she is protected against schizophrenia. It is more severe during a woman's menstrual cycle when estrogen levels are low. These findings and other evidence suggest that estrogen may have protecting properties, for example, the higher the estrogen levels in female with schizophrenia the better their mental function.

Intelligence

People with schizophrenia span the full range of intelligence. In fact, some studies reported that a higher than expected number of people who developed schizophrenia had been intellectually gifted children. Research suggested that, a decline in IQ score during childhood maybe sign of potential psychotic symptoms in adults.

Cultural and Geographic

No cultural or geographic group is immune from schizophrenia, although the course of the disease seems to be more severe in developed countries. However, the content of delusions may vary depending on a person's culture.

Socioeconomic Factors

Schizophrenia occurs twice as often in unmarried and divorced people as in married or widowed individuals. Furthermore, people with schizophrenia are eight times more likely to be in the risk of schizophrenia.

Famine and Malnutrition

Prenatal malnutrition may also play a role in the development of schizophrenia. Research studies found that people who are born during times of famine are more than twice as likely to develop schizophrenia as those born during years of adequate food. The association between famine and schizophrenia illustrates low environmental and biologic factors are connected. For example, research shown that malnourished mother may not get enough folic acid (folate) in their diet. Folate deficiency may cause genetic mutations in the developing that can lead to schizophrenia.

Other Factors Related to Schizophrenia

- *Being left or mixed handed:* The rate of left handedness or mixed handedness is significantly higher among patients with schizophrenia than the general population. This suggests that the importance new logic pattern that may be responsible for schizophrenia.
- *Obsessive-compulsive disorder:* It affects a significant number of schizophrenia climb. It is assumed that the behaviors exhibited in the disorder may actually be protective in people with schizophrenia in early stages.
- *Behavioral and motor problems in childhood:* Children who later develop schizophrenia often suffer from certain problem such as excessive shyness or minor physical and motor control problems.
- *Father's age:* According to recent research findings, the older a father is when a child is born, the greater the risk is of schizophrenia in his offspring, perhaps because of a greater chance of genetic mutations in the sperm that can be passed on.
- *Epilepsy:* A family history of epilepsy increase the chance for developing schizophrenia or similar psychotic features twine two epilepsy and schizophrenia may share similar genetic or environmental factor.

CAUSES/ETIOLOGY OF SCHIZOPHRENIA

The exact causes of schizophrenia still need research. Multiple factors play a role in the cause.

Genetics

- The research in genetics related to schizophrenia has shown a significant component. It occurs in 10% of people who have a first degree relative. People who have second degree relatives with the disease also prone for schizophrenia. The rise is greater if both biological parents have schizophrenia. The rise is higher for an identical twin of a person with schizophrenia.
- Genetic theory features that, several genres are responsible for schizophrenia. Recent findings shown that schizophrenia tend to have higher rates of rare genetic differences involve hundreds of different genes and probably decreased brain development. The current research evidence suggests there are a multiple of genetic abnormalities involved in schizophrenia, possibly originating from one or two changes in genetic expression. Probably, the genes involved are neuregulin-1 gene and the COMT gene.

Biochemical Theories

Neuroscientists postulate that an imbalance, in the complex, interrelated chemical sections of the brain involving the neurotransmitters dopamine and glutamate and possibly others, also plays a role in schizophrenia.

NEUROTRANSMITTER THEORY/DOPAMINE THEORY

- Dopamine theory postulates that hypo and hyper secretion of dopamine compound in the brain can causes positive symptoms.
- *Serotonin theory:* This theory explains the increased level of serotonin in both positive and negative symptoms of schizophrenia.
- *Norepinephrine:* Deregulation of norepinephrine exposes fundamental defects in the functioning of dopamine or other neurotransmitter systems repair increase (in paranoid) decrease in (chromic schizophrenia) or defective levels of norepinephrine.
- *GABA:* Gama amino butyric acid is believed to be inversely related to dopamine activity in the brain. The loss of inhibitory GABA neurons leads to the inadequately of the dopaminergic neurons.
- *Glutamate:* Glutamate is another important neurotransmitter implicated in schizophrenia. Research shown that the underactivity of glutamate in schizophrenic can be the cause. This evidence for dopamine theory, because dopamine receptors inhibit the release of glutamate.

Brain Abnormalities

- Individuals with schizophrenia have structural differences in their brains compared to individuals without the disorder. Enlarged brain ventricles are observed in some schizophrenia, indicating a deficit in the volume of brain tissue. There is also evidence of abnormality.
- Low activity in the frontal lobe, hippocampus and amygdalae are connected to schizophrenia positive symptoms.
- Autopsy studies of schizophrenia have revealed differences in the brain. Researchers formed small changes in the distribution or characteristics of brain cells that likely occurred before birth. Some researchers assume that problem during brain development before birth may lead to family connections. The problem may not be seem till puberty. The brain undergoes major changes during puberty and these changes could trigger psychotic symptoms.

Environmental Theory

Environmental stressors and trauma, when may include exposure to certain toxic substances, may trigger the development of schizophrenia in those who are predisposed to the disorder.

Family Theory

Double Bind Theory

- This theory explains a hypothetical family in which children receive two or more conflicting and incomplete parental messages about their behaviors, attitudes and feelings. For example, the parent who told the child to outdoors for playing and scolds the child for dirty clothes.
- Marital schism and skew: This theory describes the family pattern. In schism one parent is overly attached to child of opposite gender and in skewed relationship says power struggle between the parents and resulting dominance of one parent.
- Pseudomutual and pseudohostile families: Some families express emotional expression by consistently using pseudomutual or pseudohostile verbal communication. The child from such families may find difficulty in relating with others because child communication maybe incomprehensive to outsiders.
- *Expressed emotions:* Family members and caregivers of schizophrenic clients behave with over criticism and hostility. Many research studies reflect that replace rate is higher for schizophrenia in such families.

Social Theories

- *Low social economic status:* Low income class leads to schizophrenia caused by social conditions.
- *Social isolation:* Social withdrawal leads to disease.
- *Premorbid personality trait:* The premorbid personality of individuals who develops schizophrenia are often described as suspicious, introverted, withdrawn and eccentric.

Learning Theories

- The learning theory describes that children who late have schizophrenic learn irrational reactions and ways of thinking by imitating parents who have their own significant emotional problems.
- The poor interpersonal relations and illegal, unethical relations of persons with schizophrenia develop because of poor models for learning during childhoods.

Psychological Theories

- Sigmund Freud postulated ego defect in schizophrenic client. Ego disintegration represents a return to the time. When ego was not yet or had not begin to establish. For example, fixation at oral stage of development. This fixation produces defects in ego development and Freud postulated that such defects contributed to symptoms of schizophrenia. Defects in ego will affects reality testing and control of inner drives.
- According to Sullivan, schizophrenia is a disturbance in interpersonal relatedness. It is an adaptive method to avoid panic, terror and disintegration of his sense of self.
- Erickson's theory says schizophrenia develops when there is fixation at the stage trust vs mistrust.

TYPES/CLASSIFICATION OF SCHIZOPHRENIA

ICD–10 classifies schizotypal disorder persistent delusional disorder, acute and transient psychotic disorder, induced delusional disorder and schizoaffective disorder together with schizophrenia.

ICD–10 Classification of Schizophrenia

- F20-29 Schizophrenia, schizotypal and delusional disorders.
- F 20 Schizophrenia
- F21 Schizotypal disorder
- F22 Persistent delusional disorders
- F23 Acute and transient psychotic disorders
- F24 Induced delusional disorder
- F25 Schizoaffective disorder
- F28 Other nonorganic psychiatric disorders
- F29 Unspecified nonorganic psychosis.

DSM IVTR classified schizophrenia as

- Paranoid schizophrenia
- Disorganized schizophrenia
- Unidentified schizophrenia
- Residual schizophrenia.

Subtypes of Schizophrenia

Paranoid Schizophrenia

- It is characterized by prominent hallucination, and delusions and or in conspicuous affective symptoms.
- Delusion of persecution, references, grandeur, control, infidelity or jealousy are mainly seen symptoms.
  Delusions are well systematized.
  Disturbance of affect, volition, speech and motor behavior.
  Client maybe apprehensive and personality disorientation.
  Impairment in thinking, speech, behavioral organization and emotional expressiveness.

Disorganized/Hebephrenic Schizophrenia

- Main symptoms include disorganized speech and behavior, lack of emotional expression and difficulties in performing daily activities.
- Marked thought disorder, incoherence and severe loosening of association.
- Delusion and hallucination are fragmentary and changeable.
- Client are verbally incoherent and exhibit strange or bizarre behaviors.
- Emotional disturbances (inappropriate affects and blunted affects or senseless giggling) mannerisms, minor gazing for long period of time.
- Poor self-care and hygiene, marked impaired social and occupational functioning, extreme social withdrawal and other oddities of behaviors.

- ICD–10 recommends a period of 2 to 3 months of continuous observation for a confident diagnosis of hebephrenic schizophrenia.
- It has worst prognosis among all the subtypes of schizophrenia.

Catatonic Schizophrenia

- 'Cata' means 'disturbed', 'tonic' means 'tone', i.e. Marked disturbance of motor behavior.
- Catatonia maybe excited and stuporous catatonia.

Excited Schizophrenia

- Increase in psychomotor activity ranging from restlessness, agitation, excitement, aggressiveness to violent behavior.
- Increase in pressure of speech with increase, spontaneity, loosening of association and frank incoherence.
- The excitement, lack relationship with the environment instead inner stimuli influence excited behavior it is not goal directed behavior.
- Sometimes, excitement is accompanied by rigidity, hyperthermia and dehydration leading to death. This stage is called as lethal/pernicious catatonia.

Stuporous Catatonia

- Extreme psychomotor retardation.
- Characteristic catatonic signs are mutism, rigidity, negativism, posturing, stupor, echolalia, echopraxia, waxy flexibility and ambitendency.
- Delusions and hallucinations maybe present but not prominent.
- Not all the features are present at the same time.

Catatonia Alternatively between Excited and Stupor

Residual and Latent Schizophrenia

- Both are similar. But only difference is that residual schizophrenia is diagnosed after at least one episode has occurred.
- Mainly negative symptoms, i.e. psychomotor slowing, under activity, blunting of affect, passivity and lack of initiative, poverty of quantity or content of speech, poor nonverbal communication by facial expression, eye contact, voice modulation and posture, poor-self care and social performance.
- Marked evidence in the past of at least one definite psychotic episode fulfilling the diagnostic criteria for schizophrenia.
- A period of at least one year during which the intensity and frequency of florid symptoms such as delusions and hallucination have been minimal or substantially reduced and the negative schizophrenia syndrome has been present.

Undifferentiated Schizophrenia

- It is very common schizophrenia.
- This is characterized by episodes of two or more of the following symptoms. Delusions, hallucinations, disorganized speech or behavior, catatonic behavior or negative symptoms, but the individual does not qualify for a diagnosis of paranoid, disorganized or catatonic type of schizophrenia.

Simple Schizophrenia

- It is an uncommon disorder without hallucinations or delusions; characterized by mainly negative symptoms without preceding psychosis.
- It is very difficult to diagnose.
- Early onset (2nd decade) is very insidious and progressive course, presence of characteristic negative symptoms, vague hypochondrical feature, a drift down in social ladder, living shabbily and wandering aimlessly.
- Delusion and hallucinations are usually absent and if present, they are long lasting and poorly systematized. The prognosis is very poor.

Postschizophrenia Depression

- Some clients develop depressive clinical symptoms within a year of an acute episode of schizophrenia.
- The depressive features develop in the presence of residual or active features of schizophrenia and are associated with an increased risk of suicide.
- Depressive symptoms can occur due to side effects of antipsychotics, regaining insight after recovery is an integral part of schizophrenia.

CLINICAL FEATURES OF SCHIZOPHRENIA

- A specific characteristic of schizophrenia is deterioration from a previous level of functioning. Family or friends may note that the person is 'not the same' the person with schizophrenia experiences disturbances in thinking, feeling and behavior. Noticeable distortions occur in each of these areas. During active phase of illness, the client is usually psychotic (out of touch with reality) in behavior.
- The new research indicates that symptoms in childhood strongly predict disease in adulthood. In one prospective study, over 40% of people with schizophrenia who developed the disease in young adulthood had reported psychotic symptoms by age 11. For children with a family history of schizophrenia the following inherited traits maybe warning signs.
  - Deficits in working (short-term) and verbal memory.
  - Impairments in gross motor skills.
  - Attention deficits
  - A decline in verbal memory, IQ, and other mental functions.

Engen Bleuler is well known for describing the symptoms of schizophrenia as the 'four, as' they include the following.

- *Ambivalence:* The existing of opposing emotions, such as love and hate, at the same time.
- *Autism:* Preoccupation with self.
- *Associative looseness:* Words and thoughts shift from one subject to another in an unrelated manner.
- *Affect:* Blunting or dulling of mood in a manner that is incongruous with what is going on at the time.

Thought and Speech Disorders

Fragmented thinking is a characteristic of schizophrenia. Externally, it can be observed in the way a person speaks. Peoples with schizophrenia tend to have trouble in concentrating and maintain a train of thought. They may respond to queries with an unrelated feedback, start sentences with one topic and end somewhere with illogical thoughts.

Common clinical signs and symptoms of disorganized speech in schizophrenia include:

- *Autistic thinking.*
- *Loosening of association:* Rapidly shifting from one topic to another, with no connection between them.
- *Thought blocking*
- *Neologisms:* Cooked up words or sentences or phases that have only meaning to the client.
- *Echolalia*
- *Preservation:* Repetition of words and sentences saying the same things again and again.
- Delusion
- *Delusion of persecution:* False belief that others are out get her/him. These delusions often involve bizarre ideas and plots (e.g. My wife has put poison in lunch).
- *Delusion of reference:* A neutral environment event is believed to have a special and personal meaning. For example, a person with schizophrenia might believe a billboard or a person on TV is sending a message meant specially for them.
- *Delusion of grandeur:* A false belief that one is a famous or important figure, such as God or King, alternately. Delusion of grandeur may involve the belief that one has unusual power that no one else has (e.g. the ability to fly or forecast).

Delusion of Control

It is a false belief that one's thoughts or actions are being controlled by outsider, alien forces. Common delusions of control include thought broadcasting and thought withdrawal.

- Over inclusion
- Impaired abstraction
- Impulsiveness, violence, suicide and homicide.

Disorders of Perception

- Hallucinations
- Elementary auditory hallucination
- Thought echo
- Third person hallucination
- Voices commenting on one's action.

Auditory hallucinations (e.g. Hearing voices or some other sound) are most common in schizophrenia. Visual hallucinations are also common. The research suggests that auditory hallucinations occur when people misinterpret their own inner self-talk as coming from outside sources. Hallucinations are usually meaningful to the person experiencing them. Many times, the voices are those of someone they know. Most commonly, the voices are critical, vulgar or abusive in nature. Hallucinations also tend to worse when the person is alone.

Disorder of Affect

- Apathy
- Emotional blunting
- Emotional shallowness

- Anhedonia
- Inappropriate emotional response.

Disorders of Motor Behavior

- Increased or decreased psychomotor activity
- Mannerisms
- Stereotypes
- Decreased self-care.

Positive Symptoms

- Delusions
- Hallucinations
- Illusions
- Bizzare behavior
- An exaggeration of distortion of normal function.

Negative Symptoms

Negative symptoms are associated with disruptions to normal emotions and behaviors. These are harder to recognize as part of the disorder. These include:

- *Flat affect:* It is the reduction in the range and intensity of emotional expression, including facial expression, voice tone, eye contact and is not able to interpret body language nor use appropriate body language.
- *Anhedonia:* Lack of pleasure in everyday life.
- Lack of ability to begin and sustain planned activities.
- *Alogia:* Difficulties with speech. Inability to carry a conversation, short and sometimes disconnected replies to question and lessening of fluency.
- *Avolition:* Lack of interest or enthusiasm: no ability to pursue goal driven activities
- Attention impairment
- Lack of ability to begin sustain planned activities
- Speaking little, even when force to interact.

Disorganized Behavior

Schizophrenia disrupts goal directed activity, causing impairments in a person's ability to take care of him/her at work and interact with others. Disorganized behavior look as a decline in overall daily functioning, unpredictable or inappropriate emotional responses, behaviors that appear bizarre and have no purpose and lack of inhibition and impulse control.

Cognitive Impairments

- Impaired judgment
- Poor or absence of insight
- Partially reliable.

Other Comorbidity

- Obesity
- Diabetes mellitus

- Cardiovascular disease
- HIV
- Rheumatoid arthritis.

Diagnosis and Tests

A schizophrenia client is classified as someone who experiences two or more of the classical symptoms for a significant portion of time during a one month period. However, only one of the classical symptoms needs to be present if delusions are bizarre or hallucinations consists of a voice keeping a running commentary on the client behavior or thoughts. Beyond this, two more criteria must be met; the client also has difficulty to maintain employment, relationships or academic achievements upon the onset of the disease and continuous signs of disturbances persist beyond six months.

The tests for schizophrenia include routine investigations blood tests, MRI or CT scan, are meant to rule out physical trauma and other possible mental disorder and ascertain the clients, delusion were not induced by alcohol or other psychoactive substance. Individual response to treatment some are able to live productive lives if they stick to treatment plan, it requires hospitalization. Treatment involves a combination of medication and psychosocial intervention.

Diagnostic Evaluation

Diagnosis carried out on the basis of detailed history, MSE and psychological tests.

MANAGEMENT OF SCHIZOPHRENIA

As there is no definite cause of schizophrenia, treatment also has multiple approaches. It can help to reduce and alternate symptoms in most cases. Although each client responds to treatment differently. Some individuals respond to treatment differently, some are able to liver, productive lives if they stick to treatment plan. It requires hospitalization and psychosocial interventions.

MEDICAL MANAGEMENT

Main treatment modality requires drug/pharmacological in the form of antipsychotic medication. Drug treatment is effective in about 90% of acute cases. Positive symptoms respond better than negative symptoms to drugs.

Somatic/Drug Treatment

Antipsychotic drugs are the most commonly used drugs. These help to relieve the positive symptoms of schizophrenia by helping to correct an imbalance in the chemicals that enable brain cells to communicate with each other. It takes 3 to 4 weeks for results.

Typical Antipsychotics (Traditional/Conventional)

- Chlorpromazine (CP2) 300–1500 Mg/day
- Haloperidol 5–100 Mg/day
- Pimozide 4–12 Mg/day
- Triflupromazine 100–400 Mg/day

Atypical Antipsychotics

- Clozapine 25–450 Mg/day
- Risperidone 2–8 Mg/day
- Olanzapine 5–20 Mg/day
- Ziprasidone 40–160 Mg/day

ELECTROCONVULSIVE THERAPY (ECT)

- ECT can be a choice of treatment in case of catatonic stupor, excitement, acute exacerbation not controlled by drugs. Severe side effects of drugs in presence of untreated schizophrenia.
- Usually 8 to 10 ECTs are administered, three times a week.

PSYCHOSOCIAL REHABILITATION (PSR)

- Individual with schizophrenia often struggle in one or more of the following areas: communication, interpersonal relationships, motivation, daily routine activities, managing their illness and vocational issues.
- Psychosocial treatments include individual group or family therapy, vocational training and rehabilitation education and support or self-help groups (SHG).
- Psychoeducation.
- Milieu therapy
- Psychosocial rehabilitation is founded on the belief that people with schizophrenia or any severe mental illness are key in designing their own plan for rehabilitation. It is aim to increase the functioning of people with psychiatric disabilities and their satisfaction with their lives, with the least amount of professional interventions.

OTHER MEDICATIONS

Mood Stabilizer Medication

Lithium (lithobid), divalproex (depakote) carbamazepine (tegretol) and lamotrigine (lamictal) can be useful in treating mood swings in schizophrenia disorder. Lithium, divalproex and carbamazepine require monitoring of medication with blood levels.

Antidepressants are the primary medical treatment for the depression that can often accompany schizophrenia. These include SSRIs, that affects serotonin level like fluoxetine (prozac), sertraline (zoloft), paroxetine (paxil), citalopram (celexa) and escitalopram combination serotonergic/adrenergic medication (INRIs) like venlafaxine (effexor) and duloxetine (cymbalta) as well as bupropion, which is a dopaminergic antidepressant medication.

Family Psychoeducation

In addition to educating family members about the symptoms, course and treatment of schizophrenia, this form to treatment consist of providing family support, problem-solving skills and access to care providers during times of crisis. When this intervention is consistently provided for at least several months, it has been found to decrease the relapse rate for the individual with schizophrenia and improve the person's social and emotional outcomes. Also, the burden that family members experiences as a result of having a loved one with schizophrenia is lessened; family member tend to be more knowledgeable about the disorder and feel more supported by the health professional involved and family relationships are improved.

Assertive Community Treatment

ACT intervention consists of members of the person's treatment team meeting with that individual on a daily basis in community settings (for examples, home, work, etc.) rather than in offices. The treatment team is made up of a variety of professionals for example, psychiatric nurse, case manager, employment counselor and substance abuse counselor. It tends to be successful in reducing how often people with schizophrenia are hospitalized or become homeless.

Substance Abuse Treatment

Providing medical and psychosocial interventions that address substance abuse should be an integral part of treatment about 50% of clients with schizophrenia suffer from some kind of substance abuse or dependence.

Social Skills Training (SST)

Also caused as illness management and recovery programming, it involves teaching clients ways to handle social situations appropriately. It often involves the person scripting (thinking through /role playing). Situation that occurs in social setting in order to prepare for those situations when they actually arise. This treatment has been focused to help people with schizophrenia resist using drugs of abuse, as well as improve their relationship with health professionals and with people at work.

Supported Employment

This intervention provides supports like a work coach (someone who periodically or consistently counsels the client in the work place) as well as instruction on constructing a resume, intervention for jobs, and education and support for employees to hire individuals with chronic mental illness. Supported employment has been focused to help schizophrenia clients to secure employment, earn more money and increase the number of hours they are able to work.

Cognitive Behavior Therapy (CBT)

It is a reality based intervention that focuses on helping a client understand and change pattern that tend to interfere with his/her ability to interact with others and otherwise function. Except for people who are actively psychotic CBT has been found to help individuals with schizophrenia decrease symptoms and improve their ability to function socially. This intervention can be carried out either individually or in group sessions.

Weight Management

Educating people with schizophrenia about weight gain and related health problems that can be a side effect of antipsychotics and other psychiatric indications has been found to be helpful in resulting in a modest weight loss.

Prognosis of Schizophrenia

Individual with schizophrenia has more than twice the rate of death than those without the disorder. Almost half of people with schizophrenia will suffer from a substance use disorder, (for example, alcohol, marijuana, heroin or other substance) during their lifetime. The research findings show that people with schizophrenia or schizoaffective disorder have a better quality of life if their family members tend to be more supportive and less critical of them.

Complications of Schizophrenia

Schizophrenia has a devastating effect on all aspects of human thought, emotion and expression. Research shows that about 20% of psychiatric clients with schizophrenia can reach full recovery after a first episode; but new drugs are offering significant hope for improving quality of life.

Medical Illnesses

Research studies have reported that people with severe mental illnesses suffer more from serious health problems than those without mental disorders, and they are less likely to receive medical treatment. Substance abuse is a significant factor in this higher risk.

Research has suggested an increased risk of diabetes among people with schizophrenia. In addition, many new antipsychotic medications can elevate blood sugar levels. Clients taking atypical antipsychotic drug, such as clozapine, olanzapine, risperidone, aripiprazole, and ziprasidone, should receive a baseline blood sugar level reading and be monitored for any increase in blood sugar levels.

Depression

Research studies indicate that after 20 to 30 years, half of patients are able to care for themselves, work and participate socially, support services and appropriate hours improve this outcome. Unsurprisingly the decline in status, including the inability to earn a resources and fewer emotional disorder at the outset of symptoms. Also, on average, the later the onset of the disease, the milder the social impact. The long-term effects on work and relationships, however are usually severe and difficult to repair, even if symptoms improve.

Effect on Intelligence

Many researchers believe that a decline in IQ result after many years and it reflects early nerve damage but that it is not an inevitable consequence of the disease process.

Suicide or frightening behavior, people with schizophrenia are no more likely to behave violently than are those in the general population. In fact, these clients are more apt to withdraw from other or to harm themselves.

Suicide

Between 20 and 25% of client with schizophrenia attempt suicide and an estimated 9 to 13% commit suicide. The general risk for suicide is higher at certain times in the course of the disease. These include,

- Within the first 5 years of onset of the disease.
- During the first 6 months after hospitalization.
- Following an acute psychotic episode.

The wide spread use of antipsychotic drugs over the past decade does not appear to have had much effect on suicide rate. In fact, evidence suggests that the use of these drugs as a way of reducing hospitalization time is increasing the incidence of suicide. Depression, not delusion, appears to be the most important motive for suicide. Suicide risk is also associated with prior suicide attempts, drug abuse, agitation, poor treatment compliance, fear of mental deterioration and personal loss.

Self-Destructive Behaviors

Smoking and Other Addictions

Most people with schizophrenia abuse nicotine, alcohol, and other substance. Substance abuse in addition to its other adverse effects increases noncompliance with antipsychotic drugs in the schizophrenia client and worsen symptoms.

Obesity and Diabetes

Obesity is very common in client with schizophrenia factors that contribute to obesity and diabetes. In these clients include unstable lifestyle, low socioeconomic status and side effects of antipsychotic medications.

Effects on Family Members

Family members suffer from grief, long-term guilt and many emotional issues when faced with a schizophrenia love one. If these client commit suicide, the effects can be devastating.

NURSING MANAGEMENT

Nursing management includes nursing process assessment, nursing diagnosis, planning, intervention and evaluation are applied to client and family.

Nursing Assessment

Nursing assessment and diagnosis of the client with a schizophrenia disorder are complex processes. Primarily gathering assessment data, forming nursing diagnosis, treatment goals and interventions are carried out. Specific nursing approaches, such as openness, honestly cultural appreciation and acceptance of the unique properties of the client are essential and common to all comprehensive assessment and plan of care.

Nursing assessment includes through assessment of positive and negative symptoms. Other areas include:

- Thought disturbances.
- Affect disturbances
- Social or behavioral disturbances

Thought Disturbances

- Assessing for 'loose association' or disconnected thoughts through verbal pattern.
- Assessing delusion or fixed false belief that cannot be corrected by reasoning. They involve a misinterpretation of experience or perceptions. These maybe persecutory, grandiose, religious, somatic or referential.
- To identify a delusion, the nurse must first understand the belief characteristic of a culture, because a delusion is a belief that is not keeping with the belief accepted by a person's culture.

- Assess for type of hallucination or false sensory perceptions or sensory perception that do not exist in reality, such as seeing visions or hearing voices.
- Magical thinking is observed in a client who believes that his or her thoughts or wishes can control other people or events.
- Assess for consciousness and insight. These patients may have minimal insight.
- Clients with schizophrenia may experience depersonalization.
- For example, a man who feels that his body belongs to another person or that his something part removed from his body.
- Assess for symbolism. Symbolic words and actions can be viewed as a part of disordered thinking. Language maybe private and idiosyncratic. Client may have neologisms and may use cryptic language, which someone speaking in an abbreviated fashion, e.g. client may speak aloud only every second fourth or sixth word of each thought.
- Illusions maybe another sign of client. Thought disorder, an illusion is a misinterpretation of a real sensory experience. For example, experience of seeing a shadow in the room when making up in middle of night and immediately concluding that a thief has broken into the house. Schizophrenia clients are often disturbed and frightened by illness.

Affect Disturbances

Schizophrenia disorders are marked by an absence of affect or flat, blunted or inappropriate affect. Affective flattening is characterized by the client's face appearing static and unresponsive; with poor eye contact and no body language. The range of emotional expressiveness is reduced. The client's affect may also seem inappropriate in relation to the conversation or the context of the situation.

Social and Behavioral Disturbances

The client with a schizophrenia disorder may retreat from interpersonal contact, appearing aloof, uninterested in others and immersed with inner fantasies. Fear of himself and others prevent the client from making contact and responding to social demands. The client may fear harm from other people or fear a lack of self-control that may bring harm to others.

Assessing the client's ability to perform self-care and activities of daily living, to function in the working setting and to respond appropriately to personal physical needs is critical. At times, a client maybe unaware of safety needs and the need for food, water, rest and activity. Disordered water balance characterized by compulsion to drink, polydypsia, disturbed gait, slurred speech, confusion, disorientation and agitated behavior may occur.

The client's role in the family and community and the availability and responsiveness of a support system are important variables in the assessment process. The actual level of adaptation is strongly influenced by the presence of supportive caring and significant others. The absence of a support system reinforces a lifetime of failure and rejection and may offer the client a little hope for a satisfying future.

The psychiatric nurse needs to assess the client's relationships with the significant family members in his or her life. From these observations and objective description of family and community interaction, the nurse will formulate treatment goals and interventions for and with the client and the people who are important to him or her.

Relapse Symptoms

Relapse symptoms appear in the following order; disrupted sleep cycle, significant mood changes, most often depression; decreased appetite and somatic complaints such as headache, malaise and constipation. During relapse, client often become resistive and ambilvalent, isolative and withdrawn. They have preoccupied psychiatric symptoms.

NURSING DIAGNOSIS

Formulating nursing diagnosis of schizophrenia relies on an accurate history and clinical assessment:

- Sensory/perceptual alternations, auditory or visual related to withdrawal into the self: panic level of anxiety evidenced by poor concentration, rapid mood swings disordered thought sequencing and inappropriate response.
- Altered thought processes related to low self-esteem, repressed fear, inability to trust, possible hereditary factor, panic level of anxiety, evidenced by hypervigilence, altered attention span, distractibility, inability to concentrate, commands abstract or conceptualize.
- Social isolation related to fear of interpersonal closeness, lack of trust, regression to earlier level of development, delusional thinking evidenced by sad, dull affect, inappropriate or immature interests and activities for developmental age, preoccupation with thoughts, repetitive and meaningless actions isolating behavior.
- Risk for violence, self-directed or directed at others related to catatonic excitement, hallucination commands, panic level of anxiety, rage reaction evidenced by increased pacing overt and aggressive acts, goals directed destruction of objects in the environment; self-destructive behavior or aggressive suicidal acts hostile, threatening verbalizations, increased motor activity; excitement ; agitation and irritability.
- Impaired verbal communication related to disordered unrealistic thinking, regression, withdrawal, panic level of anxiety evidenced by loose association of ideas, use of loose association; word salad, neologisms and echolalia, verbalization reflecting concrete thinking and poor eye contact.
- Self-care deficit related to perceptual or cognitive impairment; withdrawal evidenced by impaired ability to perform hygiene tasks, dress groom, maintain appearance at satisfactory level, toilet and eating.
- Altered family processes related to presence of long-term mental illness in family member evidenced by alteration in family's goals and plans, social activities and daily activities.
- Disabled family coping related to difficulty in coping with client's illness.

Nursing Care Plan for Schizophrenia

- *Nursing diagnosis:* Altered thought processes related to inability to distinguish reality from fears and belief.
- *Outcome:* Client will communicate and behave in a social manner.

Nursing intervention	Rationale
• Accept client's delusion without agreeing or disagreeing with them.	Trust begins to develop when the client feels that he/she's beliefs are accepted.
• Establish a consistent routine	

Contd...

Contd...

Nursing intervention	Rationale
• Prepare client for daily event.	Specific instructions about what to expect and what be expected of him to decrease client suspiciousness and paranoia.
• Provide consistency of staff member.	Contact with staff who are known to him helps to diminish client' fears and build trust.
• Orient the client to reality and engage him in reality based conversation.	Reality orientation explains and reinforces to client what is happening around him to counteract his fears.

- *Nursing diagnosis:* Social isolation related to disordered thought process feeling to fear or suspension, disorientation, delusion or hallucination.

Nursing Objective

To decrease the client's withdrawal behavior, provide goal directed structured activity.

Nursing interventions	Rationale
• Spend time with the client even when he or she is unable to respond verbally or in a coherent manner. Convey your interest and caring.	• Nonverbal caring can be processed to the client even when verbal caring is not understood.
• Provide realistic promises	• Breaking promise can result in mistrust.
• Provide an opportunity for the client to learn that his or her feelings are valid and not to different from others.	• The client can begin to identify with wellness or normalness.
• Limit the environment to enhance his or her feeling of security.	• Unknown boundaries or limit can foster insecurity in the client.
• Initially assigns the same nursing staff to take care.	• Consistency can reassume the client.
• Begin with one to one interaction than progress to small group as tolerated.	• Initially the client will tolerate and deal with limited contact.
• Establish and maintain a daily routine, explain any variation in routine to the client.	• The client's ability to adapt to change is limited.

Nursing Diagnosis

- *Risk for violence:* Self-directed or directed at other related to fear of environment and others.

Nursing Outcome

Client will not injure self or others.

Intervention	Rationale
• Always approach the client while talking to him/her.	• Approaching the client without warning could frighten him/her.
• Always keep distance between client and nurse, never invade space without permission, able permission before teaching him.	• Client has fears about harm from other. Keeping distance and asking permission convey respect for the client and his belief.
• Watch for signs of escalation, such as talking to self, pacing or hostile, angry expressions while pacing or talking to self.	• Optimal interventions involves assessing and intervening in escalating behavior before it erupts into violence.
• Help the client to de-escalate by approaching calmly and distressing what you observe ask what's bothering him and whether the voices are telling him to do something.	• A calm demeanor defuses the situation and help the client to remain calm.

Contd...

Contd...

Intervention	Rationale
• Offer a calm, quiet environment and antipsychotic medication before behavior surfaces.	• Asking the client to describe his experience gives nurses information on which to plan intervention.
	• Providing a nonstimulating environment helps the client de escalate, antipsychotic medication helps to manage psychotic symptoms of delusional, paranoid thinking.

Nursing Evaluation

- Client demonstrates no aggressive, violent and angry outbursts.
- How self-esteem related to inadequate interpersonal relationships and lack of successful composing strategies. Delusions/hallucination/illusions.

Objectives

To increase the client's self-esteem and feelings of self-worth.

Nursing interventions	Rationale
• Provide attention in a sincere and professional manner.	• Flattery can be interpreted as biting by the client.
• Support any successful task, ward responsibilities, project interactions with the staff members and others clients and so on.	• Sincere and genuine praise that the client has earned can improve self-esteem.
• Avoid trying to convince the client verbally of his or her own work	• The client will recognize unfolded praise or flattery and feel worse because of it.
• Help the client improve his/her grooming assist when necessary in bathing, doing laundry work, etc.	• Attractive and good grooming can foster feeling of well-being and self-esteem.

Disturbed sensory perception related to presence of positive symptoms.

Objective

Client will not harm self or others.

Nursing intervention	Rationale
• Maintain low level of stimuli in client environment, i.e. Low illumination and noise restricted entry levels.	• Anxiety level rises in stimulation of environment they are considered as threatening for suspicious client.
• Keep client in constant observation.	• Constant observation will help in immediate interventions.
• Remove all potential dangerous object from client's surroundings	• Remove all dangerous objects prevents client from harming self and others.
• Redirect aggressive and violent behavior with physical outlets fro the anxiety.	• Physical activities are safe and effective way to reduce anxiety.
• Maintain calm attitude towards the client.	• Anxiety is contagious and can transmitted to staff to client.
• Maintain sufficient number of staff to show strength to client if it is required	• This provides some security to staff and client and evidence of control over the situation.

Contd...

Contd...

Nursing intervention	Rationale
• Administration of transquilizer medications as ordered by the doctor. If chemical restraining fails mechanical restraining can be done.	• Restraining will help to decrease aggressiveness or violent behaviors.

- Self-care deficit related to regression, withdrawn and perceptual or cognitive impairment.

Nursing Objective

Client will be able to fulfill his needs independently.

Nursing intervention	Rationale
• Provide assistance in ADL as required. Those withdrawn client require comprehensive care.	• Client's safety and comfort are primary responsibilities of nurse.
• Encourage the client to perform independency as much as possible positive reinforcement should be provided for independent accomplishment.	• Independent accomplishment and positive reinforcement enhance self-esteem and increase the frequency of desirable behaviors.
• Use concrete and firm communication to show client what is expected from him.	• Explanation which is provided to the client should be at client's concrete level of comprehension.
• Creative approaches may need to be taken with the client the who is not eating. Such as allowing client to open packed food in his own or taste client's food in front of him/her.	• These techniques maybe helpful with the client who is paranoid and maybe suspicious that he/she is poisoned with food or medication.
• If toileting needs are not being met, establish a structured schedule for the client.	• A structured schedule will help the client establish a pattern so that the client can develop a habit for toileting independency.

Disabled family coping related to difficulty in coping with client's illness.

Nursing Objective

Family will identify more adaptive coping strategies for dealing with client's illness and treatment program.

Nursing intervention	Rationale
• Identify levels of family functioning assess communication patterns. 18 R between members, role expectation, problem-solving skills and availability of support systems.	• These factors will help to determine how successful the family is in dealing with stressful situation and areas where assistance is required.
• Provide information regarding client's illness, what will be required in the treatment program and long-term prognosis to the family.	• Knowledge and understanding about what to expect may facilitate family's ability to help the client.
• Explain to the family regarding how to respond to bizarre behavior and communication patterns and in the event that the client becomes violent.	• A plan of action will assist the family to respond adaptively in the face of what they may consider to be crisis.

Nursing Planning

Planning includes a collaborative approach of mental health team, which includes client and family. Flexibility and creativity are important for holistic nursing care to achieve maximum health outcomes.

Goal Setting

The major goals for the schizophrenic client include the following:

- Promoting trusting relationship
- Establishing a safe and calm environment
- Encouraging satisfactory social relationships
- Enhancing self-esteem
- Validating perception
- Classifying and reinforcing reality
- Promoting safety
- Encouraging independency
- Care of physical needs
- Reduction of positive symptoms
- Co-coordinating treatment
- Psychoeducation

Client outcomes are more specific than goals and are measurable, attainable, realistic, time oriented and client focused.

Discharge Planning

- Discharge planning begins at the time of admission. Many schizophrenic clients suffer from both long-term effects as well as with. 'Rip van Winkel syndrome' what that is, they awaken from a long sleep to find a world with changed, technologies, cultured values and economic. It is a frightening world for discharge clients who may have been comfortable in the protected hospital climate.
- Discharge planning includes community participation or networking. Work or job skills. Confidence in dealing with problems and involvement in community.

Nursing Interventions

Recovery from severe mental illness is a tedious concepts. It is a way of living a hopeful, satisfying life and contributing to society within the limitations imposed by the illness. This recovery depends on the following factors:

- Medication
- Self-control or self-monitoring of symptoms
- Community support and mental health services
- Vocational activity
- Spirituality
- Mutual aid groups and supportive friends
- Involvement of significant people
- Knowledge and acceptance of the illness.

Nursing interventions focus on assisting the client to meet the following goals:

- Establish a trusting.
- Alleviate/reduce anxiety.
- Maintain biological integrity and,
- Establish, clear, simple, consistent and open therapeutic communication.

The psychiatric nurse must establish a therapeutic relationship in order to communicate effectively with the patient. It should be goal directed, simple and easy to understand both.

Schizophrenic client may refuse to communicate or may communicate ineffectively because of:

- Conflicting and complex statement
- Frequent changes in subject matter
- Inconsistency in verbalization
- Fragmented talk.
- Presence of hallucination, delusion and illusions.

One main point, always psychiatric nurse has to remember that all behavior is meaningful to the client, if not to anyone else.

Reality should be considered while caring. Recognizing the presence of hallucination and delusion is necessary for an appropriate response. The psychiatric nurse should consider factor for causing hallucination and attempt to intervene before they occur. The delusion can be ignored.

Consider safety measures where clients display poor judgment, disorientation, destructive behavior, suicidal ideation or agitation. Limit setting, acknowledging spatial territory and providing protective measures are the main nursing interventions.

Psychiatric nurse should plan activities to increase the client's self-concept. Positive compliments shall be given when client shows positive aspects of capabilities. Encouragement in activities is a paramount need.

The nurse must observe for extrapyramidal side effects of psychotropic drugs and monitor the client's willingness to take the drugs. Clients may refuse to take medication, pretend to take medication by keeping it or pretend to shallow the medication while retaining the pill in the mouth.

Psychoeducation should contain the primary aspects and rehabilitative measures of schizophrenia. Involvement of community resources are necessary for deinstitutionalization.

Evaluation

The evaluation process is continuous in nature by constantly examining changes in the client's behavior. The psychiatric nurse has the opportunity to change and strengthen the treatment process.

SCHIZOAFFECTIVE DISORDER

Schizoaffective disorder is a condition that causes both a loss of contact with reality and mood problem. It includes both features of schizophrenia and affective disorder. ICD-10 classifies it as a distinct entity and can be applied to client who have co-occurring mood symptoms and schizophrenia with mood incongruent psychosis.

EPIDEMIOLOGY

Prevalence

The prevalence of schizoaffective disorder is less than 1% mostly its range is 0.5–0.8%.

Age of Onset

It can occur at late adolescence or at later life. The depressive type of schizoaffective disorder is more common in older persons than in younger persons and bipolar disorder is more common flat young adults than in older individuals.

Gender

Schizoaffective disorder is believed to be less common than schizophrenia and mood disorders. Women may have the conditions more often than men. It tends to be rare in children. Men with schizoaffective disorders are likely to exhibit antisocial behavior and to have markedly flat or inappropriate affect.

Comorbidity

Schizoaffective disorder maybe associated with substance abuse. In men, nearly 25% of clients diagnosed with schizoaffective disorder have a postpsychotic depression and panic attacks.

Causes/Etiology

The exact cause of schizoaffective disorder is unknown. Changes in genes and neurotransmitters may play a role. This disorder maybe a type of schizophrenia, a type of mood disorder or the simultaneous expression of each.

Signs and Symptoms

The symptoms of schizoaffective disorder vary according to person. Often, people with schizoaffective disorder seek treatment to problem with mood, or abnormal thoughts. Psychosis and mood problems may occur at the same time or by themselves. The course of the disorder may involve cycles of severe symptoms followed by improvement.

The symptoms include:

- Changes in appetite and energy
- Disorganized speech and thought
- Paranoia and delusion
- Neglect of personal hygiene.
- **Mood:** Either too good, depressed or irritable
- Lack of concentration
- Sadness/hopelessness
- Presence of hallucination
- Social isolation
- Loud speech.

Diagnosis

DSM-IVTR diagnostic criteria include:

- An uninterrupted period of illness during which at sometime there is either a major depressive episode, a manic episode or a mixed episode concurrent with symptoms that meet criterion for schizophrenia.
  Note: The major depressive episode must include criterion A1 depressed mood.
- During the same period of illness, there have been delusion or hallucination for at least 2 weeks in the absence of prominent mood symptoms.
- Symptoms that meet criteria for a mood episode are present for a substantial portion of total duration of active and residual period of the illness.
- The disturbance is not due to the physiological effects of a substance (e.g. Drug abuse, a medication or a general medical condition).

Type

- *Bipolar type:* If the disturbance includes a manic or a mixed episode (or a manic or a mixed episode and major depressive episode).
- *Depressive type:* If the disturbance includes only major depressive episodes.

MANAGEMENT

- Antipsychotics are used to treat psychotic symptoms.
- Antidepressants/mood stabilize maybe for improving mood.
- Carbamazepine, SSRIs like fluoxetine/sertraline and haloperidol can be used.
- Combination of drugs with therapies like family therapy, SST, individual therapy and cognitive and psychosocial rehabilitative measures are considered.

SCHIZOPHRENIFORM DISORDER

Schizophreniform disorder is diagnosed when the symptom criteria schizophrenia are met, but the duration is too short with impairment in social and occupational functioning. The essential features of schizophrenia form disorder are identical to those of schizophrenia (criterion A) except for two differences, the total duration of the illness (including prodromal, active and residual phases) is at least 1 month but less than 6 months (criteria B) and impaired social or occupational functioning during some part of the illness is not required. The duration required for schizoniform disorder is intermediate between that for brief psychotic disorder and schizophrenia.

The diagnosis of schizophreniform disorder is made under two conditions. In the first, the diagnosis is applied without qualification to an episode of illness of between 1 and 6 months duration from which the individual has already recovered.

In the second case, the diagnosis is applied when a person who, although symptomatic has been so, for less than 6 month required for a diagnosis of schizophrenia. In this case, the diagnosis of schizophrenia form disorder should be qualified as 'provisional' because there is no certainty that the individual will actually recover from the disturbance within the 6 month period. If the disturbance persists beyond 6 months, the diagnosis would be changed to schizophrenia.

EPIDEMIOLOGY

The prevalence of schizoniform disorder is equally distributed between gender, with peak onset between women. Unlike schizophrenia in which prodromal symptoms may develop over several years; schizophrenia from disorder requires, among other features, a rather rapid period from the onset of prodromal symptoms to the point at which all criteria fro schizophrenia (except duration and deterioration) are met (within 6 months). According to APA, approximately two thirds of clients diagnosed with schizophrenia from disorder progress to a diagnosis of schizophrenia.

MANAGEMENT

- Hospitalization is required. The drug treatment is similar to schizophrenia.
- Atypical antipsychotics, e.g. risperidone, olanzapine, quetiapine and ziprasidone are prescribed. A new drug ariprazole maybe prescribed.
- ECT in case of catatonic and depressive symptoms.

DELUSIONAL DISORDER

Delusional disorder is characterized by presence of nonbizarre delusion which have persisted for at least one month. Nonbizarre delusions typically are belief of something occurring in a person's life which is not out of the realm of possibility. For example, the person may believe that their significant others are cheating on them, that someone close to them is about to die, a friend in reality is a government agent, etc. all of these situation could be true or possible, but the person suffering from this disorder knows them not to be (e.g. through fact checking, third person confirmation, etc).

Delusional disorder clients generally do not experience a marked impairment in their daily functioning in a social, occupational or other important setting. Outward behavior is not noticeably bizarre or objective characterized as out of the ordinary.

These delusions cannot be better accounted for by another disorder, such as schizophrenia, which is also characterized by delusions (which are bizarre). The delusion also cannot be letter accounted for by a mood disorder, if the mood disturbances have been relatively brief in duration.

EPIDEMIOLOGY

The incidence rate of delusional disorder in adults is unclear. The prevalence is estimated lower than the rates of schizophrenia. It may account for 1–2% of admission to inpatient psychiatric hospitals. Age of onset ranges from 18-90 years with a mean age of 40 years. More females than males (overall) suffer from delusional disorder, especially the late onset in elderly.

Diagnosis: It is done as per below:

- Nonbizarre delusions (i.e. involving situation that occur in real life, such as being followed, poisoned, infected, loved at a distance or deceived by spouse or lover or having a disease) of at least one months duration.
- *Criterion A for schizophrenia has never been met note:* Tactile and olfactory hallucinations maybe present in delusional disorder if they are related to the delusional theme.

Criterion A of schizophrenia requires two (or more) of the following, each present for a significant portion of time during a-1 month period (or less if successfully treated).

- Delusions
- Hallucination
- Disorganized speech (e.g. frequent derailment or incoherence)
- Grossly disorganized or catatonic behavior
- Negative symptoms, i.e. Affective flattening, alogia or avolition.
  Note: Criteria A of schizophrenia requires only one symptoms if delusions are bizarre or hallucinations consist of a voice keeping up a running commentary on the person's behavior or thoughts or two or more voices conversing with each other.
- Apart from the impact of the delusion(s) or its ramification, functioning is not markedly impaired and behavior is not odd or bizarre.
- If mood episodes have occurred concurrently with delusions, their total duration has been brief in relation to the duration of the delusional periods.
- The disturbance is not due to direct physiological effects of a substance, e.g. A drug of abuse, a medication or a general medical condition.

Types

- *Erotomanic type:* Delusions that another person, usually of higher status, is in love with the individual.
- *Grandiose type:* Delusion of inflated worth, power, knowledge identify or special relationship to a deity of famous person.
- *Jealous type:* Delusion that the individual sexual partner is unfaithful.
- *Persecutory type:* Delusion that the person (or someone to whom the person is close) is being malevolently treated in someway.
- *Somatic type:* Delusion that the person has some physical defect or general medical condition.
- *Mixed type:* Delusional characteristic of more than one of the above types, but no one theme predominates.
- *Unspecified type.*

ETIOLOGY

No single cause is identified for delusional disorders. The theories regarding causes are:

Genetic or Biological Theory

Genetic theory emphasizes on genetic make-up. Close relatives of person with delusional disorder have increased rates of delusional disorder and paranoid personality traits. They do not have higher rates of schizophrenia, schizoaffective disorder or mood disorder compared to relatives of non delusional persons. Increased incidence of these psychiatric disorders in individuals closely genetically related to person with delusional disorder suggest that there is a genetic component to the disorder. Further more, a number of research studies comparing activity of different regions of the brain in delusional and nondelusional study participants yielded data about differences in the functioning of the brains between member of the two groups. These differences in brain activity suggest that persons neurologically with delusions tend to react as if threatening conditions are consistently present certain kind of conditions where the interpretation of being threatened is more accurate. With both brain activity evidence and family heritability evidence, a strong bond exists that there is a biological aspect to delusional disorders.

Dysfunctional Cognitive Processing

An elaborate term for thinking is 'cognitive processing' delusions may arise from distorted ways people have, of explaining life to themselves. The most prominent cognitive problems involve the manner in which delusion suffers develop conclusions both about other people and about causation of unusual perceptions or negative events. Research studies in how people with delusion develop theories about reality, show that the subject have ideas which they tend to reach at an inference based on less information than most people use. This 'jumping to conclusions' bias can lead to delusional interpretations of ordinary events. For example, developing flu-like symptoms coinciding with the week new neighbors more in might lead to the conclusion, 'the new neighbors are poisoning or killing me'. The conclusion is drawn without considering alternative explanations catching an illness from a relative with the film and that a virus seems to be going around at work. Research also shows that persons prone to delusions 'read' people differently than nondelusional individuals do, whether they do so more accurately or particularly poorly is a matter of issue. They tend to view life as a continuing series of threatening events. When these two aspects of thought co-occur, a tendency to develop delusion about others wishing to do them harms likely.

Motivated or Defensive Delusion

Some predisposed persons might suffer the onset of an ongoing delusional disorder when coping with life and maintaining high self-esteem becomes a significant challenge in order to preserve a positive view of oneself, a person views others at the cause of personal difficulties that may occur. This can become an ingrained pattern of thought.

TREATMENT

Management of delusional disorder includes drugs and psychotherapy. It is highly resistant to treatment with medication alone.

Psychotherapy is the primary treatment for delusional disorder, including psychosocial treatment which can help with the behavioral and psychological problem associated with delusional disorder. Through this therapy, clients can learn to control their own symptoms, identify warning signs of relapse and develop a relapse prevention strategy.

Psychosocial therapies include:

- *Individual psychotherapy:* It can help the person to recognize and correct the underlying thinking that has become distorted.
- *Cognitive behavior therapy (CBT):* It can help the person learn to recognize and change his thought pattern and behaviors that lead to problematic feelings.
- *Family therapy:* it can help families deal more effectively with a love one who has delusional disorder, enabling them to contribute to a better outcome for the person.

Drug Management

- *Antipsychotics:* These are used to treat psychotic symptoms they act by blocking dopamine receptors in the brain. For example, thorazine prolixin, haldol, navane, stelazine trialfon, mellaril.
- *Atypical antipsychotics:* Atypical antipsychotic found to be more effective in treating the symptoms of delusional. They act by blocking dopamine and serotonin receptors in the brain. For example, Risperidol, clozaril, seroquel, geodon, zyprexa.
- *Other drugs:* Tranquilizers and anti-depressants may also be used to treat delusional disorder. Tranquilizers can be used if the client has very high level of anxiety and sleep disturbances. Anti-depressants might be used to treat depression in delusional disorder.

  Clients with severe debilitating symptoms or who are at risk of hurting themselves or other might need to be hospitalized until the condition will be stabilized.

PROGNOSIS

Clinical evidence show that 10% of cases will improve, 30 to 40% of client suffers with persistent non-improving symptoms. The prognosis is largely related to the level of conviction regarding the delusional and the openness the person has for allowing information that contradicts the delusion.

Nursing Management

Nursing care is based on symptomatology related to thought content and form, perception, affect, sense of self, volition, impaired interpersonal relationship to the external world and psychomotor behavior.

Mood Disorders

INTRODUCTION

Bipolar disorders used to be called 'manic depression' earlier. As the name denotes, these clients will have severe mood swings ranging from low to high as well as mixed. These mood swings last several weeks or months to years.

Mood refers to sustained and pervasive emotional response which is subjective in its expression. Affect denotes to short lived emotional response to an event or idea which is objective in its expression.

HISTORICAL PERCEPTIVE

- The word 'depression' is noted since antiquity. Hippocrates (400 BC) noted that black bile and phlegm influence the brain by 'darkening the spirit and making melancholy'.
- According to medical historical survey, Aretaeus of Cappadocia first recognized symptoms of mania and depression and felt they could be linked to each other. In 1650, Richard Burton wrote a book, The Anatomy of Melancholia, which focused on depression, for this he is cited with being the father of depression as a mental illness.
- In 1854, Jules Falret coined the term 'folie circulaire' (circular insanity) and established a link between depression and suicide, and in 1875 noted the term manic depressive psychosis.
- In 1913, Emil Drapeli established the term manic depressive and noted in-depth about this disorder.
- In 1980, the term bipolar disorder replaced manic depressive disorder as a diagnostic term found in DSM-III.
- In 1994, DSM-IV and most recent DSM-IVTR (DSM-IV text revision, 2000 the definition of biolar diagnosis has evolved from a monolithic disorder with a single set of criteria, to a more defined subsystem, where bipolar I and bipolar II forms of the disorder are recognized and separately diagnosed.

Myths and Facts about bipolar disorder:

- *Myth:* People with bipolar disorder cannot get better or lead a normal life.
- *Fact:* Many people with bipolar disorder have successful careers, happy family lives, and satisfying relationships living with bipolar disorder is challenging. But with treatment, healthy coping skills and a good support system helps to recover to normalcy.
- *Myth:* People with bipolar disorder swing back and forth between mania and depression.
- *Fact:* Some clients alternate between extreme episodes of mania and depression, but most are depressed more often than manic. Mania can go unnoticed. People with bipolar disorder can also go for long stretches without symptoms.

- *Myth:* Bipolar disorder only affects mood.
- *Fact:* It affects the energy level, memory, concentration, appetite, sleep patterns, sex drive and self-esteem. It is also linked to anxiety, substance abuse and general health problems such as diabetes, heart disease, migraines and hypertension.

CLASSIFICATION OF BIPOLAR DISORDERS

Bipolar disorder (affective) are classified in ICD-10 as follows:
- F30 Manic episode
- F31 Bipolar affective disorder
- F32 Depressive episode
- F33 Recurrent depressive episode
- F34 Persistent mood (affective) disorder
- F38 Other mood (affective) disorder
- F39 Unspecified mood (affective) disorder.

EPIDEMIOLOGICAL PERCEPTIVE

- Bipolar affective disorders are very common; the prevalence is up to 20% and they have a high level of morbidity and mortality.
- Major depressive disorder is a common disorder with a life time prevalence of 15% . The fundamental disturbance is a change in mood and affect; usually to depression (with or without anxiety) or elation. The mood change is usually accompanied by a change in the overall level of activity.
- Most of the time, these disorders are recurrent in nature and is often related to stressful events or situations.
- *Gender:* Male female ratio of major or depressive disorder is 2%. Bipolar disorder-I has equal prevalence. Manic episodes are more common in males.
- *Age:* The onset of-bipolar I disorder is earlier than major depressive disorder. The mean age for bipolar-I disorder is 30 and ranges from 5 to 6 years to 50 years. The mean age for major depressive episode is 40 years.
- *Marital status:* Depressive symptoms are more common in individuals without close interpersonal relationships and who are divorced and separated. More common in married and single person.
- *Socioeconomic status:* A higher than average incidence of bipolar-I disorder is found among the upper socioeconomic groups. Depression is more common in rural areas than urban areas.
- *Seasonality:* Bipolar disorder are more common in spring and winter.
- *Burden of disease:* An estimated 3 to 4% of India's population suffers from major mental disorders and about 7 to 10% of the population suffers from minor depressive disorders.
- *Suicidality:* Depression is associated with high suicidality. About 50% of suicidal deaths occur due to depression. According to official estimates in Ministry of Health India, 120000 people commit suicide every year in India and also over 400000 people attempt suicide.

ETIOLOGICAL FACTORS

No single factor is responsible for the cause of bipolar disorder. Many theorists postulated multiple causes. These are:

Genetic Theory/Genetic Factors

- Some twin research studies indicated 'substantial genetic contribution' to bipolar disorder. In first degree relatives, prevalence is nearly 20% for bipolar disorder, 10 to 15% for unipolar with 1 to 3% in general population.
- Theorists also postulated that rare copy number variants, abnormal sequences of DNA plays a major risk of onset for bipolar disorder.
- Twins: Monozygotic versus dizygotic: 68:20%.

Biologic Amine Theories

- *Norepinephrine:* Deficiency of norepinephrine causes depression. Research studies have shown that in depression, activation of Beta 2 receptors also takes place which leads to decrease in nor epinephrine levels and in manic episode norepinephrine remains in excess.
- *Serotonin:* Depletion of serotonin levels may precipitate depression. Suicidal clients impulses have low CSF concentration of serotonin metabolites.
- *Dopamine:* The data suggests that dopamine activity maybe reduced in depression and increased in mania.
- *Neuroendocrine Regulation:* The hypothalamus is central to the regulation of neuroendocrine axis and itself receive many neuronal inputs that use biogenic amines neurotransmitters. The major disturbance found in the adrenal thyroid and growth hormone axes are:
  - *Adrenal axis:* About 50% of depressed client have elevated cortisol levels.
  - *Thyroid axis:* Thyroid disorders are often found in about 5 to 10% of persons with depression. 1/3rd of depressive clients have bluented release of thyropentin. TSH, TRH and prolactin. In bipolar-I disorders, antithyroid antibodies are also detected, growth hormone: Depression has been associated with dysregulation of release of growth hormone.

Sleep Abnormalities

The following findings show a link between sleep and mood disorders:

- Increased duration and intensity of REM during sleep in people with depression.
- Sleep deprivation leads to temporary improvement in mood.
- Seasonal affective disorders suggests the involvement of circadian rhythms.
- Extended bouts of insomnia have been linked to MDP.
- *Brain imaging:* Clients with bipolar-I disorder mainly men have enlarged cerebral ventricles. Research shown that clients with major depressive disorder have similar caudate nuclei and smaller frontal lobes.
- *Hormonal changes:* Hormonal imbalances are thought to possibly trigger or cause bipolar disorder.

Psychological Theories

Psychodynamic Factors in Depression

According to Freud and Abraham, it consists of four components.

- Disturbance in infant-mother relationship during oral phase of development, often the loss or threatened loss of a parent.

- Depression can be linked with real or imagined object loss. Adult relationships are unconsciously constructed in a way that reflects this loss, e.g. loss of early attachment—dependence or avoidance in current relationships.
- Introjections of the departed objects is defense mechanism involved to deal with distress connected with object loss.
- Depression rooted in an early defect in the attachment relationship with the caregiver. Any present event.
- Involving loss reactivates the primal loss and the person regresses to the childhood trauma. Because lost object is regarded with the mixture of love and hate, feelings of anger are directed inwards at self-resulting in depression.

Psychodynamic Factors in Manic Episode

Many theories related to mania view manic episode as a defences underlying depression. The manic episode may result from tyrannical super ego which produces intolerable self-criticism that is then replaced by euphoric self-satisfaction. Lewin's theory regards that the manic client's ego as overwhelmed by pleasurable impulses such as sex by feared impulses such as aggression.

Cognitive Theory

- Beck postulated a cognitive triad of depression that consists of belief about the world, oneself and the future.
- *Views about self:* A negative self-concept.
- *About the environment:* A tendency to experience the world as hostile and demanding.
- *About the future:* The expectation of suffering and failure.

Biological Trait Theory

Theorists say that clients with bipolar disorder often have physical changes that occurred in their brains. It is ensure that how change can lead to the disorder.

Learned Helplessness Theory

Learned helplessness theory is derived from Seligman's experiment with dogs. The dogs were exposed to electrical stimulation from which they could not escape. Later when, they were given the opportunity to avoid the trumatic experience, they reacted with helplessness and made no attempt to escape. A similar state of helplessness exists in humans who have experienced multiple failure (real or perceived). The individual avoids any further attempts for success.

Environment Theory

Environment a-lists stresses abuse as well as mental trauma, a significant loss, may contribute towards bipolar disorders.

Different Faces of Bipolar Disorder

- *Bipolar I disorder (mania or mixed episode):* The classic manic-depressive form of the illness, characterized by at least one manic episode or mixed episode. Usually but not always—bipolar I disorder also involves at least one episode of depression.

- *Bipolar II disorder: (hypomania and depression):* In bipolar II disorder, the person does not experience full blown manic episodes. Instead, the illness involves episodes of hypomania and severe depression.
- *Cyclothymia: (Hypomania and mild depression):* Cyclothymia is a milder form of bipolar disorder. It consists of cyclical mood swings. However, the symptoms are less severe than full blown mania or depression.

CLINICAL FEATURES OF BIPOLAR DISORDER

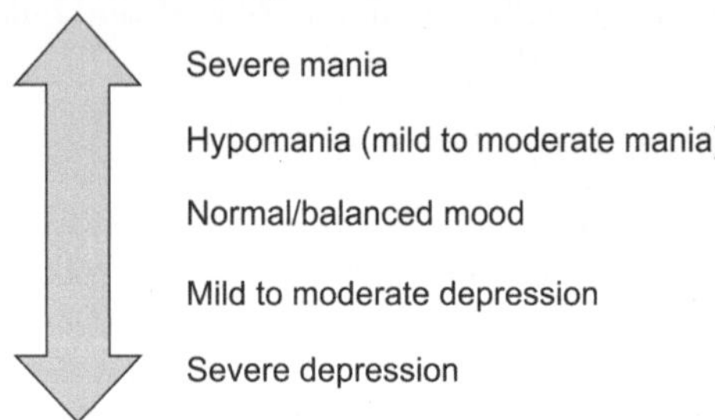

Fig. 7.1: Clinical features of mood disorder

Bipolar disorder can present very different in different individuals. The symptoms vary widely in their pattern, severity and frequency. Some individuals are more prone to either mania or depression, while others alternate equally between the two types of episodes. Some have frequent mood disruptions, while others experience only a few over a lifetime.

There are four types of mood episodes in bipolar disorders mania, hypomania, depression and mixed episodes (Fig. 7.1). Each one has it own unique features.

Clinical Features of Mania

- In the manic phase of bipolar disorder. Feelings of heightened energy, creativity and euphoria are very common. People experiencing a manic episode often talk a lot, sleep very little and are hyperactive. They may also feel like they are all powerful, invincible or destined for greatness.
- Main ionic clinical feature is elevated, expansive/irritable mood. Mood can pass through the following stages:
  - *Euphoria:* Mild elevation of mood.
  - *Elation:* Moderate elevation of mood.
  - *Exaltation:* Severe elevation of mood
  - *Ecstasy:* Very severe elevation of mood.
- *Enhanced psychomotor activity:* It ranges from over activeness and restlessness to manic excitement where he feels, on the to on the go' (i.e. involves in many useless activities). It may lead to physical exhaustion.
- *Speech and thought:* Talkative and irritable. The client describes thought racing in mind, develops pressure of speech, users playful language with punning, rhyming, joking, teasing and speaking loudly. Later they may be incoherent. Delusions of persecution and grandeur maybe an iconic features. Speech will be distractible and changes in speed.

- *Goal diverted activity:* In initial stages, may function better but later on client shows impulsiveness, disinhibition, sexual indiscretion and usually becomes hypersexual and promiscuous.
  - Sleep disturbances are much marked. Appetite will be lost. Loss of insight and vague physical appearance in later stages.

Hypomania Symptoms

Hypomania is a less severe form of mania. People in a hypomanic state feel euphoric, energetic and productive, but they are able to carry on with their day-to-day lives and they never lose touch with reality. To others, it may seem as if people with hypomania are merely in an unusually good mood. However, hypomania can result in bad decisions that harm relationships, careers and reputations. In addition, hypomania often escalates to full blown mania or is followed by a major depressive episode.

Common clinical features of mania are:

- Feeling usually 'high' and optimistic or extremely irritable.
- Unrealistic, grandiose beliefs about one's abilities or powers.
- Sleeping very little but feels very energetic.
- Talking so rapidly that other's cannot keep-up.
- Racing thoughts, jumping quickly from one idea to the next.
- Highly distractible, unable to concentrate.
- Impaired judgment and impulsiveness.
- Acting recklessly without thinking about the consequences.
- In severe cases, delusion and hallucinations.

Clinical Features of Bipolar Depression

The typical depressive episode is characterized by the following features:

Depressive Mood

The most important and prominent feature is the sadness of mood or loss of interest in life (anhedonia), present throughout the day (persistent sadness). The sadness of mood is quantitatively as well as qualitatively differs from normal sadness. The depressive mood is often not responsive to environment stimuli. The loss of interest results in social withdrawal, decreased ability to function in work and interpersonal areas and decreased involvement in previously pleasurable activities.

Depressive Ideation

Sadness of mood is associated with pessimism. It results in three types of depressive ideas.

1. Helplessness
2. Hopelessness
3. Worthlessness

The ideas of worthlessness can be lead to guilt feeling. Other clinical features include difficulty in thinking, concentration, indecisiveness, slowed thinking, subjective poor memory, lack of initiative and energy. Often, ruminations of pessimistic ideas, thought of death/suicide and preoccupation with death are not uncommon. Nihilistic delusions maybe seen in severe cases.

Psychomotor Activity

In younger adults retardation is more common, characterized by slowed thinking and activity, decreased energy and monotonous voice. In severe form, client becomes stuporous (depressive stupor). In older clients agitation is more common with marked anxiety, restlessness and subjective uneaseness.

Biorhythm Function

Disturbance in biorhythm is seen with insomnia, loss of appetite and weight (sometimes gain) and loss of sexual energy and drive. ICD-10 denotes these symptoms as somatic syndrome. If patient complains of hypersomnia increased appetite and weight gain in DSM-IVTR. It is know as depression with atypical features.

Physical Symptoms

These vary according to age of the client. Usually client manifests multiple physical symptoms like heaviness of head, vague bodyaches, etc.

Psychotic Features

Nearly 20 to 25% of depressive clients have delusions, hallucination, grossly inappropriate behavior or stupor. Psychotic features can be mood-congruent (e.g. Delusion of guilt, delusion of nihilism) which are understandable in the light of depressive mood or can be mood incongruent (delusion of control).

Suicide

Suicidal thoughts/ideas in depression if expressed should be taken seriously. There is high-risk for suicide in every depressive client. The risk is more in the presence of hopelessness, males > 40 years, single/divorced/widowned women. Written or verbal communication of suicidal intent and or plan in elderly stage in recovering from depression and period of three to four months after recovery.

Reactive Depression

Reactive depression spurts from some event or some outstanding stress. It may due to problems in relationships, death of closed one, loss of loved one, changing job, etc. In this type of depression, sleep problems are mainly observed. People who do not respond to antidepressant medication suffers from reactive depression.

Endogenous Depression

Here, there is no exact cause. It appears to come from nowhere. It has a strong genetic link, so it is manifested by altered sleep pattern, poor concentration and loos of interest in activity. The symptoms are marked by feeling tiredness, hopelessness, sadness, memory problems, and disturbances in sleep pattern.

Signs and Symptoms of Mixed Episode

A mixed episode of bipolar disorder features symptoms of both mania or hypomania and depression. Common signs of mixed episode include depression combined with agitation, irritability, anxiety, insomnia, distractibility and racing thoughts. This combination of high energy and low mood makes the individual for a high-risk of suicide.

Diagnostic Criteria for Major Depressive Episode (DSM-IVTR)

Five or more symptoms have been present during the same two weeks period and represent a change from previous functioning at least one of the symptoms is:

Depressed mood or loss of interest/pleasure (anhedonia).

- Depressed mood most of the day, nearly everyday, as indicated by subjective assessment (e.g. Feels sad or empty) or observation made by others (e.g. appears tearful) (Note: Children and adolescents can have irritable mood) and adolescents can have irritable mood.
- Markedly diminished interest or pleasure in almost all activities most of the day, nearly everyday.
- Significant weight loss when not dieting or weight gain (e.g. Change of more than 5% of body weight in a month), or a decrease or increase in appetite nearly everyday.
  Note: In children consider failure to make expected weight gains.
- Insomnia or hypersomnia nearly everyday.
- Psychomotor retardation or agitation nearly everyday (observable by others, not merely subjective feelings of restlessness or being slowed down).
- Fatigue, loss of energy or sexual problems nearly everyday.
- Feeling of worthlessness or excessive or inappropriate guilt. (which maybe delusional) nearly every day.
- Decreased ability to think or concentrate or indecisiveness nearly everyday (by subjective assessment).
- Recurrent thoughts of death (not just fear of dying), recurrent suicidal ideas without a specific plan or a suicidal attempt or a specific plan for committing suicide.
  - There has never been a manic episode, a mixed episode, or a hypomanic episode that was not substance or treatment induced or due to the direct physiological affects of general medical condition.
  - The symptoms cause clinically significant distress or impairment in social, occupational or other important area of functioning.
  - The symptoms are not due to the direct physiological effects of a substance, e.g. a drug of abuse or a medication) or a general medical condition (e.g. hypothyroidism).
  - The symptoms are not better accounted for bereavement (i.e. after the loss of a loved one), the symptoms persist for longer than two months or are characterized by marked functional impairment, morbid preoccupation with worthlessness, suicidal ideation, psychotic symptoms or psychomotor retardation.

DIAGNOSTIC CRITERIA FOR MANIC EPISODE (DSM–IVTR)

- A distinct period of abnormally and persistently elevated, expansive or irritable mood, lasting for at least 1 week (or any duration if hospitalization is necessary).

- During the period of mood disturbance, three or more of the following symptoms have persisted (four if the mood is only irritable) and have been present to a significant extent:
  - Inflated self-esteem or grandiosity.
  - Decreased need for sleep.
  - More talkative than usual or pressure of speech.
  - Flight of ideas or subjective experience that thoughts are racing.
  - Distractibility (i.e. Attention too easily drawn to unimportant or irrelevant external stimuli).
  - Increase in goal-directed activity (socially at work or school or sexually) or psychomotor agitation.
  - Excessive involvement in pleasurable activities that have a high potential for painful consequences (e.g. Engaging in unrestrained buying sprees, sexual indiscretions or foolish investments).

c. The mood disturbance is sufficiently severe to cause marked impairment in occupational functioning or in usual social activities or relationships with others or to necessitate hospitalization to prevent harm to self or others or there are psychotic features.
d. The symptoms are not due to direct physiological effects of a substance (e.g. a drug of abuse, a medication or other treatment) or a general medical condition (e.g. hyperthyrodism).

Bipolar Disorders

- Bipolar disorders are characterized by mood swings from profound depression to extreme euphoria (mania) with intervening periods of normalcy. Delusions or hallucination may or may not be a part of the clinical picture and onset of symptoms may reflect a seasonal pattern.
- Manic episode is present with the symptoms of mania discussed above.
- A somewhat milder representation of this clinical symptoms picture is called hypomania. Hypomania is not severe enough to cause marked impairment in social or occupational functioning or to require hospitalization and it does not include psychotic features.
- The diagnostic picture for depression associated with bipolar disorder is identical to that described above with one addition that the client must have a history on one or more manic episodes.
- When symptoms presentation includes rapidly alternating moods (sadness, irritability, euphoria) accompanied by symptoms associated with both depression and mania, the individual is given a diagnosis of mixed bipolar disorder. The disturbance is severe enough to cause marked impairment in social or occupational functioning or to require hospitalization. Psychotic features maybe evident.

Bipolar I Disorder

Bipolar I disorder is diagnosed when an individual who is experiencing or has experienced a full syndrome of manic or mixed symptoms. The client may also have experienced episodes of depression.

Bipolar II Disorder

The diagnosis is done when the client experiences recurrent bouts of major depression with episodic occurrence of hypomania.

DYSTHYMIC DISORDER

Definition

Dysthymic disorder is a chronic disorder characterized by the presence of depressed mood that lasts most of the day and is present almost continuously, i.e. Low grade depression with accentuation of depressive temperament for at least two years (one year for children and adolescents).

Epidemiological Factors

- *Onset:* Childhood and adolescence
- Five to six percent of all persons.
- *Gender:* Equal in both gender.
- More in unmarried and low socioeconomic people.
- Coexists with medical illness, anxiety disorders especially panic, substance abuse and borderline personality disorders.
- *Causes:* Same as in depressive disorders.

CLINICAL FEATURES

- Two years duration (continuous)
- More features seen as subjective than objective
- Depressed mood
- Habitual gloom, brooding, lack of joy, preoccupation with inadequacy
- No severe disturbance in appetite, libido, psychomotor retardation

Diagnostic Criteria

- Depressed mood for most of the day, more days than not as subjective accounts or observation by others, for at least two years.
  Note: In children and adolescents mood can be irritable and duration must be at least one year.
- Presence while depressed of two or more of the following.
  - Poor appetite or overeating
  - Insomnia or hypersomnia
  - Low energy or fatigue
  - Low self-esteem
  - Poor concentration or difficulty in making decisions
  - Feeling of hopelessness.
- During the one years period (one year for children or adolescents) of disturbance, the person has never been without the symptoms in A or B for more than two months at a time.
- No major depressive disorder has been present during the first two years of the disturbance (one year for children).
- There has been a manic, mixed or hypomanic episode and criteria has never been met for cyclothymic disorder.
- The disturbance does not occur exclusively during the course of a chronic psychotic disorder such as schizophrenia or delusional disorder.

- The symptoms are not due to the direct physiological effect of a substance (e.g. a drug of abuse, a medication) or a general medical condition (e.g. hypothyroidism).
- The symptoms cause clinically significant distress or impairment in social, occupational or other important areas of functioning.

MANAGEMENT

It includes several goals. Primarily, client's safety and diagnosis. Treatment includes reducing the symptoms and follow-up.

CYCLOTHYMIC DISORDER

Definition

It must be chronic in nature (two years) fluctuating disturbance including periods of hypomania and depression in milder form than bipolar I, shorter duration than bipolar II.

EPIDEMIOLOGICAL ASPECTS

- Lifetime prevalence: 1%.
- Coexist with border line personality disorder and substance abuse.

CLINICAL FEATURES

- *Presentation:* Marital conflicts, instability of interpersonal relationships.
- Changes in mood are irregular and abrupt sometimes occurs within hours.
- Client may be achiever if controlling his symptoms or may have professional and social difficulties.

Diagnostic Criteria

For at least two years, the presence of numerous periods with hypomanic symptoms and numerous periods with depressive symptoms that do not meet criteria for major depressive disorder (in children and adolescents the duration must be at least one year). The clinical features are that of minor depressive episode, hypomanic episode or mixed and irritability. The client may present with marital difficulties and unprovoked disagreement with friends, family or co-workers.

Treatment

- Drug/pharmacotherapy.
  - Mood stabilizers (lithium, carbamazepine, depakote, clonazepam, gabapentin).
  - Use of antidepressants with caution to avoid antidepressant induced hypomania.

Psychotherapy

- *Individual therapy:* Psychoeducation to enhance client's awareness to his disease condition and help positive coping methods for mood swings.
- Family and group therapy.

MANAGEMENT OF DEPRESSIVE DISORDER

Assessment

- Depression can be viewed as a continuum according to severity of illness. Every individual becomes depressed one time or other in their lifespan due to various causes.
- Mild depression occurs when the grief processes is triggered in response to the loss of a valued object. This can occur with a loss of loved one, friend, pet or significant other. As individual progresses with the acceptance of loss then symptoms are subsided and activities of daily living are resumed within few weeks. If this does not occur grief is prolonged or exaggerated and symptoms are intensified.
- Moderate depression occurs when grief is prolonged or exaggerated. The individual is fixed in anger and this is turned inward on the self and the individual feels difficulty in functioning. Dysthymia is an example of moderate depression.
- Severe depression is a form of chronic depression where the individual is severely depressed and loses touch with reality. Client is manifested with anhedonia, suicidal ideation with delusions.
- The Beck Depression Inventory and The Zung Rating Scale are self-report methods to assess the depressive symptoms. The Hamilton Rating Scale is an observer rated tool to assess depressive symptoms.

DRUG MANAGEMENT

In acute phase of depression (4–6 weeks)

- Major depressive disorder (mild, moderate): pharmacotherapy + psychotherapy.
- Severe without psychotic features: pharmacotherapy + psychotherapy + ECT.
- Chronic with psychotic features pharmacotherapy + ECT + antipsychotic.
- Major depressive disorder with catatonia pharmacotherapy + ECT + antipsychotic + benzodiazepines.
- Major depressive disorder in bipolar type mood stabilizer + antidepressants.
  - Mostly depressive cases (Mild to Moderate).
  - Can be managed at OPD basis, hospitalization is required when symptoms are associated with suicidal ideation or attempts.

Criteria for Hospitalization

- Suicide or homicide
- Progressive symptoms and severe retardation
- Catatonic
- Refusal of treatment and food
- Lack of social support
- Psychotic depression
- Impaired insight.

Pharmacotherapy

Tricyclic Antidepressants (TCAs)

Drug	Dosage
• Amitryptyline (AMT)	75–300 mg/day.
• Imipramine	75–150 mg/day
• Clomipramine	75–250 mg/day
• Amoxapine	75–300 mg/day
• Desipramine	75–300 mg/day
• Doxepin	75–300 mg/day
• Nortriptyline	50–200 mg/day

Side Effects

- Anticholinergic: Dry mouth, blurred vision, urinary retention, constipation, palpitation, sedation and dizziness
- Fine tremors
- Postural hypotension
- Weight gain:
  - Change in sexual functioning like loss of libido and anorgasmia in both genders
  - Loss of erectile or ejaculatory dysfunction in males
  - Insomnia and anxiety.

SELECTIVE SEROTONIN REUPTAKE INHIBITOR (SSRI)

Drug	Dosage
• Escitalopram (cipralex)	20–60 mg/day
• Fluoextine (prozac)	20–60 mg/day
• Sertraline (Instral)	50–200 mg/day
• Fluvoxamine (faverin)	50–300 mg/day
• Paroxetine (seroxat)	20 mg/day

Side Effects

- GI upset, insomnia, agitation, headache, sexual dysfunction.
- Serotonin syndrome especially in combination of drugs are manifested as abdominal pain, fever, sweating and flushing.

Other Drugs

- Tetracyclic antidepressant as Maprotiline (Ludiomil) 150 to 300 mg
- MAOI in atypical features
- Serotonin noradrenergic reuptake inhibitor as venlafaxine (Effexor) 15 to 75 mg
- Serotonin modulator as trazodone 150 to 600 mg.
- Bupropion

- Norepinephrine, serotonin modulator as Mirtazepine (remeron) 30 mg/day
- Lithium (Lithium carbonate) camcolit
- Anticonvulsant (sodium valproate) Depakote
- Antipsychotic (olazapine, risperidone).

Electroconvulsive Therapy (ECT)

- ECT is effective with client who are not well responding to drugs. Other factors such as catatonic features and suicidal symptoms.
- To minimize the cognitive impairment, ECT maybe administered unilaterally on the non-dominant hemisphere. ECT is a major treatment choice in major depression.
- Side effects of ECT include temporary amnesia, confusion and rarely fractures.

PSYCHOTHERAPEUTIC TREATMENT MODALITIES

Psychotherapy

It is the use of various psychological approaches to treat emotional and effective disorder. It is very helpful in the treatment of bipolar disorder to prevent relapses.

Goal of Psychotherapy

- Gain in understanding of the emotions and ideas that contribute to exaggerated mood swings
- Identify and understand life problems or events
- Learn coping techniques and problem-solving skills
- Regain a sense of control and pleasure in life.

INDIVIDUAL THERAPY

Therapist meet the client on the basis to discuss issues that are disturbing them.

SUPPORTIVE PSYCHOTHERAPY

It is effective therapist—client relationship with gaining confidence. Documentation is maintained regarding destructive impulses directed toward self and an explanation of symptoms. It is a ongoing psycho education program, involving knowledge and feedback are provided regarding client's illness and prognosis. Client's morale is improved by provoking, strengthening expectations of help and hopefullness, realistic and attainable goals are set and client is guided regarding daily schedule and meetings.

PSYCHODYNAMIC THERAPY

Psychodynamic psychotherapy is based on the assumption that a person is mentally ill because of unresolved, unconscious conflicts, often arises from childhood. The goal of this therapy includes for clients to understand the emotions they experience and to learn how to manage them more effectively. It lasts many months to even years.

INTERPERSONAL THERAPY

This therapy focuses on the behaviors and interactions a client has with other individuals and family members. It attempts to recognize and explore interpersonal stressors, role disputes and transitions and social deficits. It is useful in the treatment of moderate unipolar depression with or without antidepressants. In this the client is helped in resolving ambivalence with the lost relationship, serving as temporary substitute for the lost relationship and assisting in establishing new relationship.

BEHAVIOR THERAPY

It is based on learning theories involving various activity scheduling, self-control therapy, social skill training and problem-solving.

FAMILY AND MARITAL THERAPY

The ultimate objective of working with family of client with affective disorders is to synthesize the available data to formulate a therapeutic plan with two key goals—resolution of the symptoms and restoration or creation of adaptive family function. Marital and family stressors maybe consequences of depression but may also increase vulnerability to depression.

COGNITIVE BEHAVIOR THERAPY

Cognitive behavior therapy (CBT) helps to control thought distortions that are considered a factor in the development and maintenance of mood disorders. In cognitive model, depression is characterized by a triad of negative distortions related to expectations of the environment, self and future. The general goals in cognitive therapy are to obtain symptoms relief as early as possible, to assist the client in identifying dysfunctional patterns of thinking and behavioring and to guide the client to evidences and logic that effectively test the validity of dysfunctional thinking. Therapy focuses on charging 'automatic thoughts' that occur spontaneously and contribute to the distorted effect.

GROUP THERAPY

It is an important dimension of multi model treatment plan of the manic and depressive clients. Once the acute phase is passed, group can provide an atmosphere in which individuals may discuss issues in their lives that cause, maintain or arise out of having a serious affective disorder. Support group members gain a sense of perspective on their conditions and tangibly link-up with others who have similar problems.

MEDICATION AND MINDFULNESS THERAPY

These therapies focus on inner peace, serenity, relaxation and awareness of the divine self of life. These therapies are usually conducted in groups when individuals gather together to share life experiences. There is no limit time frame for therapies. They may continue through life.

Psychoeducation

It should focus on the following objectives:

- Identify the early signs of relapse of mania and depression
- Discuss the importance of support groups and how to find them
- State the need for and benefits of follow-up
- Participate in support groups and personally satisfying activities

- Discuss the issue of alcohol and substance use–abuse.
- Identify the action, side effects and special instructions of prescribed drugs.
- Describe ways to manage the side effects of medication such as weight gain, sleep, and lowered blood pressure.

MANAGEMENT MODALITIES OF BIPOLAR DISORDER

In Acute phase (4–6 weeks)

- Hospitalization
- ECT in acute and catatonic features
- *Drugs:* Mood stabilizers + sedatives + antipsychotics.
- Psychotherapy.
- Psychosocial rehabilitative measures.

In case of typical clinical features:

- Lithium carbonate (comcolt) 400 mg, 2 tablets/day
- Divalproex 500 mg. 1–3 times/ day
- Olanzapine
  - Atypical features. (mixed episode, rapid, dyphoric mania), car Carbamazepine (Tegretol) (tegretol) 200 tab. 3–6 times/day
  - Anxiolytics
    - Benzodiazepines, e.g. Clonazepam
    - Antipsychotics may be discontinued after 2–3 weeks.
    - Antipsychotic, e.g. CP 2, haloperidol.
  - *Drugs:* lithium carbonate 800–1200 mg/day.
  - Maintain serum level in the range 0.8–1.2 mEq/L.
  - Carbamazepine and Divalproex.
  - Lamotrigine and Gabapentin.

SIDE EFFECTS AND LITHIUM TOXICITY

- These are related to plasma concentration levels, so needs constant and ongoing monitoring of the level
- Lithium high levels (1.0 mEq/L and more) higher than 2 mEq/L can be threatening or fatal in outcome.
- Symptoms can be neurological, gastrointestinal, enlarged thyroid, weight gain, memory difficulty, kidney dysfunction cardiovascular and renal dysfunction, polyuria, tremors, hypothyroidism, hypokalemia, seizures, and changes in ECG.
- Contraindicated during pregnancy.
- If lithium carbonate fails to action, look for alternate agents.

Valproic Acid (Depakote)

- *Action:* Antiepileptic and antimanic.
- Augments the post synaptic action of GABA at its receptors
- Best of rapid cycling and acute mania
- *Therapeutic blood levels:* 50-100 mg/L
- *Side effects*: GI upset, lethargy, fine tremors, metabolic liver changes and alopecia
- It can be a drug of choice in anxiety, mood and personality disorder.

Carbamazepine (Tegretol)

- Acts superior to lithium for rapid cycling, regarded as a second line treatment for mania.
- Correlation between therapeutic and plasma levels.
- Side effects include sedation, stomach upsets, ataxia and sociocognitive effects.

Gabapentin

- Primarily an anticonvulsant. Used in bipolar disorders and in pain disorders
- GABA Analogue
- Not bound to plasma proteins
- Half-life period in 5–7 hours.
- Side effect include dizziness, ataxia, double vision and changes in sleep cycle.

Atypical Antipsychotics

- Common atypical antipsychotics, e.g. clozapine, risperidone and olanzapine
- Clozapine is effective, yet not readily used due to potential serious side effects
- Olanzapine can be given in acute mania.

NURSING MANAGEMENT

The client who suffers from depressive disorders maybe difficult to communicate. Isolation, withdrawal, ambivalence, hostility, guilt or impaired thought and psychomotor activities can interfere in therapeutic relationship. The manic clients hyperactivity, pressured speech and manipulation also interfere in maintaining relationship.

The psychiatric nurse must be aware of personal vulnerability to depressive behavior. Working long with such persons may cause one to react to the depressed atmosphere and in turn experience symptoms of depression. The following is a list of attitudes that the nurse should display toward depressed and manic clients.

- *Acceptance:* The psychiatric nurse should spend time with the client and accept the client as he or she is. Depressed individuals are not always able to express feelings and may exhibit complex behavior. They exhibit a low self-esteem and hopelessness the care given should avoid acting in any manner that could be interpreted as rejection or criticism. The manic person's manipulative demanding and irritable behavior may elicit feelings of disgust and nonacceptance. The nurse should make the manic person aware that the nurse will accept the person but not the behavior. Limit setting is one-way of displaying acceptance.
- *Honesty:* The psychiatric nurse should be truthful, not to make promises that she or he is unable to keep, and not provide false reassurance. The depressed person is less able to tolerate disappointment.
- *Empathy:* Any attempts is to cheer up a depressed person will be viewed as an inability to understand his or her feelings or problems. Such an approach may cause further withdrawal, isolation and depression. The caregiver should provide the person with an opportunity to express negative, painful feelings and respond in such a way as to convey the message that one recognizes and emphasizes with the emotions, thoughts or feelings of another person.
- *Patience:* Depressed individuals maybe unable to make correct decisions as simple as like what to eat for breakfast or what to wear? The nurse should be aware of the impact of psychomotor retardation on decision-making psychomotor agitation also requires patience. Underlying anxiety in the depressed person may cause hyperactivity, anger and hostile behavior.

The psychiatric nurse also must demonstrate patience while setting limits with the demanding manipulative manic client. Such clients can test and try one's patience, resulting in feelings of frustration, irritation and anger on the part of the caregiver.

Nursing assessment focuses on mood, affect, behavior and appearance. Body language replaces communication skills because the person is unable to convey feelings of anger, hostility and ambivalence.

The nurse can ask questions to assess the level of depression, while observing facial expressions, body posture, tone of voice, mood and overall appearance, include the following:

- Do you have difficulty falling asleep at night?
- Do you experience middle of the night awakening?
- If so, are you able to sleep take?
- Do you wake-up very early in the morning?
- Are you alert or depressed when you get-up in the morning?
- Do you sleep excessively?
- Have you been experiencing feelings of worthlessness, self-reproach or inappropriate guilt?
- Do you have difficulty concentrating or making decisions?
- Can you watch full movie or TV show?
- Does your mood charge or fluctuate during the day?
- Has your sexual desire decreased?
- Are you frequently constipated?
- Has your energy level decreased?
- Have you lost interest in life?
- Do you feel alienated from those around you?
- Has there been change in your appetite?
- Have you ever considered or attempted suicide?

Nursing intervention includes assisting the person in meeting basic human needs. The most severe the depression, the more important becomes physical care since the person losses interest in self-care. Clients who exhibit manic behavior also may neglect personal hygiene. The caregiver may need to assist the person with bathing, brushing and grooming as well as with personal hygiene. Because appearance is neglected, the client may need help in selecting the clothes to wear as well as washing and ironing the desired clothes.

Dietary needs should be monitored. The depressed client may avoid to eat whereas manic maybe too hyperactive to eat. Monitoring the intake and output (I and O) is significant.

Periods of rest and activity need to be evaluated because depressed client may sleep contiuoulsy to avoid anxieties of real world. Neurotic depression or dysthymic is characterized by increased feelings of depression as the day progresses. Such persons generally 'feel better in the morning'. Persons with major depressive disorder or psychotic depression fall asleep easily, awaken early and feel better as the day progresses.

Simple activities are most effective for a person with a short attention span or an inability to concentrate. Completion of such tasks enhances one's self-concept because the person feels more worthwhile after the job is done. One also must consider the person's energy level: the more energy the task requires, the less energy the person will have to engage in hostile, aggressive behavior.

Protective care maybe necessary for the manic as well as for the depressed person. Persons who exhibit manic behavior may injure themselves owing to excessive motor activity, inability to concentrate, distractibility and poor judgment. Their destructive tendencies may include self-inflicting behavior and accidental injury. They may also provoke self-defensive actions unintentionally from others who fear injury.

Depressed persons may attempt self-inflicted harm or suffer injury owing to severe depression; lack of interest, psychomotor retardation, the inability to concentrate or the inability to defend themselves against aggressive persons. The psychiatric nurse should be aware of the potential for self-destructive behavior. Such an action may occur as the person's psychomotor retardation lessons, the ability to concentrate returns and the person is able to formulate a plan of action.

Assisting with electroconvulsive or electroshock therapy is another nursing intervention while caring for depressed client. Carrying to through physical examination before treatment is necessary. The nurses, role before treatment is to withhold breakfast and to administer all premedication. The nurse must be available to answer any questions the client may have, to provide supportive care, and to assist with the treatment and monitor the person's responses during a recovery period that usually lasts from a half hour to one hour.

Observing for side effects of psychotropic drugs is another responsibility of the nurse. Tricyclic antidepressants may cause dry mouth, blurred vision, drowsiness, difficulty with urination and constipation. Antipsychotics may produce extrapyramidal side effects.

If the client is on MAOI's, they require strict dietary adherence. Foods to be avoided include yoghurt, cheese, wine, beer, yeast and chocolate. Hypertensive crisis may occur after the administration of such drugs if the person combines the drug with food containing tyramine.

Monitoring lithium in blood is very necessary. It is frequently monitored in an acute phase of bipolar disorder and on a routine basis during the maintenance phase because of toxicity in case of excess dose of the drug or in the presence of a decreased serum sodium level. The therapeutic level is usually between 0.8 and 1.5 mEq/L. Diuretics, profuse diaphoresis, a low salt diet or diarrhea may result in lowered serum sodium levels and higher lithium levels. Symptoms of lithium toxicity include vomiting, diarrhea, twitching, weight loss, excessive thirst, abnormal muscle movement, muscle twitching, slurred speech, blurred vision, dizziness, stupor and an irregular heart rate.

Client psychoeducation is another important nursing intervention for depressed and manic clients. Such clients should be informed about the importance of outpatient treatment as well as the continuation of prescribed medications.

They maybe placed on long-term maintenance level of medication and could suffer a relapse if they discontinued the drugs. They should be taught to recognize the onset of side effects, as well as the recurrence of symptoms to avoid rehospitalization.

Manic clients should be cautioned not to take on too many responsibilities or to overextend themselves. Depressed individuals should be instructed to contact health care provider or agency if symptoms reappear.

Another aspect of nursing care is that of being supportive during psychotherapy sessions. The person may have difficulty expressing feelings of hostility, ambivalence and guilt. Feelings of anxiety may occur or increase as the person begins of the therapy sessions. Such sessions maybe directed at exploring feelings about self to improve the person's self-esteem and decrease feeling of helplessness, hopelessness and powerlessness. The nurse can be supportive in identifying the symptoms such as anxiety.

Nursing Diagnosis and Care

- *Nursing Diagnosis:* High-risk for injury related to extreme hyperactivity, restlessness, hostile behavior and suicidal ideation.
- *Goal:* The client will remain free of injury during hospitalization.

Nursing Intervention	Rationale	Outcome criteria
• Decrease environmental stimuli. Provide quiet and calm surrounding with low level of light and noise.	Client is extremely distractable to even slightest stimuli. A nontherapeutic environment can be very stimulating.	Client understands the importance of calm environment.
• Remove all potential hazardous objects and substances.	Client can use those object for hearming self or others.	Feels safe and secure.
• Administer medications as ordered.	Antipsychotics are usually prescribed to calm the client.	Demonstrate an understanding of the purpose of antipsychotics and other drugs.
• Provide physical facilities.	Physical activities are helpful to vent up emotions and to channelize energy.	Begin to verbalize thoughts and feelings.

- *Nursing diagnosis:* Risk for violence directed to self or others related to manic excitement, delusions and hallucinations.

Nursing intervention	Rationale
• Observe the client every 15 minutes.	Important to control unwanted behavior timely.
• Maintain low level of stimuli in client's environment.	This will helpful to minimize anxiety and suspiciousness.
• Redirect violent behavior with physical activities, tension and hostility.	Physical activities are helpful to relieve anxiety.
• Ensure that all sharp objects, glass and harmful subjects have been removed from his room.	These objects maybe used to harm self and others.
• Maintain a calm attitude to client. Clear handle conflicts.	Anxiety is contagious and can be transferred from one to another.
• Have one to one interaction with the client, assign the same staff as much as possible and have sufficient staff of indicate a show of strength to client if necessary.	This conveys evidence of control over the situation and provides some physical security to the staff.
• Administer tranquilizers as prescribed. If client refuses go for mechanical restrints after prescription.	Helps to avoid violent behavior.
• Client can be given medication after restraining. Observe the client every 15 min.	Client's safety is priority. Observation helps to ensure nutrition and elimination needs.
• Restraints can be removed gradually one at a time.	Gradual removal of restraints reduces the risk for injury to client and the staff.

- *Nursing diagnosis:* Altered nutrition less than body requirement related to refusal and inability to sit long enough to eat.
- *Nursing goal:* Client is free from signs and symptoms of malnutrition.

Nursing intervention	Rationale
• Client should be provided with high protein, high calorie and nutritious food and drinks that can have.	• Client is unable or unwilling to sit and eat, highly nutritious food that require little effort to eat is effective.
• Monitor client's eating pattern and food intake. Recording of client intake and output calorie count and protein intake should be documental.	• The client maybe unaware of physical needs or may ignore feelings of thirst and hunger.
• Client should be provided foods according to his/her taste.	• This enhances eating pattern.
• Additional supplements of vitamins and minerals can be provided along with diet.	• It will increase nutritional status of client.

- *Nursing Diagnosis:* Bizarre and inappropriate behavior, dress or appearance related to low self-esteem, delusions and disordered thought.
- *Nursing outcome:* Client will try to maintain interaction with other.

Nursing intervention	Rationale
• Recognize the manipulative behavior, help to reduce feelings of insecurity by increasing feelings of power and control.	• Understanding the motivation behind the behavior may facilitate greater acceptance.
• Decrease environmental stimuli whenever possible. Respond to cues of increased restlessness or agitation by removing stimuli and perhaps isolating the client a single accompany room maybe beneficial.	• The client's ability to deal with stimuli is impaired.
• Set limit on manipulative behavior explain what is expected and consequences if limit are violated. Terms of limitations must be agreed on by all staff who are caring the client.	• Consequences for violation of limits must be consistently administered or behaviors will not be eliminated. Nursing management of depressed client.
• Limit group activities in terms of size of group and frequency of activities based on the clients level of tolerance.	• The client's ability to respond to others and to deal in the increased amounts and complexing of sentiments is threatening.
• Ignore or withdraw attention from bizarre dress, behavior and sexual acting out as much as possible.	• It is important to minimize attention given to unacceptable behaviors withdrawing attention can be more effective then negative reinferent in decreasing unacceptable behaviors.
• Simple and direct open explanation for routine actions, procedures, tests should be given. Do not argue with the client.	• The client has limited ability to perceive and respond to complex stimuli. Arguing with the client interjects doubt.
• Client should be encouraged to verbalize his/her feelings of anxiety, anger and fear, dizziness the wags of management of stress.	• Ventilation of feelings may help relieve anxiety and anger. These will relieve tension.
• Physical activities should be provided as an outlet for negative energy.	• Physical activities can channelize energy and stress in a healthy manner.
• Avoid highly competitive activities.	• Competitive situation can exacerbate the clients, hostile and aggressive feelings or can reinforce the clients, low self-esteem.
• Help client identify positive aspects about self, recognize accomplishments and feel good about them.	• As self-esteem is increased, client will feel less need to manipulate others for gratification.

NURSING MANAGEMENT OF DEPRESSED CLIENT

- *Nursing Diagnosis:* Risk for suicide related to depressed mood, feelings of worthlessness and anger toward self.
- *Nursing outcome:* Client will not harm self and others.

Nursing intervention	Rationale
• Talk to client directly. Ask have you thought about harming yourself in anyway? If so what do you plan to do? Do you have the means to carry-out this plan?	• The risk of suicide is greatly increased if the client has developed a plan and particularly if means exist for the client to execute the plan.
• Determine the appropriate level of suicide precaution for the client. Create a safe environment; remove all potentially harmful objects from the client's access. Supervise client closely during meals and drug administration.	• Physical safety is prime priority.
• The client has one to one contact with staff members at all the times even when going to washroom.	• A client who is at high-risk for suicidal behavior needs constant supervision and limitation of opportunities to harm himself or herself.
• Maintain special care in administration of drugs.	• Prevents hoarding for overdose or discarding the drug.
• Make irregular frequent checking at night and early morning.	• It prevents staffs surveillance from being predictable.
• Encourage client to express honest feelings including violent behavior.	• Depression and suicidal behavior can be prevented by verbalization.

- *Nursing diagnosis:* Low self-esteem related to feelings of worthlessness, hopelessness and helplessness.
- *Nursing outcome:* Client will be able to attempt new activities without the fear of failure.
- Client will express feelings directly and openly.

Nursing interventions	Rationale
• As necessary help the client have good personal hygiene and appearance.	• The client maybe unaware of or lack of interest in personal hygiene. Good personal hygiene is helpful to enhance clients self-esteem.
• In the beginning, provide simple activities that can be easily and quickly completed. Start with the client alone and gradually progress to group, occupational and recreational therapy sessions.	• The client maybe limited in his or her ability to deal with complex tasks or stimuli. Success and independence promotes feelings of self-worth.
• Provide the client honest positive reinforcement after successful completion of tasks.	• Client with low self-esteem do not benefit from undue flattery. Positive reinforcement will enhance the frequency of desired behavior.
• Gradually increase the complexity of activity or responsibilities. Provide positive feedback after every successful accomplishment.	• As client's self-esteem increases he/she can carry-out complex and multiple tasks.
• Encourage the client to recognize areas of change and provide assistance toward his effort.	• Client will need assistance and help in problem-solving.
• Client should be taught assertiveness and communication techniques.	• Effective assertiveness and communication techniques promote self-esteem.

- *Nursing Diagnosis:* Disturbance in interpersonal communication related to helplessness and low self-esteem, disordered thought process.
- *Nursing Outcomes:* The client will communicate with others and participate in group activities

Nursing intervention	Rationale
• Encourage the client to verbalize his/her feelings in whatever ways he/she licks verbal or nonverbal. Let the client known that you will listen and accept what he/she is expressing.	• Ventilation of feelings may help to relieve feelings of despair hopelessness, sadness and so forth. Nurse should remain nonjudgmental about the client's feelings and express this to the client, directly or indirectly.
• Be comfortable sitting with the client in silence let the client know that you are available to verbalize.	• Sitting silently bedside the client reflect nurse's interest in client and motivates client to verbalize.
• Provide expression of hope to client in positive manner.	• Even if the client feels hopelessness, it is helpful to hear positive expression from others.
• Help the client identify areas of life that can be controlled and that cannot be controlled.	• Client's emotional conditions may interfere understanding problem realistically.
• Help the client to solve problems, change behavior and make plan for discharge and follow-up.	• The client needs to resume responsibility for him/herself as his/her ability increase.

Other Modes of Treatment

Many different alternative and complementary therapies are used to deal with depression. These are:

- *Meditation:* Practiced regularly in the form of chanting transcendental meditation is very useful
- Life style changes such as adopting a healthy diet, exercise and stress reduction measures
- Biofeedback and relaxation therapies, such as humor therapy, flower therapy, hydrotherapy, hypno therapy and magnetic therapy are useful.
- Physical therapies such as massage, reflexology and acupuncture.
- Environment therapies such as music, aroma therapy.
- Interaction with outside world—nature and animals.
- Limiting the intake of alcohol and other illicit drug.

Psychosocial Rehabilitation

Day Centers

Day centers, day hospitals and drop-in-centers can vary widely in their functions. Services may include therapy groups, counseling, information or advice. Some centers may offer a chance to learn new skills such as music, cooking or crafts, some organize trips and provides an opportunity for social networking.

Follow-up

- Depending on the severity of depression, the client should approach health provider regularly, at least once in a week.
- Notify the side effects and if any changes to be done.

Preventive Strategies for Depression

Identifying the high-risk factors in community is paramount need. People should be screened regularly by conducting surveys regularly.

Depression Diagnosis

- Untreated episodes of clinical depression typically lasts from six to twenty four months of duration.
- Proper treatment reduces relapses.
- About 75% of people will recover and return to their usual normal daily activities within few days to weeks.
- Around 25% of client will exhibit some residual symptoms for a significant time.
- Nearly 10% of people with depression will have continuous or intermittent symptoms for two or more years. A person who has one episode of depression should be on the lookout for recurrent episodes of depression, since these occur about 50% of the time. However, prompt treatment will usually be effective for these recurrent depressions.

Follow-up for Bipolar Disorder

- It is mandatory for clients to take medications regularly without discontinuance. The client will be tempted to stop medication. Abrupt stopping will give rise to complications, so, tapering of the drug is must. It maybe possible to reoccur the symptoms.
- Depending on the drug used, client needs regular blood tests to monitor levels and to check for side effects of the drug.
- Regular meetings with health personnel and doctor is necessary for detecting any abnormality in mood.
- Ongoing psychoeducation for client and his/her family is crucial to help everyone deal with the disease.
- Family teaching is necessary to detect the early symptoms of disease and its preventive and promotive measures.
- Coping with his/her own feelings is necessary. It needs psychosocial support from within and environment. Social networking helps to build confidence.
- Psychoeducation, social skill training, cognitive remediation, family education, vocational rehabilitation and case management programs are essential for rehabilitation of mood disorders.

8 Nursing Management of Patient with Neurotic, Stress Related and Somatization Disorders

INTRODUCTION

In this modern era, it has become natural to worry and feel tense or scared to live under pressure. This has given rise to anxiety. Anxiety is the body's natural response to danger, an automatic alarm that goes off when we feel threatened.

In moderation, anxiety is not always a bad thing. In fact, anxiety can help to stay alert and focused, spur to action and motivates to resolve the problem situations. But when anxiety level is constant or overwhelming, when it interferes with interpersonal relationships and activities it stops being functional, then it gives rise to anxiety disorders.

DEFINITIONS AND MEANING

The concept of anxiety was first introduced by Freud. He referred to it as a danger signal a person exhibit in response to the perception of physical pain or danger. The term anxiety is used to describe feelings of uncertainty, uneasiness, apprehension or tension that a person experiences in response to an unknown object or situation. A 'fight or flight' decision is made by the person in an attempt to overcome conflict, stress trauma or frustration.

According to Walker (1982), refers to anxiety as 'butterflies and nuisance' which can be constructive when present in a moderate degree because it increase one's alertness and ability to perform in a positive manner. Anxiety also can be a painful reaction to internal conflict as the conflict lingers and produces physical and emotional symptoms. People who exhibit symptoms of increased anxiety when unable to cope with existing conflict or frustration may develop an anxiety disorder.

An anxiety state consists of feelings of tension, apprehension, nervousness, worry and activation of the autonomic nervous system. The physiological manifestations generally include increased blood pressure, rapid heart rate, sweating, dryness of mouth, vertigo, irregularities in breathing and musculoskeletal disturbances.

Fear differs from anxiety in that it is the body's physiologic and emotional response to a known or recognized danger.

EPIDEMIOLOGICAL DATA

According to WHO survey, the overall average prevalence estimates for any type of anxiety disorders ranges from 10.6 to 16.6%, but rates for individual disorders varies widely. Women had generally higher prevalence rates than men, but the magnitude of the difference varies a lot.

TYPES OF ANXIETY

Types of anxiety are described as signal anxiety, anxiety trait, anxiety state and free floating anxiety.

Signal Anxiety

It is a response (anxiety) to an anticipated event. For example, a mother who normally is relaxed exhibits tachycardia, dizziness and insomnia when her child attends school for the first time.

Anxiety Trait

It is a part and parcel of personality that has been present over a long period of time and is measurable by observing the person's physiological, emotional and cognitive behavior. The person who responds to various nonstressful situations with anxiety is said to have an anxiety trait. For example, a 30-year-old watchman frequently complains of blurred vision, dizziness, headaches and insomnia in relatively stress free job.

Anxiety State

It occurs as the result of a stressful situation in which the person loses control of her or his emotions. For example, a mother who is told her son has been injured while driving a motorcycle and has been admitted in emergency may exhibit an anxiety state by becoming hysterical, complaining of tightness in the chest and eagerly waiting to see him.

Free Floating Anxiety

It is always present and accompanied by a feelings of dread. The person may exhibit ritualistic and avoidance behavior.

SEVERITY OF ANXIETY

Severity of anxiety is described as normal, acute, chronic and panic. Normal anxiety is anxiety that is present in a low degree, can motivate individual and is necessary for survival. Acute anxiety interferes with one's ability to think and is referred to as extreme nervousness. It usually occurs suddenly and lasts a short period of time. Chronic anxiety may be present over a period of months or years. The person appears to be stable but exhibits tremulous motor activity and rigid posture. Panic anxiety is a severe form of anxiety that causes disintegration of the personality, resulting in the inability to function normally. The individual looses touch with reality.

CHARACTERISTICS OF ANXIETY

The chief characteristics of anxiety include the following:

- Anxiety is a negative emotions.
- It is very communicable in nature.
- Varies from mild to panic. Mild anxiety serves as a motivational force behind to fulfill tasks. Its very high degree may cause incapacity or a panic state.

ANXIETY AS A CONTINUOUS PROCESS

Mild Anxiety

It is 'spice of life' and motivational in nature. The symptoms include:
- Enhanced perceptual field.
- Increased level of energy.
- Produces productivity, growth and creativity.
- Increase awareness and motivation.
- Increase problem solving and learning.
- Irritability and restlessness.
- Feeling of 'butterflies in stomach'.
- Enhanced sleep disturbances.
- More sensitive to noise.

Moderate Anxiety

Periphery is blocked out:
- Narrow perceptual field.
- Selective inattention.
- Immediate task oriented.
- Attentive to immediate task.
- Difficulty in concentration.
- Frequent urination.
- Dry mouth/muscle tension.
- Increase rate of speech.
- Diaphoric.

Severe Anxiety

- Can focus on only specific subjects.
- Learning and problem solving not possible.
- Narrowed perceptual task or solving problems.
- Feeling of dread/doom.
- Crying without reason.
- Ritualistic behaviors.
- Headache/nausea and vomiting.
- Vertigo.
- Tachycardia.
- Complain in stomach and chest.
- Rigid stance.

Panic Anxiety

- Disorganized personality totally out of control.
- Unable to fulfill task even with direction.
- Inability to process environment stimuli.
- Can only focus on self.

- Self harm.
- Irrational thoughts/behaviors.
- Possible delusions/hallucinations.
- Dilated pupils.
- Increased vital signs.

Symptoms of Anxiety Disorders

Actually, anxiety disorders are culmination of many related conditions and manifests differently in persons. Despite their different forms, all anxiety disorders share one major symptoms; persistent or severe fear or worry in situations where most people would not feel threatened.

Emotional Symptoms of Anxiety Disorders

In addition to the primary symptoms of irrational and excessive fear and worry, other common emotional symptoms of anxiety include:
- Feeling of apprehension or dread
- Trouble concentrating
- Feeling tense and jumpy
- Anticipating the worst
- Irritability
- Restlessness
- Watching for signs of danger
- Feeling blank in mind.

Physical Symptoms of Anxiety

Anxiety is more than just a feeling. As a product of the body's fight or flight response, anxiety involves a wide range of physical symptoms. Because of numerous physical symptoms, client visits many doctors.

Very Common Physical Symptoms of Anxiety include:
- Pounding heart
- Sweating
- Shortness of breath/difficulty in breathing
- Fine tremors and twitches
- Muscle tension
- Fatigue
- Insomnia
- Restlessness
- Watching for signs of danger
- Feeling like your's mind's gone blank.

Physical symptoms of anxiety

- Pounding heart
- Insomnia
- Sweating
- Tremors and twitches

- Shortness of breath
- Feeling detached/unreal
- Headaches
- Fatigue.

Etiology

The exact cause of anxiety disorders is unknown. These are caused by a multiple factors, including changes in brain and environmental stress. The psychophysiological theories have classified causes of anxiety as stress, childhood conflicts, faulty learning and social and cultural factors.

Psychodynamic theory postulates that unconscious conflicts of childhood, such as fear of losing a parent's love or attention, fear of losing security, competition with a parent of the same gender, resentment and anger or fear of being considered a 'bad person' may emerge and result in feelings of discomfort or anxiety in childhood, adolescence or early adulthood.

Selye's biological theory (1956) focuses on the effect of stress on the body and is referred to as the General Adaptation Syndrome (GAS). Stress causes wear and tear of the system (structural and clinical changes) on the body and requires some type of coping behaviors by the individual. Such behaviors may be adaptive (positive) or maladaptive (negative) resulting in exhaustion and integration of the mind or body or both.

Behavioral theorists state that an individual's response to a stressful event is often the result of learned or conditioned behavior. If one experiences too many life changes over a short period of time, one does not have enough time to adjust or condition one self to each change and may exhibit dysfunctional or maladaptive behavior.

Social and cultural theorists believe factors cause anxiety explain that as a person's personality develops, his or her impression of self may be negative (low self concept). The person experiences difficulty adapting to everyday social problems owing to this self concept and inadequate coping mechanisms. The stressful stimuli of modern society pose a psychological threat for such a person and can result in the development of maladaptive behavior and the onset of an anxiety disorder.

Carpenito (1992) lists the following contributing risk factors or etiology for the nursing diagnosis of anxiety.

- Pathophysiological factors, which interfere with the basic human needs.
- Situational factors, which result in an actual or perceived threat or loss of significant others; actual or perceived change in the environment or one's socio economic status, or the transmission of another persons' anxiety to the individual.
- Maturational factors, which include a threat to the development task (s) of infants, children, adolescents, adults or the elderly.
- According to Mc Farland and Wasli (1992) list 16 contributing or causative factors in the development of anxiety including threats to:
  - Self concept
  - Personal security system
  - Beliefs
  - Stable environment
  - Role functioning
  - Meaningful interpersonal relationship and
  - Health status.

CLASSIFICATION OF ANXIETY DISORDERS

ICD-10 classifies anxiety disorders as follows:
- **F40-F48:** Neurotic, stress related and somatoform disorders
- **F40:** Phobic anxiety disorders
- **F41:** Other anxiety disorders
- **F42:** Obsessive compulsive disorders
- **F43:** Reaction to severs stress and adjustment disorders
- **F44:** Dissociative (conversion) disorders
- **F45:** Somatoform disorders
- **F46:** Other neurotic disorders.

  Neurosis is considered to be an emotional disturbance in which the person experiences increased subjective psychological pain or discomfort. As a result of stress, the persons handles anxiety or internal conflict in a maladaptive way, such as by developing a phobia or by experiencing a state of panic.

Neurosis is differentiated by psychosis as follows:

Neurotic behavior	Psychotic behavior
• Reality oriented	Out of contact with reality or denies reality.
• Demonstrates socially acceptable behavior	Demonstrates bizarre, inappropriate and abnormal behavior.
• Interacts with the reality	Creates a new world or environment and withdraws from reality in an effort to seek security in the newly created world.
• Absence of positive symptoms	Presence of positive symptoms such as delusions, hallucinations, illusion and mutism.
• Uses coping mechanisms in an attempt to decrease anxiety (primary gain).	Coping mechanisms are ineffective resulting in disintegration of one's personality.

Primary gain is defined as the relief from emotional conflict and freedom from anxiety that a person achieves by using defence or coping mechanisms. For example, a client refuses to talk about her mastectomy, because she becomes 'anxious' when the surgery is discussed. The client is using the mental mechanism 'suppression' to decrease her anxiety.

Secondary gain is an external gain derived from an illness, such as attention, disability benefit, monetary gain or the release from responsibility. For example, a 30 year old man injured his back while lifting bricks at work a year ago. He asks the company doctor to place him on sick leave so that he may collect disability benefits because he feels that he has never recovered from the injury.

Classifications of anxiety disorders include panic disorders, phobic disorders, generalized anxiety disorders, obsessive compulsive disorder and post traumatic stress disorder.

PANIC ANXIETY DISORDER

It is a real illness with both a physical and a psychological component. It begins during late teens or early 20s and although it can occur in both men and women, most individuals with panic disorder are women (more than 75%). It may last between a minute to an hour. The intensity of the attacks may fluctuate in the same person also.

The diagnostic criteria for this category require that at some time during the disturbance, one or more panic attacks have occurred that were unexpected and not triggered by situations in which the person was the focus of other's attention. The individual also experienced four or more attacks within a four week period or one or more attacks followed by a period of at least a month of persistent fear of having another attack.

According to the DSM III-R, at least four of the following symptoms must be present to diagnose a panic disorder.

- Dyspnea or shortness of breath
- Palpitations
- Chest pain or discomfort
- Choking or sympathizing sensation
- Vertigo or unsteady feelings.
- Diaphoresis
- Feelings of unreality or depersonalization.
- Trembling or shaking
- Syncope
- Nausea or abdominal distress
- Hot and cold flashes
- Tingling in hands or feet (paresthesia)
- Fear of losing control or dying.

People with panic state condition have feelings of terror that strike suddenly and repeatedly with no warning.

Symptoms of a panic attack develop suddenly and increase in intensity within ten minutes of awareness of the first sign. For example, chest pain occurs followed by three other symptoms that increase in intensity within ten minutes of the onset of chest pain.

Panic Disorder with Agoraphobia

Here, the individual has symptoms of panic attack and he/she experiences a fear of being in places or situations from which escape might be difficult or in which help might not be available. The fear severe strictly the individual to be homebound. The common agoraphobic situation are being in crowded places, out from home alone, standing in a line, visit to a shopping mall, traveling in a bus or train or aeroplane.

Generalized Anxiety Disorder

Generalized anxiety disorder (GAD) is a chronic disorder characterized by excessive, long lasting anxiety and worry about nonspecific life events, objects and situations. The individuals often feel a afraid and worried about health, money, family, work or school but they have trouble both in identifying the specific fear and controlling the worries. Their fear is usually unrealistic or out of proportion with what may be expected in their situation. The suffers expect failure and disaster to the point that interferes with daily functions like work, school and also relationships.

The DSM-IIIR classifies the symptoms according to three categories. They are:

- Motor tension, such as muscle aches, inability to relax, fidgeting, restlessness and being easily started.
- Autonomic hyperactivity, including cold and clammy hands, dry mouth, dizziness, frequent urination, flushing, increased pulse rate while resting and frequent stomach upset.

- Vigilance and scanning, a state in which the person is hyperactive, easily distracted, has difficulty concentrating experiences insomnia and is irritable or impatient.
  - The individual exhibits unrealistic or excessive anxiety and worry about two or more life circumstances during the six month period and may be mildly depressed. Symptoms rarely interfere with social or occupational functioning.

Etiology

Generalized anxiety disorders may be caused by environment factors, genetics, brain chemistry, substance abuse or a combination of these all. It is most commonly triggered by the stress in our lives. Usually, anxiety is a response to outside forces, but it is possible that we make ourselves anxious with 'negative self talk' a habit of always telling ourselves the worst will happen in future.

Psychodynamic Theory

According to Freud, anxiety is an inability of ego to intervene when conflicts occur between id and superego. When developmental defect in ego function is unable to resolve the conflict the individual will use defense mechanism to solve the conflict. Over use or ineffective use of ego defense mechanism result in maladaptive response to anxiety.

Cognitive Theories

According to cognitive theorists, anxiety erupts because of faulty or distorted thinking patterns accompanying maladaptive behaviors and emotional disorders. When there is disturbance in cognition there is subsequent disturbance in feeling and behavior. Because of faulty cognition there is a loss of ability to reason regarding the problem whether it is physical on interpersonal.

BIOLOGICAL THEORIES

Genetic Theory

Many researchers postulated that a family history of anxiety increases the likelihood that a person will develop. That is, some individuals may have a genetic predisposition to get anxiety disorders.

Familial studies support a genetic model (15-20% of the first degree relatives of those with GAD display it themselves–incidence is 4% in general population). The concordance rate in the monozygotic twins of clients with panic disorders is as high as 80%.

Biochemical Theories

Abnormal increase of blood lactate has been recorded in clients with panic attacks. Infusion of sodium lactate in clients with anxiety produces panic symptoms in individuals. Enhanced levels of norepinephrine are associated with physical signs of hyper arousal such as higher heart rate, palpitation and tachycardia.

It is also observed that undefined abnormality in serotonin system leads to panic attacks can be corrected by administering of SSRIs. GABA is the most prevalent inhibitory neurotransmitter in the CNS. It has been suggested that an alteration in GABA levels may lead to production of anxiety. Anxiolytics, such as benzodiazepines are effective in the treatment of panic disorder by facilitating GABA transmission and preventing anxiety.

Substance Use and Abuse

It is estimated that about half of clients who utilize health services for anxiety disorders, such as GAD, panic disorders or social phobia are consuming alcohol or benzodiazepine dependence. More generally, anxiety is known to result from:

a. Intoxication from an illicit drug, such as cocaine or amphetamine.
b. Withdrawl from an illicit drug, such as heroin or from prescription of drugs like benzodiazepines or barbiturates.

Medical Causes

Anxiety is associated with medical factors, such as anemia, asthma, infections and several cardiac conditions.

Causes of anxiety related to medical include:

- Stress from a debilitating disease
- Side effects of medications
- Signs and symptoms of diseases
- Lack of oxygen from emphysema or pulmonary embolism.

Environmental and External Factors

Environment factors that are known to cause several types of anxiety include:

Trauma from stressful events, such as abuse/ rape victimization or death of a loved one.

- Unhealthy relationships
- Job stress
- Financial and home stress.

MANAGEMENT OF GAD

The treatment of GAD includes many psychotherapeutic strategies. Before any intervention, self assessment plays an important role, every one who worries will not be having GAD. It may be because of overly demanding schedule lack; of exercise or sleep, pressure at home or work or even too much consumption of beverages.

The main cause for anxiety is unhealthy life style and being stressful. So, if you feel like you worry too much, take some time to evaluate how well you are caring for yourself. Consider the following questions.

- Do you make time each day for relaxation and fun?
- Are you getting the emotional support?
- Are you taking care of your body?
- Are you overloaded with your responsibilities?
- Do you ask help when you need it?

If your stress levels are through the roof, think about now you can bring your life back into balance. There may be responsibilities you can give up, turn down or delegate to others. If you are feeling isolated or unsupported, find someone to ventilate it. Just talking worries can be less frightening.

Self-help for Anxiety Attacks and Disorders

Self-help for anxiety attacks and anxiety disorder negative thoughts.

To overcome negative thoughts, practice the following:

Write Down Your Worries

Try to write down the worries on paper. Whenever you experience anxiety, write down and list out the worries on priority basis. Writing down is a harder work than simply thinking about them, so the negative thoughts are likely to disappear sooner. Writing down plays a significant role in calming the mind.

Create an Anxiety Worry Period

Choose one or two session of ten to fifteen minute schedule of 'worry periods' every day; time you can devote to anxiety. During this period, focus only on negative, anxious thoughts without trying to correct them. The rest of the day, however, is to be designated free of anxiety. When anxious thoughts occur during the day, write them down, and 'postpone' them to worry period.

Accept Uncertainty

Unfortunately, worrying about all the things that could go wrong does not make life any more predictable–it only keeps you from enjoying the good things happening in the present. Learn to accept uncertainty and not require immediate solutions to life's problems.

SELF-HELP FOR ANXIETY ATTACK AND ANXIETY DISORDERS TO TAKE CARE OF YOURSELF

- *Practice relaxation technique:* When practiced regularly, relaxation techniques, such as mindfulness meditation, progressive muscle relaxation and deep breathing exercises can reduce anxiety symptoms and increase feelings of relaxation and emotional well being.
- *Adopt healthy eating habits:* Start the day right with breakfast, and continue with frequent small meals throughout the day, going too long without eating leads to low blood sugar, which can make you feel more anxious.
- *Reduce alcohol and nicotine:* They lead to more anxiety not less.
- *Exercise regularly:* Exercise is a natural stress buster and anxiety relievers. To achieve the maximum benefit, aim for at least 30 minutes of aerobic or exercises on most days.
- *Get enough sleep:* A lack of sleep can exacerbate anxious thoughts and feelings. So try to get 7 to 9 hours of quality sleep at night.

TREATMENT OPTIONS FOR ANXIETY DISORDER

Treatment of anxiety disorders involves multiple combinations. Anxiety disorders respond very well to treatment and often in a relatively short amount of time. The specific treatment approach depends on the type of anxiety disorder and its severity. But in general, most anxiety disorders are treated with behavioral therapy, medication or combination of both. Sometimes complementary or alternate therapies will also be helpful.

Psychotherapy

- Psychodynamic psychotherapy is a general term which denotes therapeutic treatment modalities to bring feelings to the surface, so that client can understand them. It uses the basic assumption that everyone has feelings held in the subconscious which are too painful to be faced. To protect these, client uses defenses or defense mechanisms.

- Psychodynamic psychotherapy assumes that these defenses were worked wrong and causing more harm than use, making the client to seek medical care. It tries to subdue them with the intention that once the client is aware of what is really going on in his/her mind the feelings will not be as painful. It consumes more time and is labor intensive.
- Supportive psychotherapy is usually used either alone or in combination with drug treatment. The establishment of good rapport and therapist client–relationship is often first step in psychotherapy.

Cognitive Behavioral Therapy (CBT)

It aims to recognize and change the client's thinking pattern that are associated with the anxiety and troublesome and irritable feelings. It has two parts: a cognitive part designed to limit distorted thinking and a behavioral part designed to change the way people react to the objects or situations that trigger anxiety.

Cognitive behavior therapy imparts clients to react differently to situations and bodily sensations that trigger anxiety and teaches client to understand how thinking patterns contribute to symptoms. For example, a client underlying CBT for panic disorder might work on learning that panic attacks are not really heart attacks.

Relaxation Therapies

Relaxation therapies are used as psychotherapeutic interventions in a variety of situations. These techniques are self used as a routine on a daily basis. These include:

Visual Imagery

This technique is used effectively to reduce anxiety experienced by cancer clients. As clients relax they engage in a fantasy in which they visualize the identified cause of anxiety, such as pain due to cancer or the cancer itself. A person who has an unresolved conflict, such as not attending the funeral of a near and dear one, could utilize this techniques in an attempt to work through guilt feelings or unresolved grief.

Change of Pace or Scenery

Walking in the forests/woods or along the beach, listening to music, caring for a pet, crafting/sewing, or engaging in a hobby are iconic examples of ways to change pace or scenery in an attempt to decrease anxiety by removing oneself from the source or cause of stress.

Exercise or Massage Therapy

Exercise can be a release or outlet for pent up tension or anxiety. Massage is soothing and helps to relax one's muscles.

Progressive Muscle Relaxation

When anxiety takes hold, progressive muscle relaxation can help in releasing muscle tension and takes a 'time out' from worries. The technique involves systematically tensing and then releasing different muscle groups of body, as body relaxes mind will also relaxes.

Meditation

Meditation has psychotherapeutic effects on anxiety reduction. Mindful meditation, in particular, shows a good promise for relief of anxiety. The yogic research studies show that mindfulness meditation can actually change the brain neurocircuit with regular practice, it boosts activity on the left side of the prefrontal cortex, the area of the brain responsible for serenity and happiness/joy. Transcendental meditation (TM): This technique was propagated by Maharishi Mahesh Yogi. It has 4 components, these include (a) a quiet environment (b) a passive state of mind (c) a comfortable position (d) and the ability to focus on a specific word or object. Physiological, psychospiritual relaxation occur. Transcendental meditation is very effective in treating anxiety disorders.

Biofeedback

The person is able to monitor various physiologic processes by auditory or visual signals. This technique has proven effective in the management of conditions such as migraine headaches, essential hypertension and pain that is the result of enhanced stress and anxiety.

Systematic Desensitization

This technique refers to the exposure of a person to a fear–producing situation in a systematized manner to decrease a phobic disorder.

Relaxation Exercise

Many methods are used to help people learn to relax. The common steps to relaxation include taking a deep breath and exhaling: tensing and then relaxing individual muscles, starting with the head and progressing to the toes and finally relaxing all parts of the body simultaneously. Some methods suggest that the person imagine a peaceful scene before doing the exercise.

Therapeutic Touch or 'Laying on of Hands'

Many alternative practitioners use this method to heal the client. Reiki and pranic healing are examples.

Hypnosis

This is used to enhance relaxation or imagery. Client has been taught self hypnosis to decrease anxiety.

Other techniques utilized to treat anxiety disorders induce behavioral modification, cognitive therapy, exposure therapy, psychoanalysis, group therapy and environmental modification.

Pharmacotherapy

- Drugs are used to treat pain or any physical ailment in anxiety disorders. Usually, medicines include antidepressants, benzodiazepines, tricyclis and beta blockers are used.
- Very commonly, anxiety is treated by benzodiazepines. Because of their addictive nature, use has reduced. These show side effects.
  - Diazepam; 5–10 mg.
  - Lorazepam

- Alprazolam
- Clonazepam

Antidepressants

These are SSRIs (selective serotonin reuptake inhibitors) are commonly used to treat anxiety. These have very few side effects than older antidepressants, but still they show symptoms like nausea, sexual dysfunction and jittersness.

Example: Sertraline
Paroxetine
Fluxetine
Escitalopram
Citalopram
Venlafaxine

- Tricyclics (TCAc) are very helpful to treat anxiety except obsessive compulsive disorder. These drugs are known to cause side effects such as dizziness, drowsiness, dry mouth and weight gain. Two types of tricyclis include:
  - Imipramine
  - Clomipramine
- Other drugs used to treat anxiety include monoamine oxidase inhibitors (MAOIs), beta blockers and buspirone. MAOIs, such as phenelzine (Nardil), tranylcypromine (parnate) and isocarboxazid (Marplan) are used to treat some kind of anxiety disorders.
- Beta blocker such as propranolol (inderal) are usually used to treat cardiac conditions but also used in anxiety. Buspirone (Buspar) is another type of medication that affects neurotransmitters to control anxiety disorders, but lacks the side effects of sleepiness and dependency. However, it has been associated with dizziness, headaches, nausa and vomiting.

Nursing Management

People who exhibit signs of acute anxiety or a panic state may harm themselves or others and need to be supervised closely until the anxiety subsides. Such people may be admitted in general hospitals or specially psychiatric units. The main aim is to ensure a safe, protective environment.

The person may be in severe distress or immobilized or may be engaged in purposeless, disorganized or aggressive activity. Feelings of intense awe, dread, horror or terror may occur. The client may express the fear that he or she 'losing control'.

The assessment includes the following factors:

- Monitoring physiological signs and symptoms and complaints.
- Irritability
- Restlessness
- Attention deficits
- Feelings of discomfort, apprehension or helplessness
- Poor impulse control
- Insomnia.

GOALS OF NURSING A PERSON EXPERIENCING AN ANXIETY DISORDER

Appropriate goals for caring for a person with anxiety include:

- Develop a therapeutic relationship with the person based on empathy and trust.
- Promote an understanding of the features of an anxiety disorders.
- Promote effective strategies for coping with anxiety.
- Promote positive health behaviors, including medication compliance and healthy lifestyle cloices (for example diet, exercise, non smoking).
- Promote the person's engagement with their social support network.
- Ensure effective collaboration with other health care providers through development of effective working relationship and communication.
- After the client is examined, a nursing care plan is initiated to correspond to the physician's treatment plan for an acute anxiety attack or panic state.

During the panic state the nursing interventions include:

- Staying with the client at all times and caring.
- Remaining calm. The client will perceive any anxiety exhibited by the nurse.
- Speaking therapeutically, short and simple sentences.
- Displaying firmness to provide external controls for the client.
- Maintaining quiet environment to minimize internal stimuli.
- Providing protective care because the client may harm self or others. The client's behavior also may elicit responses from other clients who are unable to tolerate her or his anxiety state.
- Attempting to channel the client's behavior by engaging the client in physical activities that provide an outlet for tension or frustration.
- Administering anxiolytics and other prescribed drugs to decrease anxiety.

Persons who exhibit symptoms of mild or moderate levels of anxiety may be treated as outpatients if the anxiety does not interfere with the ability to function normally.

Nursing interventions for mild to moderate anxiety levels, include assessing the clients, anxiety level, reducing anxiety, providing protective care, encouraging verbalization of anxiety, meeting basic human needs and setting achievable goals for care.

The nurse provides supportive and collaborative care by:

- Recognizing the client's anxiety and helping him or her identify the anxiety and describe feelings.
- Reassuring the client.
- Accepting the client unconditionally. Do not pass judgement or respond emotionally to the client's behaviors.
- Listening to the client's concerns. Be available but respect the client's need for personal space.
- Protecting the client's defenses (e.g. ritualistic behavior). Any attempt to stop such behavior increase anxiety because the client has no other defenses.
- Encouraging verbalization of feelings. Answer questions openly and in a direct way.
- Allowing the client time to respond to nursing interventions. Set realistic goals for improvement. Allow the client to set the pace.
- Exploring alternative ways of coping strategies to decrease the present anxiety to a minimum level. Assist the client in learning new methods to cope with anxiety.

- Identifying the client's developmental stage and helping the client to work through unmet developmental tasks.
- Administering prescribed medications and other therapeutic treatment to reduce anxiety or discomfort.

If hospitalization is required, it is generally short-term and intensive in duration. Out patient follow-up care usually is recommended to continue with supportive therapeutic measures. Discharge planning will include an evaluation of the client's present status, recommendations for further referral and guidelines for drug therapy. The client should be instructed about whom to contact if anxiety increases and panic or a crisis like situation occurs.

Nursing diagnoses utilized to develop nursing care plans for individuals experiencing anxiety and stress include:

- Anxiety
- Ineffective individual coping
- High risk for injury
- Impaired verbal communication
- Impaired social interaction
- Sleep pattern disturbance
- Post trauma response
- Rape trauma syndrome
- Hopelessness
- Altered health maintenance and knowledge deficit regarding illness.

Examples of nursing diagnosis and interventions, the client with an anxiety disorders.

- *Nursing Diagnoses:* Anxiety related to relocation.

Nursing interventions	Outcome criteria
	Within 24 to 48 hours the client will be able to do the following.
• Educate regarding symptoms and causes of anxiety.	Identifying physiological signs and symptoms of anxiety.
• Encourage verbalization of feelings.	Describe own anxiety. Identify one or two stressors contributing to anxiety.
• Explore coping skills.	Describe own coping patterns. Identify one or two alternative coping patterns.
	Relate an increase in physiological and psychosocial comfort.

- *Nursing Diagnosis:* Powerlessness related to impaired cognition.
- *Nursing Outcome:* Client will be able to effectively solve problem, take over life situation thereby lessening the feelings of anxiety and powerlessness.

Nursing interventions	Outcome criteria
• Allow client to take as much responsibility as possible for self care practices, such as:	• Providing choice will increase client's feelings of control.
a. Allow client to plan her/his own day schedule for ADL. b. Include client in setting goal for his/her care. c. Provide privacy to client as per need. Provide positive reinforcement for the decision made by the client. Respect client's right to make those decisions independently.	

Contd...

Contd...

Nursing interventions	Outcome criteria
• Assist client to set realistic goals.	• Unrealistic goals set the client up for failure and reinforce feelings of powerlessness.
• Help identify areas of life situation that client can control and do by himself/herself.	• Client's emotional condition interferes with the ability to solve the problems. Assistance is required to perceive the benefits and consequences of available alternatives accurately.
• This will assist the client to deal with unresolved issues and to learn to accept what can not be changed. This encourages a new coping method.	• Help the client to identify areas of life situation that are not within his/her ability to control. Encourage verbalization of feelings related to this inability.

- *Nursing Diagnosis:* Limited ability or inability to use the problem solving process related to feelings of apprehension, helplessness and disorganized thought processes.
- *Nursing Outcome:* Client will use problem solving process to deal with day to day problems.

Nursing intervention	Rationale
• Teach the client step by step approach for solving problem, identifying problems, exploring alternatives, evaluating consequences of alternatives and making decision.	• The client may be unaware of logical process for examining and resolving problems.
• Support the client's positive action in viewing him or herself and his or her abilities realistically.	• Enhancing the client's confidence and abilities to self evaluate problems his/her sense of self reliance.
• Encourage the client to use methods to reduce anxiety prior to approaching problems when possible.	• The client will be able to use problem solving skills when anxiety persists.
• Encourage the client to evaluate the success of the chosen method to reduce anxiety. Help the client continue to try alternatives if her/his initial choice may fail.	• The client needs to know that he/she can survive making a mistake and making mistakes is a part of learning.
• Help the client to view mild anxiety as a positive catalyst for change.	• A frequent misconception is that anxiety itself is bad and not useful.

Preventive Measures of Anxiety Disorder

Anxiety cannot be eradicated but can be controlled by number of factors. These include:

- Reducing the intake of carbonated drinks, tea, coffee and chocolate consumption.
- Try to avoid taking medicines by own.
- Practicing regular exercise schedule.
- Eating healthy foods.
- Maintaining regular sleep pattern.
- Avoiding alcohol and using multiple drugs.
- Practicing relaxation techniques like yoga, meditation and deep breathing exercises.
- Involving in social activities and social groups.

Coping with Anxiety

The mnemonic 'AWARE' is used to practice to cope with anxiety. The key to switching out of an anxiety state is to accept it fully. Remaining in the present state and accepting anxiety causes it to disappear.

Accept the Anxiety

Welcome it. Do not fight it. Replace rejection, anger and hatred with acceptance. By resisting, one is prolonging the unpleasantness of anxiety. Instead, flow with it. Do not make it responsible for how you think, feel and act.

Watch your Anxiety

Look at it without judgment not good bad. Rate it on a 0 to 10 scale and watch it go up and down. Be detached. The more you can separate yourself from the experience, the more you can just watch it.

Act with the Anxiety

Act as if you are not anxious. Function with it. Slow down if you have to, but keep going. Breath slowly and normally. If you do away from the situation your anxiety will go down, but your fear will go up. If you stay, both your anxiety and your fear will go down.

Repeat the Steps

Continue to accept your anxiety, watch and act with it until it goes down to a comfortable and manageable level. And, i.e. just keep repeating these three steps: accept, watch and act with it.

Expect the Best

What you fear the most rarely happens. Recognize that a certain amount of anxiety is normal for optimal functioning. By expecting future anxiety, you are putting yourself in a good position to accept it when it reappears.

PHOBIC DISORDER

Phobia

Phobias are the most common form of anxiety disorders. It is defined as an unrelenting fear of a situation, activity or thing that causes one to avoid it. Phobia is described as 'an irrational fear' of an object, activity or situation that is out of proportion to the stimulus and results in avoidance of the identified object, activity or situation. The person has unconsciously displaced the original internal source of fear or anxiety, such as an unpleasant childhood experience to an external source. Avoidance of the object or situation allows the person to remain free of anxiety.

Differences Between a Normal Fear and Phobia

Fear	Phobia
• Feeling anxious when flying through turbulence or taking off during a storm.	• Not joining a good job because he/she has to work on the 15th floor of the office.
• Experiencing butterflies when peering down from the top of a skyscraper or climbing a tall ladder.	• Not going to attend near and dear one's marriage in America because of fear of flying high.
• Getting nervous on seeing a dog.	• Running away on seeing a dog.
• Feeling squeakys when getting an injection or when blood is being drawn.	• Avoiding necessary medical treatments or doctors, check ups because of fear of needles.

Types of Phobia

There are mainly three types of phobia:

Agoraphobia

- **Agoraphobia:** Agoraphobia is a most common phobic disorder. It is a fear of being outside or of being in a situation from which easy escape would be impossible.
- Agoraphobia is the fear of being alone in public places from which the person, thinks escape would be difficult or help unavailable if the person were incapacitated. Normal daily activities become restricted and victims refuse to leave their houses. Two-thirds of those exhibiting clinical symptoms are women who develop symptoms between ages 18 and 35. Onset may be sudden or gradual. These people are likely to develop depression, fatigue, tension and spontaneous obsessive or panic disorders.
- **Social Phobia:** In social phobia, there is a compelling desire to avoid situations in which a person may be criticized by others. The person experiences persistent, irrational fear of criticism or embarrassment. The person does realize that fear is excessive or disproportionate to the activity or situation. Social phobia rarely is dangerous but may cause considerable inconvenience. The abuse of alcohol and drugs may occur as the person with social phobia attempts to reduce anxiety. Examples of social phobia are fear of public speaking, using public utilities or using public transportation.
- **Simple Phobia:** A simple phobia is defined as an excessive fear of an object, activity or a situation, which leads a person to avoid the cause of that fear. Such a phobia can seriously disrupt a person's lifestyle.
- It is characterized by irrational fear of objects or situation. Anticipatory anxiety leads to persistent avoidant behavior.
- It is diagnosed only when there is marked distress/or disturbance in daily functioning, in addition to fear and avoidance of specific objects or situation. There are approximately 700 identified phobias. Some of the common are listed below.

Acrophobia	:	Fear of heights
Androphobia	:	Fear of men
Amathophobia	:	Fear of dust
Astraphobia	:	Fear of storms, lightening, thunder
Aviophobia	:	Fear of flying
Belonephobia	:	Fear of needles, pins or other sharp objects
Brontophobia	:	Fear of thunder
Claustrophobia	:	Fear of confined spaces
Ceraunophobia	:	Fear of lighting
Eurotophobia	:	Fear of female genitals
Gephyrophobia	:	Fear of crossing bridges
Hematophobia	:	Fear of blood
Hydrophobia	:	Fear of water
Iatrophobia	:	Fear of doctors
Odontiatophobia	:	Fear of dentist
Nyctophobia	:	Fear of night
Ochlophobia	:	Fear of crouds
Phartophbia	:	Fear of passing gas in a public place

Phasmophobia	:	Fear of ghosts
Phobophobia	:	Fear of having fears or developing a phobia.
Pyrophobia	:	Fear of fire
Scoleciphobia	:	Fear of worms
Trikaidekaphobia	:	Fear of all things associated with the number 13
Trypanophobia	:	Fear of injections
Zoophobia	:	Fear of animals (usually spiders, snakes or mice).

Etiology

The exact cause for phobias are unknown. It is assumed that phobias run in families, are influenced by culture. More stress and fear may be the cause for phobia. Different theories postulate different views.

Psychodynamic Theory

According to Freud, the mental mechanism repression is used. When repression fails to function adequately, other secondary defense mechanism of ego come into play. In phobia, the secondary defense mechanism include displacement. By displacement the anxiety is transferred from really dangerous or frightening object to neutral object. These two objects have symbolic association. The neutral object chosen is easily avoided in day to day activity.

Behavioral Theories

According to behaviorists, phobia is considered as a conditioned reflex. Specific phobias may result from pairing of a specific object or situation with the emotions of fear and panic. A stressful stimulus produces the 'unconditioned response' of fear. When the stressful stimulus is repeatedly paired with a harmless object, eventually the harmless object alone produces a 'conditioned' response fear. This fear will convert in phobia when the individual consciously avoids the harmless object to escape fear.

Biological Theories

Specific phobias tend to run in families. Children whose parents are affected with panic disorder show a trait characterized by consistent pattern of behavioral inhibition and it may develop into severe shyness as children grow older.

Clinical Manifestations

The symptoms of phobia can range from mild feelings of apprehension and anxiety to a full blown panic attack. Panic symptoms include feeling dread or terror, despite recognition that those feelings are excessive in relationship to any real danger... as well as physical symptoms like shaking, sweating, nausea, rapid heart beat, chest pain or tightness, hot or cold flashes, tinging sensation, feeling dizzy or light-headed and an over whelming desire to escape the situation that causes phobic reaction. Sometimes extreme measures are taken to avoid or escape the situation.

Differential Diagnosis

A phobic may be associated with a number of other mental health conditions, including schizophrenia and anxiety disorders.

Management

- *Psychotherapy:* It is indicated when phobia is combined with personality disorders. Supportive psychotherapy is helpful with behavior therapy and drug treatment.
- *Behavior Therapy:* Cognitive behavior therapy is mostly used either desensitization or exposure; i.e. the phobic client is exposed in a hierachial way. This concept was developed by Joseph Wolpe in 1958. With the use of tranqualizers, hypnosis and relaxation techniques patient are taught how to induce in themselves both physical and mental response. When mastery occurs, exposure to phobic stimulus is initiated. As clients became desensitized with lower anxiety producing stimulus they are moved to the next level of hierarchy until and ultimately what previously produced the most anxiety no longer elicits the painful affect. Sessions may be executed in fantasy, in real life (in vivo) situation or sometimes both.

Other behavioral technique used is flooding or implosive therapy. In this procedure, the client must imagine a situation or participate in real life situation that he/she finds extremely frightening for a prolonged period of time without relaxation or medications.

- *Drug Management:* SSRIs are used to treat phobias, particularly when desensitization and CBT are inadequately effective. These affect levels of serotonin in the brain.
  Example: Paroxetine, Sertraline, Fluoxetine, Flu voxamine, Citalopram, Escitalopram.
- The possible side effects of these medications vary greatly from individual to individual. Common side effects include dry mouth, sexual dysfunction, nausea, fine tremors, sleep disturbances, blurred vision, soft stools and dizziness.
- Beta blockers are also used to treat phobias. Beta blockers block adrenaline which reduces the intensity of the attack.
  Example: Propranolol.
- Benzodiazepines are used to calm down the client.
  Example: Diazepam, Alprazolam, Lorazepam, Clonazepam.

Nursing Management

- *Nursing Diagnosis:* Fear related to an irrational feeling towards objects/things.
- *Nursing Outcome:* Client will be able to function in presence of phobic object or situation without experiencing panic anxiety.

Nursing interventions	Rationale
• Reassure the client that he/she is safe.	• In extreme anxiety, client may fear for his/her own life.
• Explore client's perception of the threat to physical integrity or threat to self concept.	• To understand client's perception to phobic object is important to implement desensitization program.
• Discuss reality of the situation with client to understand aspects that can be changed and those that cannot.	• Client must accept the reality of the situation before applying treatment program.
• Involve client in making decisions regarding selection of alternative coping skills.	• Allowing the client to make choices provide a measure of control and serves to increase feelings of self worth.
• If client elects to work on elimination of fear techniques of densensitization and flooding may be employed.	• Fear is decreased by using various psychological therapies.

Contd...

Contd...

Nursing interventions	Rationale
• Encourage client to explore underlying feelings that may be contributing to irrational fears and to face them rather than suppress them.	• Exploring underlying feelings may help the client to confront unresolved conflicts and develop more adaptive coping abilities.

- *Nursing Diagnosis:* Social isolation related to self–protected avoidance.
- *Nursing Outcome:* Client will voluntarily participates in all group activities.

Nursing interventions	Rationale
• Convey an accepting attitude and unconditional positive regards. Make brief, frequent contacts. Be honest and keep all promises.	• These intervention increase feelings of self worth and facilitate a trusting relationship.
• Help the client to attend group activities if it is frightening to the client.	• The presence of the trusted individual provides emotional security.
• Be cautious to touch. Allow client extra space and an avenue for exit if anxiety becomes uncontrollable.	• A person in panic anxiety may perceive touch as threatening.
• Administer tranqualizer as prescribed.	• Tranqulizer reduces anxiety.
• Discuss with client signs and symptoms of anxiety and techniques to interrupt the response.	• Maladaptive behaviors are manifested during excess anxiety.
• Provide recognition and positive reinforcement for voluntary interactions with others.	• It enhances self–esteem and encourages repetition of acceptable behaviors.

FAMILY AND CLIENT PSYCHOEDUCATION

Client and family are taught to manage anxiety and fear by learning to use relaxation techniques. Deep breathing, meditation, and muscle relaxation are powerful antidote for anxiety. Regular practice can improve client's ability to control the physical symptoms of anxiety, which makes phobia less intimidating. Relaxation techniques will also help to cope more effectively with stress and anxiety.

Conversion and Dissociative Disorder

Introduction

Conversion and dissociative disorders are characterized by physical or psychological symptoms in the absences of physical pathology. Instead, the causative factors are likely to be psychological, in the form of stressful events and or problems with relationships. These disorders may appear to mimic neurological condition, e.g. paralysis, speech, hearing or visual disturbances, the symptoms are not deliberately produced but conformed to the client's ideas about a particular illness.

Certain phenomena are associated with conversion and dissociate disorders, viz.

Primary and Secondary Gain

- The symptoms of conversion and dissociation bring about a reduction of anxiety. For example, a man developed paralysis of the lower limb upon receiving news that he was required to take part in a 20 km running race. As a result of being excused from taking part in the race, his primary gain was that of anxiety reduction.
- Secondary gain refers to the care, attention and sympathy received from others as a result of the physical symptoms.
- The effects of primary and secondary gain severe to prolong disability.

La Belle Indifference

An apparent lack of distress in clients with conversion and dissociative symptoms is termed as la belle indifference.

 HISTORICAL PERSPECTIVE

Conversion and dissociative disorders were previously referred as 'hysteria'; a term derived from the Greek, 'hysteria' meaning 'uterus'. The concept could be tracked back to 1900 B. C when Egyptian physician explained multiple somatic symptoms due to a wandering of the uterus with the body. In the 17th century, these symptoms were first attributed to a disorders of the brain rather than any uterine dysfunction.

Charcot, an eminent neurologist in the 19th century, believed that hysteria was caused by a functional disorder of the brain and that the–so called hysterical patient could respond to hypnosis. His views were further developed by his pupil Pierre Janet who proposed that hysterical patients experienced a process of dissociation, i.e. they did not have sufficient mental energy to integrate the various aspects of mental functions, e.g. sensations, memories and volition, such that the individual then suffered a restriction of personal awareness, including insight into his own feelings.

Freud opined that 'conversion' was the means whereby distressing feelings were converted into somatic symptoms. He explained that hysteria was a result of repression of painful memories such that these memories become lodged in the patient's unconscious mind and thus psychotherapy was excluded from conscious awareness. He subsequently developed a technique of in which by describing one's painful feelings in words, much of the emotional pain hidden in one's unconscious (subconscious mind) would surface into conscious awareness. This would cause conversion symptoms to disappear.

Dissociative Disorders

- Dissociative amnesia may occur suddenly where clients unable to recall periods of their waking lives. Clients with dissociative fugue often wander away from their homes and have no recollection of their activities during the period of their wanderings. During this period they may also deny knowledge of their identify. In dissociative stupor, clients are motionless, do not respond to their environment and make no verbal responses to any clues.
- Dissociative identity disorder (multiple personality disorder) is characterized by an individual having two or more personalities coexisting in the same person. Each of the personalities is almost always unaware of one personality to the other, but usually in response to severe stress. Each of the personalities has it own set of responses, behaviors, attitudes and memories, markedly different from the client's visual personality.
- Dissociative trance or trance and possession disorder is characterized by a temporary loss of both sense of personal identity and full awareness of one's surroundings. The person acts as if a force, spirit or deity possesses him. There is a reduced awareness of one's surrounding or alternatively a selective focusing of attention on certain aspects of the external environment. The person in a trance may display repetitive movements, adopt postures or make utterances. Such behaviors are not a part of a religious ceremony for that particular culture.

Epidemic Hysteria

Dissociative disorder may start with a person in a group and the symptoms spread to the other members of the group. It is usually the more suggestible, histrionic member who is the first to manifest the condition, usually with dizziness and or fainting spells and with considerable anxiety.

Ganser Syndrome

The clinical features include the giving of approximate answers, clouding of consciousness, conversion symptoms and hallucinations. The approximate answer to question, e.g. saying that a dog has five legs, that the sum of three and two is six, suggest that the subject knows the correct answers but persists in giving the wrong ones. Clouding of consciousness may be reflected in the therapy to the extent of being semi-stuporous. They may show the symptoms like poor attentions, bewilderment, disorientation and impaired grasp of events together with amnesia for the episode. Conversion symptoms, such as paralysis, rigidity of limbs, ataxia or sensory loss may be elicited. Visual and or auditory hallucinations may be present.

Conversion Disorder

Conversion disorders involve motor or sensory altered symptoms that can be explained by any known medical or pathophysiological theory.

Epidemiology

The ratio of women to men among adult client is 2:1 and as much as 10:1 more seen in adolescent and young adults, real populations, individual with very low socioeconomic status and in military forces.

Etiology

Psychoanalytic Theory

According to Freud, conversion disorder is caused by repression of unconscious intrapsychic conflict and conversion of anxiety into physical symptoms. The conflict is between instinctual impulses (e.g. aggression or sexuality) and the prohibitions against its expression. The symptoms allow partial expression of the forbidden wish or urge but in disguise, so that clients can avoid consciously, confronting their unacceptable impulses, conversion disorder symptoms has a symbolic relation to the unconscious conflict for e.g. vaginismus protects the client from expressing unacceptable sexual wishes.

Learning Theory

According to conditioned learning theory, conversion symptoms can be seen as a part of classically conditioned learned behavior like symptoms of illness learned in childhood as a means of coping with an otherwise impossible situation.

Biological Theory

The new research findings implicated that biological and neuropsychological factors in the development of conversion disorder symptoms. Preliminary brain imaging studies have found hypometabolism of the dominant hemisphere and hyper metabolism of the non dominant hemisphere and have implicated impaired hemispheric communication in the cause of conversion disorders.

Clinical Features

Very common conversion symptoms include involuntary movements, tics, seizures, paralysis, aphonia, anesthesias, blindness, deafness, psychogenic vomiting, pseudocysts (false pregnancy) and others. Despite claiming to have a loss of sensations in the lower limbs, clients can walk in the dark without knocking into objects, those with conversion blindness have pupil equal and reactive to light and have visual evoked potentials on their electroencephalograms similar to those with norms vision.

Anesthesia and paresthesia are common symptoms, especially of the extremities. It may also involve organs of special sense and produce deafness, blindness, tunnel vision, etc. pseudo seizures also may occur.

Other Features

- *Primary Gain:* Conversion clients achieve primary gain by keeping internal conflicts outside their awareness. Symptoms have symbolic value, which represent unconscious psychological conflict.
- *Secondary Gain:* Clients take advantages and benefits as a result of being sick.
- *Labelle Indifference:* In this, the client seems to be unconcerned about what appears to be a major impairment.
- *Identification:* Clients with conversion disorders may unconsciously model their symptoms on those of someone important to them.

Marked emotional stress is usually present, e.g. physical abuse, sexual abuse or grief reaction.

Fictitious Disorders

Fictitious disorders are distinguished from malingering in that the former symptoms are intentionally produced in order to assume the sick role. In malingering, symptoms are intentionally produced to derive gain, which could be in the form of financial compensation or the avoidance of having to perform some unpleasant duties. By assuming the sick role, the subject is exempt from attending work, college or in carrying out social obligations. They are entitled to seeking help and receiving sympathy. Sick role reflects society's expectations of a person who is sick. Illness behavior refers to how a person behaves when he perceives he is ill, which includes seeking medical help, taking medications and the like. Illness behavior serves an adaptive function. When the person continues to display illness behavior even when he has recovered from illness, such behavior become maladaptive.

Munchausen Syndrome

This syndrome is also known as 'hospital addiction syndrome'. Here, the client typically injures self, inserts objects into vaginal, anal or nasal orifices, swallows test tubes, thermometers or even a spoon and then seeks treatment at casualties. Apparently, such dramatic behaviors are serious attempts to gain admission into hospital. The client has a multi-scarred appearance, testimony of numerous surgical operations to remove foreign bodies. Turning up late at night at casualty departments, they give incredible stories about their life circumstances to the staff, who feel manipulated by the client, and having no other choice than to admit them for surgery. Clients are prone to lying, often giving false names or if their identifies have been exposed, seeking treatment from different hospitals. Such clients also suffer from personality disorders for which prognosis is very poor.

Management

A detailed history corroborated by information from suitable informant is necessary. Careful physical examination to detect for physical causes should be carried out to detect underlying signs, for example, the presence of intact tendon reflexes, a lack of muscle fasciculation, and a so–called paralysed arm that does not land on the client's face when dropped, help to confirm the diagnosis. Discrete observation over time allow staff to record symptoms which seem to improve when the client thinks no one is watching but conversely worsen when he thinks he is being watched.

Laboratory investigations showing a lack of rise in serum prolactin after it is evident that a fit did not occur and normal visual and auditory evoked potentials would suggest normal vision and hearing. EEG and computerized scan or magnetic resonance imaging may be necessary to exclude organic brain disorders.

Alternative and Complementary Therapies

Alternative and complementary therapies which are also used and helpful in the treatment of conversion disorder include hypnosis, relaxation techniques, visualization and biofeedback.

Prognosis

The prognosis for recovery from conversion disorder is highly favorable client who have clearly identifiable stressor in their lives, acute onset of symptoms and a short interval between symptom onset and treatment, have the best prognosis. Between 20% to 25% of clients will relapse within a year. The individual symptoms of conversion disorder are usually self limited and do not lead to lasting disabilities; however, clients with hysterical aphonia, paralysis or visual disturbances, have better prognoses for full recovery than those with tremor or pseudoseizures.

Prevention

Educating about human physiology and psychology can help to prevent these disorders in adults.

Treatment

Most conversion and dissociative symptoms are self limiting. A caring, supportive therapy is more likely to bring about early symptom resolution than one who is confrontational. The client should be reassumed that the symptoms should subside completely, and be given encouragement to regain control of their disabilities. He/she should be referred for physiotherapy to help to achieve complete recovery. Care should be taken to avoid achieve complete recovery. Care should be taken to avoid reinforcing the symptoms, for example, paying a great deal of attention to the symptoms. Stress factors should be dealt with and the client is encouraged to talk about psychological issues rather than physical factors. Others therapies like onsight oriented supportive or behavior therapy, hypnosis and anxiolytics are prescribed.

EPIDEMIOLOGY SOMATOFORM DISORDERS

The life time prevalence of somatization disorder in the general population is estimated to be 0.2–2% in men. It usually begins before the age of 30. Male female ratio is 1:5. It coexists with mental health conditions.

Causes

- *Psychological factors:* The exact cause is not known. The psychological configuration of the cause involve interpretation of the symptoms as social communication whose result is to avoid obligations (e.g. going to a job a person does not like to do) to express emotions (e.g. Anger towards spouse) or to symbolize a feeling or a belief (eg. A pain in the gut).
- *Biological factor:* Research studies refer to have characteristics of attention and cognitive impairments those results in the faulty perception and assessment of somatosensory inputs.
- *Genetic factors:* These disorders run in families. The transmission of somatization disorder in 10–20% of the 1st degree female relation of probands of clients with somatization disorders within these families first degree male relatives are prone to substance abuse and antisocial personality disorders.

Somatoform Disorder

The term somatoform derives from the Greek word 'soma' for body and the somatoform disorders are a broad group of illness that are characterized by a concern with the body. These symptoms are characterized by repeated presentation with physical symptoms which do not have any adequate physical basis and a persistent request for investigations and treatment despite repeated assurance by health personnel. These clients experience the anxiety as fatigue, loss of appetite, body aches, headaches, gastrointestinal problems and so on.

DSM IV–TR recognizes five specific somatoform disorders. They are:

- Somatization disorder characterized by many physical complaints affecting many organ systems.
- Conversion disorder characterized by one or two neurological complaints.
- Hypochondrias characterized by patient's beliefs that they are having a noncurable disease.
- Body dimorphic disorder, characterized by a false belief or exaggerated perception that a body part is defective.
- Pain disorder, characterized by symptoms of pain that are either solely related to or significantly exacerbated by psychological factors.

Somatization Disorder

Somatization disorder is characterized by multiple somatic symptoms that cannot be explained adequately on the basis of physical and laboratory investigations. These disorders were recognized since Egyptian civilization. Earlier it is called as 'hysteria' means 'wandering uterus'. Paul Briquette, identified multiplicity of symptoms and later it was known as Briquette's syndrome.

Epidemiology: Clinical Features

- Clients with somatization disorder have a multitude of somatic complaints and long, complicated medical history like nausea and vomiting, difficulty swallowing, pain in the arms and legs; shortness of breath unrelated to exertion, amnesia, complications of pregnancy and menstruation are the most common symptoms. The belief that one has been sick most of one's life is also common.
- Psychological distress and interpersonal problems are prominent with anxiety and depression being the most prevalent psychiatric conditions. Suicidal threats are more seen if suicide fails, it is usually associated with substance abuse.

- The client medical histories are circumstantial vague, imprecise, inconsistent and disorganized. They describe their complaints in a dramatic, emotional and exaggerated way, with vivid and colorful language. They are often dressed in an exhibitionistic manner and may be coy or seductive. They are described as dependent, self centered, craving for admiration, praise and very manipulative in characteristics.
- This disorder is commonly associated with other psychiatric diagnosis, most often with antisocial and histrionic personality disorders, substance abuse (alcohol and other multiple drugs) include the conviction and fear of disease.

Treatment

- Somatization client needs a long-term, ampathetic relationship with a single handed consultant. Psychotherapy is helpful to clients with somatization disorder. In these, clients are helped to cope with their symptoms and possibly to eliminate them.
- Anxiolytics and anti-depressants are also used.

HYPOCHONDRIASIS

The term 'hypochondriasis' is derived from the term 'hypochondrium' meaning 'below the ribs'. It is defined as a person's preoccupation with the fear of contracting a serious disease.

Hypochondria is a belief that physical symptoms are signs of a serious illness, even when there is no medical evidence to support the presence of an illness.

Epidemiology

- It is found 4 to 6% in general medical population. Both genders equally affected. Commonly appears in 20–30% years of age group.
- Hypochondriacal complaints reportedly occur in about 3% of medical students.
- An estimated 75–85% of people who have hypochondrias also have anxiety, depression or another mental disorder.

Etiology

The exact cause of hypochondriacs is not known. Factors that might be involved in the development of the disorder include.

- A history of physical or sexual abuse.
- A history of having a serious illness as a child.
- A poor ability to express emotions.
- A parent or close relative with the disorder, children might learn this behavior is overly concerned about disease and/or over reacts to even minor illness.
- An inherited susceptibility for the disorder.
  - DSM-IV TR indicates that the symptoms reflect a misinterpretation of bodily symptoms. A reasonable body data indicate that person with hypochondriacs argue and amplify their somatic sensation, they have low thresholds for tolerance of physical discomfort.
- According to Social learning theory, it is a learned phenomena. Sick role made by the clients to postpone unwelcome challenges and to be excused from usual duties and obligations.
- It may be related to another psychiatric disorder, such as anxiety or OCD. In other words, hypochondriacs may develop from or be a sign of one of these other disorders.

Signs and Symptoms

- Preoccupation with a serious illness for at least 6 months.
- Misinterpreting normal body functions.
- Persistent fear of illness despite being reassumed by health care providers that you are not ill.
- Difficulty to maintain a job, keeping relationships and performing normal daily activities.

Warning Signs

- The person has a history of consulting too many doctors. He or she may even ' shop around' for a doctor who will agree that he or she has a serious illness.
- The person recently experienced a loss or stress event.
- The person is overly concerned about a specific organ or body system, such as the heart or the digestive system.
- The person's symptoms or area of concern might shift or change.
- A doctor's reassurance does not calm the person's fears; he or she believes the doctor is wrong or made a mistake.
- The person's concern about illness interferes with his or her work, family and social life.
- The person may suffer from anxiety, nervousness and/or depression.

Diagnosis

The DSM-IVTR indicates diagnostic criteria for hypochondriasis require that client is preoccupied with the false beliefs that they have a serious disease, based on their misinterpretation of physical signs or sensation. The belief must last atleast for 6 months despite the absence of pathological findings on medical and neurological examinations.

Treatment/Management

- A main goal of hypochondria treatment is to help client's live and function as normally as possible, even if they continue to have symptoms. Treatment also aims to alter the thinking and behavior that leads to the symptoms.
- Hypochondria can be very difficult to treat. This is due, in part, to the fact that people with this disorder refuse to believe their symptoms as the result of mental or emotional rather than physical causes.
- Treatment for hypochondria mostly includes a combination of the following options.

Supportive Care

In most cases, the best course of action is for the person to stay in regular contact with a trusted health care provider. Within this doctor/nurse-patient relationship; the doctor can monitor the symptoms and stay alert to any changes that might signal a real medical illness. The doctors main approach is likely to focus on reassuming and supporting the person and preventing unnecessary tests and treatments. Medications are used when necessary.

Medications

Drugs are generally not used to treat hypochondriacs specifically, but for associated mental health conditions. They may improve symptoms of hypochondriacs. SSRIs, such as fluoxetine, sertraline, fluvoxamine or paroxetine are used.

Psychotherapeutic Interventions

- **Cognitive behavior therapy:** CBT helps to identify thoughts that contribute to fears about illness and to correct the misinterpretation of body sensations. It teaches people to concentrate less on thoughts and fears of illness and to use relaxation and distraction techniques.
- Behavioral stress management therapy teaches stress management and relaxation exercises to help people avoid becoming focused on illness during stressful situations. It may be used together with cognitive behavior therapy.

Alternative Therapies

Homeopathy: Drugs used are aconitum, aresenicum album, lycopodium, and phosphorus.
Acupuncture: May be useful in treating hypochondiasis. It balances the flow of energy (qi) in the body. This balancing effect may be particularly helpful for people who have distorted perceptions of normal body sensations.

Complications Associated with Hypochondriacs

A person with hypochondria is at risk for repeated episodes of symptoms. He or she also might suffer from reactions or health problems related to multiple tests, procedures and treatments. In addition to the pain and frustration, this disorder often causes to the person and his or her family, repeated episodes also can lead to unnecessary and risk procedures, as well as high medical expenditure. Further genuine medical problems can be missed in a person with a long history of having tests with negative results, because doctor's may assume the person's complaint is caused by hypochondriacs, not a real illness.

Prognosis and Follow-up

Hypochondria is a long-term/chronic condition that can last for years. The symptoms recover frequently. Only a small percentage of clients recover completely. To that reason, the focus of treatment is on learning to manage and control symptoms and on minimizing functional problems associated with his disorders.

Body Dysmorphic Disorder

Clients with body dysmorphic disorder (BDD) have a pervasive subjective feelings of ugliness of some aspect of their appearance despite a normal or nearly normal appearance. The cause of the disorder is the person's strong belief of fear that he or she is unattractive or even repulsive. Earlier this disorder was called as 'dysmorphophobia'.

Epidemiological Concepts

- Age of onset 15–30 year.
- Females are more affected than males.
- Affected client is likely to be unmarried.
- Commonly coexist with mental disorders.

Characteristics of BDD

- BDD is a body–image disorder characterized by persistent and intrusive preoccupations with an imagined or slight defect in one's appearance.

- People with BDD can dislike any part of their body, mostly found faulty with their skin, hair, nose, chest or stomach. In reality, a perceived defect may be only a slight imperfection or nonexistent. But for someone with BDD, the flaw is significant and prominent often causing severe emotional distress and difficulties in daily functioning.

Etiology

- Cause is unknown, but certain biological and environmental factors may contribute to its development, including genetic predisposition, neurobiological factors, such as malfunctioning of serotonin in the brain, personality traits and life experiences.
- Stereotyped concepts of beauty emphasized in families.
- The high comorbidity with depressive disorder.
- Seen in reflecting the displacement of a sexual or emotional conflict onto a non related body part, such as an association occurs through the defense mechanisms of repression, dissociation, distortion, symbolization and projection.

CLINICAL FEATURES

- People with BDD suffer from obsessions about their appearance that can last for hours or up to entire day. Hard to resists or control, these obsessions make it difficult for people with BDD to focus on anything but their imperfections. This can lead to low self-esteem, avoidance of social situations and problems at work or school.
- People with severe BDD may avoid leaving their homes altogether and may even have thoughts of suicide or make a suicide attempt.
- BDD suffers may perform some type of compulsive or repetitive behavior to try to hide or improve their flaws although these behaviors usually give only temporally relief. These may be:
  - Camouflaging (with body position, clothing, make up, hair, hats, etc.)
  - Comparing body part to other's appearance
  - Seeking surgery
  - Checking in a mirror
  - Avoiding mirrors
  - Skin picking
  - Excessive grooming
  - Excessive exercise
  - Changing clothes extensively.
- Other symptoms include depression, insomnia and severe anxiety.

Treatment

- *Cognitive Behavior Therapy:* CBT teaches clients to recognize irrational thoughts and change negative thinking patterns. Clients learn to identify unhealthy ways to thinking and behaving and replace them with positive ones.
- *Antidepressant medications:* Including SSRIs, can help relieve the obsessive and compulsive symptoms of BDD.

PAIN DISORDER

DSM-IV-TR defines pain disorder as the presence of pain that is predominant focus of clinical attention. Primary symptoms are pain in one or more sites in not fully accounted for a non-psychiatric medical or neurological condition. The pain is associated with emotional distress and functional impairment.

Incidence

- Pain disorder is diagnosed twice as frequently in women than in men.
- The peak age or onset is in the fourth or five decades.

Etiology

Psychodynamic Factors: Clients who experience bodily aches and pains without identifiable and adequate physical causes may be symbolically expressing intrapsychic conflicts through the body. The symbolic meaning of body disturbances may also relate to atonement for perceived sin or to suppress aggression. Pain can function as a method of obtaining love, a punishment for wrong doing and of atoning for an innate sense of badness.

Neurological Causes

- Serotonin is probably the main neurotransmitter in the descending inhibitory pathways.
- Endorphin deficiency seems to correlate with augmentation of incoming sensory stimuli.

Behavioral Factors

Pain behavior is reinforced when rewards are inhibited when ignored or punished. For example, pain symptoms may become more intensive when followed by the solicitous and attentive behavior or others, monetary gain or the successful avoidance of distasteful activities.

Interpersonal Factors

Intractable pain has been conceptualized as a means for manipulation and gaining advantages in interpersonal relationships, for e.g. to ensure the devotion of family members or to stabilized a fragile marriage. Such secondary gain is important to client with somatoform pain disorder.

Clinical Symptoms

- The predominant feature of somatoform pain disorder is a preoccupation with severe and continuous pain of at least six months duration that has no medical explanation.
- Symptoms vary depending on the site of pain. These are:
  - Negative distorted cognition, such as feeling helpless or hopeless with respect to pain and its management.
  - Inactivity, passivity and/or disability.
  - Increased pain requiring clinical intervention.
  - Insomnia and fatigue.
  - Disrupted social relationships at home, work or school.
  - Depression/anxiety.

Treatment

- Pharmacological treatment:
  - Acetaminophen or non steroidal anti–inflammatory drugs.
  - Opioids and analysis.
  - *Antidepressants:* TCA's/SSRI.

- *Psychotherapy:* Individual or group therapy. Family, behavioral, physical, hypnosis, biofeedback.

Prognosis

The prognosis for total remission of symptoms is good fro acute pain disorder than chronic pain disorder. The typical pattern for chronic pain entails occasional flare-ups alternating with periods of low to moderate pain. The prognosis for remission of symptoms is better when clients are able to continue working.

OBSESSIVE COMPULSIVE DISORDER

Introduction

Normally, the people do on occasion, to go back and double check the iron box is put off or the car is locked or not. But the suffers from OCD, obsessive thoughts and compulsive behaviors become so excessive that they interfere with daily living activities.

Definitions

- Obsessive compulsive disorder (OCD) is an anxiety disorder characterized by thoughts or actions that are repetitive, distressing and intrusive. OCD suffers usually know that their compulsions are unreasonable or irrational, but they serve to alleviate their anxiety.
- An obsession is a persistent, painful, intrusive thought, emotion or urge that one is unable to suppress or ignore.
- Obsessions are involuntary, seemingly uncontrollable thoughts, images or impulses that occur over and over again in the mind. Really, the person does not want to have these ideas but he/she cannot stop them. Unfortunately, these obsessive thoughts are often disturbing and distracting.
- Compulsions are behaviors or rituals that the person feel driven to act out again. Usually, compulsions are performed in an attempt to make obsessions go away.
- A compulsion is the performance of a repetitious, uncontrollable but seemingly purposeful act to prevent some future event or situation.
- Common obsessive thoughts include topics, such as religion, sexuality, violence and contamination. Obsessions are considered senseless or repugnant and they cannot be eliminated by logic or reasoning. A repetitive thought of killing one's mate is an example of a violent obsession.

  Typical obsessions include:
  - Contamination
  - Fear of shameful misbehavior
  - Symmetrical arrangements
  - Lucky or unlucky numbers
  - Death and disaster
  - Perverted sexual thoughts
  - Intrusive thoughts and images
  - Unsatisfactory body images.

Typical compulsion acts include:

  - Cleaning
  - Counting

- Washing
- Checking
- Measuring
- Hoarding things
- Repeating ritual actions
- Confessing imaginary 'sins'.

Majority of OCD cases involve both obsessions and comulsious so, most people with OCD fall into the following categories.

- *Washers:* Washers are afraid of infection or contamination. They usually have cleaning or hand washing compulsions. These are mostly seen in women than men. They tend to react to things that make them anxious by performing complicated or endlessly repeated rituals of washing hand, hair, clothing, bedding, floors-almost anything may be involved. It may develop rapidly also.
- The rituals are a response to an obsessive fear of contamination and the choice of what contamination to fear is often highly illogical. For instance, some obsessive compulsives have a deep fear of dog feces, but are not particularly worried about human feces or those of cats and other animals.

Washing and Cleaning

Obsessive compulsives commonly feel threatened by germs, asbestos, radiation and even with fiber glass. Those who are associated with dog feces often worry about the invisible organism called toxicara canis, which is said to infect many dogs.

- *Repeating:* Client with OCD, may feel compelled to repeat a series of actions many times, before doing some perfectly simple things, such as going to bed. The repeating act comes in because they feel that the ritual has to be absolutely 'correct' before it is safely proceed. It has been known to take two hours for a 'repeated' act to get out from the care into the house. Other cases involve number rituals-counting and touching the trees or lamp posts, for example–there is a strong element of superstition in these rituals, especially in the kind where a person feels obliged to repeat the actions they were performing at the moment when some anxious thought entered their minds, and to do so a given number of times.
- *Checkers:* This involves repeatedly checking the things (e.g. oven turned off, door locked, computer turned off…) that they associated with harm or danger. Checking in OCD is usually with the thought that something dreadful may happen due to their carelessness or misbehavior. 'Did they switch that light off ? or the gas or the, water taps. Did they look the doors and catch the window properly? They go and check, frequently, mostly home after an hour.'
- Another type to checking takes place where someone fears he or she has done something dreadful or might do. In some cases, they repeatedly check that all larives are hidden away, in case they should stab someone. Others retrace the route they have just driven over, obsessed with the thought that they have run someone over and left them injured. Some may even repeatedly phone the police and registers false cases.
- *Order and Symmetry:* These are obsessions which go way beyond normal tidiness, and involve time consuming rituals. For example, one manager cannot start work until he has sharpened all his pencils to exactly the same length and fineness with a blade. This takes at least an hour each day.
- Doubters and Sinners are afraid that if everything is not perfect or done just right then something terrible will happen or they may be punished.

- Hoarders fear that something bad will happen if they throw anything away. They compulsively hoard things that they do not need or use. People who have this form of OCD find it next to impossible to throw anything away–including rubbish or even kitchen waste. They may buy vast quantities of food or other thins that will never be used. The consequences of these acts yield in multiple problems.
- **Obsessional thoughts:** (*without obvious rituals*)
- Many obsessive compulsives are present with 'endless ruminations' thoughts that go round and round in their heads. They often comment on how long it takes them to make decisions and not just important or difficult ones.
- Unfortunately, ruminations of this kind are not the whole story. There are many reports of obsessive compulsives having dark and brooding thoughts, about things which are inevitable but not necessarily imminent; the passing of time, growing old, death and the loss of loved one.
- *These thoughts can become intrusive:*
  - They suddenly enter the mind and refuse to leave. Sometimes they are not merely depressing but frightening in thoughts out;
  - Harming people, especially their loved ones, contaminating people in some way or attacking them or running them over.
  - Doing something they consider wicked or disgusting; taboo, sexual acts, perversions, incest, child abuse, rape, bestiality and many more.
- The frequency and persistence of these intrusions can be terrible filling the person concerned with confusion and guilty feelings.
- A smaller group of obsessive compulsives find their thoughts 'haunted' by intrusive images or sounds which are disturbing without being particularly threatening–a cat, for example, or a ringing phone. People in these group may start to develop rituals as a means of putting the disturbing thoughts or images out of their minds.
- Just because one has obsessive–thoughts or perform behaviors does not mean that he/she has OCD (Fig. 8.1). With OCD, these thoughts and behaviors cause tremendous distress, take up a lot of time, and interfere with daily life and psychosocial relationships. Their compulsions are so strong that ritual behavior swallows up great chunks of their day, putting jobs at risk, relationships under stress and strain, and generally making life a kind of living burden and hell. Obsessive compulsives can also damage themselves physically with constant washing.

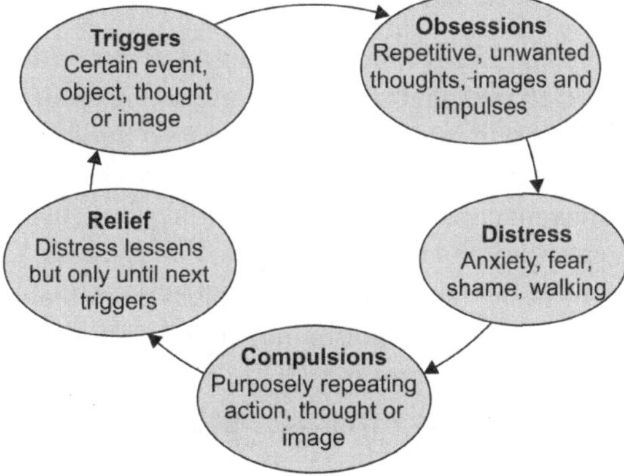

Fig. 8.1: The obsessive compulsive cycle

Epidemiology of OCD

- 1% of young people adults often report experiencing first symptoms in childhood.
- Onset can be at any age. Mean age is late adolescence for men and early twenties for women.
- 2–3% of the population will suffer from OCD in the lifetime. It is equally common in males and females. In children, washing, checking and ordering are common clinical presentations.
  - These course are usually chronic and may be complicated by depression and substance abuse. OCD usually starts in late adolescence or the early adult years. It affects both genders equally in numbers.
  - Around half of those who seek help are unmarried and in most cases the disorder seems to have developed gradually over the years. Sometimes a traumatic event can trigger. If off or turn minor obsessions into the full blown symptoms.

Causes/Etiology

The cause of OCD is not fully understood. The main theories include:

Biological Theories

Neuroanatomy

- Abnormalities in various regions of the brain have been implicated in the neurobiology of OCD. Biological causes of OCD have focused on a circuit in the brain which regulates primitive aspects of behavior, such as aggression, sexually and bodily excretions. This circuit relays information from a part of the brain called the orbitofrontal cortex to another area called the thalamus and includes other regions such as the caudate nucleus of the basal ganglia. When this circuit is activated, these impulses are brought to one's attention and cause to perform a particular behavior that appropriately addresses the impulse.
- It has been suggested that if one has OCD, then the brain has difficulty turning off or ignoring impulses from this circuit. This in turn, causes repetitive behavior called compulsion and/or uncontrollable thoughts called obsessions. For instance, brain may have trouble turning off thoughts of contamination after learning the restroom, leading one to wash his/her hands again and again.
- In support of this theory, the obsessions and compulsions associated with OCD often have themes which are related to sexuality, aggression and contamination–the very thoughts and impulses this circuit controls. In addition, neuro–imaging studies have confirmed abnormal activity in the brain circuit among people with OCD. Specifically, people with OCD show abnormal activity in different parts of this circuit including the orbitofrontal cortex, cingulated cortex and caudate nucleus of the basal ganglia.
- Brain injury, damage to basal ganglia and connections to frontal lobes caused by anoxia, toxic exposure (e.g. Co poisoning, Pb poisoning) brain infection (e.g. viral encephalitis) and substance abuse can lead to symptoms like OCD.
- Animals research studies have shown that damage to basal ganglia can lead to repetitive behaviors.
- Hyper excitability of basal ganglia pathways seen in OCD.

Biochemical Theories

- Many studies have implicated the neurotransmitter serotonin as influential in the etiology of OCD. Study findings correlated between insufficient levels of serotonin with OCD symptoms.
- Serotonin is one of the brain's chemical messengers that transmit signals between the brain cells.
- Serotonin plays a role in the regulation of mood, aggression, impulse control, sleep, appetite, body temperature and pain. All of the drugs used to treat OCD raise the levels of serotonin.

Infection

- A streptococcal infection of the throat is known to occasionally result in the body, confusing healthy cells with the infected one and causing cellular damage. If this has happened with the brain, the body's infection fighting system can attack the outside of the nerve cells in the Basal Ganglia part of the brain with the result that OCD symptoms occur. Few research study findings suggest that these symptoms do not seem to last very long and the occurrence of this 'infection OCD' seems to be very rare cases.

Genetic Theory

- OCD often runs in families. Research studies report that parents, siblings and children of a person with OCD have a greater chance of developing OCD than someone with no family history of the disorder. In one twin has OCD, the other twin is more likely to get OCD if the children are identical twins rather than fraternal twin pairs.
- Genetic researchers have looked for certain genes that may be linked to OCD, but have not been able to find any, however there may be genes that are involved in regulating serotonin and passed on through the generations.

Psychodynamic Theory

Psychodynamic theories of OCD stress that obsession and compulsions are signs of unconscious conflict that the individual might be trying to suppress or cope with. These conflicts arise when an unconscious wish (usually related to sexual or aggressive urge) is at odds with socially acceptable behavior. These are extremely repulsive of distressing the individual and can only deal with them indirectly by transferring the conflict to something more manageable, such as hand washing, checking or ordering.

Learning Theories

- Learning theories postulate the cause of obsessive compulsive behavior as a conditioned response to a traumatic event. These events produce anxiety and stress after which the individual tries to avoid the stress and anxiety by avoiding the situation with which anxiety is associated. This is known as passive avoidance. When it is not successful, the person tries to get rid of anxiety by engaging himself in various activities (behavior) associated with traumatic events (active avoidance). This leads to compulsive behaviors.
- Compulsions such as hand–washing may be a learned phenomenon. For example, in response to feeling contamination, person may wash hands. This act reduces anxiety which make to feel good and in turn reinforces the hand washing behavior. Because of this reinforcement, every time one experiences the obsession (such as contamination), he/she tries out the computation (such as washing their hands) to reduce anxiety.

Diagnostic Criteria

Either Obsessions or Compulsions

Obsession as defined by 1,2,3, and 4 points as such:
- Recurrent and persistent thoughts, impulses or images that are experienced at some time during the disturbance as intrusive and inappropriate and that cause marked anxiety or distress.
- The thoughts, impulses or images are not simply excessive worries about real like problems.
- The person attempts to ignore or suppress such thoughts, impulses or images or to neutralize them with some other thoughts or action.
- The person recognizes that the obsessional thoughts, impulses or images are a product of his own mind (not imposed from without as in thought insertion).

Compulsions are defined by 1 and 2:
- Repetitive behavior (e.g. Hand washing, ordering, checking or mental acts) (e.g. praying, counting, repeating words silently) that the person feels driven to perform in response to an obsession or according to rules that must be applied rigidly.
- The behaviors or mental acts are aimed at preventing or reducing distress or preventing some dreaded event or situation however these behaviors or mental acts either are not connected in a realistic way with what they are designed to neutralize or prevent or are clearly excessive.
- At some point of during the course of the disorder, the person has recognized that the obsessions or compulsions are excessive or unreasonable; note: This does not apply to children.
- The obsessions or compulsions cause marked distress, are time consuming (take more than 1 hour/day) or significantly interfere with the person's normal routine, occupational (or academic) functioning or usual social activities or relationships.
- If another axis–I disorder is present, the content of the obsessions or compulsion is not restricted to it (e.g. preoccupation with food in the presence of body dysmorphic disorder, preoccupation with drugs in the presence of a substance use disorder, preoccupation of having a serious disease in the presence of hypochondriasis, etc.).
- The disturbance is not due to the direct physiological effects of a substance (e.g. a drug of abuse, a medication).

Clinical Manifestations

Common obsessive thoughts in OCD include the following:
- Fear of being contaminated by germs or dirt or contaminating others.
- Fear of causing harm to yourself or others.
- Intrusive sexually explicit or violent thoughts and images.
- Excessive focus on religious or moral ideas.
- Fear of losing or not having things you might need.
- Order and symmetry; the idea that everything must line up 'just right'.
- Superstitions, excessive attention to something considered lucky or unlucky.

OCD Signs and symptoms: compulsive behaviors:

Common compulsive behaviors in OCD include:
- Excessive double checking of things, such as locks, appliances and switches.
- Repeatedly checking in on ones to make sure they are safe.
- Counting, tapping, repeating certain words or doing other senseless things to reduce anxiety.

- Spending a lot of time in washing or cleaning.
- Ordering or arranging thins 'just so'.
- Praying excessively or engaging in rituals triggered by religious fear.
- Accumulating 'junk', such as old newspapers or empty food containers.

Risk Factors

Factors that may increase the risk of developing or triggers OCD include:
- *Family history:* Having parents or other family members with the disorder can increase the risk for OCD.
- *Stressful life events:* Response to stress, may contribute for developing OCD.

Complications of OCD

Complications that OCD may cause or be associated with includes:
- Suicidal thoughts and behavior
- Alcohol or substance abuse
- Other anxiety disorder
- Depression
- Eating disorders
- Contact dermatitis from frequent hand washing
- Inability to attend work or school/absentee
- Troubled relationships
- Overall poor quality of life.

MANAGEMENT OF OCD

Treatment modalities for OCD are multimodal. But the most effective way of treatment for OCD is often cognitive behavioral therapy. Antidepressants are sometimes used in conjunction with therapy, although medication alone is rarely effective in relieving the symptoms of OCD.

Cognitive Behavioral Therapy

It involves two components:
- *Exposure and response prevention:* This process involves repeated exposure to the source of obsession. Then the client is asked to refrain from other compulsive behavior you would usually perform to reduce the anxiety. For example, if the client is a compulsive hand washer, he might be asked to touch the door handle in a public restroom and then be prevented from washing. As the client sit with the anxiety, the urge to wash the hands will gradually begins to go away on its own. In this way, you learn that you do not need the ritual to get rid of your anxiety–that you have some control over your obsessive thoughts and compulsive behaviors.
- *Cognitive Therapy:* It focuses on the catastrophic thoughts and exaggerated sense of responsibility. A big part of cognitive therapy for OCD is teaching the healthy and effective way of responding to obsessive thoughts without resorting to compulsive behavior.

Steps for Conquering Symptoms of OCD

Psychiatrist Jeffery Schwartz, author of the book 'Brain lock; Free Yourself from Obsessive–Compulsive behavior, offers the following four steps for dealing with OCD.

- *Reliable:* Recognize that the intrusive obsessive thoughts and urges are the result of OCD. For example, train yourself to say, I do not think or feel that may hands are dirty, or, I do not feel that I have the need to wash my hands. I am having a compulsive urge to perform the compulsion of washing my hands.
- *Reattribute:* Realize that the intensity and intrusiveness of the thought or urge is caused by OCD; it is probably related to a biochemical imbalance in the brain. Tell yourself 'it is not me–it is my OCD', to remind you that OCD thoughts and urges are not meaningful; but are false messages from the brain.
- *Refocus:* Work around the OCD thoughts by focusing your attention on something else, at least for a few minutes. Do another behavior. Say to yourself, I am experiencing symptoms of OCD, I need to do another behaviors.
- *Revalue:* Do not take the OCD thought to face value. It is not significant in itself. That is just my stupid obsessions. It has no meaning, that is just my brain. There is no need to pay attention to it. Remember. You cannot make the thought go away, but neither do you need to pay attention to it. You can learn to go on to the next behavior.

Cognitive Restructuring

This process is used to challenge the faculty beliefs that underlie OCD behaviors and maintain obsessions and compulsions:

- Clients with OCD possess strong beliefs about the likelihood of a given situation being dangerous to them or others.
- Often the belief is not supported by facts.
- Client is taught a series of techniques to correct negative and irrational thoughts which underline their obsessions and compulsions. This reduces their fear and reduces the need to engage in the compulsive ritual.

Family Therapy for OCD

OCD often causes problems in family life and social adjustment, family therapy can often be beneficial. It promotes understanding of the disorder and can help reduce family conflicts. It can also motivate family members and teach them how to help their loved one.

Group Therapy for OCD

Through interaction with fellow OCD suffers, group therapy provides support and encouragement and decreases feelings of isolation.

Drug Treatment

Many multiple varieties of drugs are used to treat depression have proven effective in OCD.

Tricyclic antidepressants

- Clomipramine
- SSRIs–Selective Serotonin Reuptake Inhibitors. Example:
  - Fluoxetine
  - Sluvoxamine

- Sertraline
- Paroxetine
- Citalopram
- Escitalopram

Other medications are also combined with SSRIs. Atypical antipsychotic medications are used as adjuvant to treat OCD symptoms.

Watch for Side Effects of the Above Drugs

- *Teratogenetic concerns:* Avoid or stop all medications during pregnancy unless symptoms are disabling. All SSRIs are excreted in breast milk and therefore should not be used by nursing mothers.
- *Hepatic disease and Hepatic Metabolism:* SSRIs should be used cautiously in clients with chronic helpautism diseases. Clinical monitoring and dose reductions are recommended to prevent drug interactions and undesirable side effects.
- *Sexual dysfunction:* Although most side effects associated with SSRIs are well tolerated over time, sexual dysfunction is perhaps the most troubling adverse effects and can lead to discontinuation or non-compliance with drug therapy.
- *Cessation of treatment:* Abrupt discontinuation of SSRIs can lead to development of the interruption discontinuation syndrome. This is manifested by emergence of adverse effects and worsening of obsessive compulsive symptoms. So, gradual tapering of doses or shifting among various SSRIs is recommended.
- *Adjunctive Treatment:* Buspirone hydrochloride, a specific nonbenzodiazepine anxiolytic medication, has shown benefit.
- Mood stabilizers (e.g. Lithium, carbamazepine, valporic acid) can be used to augment the efficacy of SSRIs or to treat obsessive compulsive clients with comorbid bipolar disorders.

SELF-HELP THERAPY FOR OCD

These are some tips to combat obsessive compulsive thoughts by itself.

- *Tip:* 1 Challenge obsessive thoughts and compulsive behaviors. It you have OCD, there are many ways you can help yourself in addition to seeking therapy.

Refocus Your Attention

- When you are experiencing OCD thoughts and urges, shift your attention to something else.
- You could exercise, jog, walk, listen to music, read, surf, the web, play a video game, phone call or knit. The important thing is to do something you enjoy for at least 15 minutes, in order to delay your response to the obsessive thoughts or compulsion.
- At the end of the delaying period, reassess the urge. In many cases, the urge will no longer be quite as intense. Try delaying for a longer period. The longer you can delay the urge, the more it will likely change.
- *Write down the obsessive thoughts or worries:* Keep a pad and pencil with you and write down all your thoughts or compulsions.

Anticipate OCD Urges

- By anticipating you have compulsive thoughts before they arise, you can help to ease them. For example, if your compulsive behavior involves checking that doors are locked, windows closed, or appliances turned off, then lock the door or turn off the appliance with extra attention the first time.

- Create a solid mental picture and then make a mental note. Tell yourself, 'The window is now closed and I can see that the oven is turned off'.

Create an OCD Worry Period

- Rather than trying to suppress obsessions or compulsions, develop the habit of rescheduling them
- Choose one or two 5–10 minutes worry periods each day; time you can devote to obsessing. Choose a set time and plan (e.g. in the living room from 7 to 7:10 am and 5 to 5:10 pm) that is early enough and it would not make you anxious before bedtime.
- During your worry period, focus only on negative thoughts or urges. Do not try to correct them. At the end of the worry period, take a few calming breaths, let the obsessive thoughts or urges go and return to your normal activities. The rest of the day, however is to be designated free of obsessions and compulsions.
- When thoughts or urges come into your head during the day, write them down and 'post-pone' them to your worry period. Save it for later and continue to go about the whole day.
- Go over your 'worry list' during the worry period. Reflect on the thoughts or urges you wrote down during the day. If the thoughts are still disturbing, allow yourself to obsess about them, but only for the amount of time you have allotted for your worry period.

Create a Tape of the OCD Obsessions

- Focus one specific worry or obsession and record it to a tape recorder, computer or on phone.
- Recount the obsessive phrase, sentence or story exactly as it comes into the mind.
- Play the tape back to yourself, over and over for a 45 minutes period each day, until listening to the obsession no longer causes you to feel highly distressed.
- By continuously confronting your worry or obsession you will gradually become less anxious. You can then repeat the exercise for a different obsession.
- *Tip: Take care of yourself:* A healthy, balanced lifestyle plays a big role in keeping OCD behavior, fears and worry at day.

Practice Relaxation Exercises

While stress does not cause OCD, a stressful event can trigger the onset of obsessive and compulsive behavior and stress can often make obsessive compulsive behavior worse.

- Mindful meditation, Yoga, Deep breathing exercise and other stress–relief techniques may help reduce the symptoms of anxiety brought on by OCD.
- Try to practice a relaxation technique for at least half an hour a day.

Adopt Healthy Eating Habits

- Start the day right with breakfast, and continue with frequent small meals throughout the day. Going too long without eating leads to low blood sugar level, which can trigger to feel more anxious.
- Eat plenty of carbohydrates, such as whole grains, fruits and vegetables. Not only do complex carbohydrates stabilize blood sugar, they also boost serotonin, which acts to calm the symptoms.

Exercise Regularly

- Exercise is a natural and effective antianxiety treatment that helps to control OCD symptoms by refocusing the mind when obsessive thoughts and compulsions arise.
- For maximum benefit, try to get 30 minutes or more of aerobic exercises on most days. It relives tension and stress, boosts physical and mental energy and enhances well being through the release of endorphins, the brain's feel–good chemicals.

Avoid Alcohol and Other Drugs

Alcohol temporarily reduces anxiety and worry, but it actually causes anxiety symptoms as it wears off. Similarly, while it may seem that cigarettes are calming, nicotine is actually a powerful CNS stimulant. Smoking leads to higher not lower, levels of anxiety and OCD symptoms.

Get Enough Sleep

Not only can anxiety and worry cause insomnia; but a lack of sleep can also exacerbate anxious thoughts and feelings. When you are well rested, it is much easier to keep your emotional balance, a key factor in coping with anxiety disorders such as OCD.

- *Tip: Reach out for Support:* OCD can get worse when you feel powerless and alone, so its important to build a strong support system. The more connected you are to other people, the less vulnerable you will feel. Just venting off your worries and urges can make them seem less threatening.

Stay Connected to Family, Friends and Support Groups

Obsessions and compulsions can consume the life to the point of social isolation. In turn, social isolation can aggravate the OCD symptoms. It is important to have a good network of family and friends and support system. Involving others in the treatment strategy can help guard against setbacks and keep the client motivated.

NURSING MANAGEMENT

- **Nursing Diagnosis:** Increased anxiety, fears or guilt related to obsessive thoughts, internal conflicts and compulsive acts.
- **Nursing outcome:** Client will be free from anxiety and fears related to disease.

Nursing interventions	Rationale
• At the beginning, do not attempt to prevent or call attention to the client's compulsive acts.	• Preventing or attending to compulsive acts may enhance the anxiety.
• Encourage the client to verbally identify his/her concerns, life stressors, anxieties.	• Addressing feelings directly may help diminish the client's anxiety and thus diminish obsessive thoughts, rumination and compulsive acts.
• Encourage the client to vent his/her feelings in ways that are acceptable to the client (through talking, crying, physical activities, play).	• The client may be uncomfortable with some ways of expressing emotions or find them unacceptable.
• At first allot specific time period, such as 10 minutes every hour, when the client's can focus on his/her obsessive thoughts or ritualistic behaviors. • Gradually decrease the time allotted to the client.	• Setting the limits recognizes the significance of there thoughts and acts in the client's life; but still encourage him/her to focus on other feelings and problem.

Contd...

Contd...

Nursing interventions	Rationale
• Provide structured schedule of activities for client's including adequate time for completion of rituals.	• Structure provides feelings of security for the anxious client.
• Support the client's effort to explore the meaning and purpose of the behavior.	• Client may be unaware of the relationship between emotional problems and compulsive behaviors.
• Give positive reinforcement to non ritualistic behaviors.	• Positive reinforcement enhance self-esteem and encourages repetition of desired behaviors.

- **Nursing diagnosis:** Ineffective role performance related to need to perform rituals.
- **Nursing outcome:** Client will be able to resume role related responsibilities.

Nursing interventions	Rationale
• Determine the client's previous role in family and extent to which this role is altered by the illness. Identify role of other family members.	• This is an important assessment data for formulating an appropriate plan of care.
• Discuss client's perception of role expectations.	• Determine whether client's role perception are realistic.
• Encourage the client to discuss conflicts present within the family systems. Identify how client and other family members have respond to the conflict.	• Identifying specific stressors as well as adaptive and maladaptive responses.
• Explore available options for changes or adjustments in role. Practice through role play.	• Playing and rehearsal of potential role transitions can reduce anxiety.
• Encourage family participation in the development of plan to effect positive change and work to resolve the cause of the anxiety from which the client seeks relief through use of ritualistic behaviors.	• Input from the individuals who will be directly involved in the change will increase the likelihood of a positive outcome.
• Give client lots of positive reinforcements for ability to resume role responsibility by decreasing need for ritualistic behavior.	• Positive reinforcement enhances self-esteem and promote repetition of desired behavior.

Prevention of OCD

- It is not possible to prevent OCD from the beginning. But the best way to prevent a relapse of OCD symptoms is by staying with the therapy and taking any medicine exactly as they have been prescribed.
- It is also important to involve family members and loved ones in treatment, especially if the doctor has suggested the client to participate in therapy together. Keeping lines of communication open may help the client to deal with relationships that have become strained during illness.
- Reducing overall stress in one's life; although not proven treatment for OCD symptoms, may help to cope up stress and anxiety relieving methods include:
  - Taking slow, deep breaths.
  - Soaking in a warm bath.
  - Listening to shooting music.
  - Taking a walk or doing some other exercises.
  - Practicing yogic exercises.

- Having a massage or back rub.
- Drinking a warm, non alcoholic, non caffeinated beverage.
- Eating a healthy, balanced diet and avoiding junk foods.

POST-TRAUMATIC STRESS DISORDER (PTSD)

Introduction

Alter a dreadful experience in life, it is normal to feel sad, frightened, anxious and disconnected. But, if the upset does not fade and feelings stuck with a constant sense of danger and painful memories, we can be confirmed that he/she is suffering from post-traumatic stress disorder.

It is a type of anxiety disorder. It can occur after the individual sees, hears or experiences a traumatic event that involved the threat of injury or death which is unimaginable in a normal way. It is also known as 'soldiers heart'. PTSD sufferers re-experience the traumatic event or events in some way, tend to avoid places, or other things that remind them of the event (avoidance) and are exquisitely sensitive to normal life experiences (hyperarousal).

Epidemiological Factors

The lifetime prevalence of PTSD is considered about 8% of the general population. The lifetime prevalence for women is higher than men, i.e. 10–12% in females and 5–6% in males.

Etiology

PTSD is probably caused by a complex mix of factors.

Stressors

- Stress/stressor is the major factors in development of PTSD. Along with the stressors the stressors psychological, social and biological factors and events that happened pre and post trauma events are more important.
- Post-traumatic disorder is especially common among those who have served in battle field. It is sometimes called 'shell shock', 'battle fatigue' or 'combat stress'. The most common stressors leading to the of PTSD include:
  - Combat exposure
  - Rape, physical abuse or child neglect
  - Sexual molestation
  - Physical abuse/attack
  - Being threatened with a weapon.

Other many traumatic events also can lead to PTSD, including fire, natural disaster, mugging, robbery, assault, civil conflict, plane crash, torture, kidnapping, life threatening medical diagnosis, terrorist attack and other extreme life threatening events.

Risk Factors

All individuals who have encountered with certain traumatic events do not develop PTSD, there are certain risk factors which make individual prone to this disease. These are:

- Presence of childhood trauma.
- Borderline/paranoid/dependent/ antisocial personality.

- Lack of family and social support.
- Genetic vulnerability.
- Stressful life changes.
- Being female
- Experiencing intense or long lasting trauma
- Having 1st degree relatives with depression.

Sign and Symptoms of PTSD

- The classical clinical features of PTSD include reexperience of the event, pattern of avoidance and emotional numbing.
- PTSD symptoms typically start within three months of a traumatic event. PTSD symptoms are generally grouped into three types: intrusive memories, avoidance and numbing and increased anxiety or emotional arousal.
- *Symptoms of intrusive memories may include:*
  - Flash backs, or relieving the traumatic event for minutes or even days at a time.
  - Upsetting dreams about the traumatic event.

Symptoms of avoidance and emotional numbing include:

- Trying to avoid thinking or talking about the traumatic event
- Feeling emotionally numb
- Avoiding enjoyable activities
- Hopelessness
- Memory problem/amnesia/flashbacks
- Trouble in concentrating
- Difficulty in maintaining relationships.

Symptoms of anxiety and increased emotional arousal include:

- Irritability or anger
- Overwhelming or shame
- Self destructive behavior
- Sleep disturbance
- Being easily startled or frightened
- Hallucinations/illusions.

Other associated symptoms

- Avoidance to the point of having a phobia of places, people and experiences that remind the sufferer of a trauma or a general numbing of emotional responsiveness.
- Chronic physical signs of hyperarousal, including sleep problems, irritability, anger, poor concentration, black outs or difficulty remembering things, increased tendency and reaction to being startled, and hypervigilance to threat.

Traumatic events that can lead to PTSD include:

- War
- Natural disasters
- Plane/car clashes and accidents
- Terrorist attacks
- Sudden death of a loved one
- Rape/kidnapping

- Assault
- Sexual or physical abuse
- Childhood neglect.

Symptoms of PTSD in children

In children especially those who are very young the symptoms of PTSD can be different than the symptoms in adults. Symptoms in children include:

- Fear of being separated from parent
- Losing previously acquired skills (e.g. toilet training)
- Sleep problems and nightmares without recognizable content
- Sombre, compulsive play in which themes or aspects of the trauma are repeated
- New phobias and anxieties that seem unrelated to the trauma
- Acting out the trauma through play, stories or drawings
- Aches and pains with no apparent cause
- Irritability and aggression.

Risk Factors for PTSD

No one knows who will get PTSD at what moment. It is impossible to predict who will develop PTSD in response to trauma, but there are certain risk factors that increase for vulnerability.

Many risk factors revolve around the nature of the traumatic event itself. Traumatic events are more likely to cause PTSD when they involve a severe threat to the life or personal safety. The more extreme and prolonged to threat, the greater the risk of developing PTSD in response. Intentional, human inflicted harm, such as rape, assault and torture–also tends to be more traumatic than 'acts of god' or more impersonal accidents and disaster. The extent to which the traumatic event was unexpected, uncontrollable and inescapable also plays a role.

Apart from these, other factors include:

- Previous traumatic experiences, especially in early life.
- Family with PTSD or depression
- History of physical or sexual abuse
- History of substance abuse
- History of depression, anxiety or another mental illness
- High level of stress in life
- Lack of psycho-socioeconomic support after trauma
- Lack of coping skills.

Management of PTSD

Post-traumatic stress disorder management/treatment can help the person to regain a sense of control over the life. The treatment often includes both medication and psychotherapy. Combining these treatments can help improve the symptoms and teach the person to adopt skills to cope better with the traumatic event and life beyond it.

Medications

- Antipsychotics to relieve anxiety and related psychophysical problems, such as anhedonia, or emotional outbursts.

- Antidepressants can help to reduce anxiety and depression. They can also help improve sleep problems and to improve the concentration. SSRIs like sertraline, paroxetine are used.
- Other medications, such as bupropion and venlafaxine are also used to treat PTSD.

Psychotherapy

Many types to psychotherapies are used to treat both children and adults with PTSD. These include:
- *Cognitive Therapy:* It helps to recognize the ways of thinking (cognitive pattern) that are keeping the person stuck; for example, negative or inaccurate ways of perceiving normal situations. In PTSD, cognitive therapy often is used along with a behavioral therapy known as exposure therapy.
- *Exposure Therapy:* It helps to face everything that finds frightening; so that he/she can learn to cope with it effectively. A new approach to exposure therapy uses 'virtual reality' programs that allow the person to re-enter the setting in which the person experienced trauma, e.g., a 'virtual exposure to dogs'.
- *Eye movement desensitization and reprocessing (EMDR):* This combines exposure therapy with a series of guided eye movements that help to process traumatic memories.
- Families of PTSD individuals, as well as the sufferer may benefit from family counseling, couple counseling, parenting classes and conflict–resolution education. Family members may also be able to provide relevant history about their loved one (for example, about emotions and behaviors, drug abuse, sleeping habits and socialization) that people with the illness are unable or unwilling to share.

Alternative Medicine

Acupuncture is effective in PTSD symptoms resolution.

Nursing Management

Clients who exhibit signs of acute and severe anxiety or panic anxiety may harm themselves or others and need to be supervised closely until the anxiety is reduced. Such clients are placed in wards/special wards to ensure a protective environment.

During severe anxiety and stress the nursing interventions include:
- Staying with the client at all times.
- Remaining calm. The client will sense any anxiety, exhibited by the nurse.
- Speaking in short, simple sentences.
- Displaying firmness to provide external controls over the client.
- Maintaining quiet and calm environment.
- Providing protective care.
- Verbalizing the emotions and feelings by psycho therapeutic talk.
- Administering medications and monitoring for adverse effects.
- Help the client in tolerating the intense memories and emotional pain.
- Nurse should use simple, reassuring statement while talking with the client.
- Development of trusting relationship and teaching client new ways of coping strategies.
- Protecting the client's defenses (e.g. ritualistic behavior).
- Monitoring the client for follow-up.

Substance Use Disorders and its Management

INTRODUCTION

In most societies, use of substances to alter mood, behavior, perceptions, etc. is accepted. In our culture also, use of alcohol, caffeine and nicotine is widely accepted as normal. Nevertheless, these substances can lead to all sorts of problems for the user. There are many other substances that people take which have even clearer risks associated with that, e.g. cocaine, LSD, heroin, PCP, barbiturates, etc.

Substance use disorder commonly known as drug abuse/drug addiction refers to a maladaptive patterned use of a substance in which the user consumes in amounts or with methods not advised by health personnel. Substance abuse is not limited to mood altering or psychoactive drugs. It is also considered substance abuse when inappropriately used such as in sports and clubs. Substance abuse is described in Vedic literature, Biblical, Greek and Roman. Accounts of use of substance are as old as civilization.

DEFINITIONS

- *Psychoactive substance:* Chemicals which affect the central nervous system, therapy altering mental functioning.
- *Substance abuse:* Abuse is the use of any substance to that extent when it interferes with individual's normal functioning. It can be distinguished by following criteria.
- *A pattern of pathological use:* It is manifested by intoxication throughout the day, inability to cut down or cease the use, repeated efforts to control use through periods of temporary abstinence or restriction of use to certain times of the day, continuation of substance use despite of a serious physical disorders.
- *Impairment in social or occupational functioning due to pathological use:* Social relations are disturbed maybe because of individuals failure to meet his roles and responsibilities towards his family, friends and society or by irrational, aggressive, impulsive, erotic and criminal behavior. Individual's occupational functioning is also impaired because of individual's inability to carry-out his duties, targets and code of conduct. Duration of disturbance at least one month.

Substance Dependence

It is more severe form of substance abuse. Dependence is of two types and is evident by tolerance and withdrawal.

- Physical dependence refers to need of a particular substance to function normally or to carry-out daily activities. The user's body system becomes so accustomed to a particular substance that without that substance in the body, the person is unable to carry-out daily activities.
- *Psychological dependence:* It is that, when in the absence of the particular substance, the user's cognitive functioning is impaired. The thought of that substance is the main focus of person's thought process. It is difficult to stop thinking about that substance and it produces strong desire to have that substance and its effect.
  - *Tolerance:* Tolerance is failure of same amount of drug to produce desired effect and a larger dose is required to produce the same degree of substance effects.
  - *Withdrawal:* Withdrawal is a reversible set of substance specific symptoms that are caused by the cessation or reduction in heavy and prolonged substance use.
  - *Habit:* It is characterized by only desire to take the drug. There is no need to increase the dose or frequency and is usually not followed by physical withdrawal.
  - *Addiction:* It is a state of periodic or chronic intoxication, harmful for individual and to the society produced by repeated consumption of the drug. It involves both dependence and habit.
  - *Loss of control:* It is an inability to control over the quantity of substances consumed and length of substance use episodes.
  - *Inability to abstain:* It is inability to maintain long-term abstinence.

Biopsychosocial Deterioration

It is progressive physical, psychological and social deterioration as long as substance use continues which ends in serious physical illness. It includes serious psychiatric illness, suicide, death or involvement in treatment.

Examples of Common Substance Abused

	Class	Example	Route/via
1.	Alcohol	Beer, Rum, Whiskey, Brandy, Vodka.	Oral
2.	Cannabis	Bhang, Charas, Ganja	Oral/smoking
3.	Cocaine	Hashish, Marijuana, Crash2	Orally, nasal, IV
4.	Hypnosedatives	Barbiturates, Benzodiazepines	Orally/injection route.
5.	Opioids	Smack, Heroine, Morphine, Pethidine, Opium	Sniffing, orally.
6.	Hallucinogens	LSD, Mescaline	Orally, snuffing, smoking.
7.	Inhalants	Glue, Thinner, Paints, Varnish, Acetone, Amphetamines	Snuffing
8.	Psychostimulants	Methylphenidate	Injections

Contd...

Contd...

	Class	Example	Route/via
9.	Nicotine	Chewing tobacco, cigarettes, pipes.	Chewing, smoking
10.	Caffeine	Coffer powder, soft drinks, tea, coffee.	Orally

Mann's 'index of addictability': List of mood altering substances arranged according to the potential each has for causing addiction.

Heroin
Morphine
Demerol
Cocaine
Barbiturates
Amphetamines
Alcohol
Minor tranquilizers
Sleeping pills
Codeine
Bromides
Nicotine
Marijuana
Caffeine

High ◄———— Addictability ————► Low

ETIOLOGY OF DRUG ABUSE

The exact cause for drug abuse is still unknown. It can be explained on the basis of multiple theories.

Genetic Theory

This theory mainly focuses on alcoholism. Twin, adoption and family findings show the importance of genetics in causation of alcoholism. Children of alcoholics develop alcoholism four times more than children of nonalcoholic. Twin studies have suggested that the concordance late for alcoholism in monozygotic twins was almost double of that in dizygotic twins (58 v/s 28%). Genetic factors also have role in causation of cigarette smoking.

Neurobiological Theory

These theories postulated the cause of dependence and repetitive drug use behavior. Animal experiments have shown that the reinforcing effects of substance of abuse are mediated by increased dopamine release in the subcortical regions. It is also believed that these substances act on brain circuits that promote the normal reinforcement function of the central nervous system like behavior of feeding. It has been suggested that substance abuser have a defect in their ability to capture reward and pleasure from everyday life experiences.

It is also seen that chronic administration of opiate agonists leads to decrease in the synthesis and or release of endorphins in the brain, and these endorphins have important role in relieving pain and stress in day-to-day life.

It is also postulated that craving is linked with changes in the concentration of neurotransmitter in brain like that of dopamine and endorphins in hippocampus and nucleus accumbens regions of the brain. Changes in dopamine are concerned with craving of cocaine and stimulants and changes in endorphins is linked with craving of alcohol.

Learning Theory

The external environmental cues and internal cues of an individual get conditioned with pleasurable effects of substances. This conditioning can lead to dependence of substances. External environmental cues are advertisement, role model and drug abuser friend and internal cues are individual's own anxiety, frustrations, failure and depression. This conditioning occurs not only to pleasurable effects but other substances related experiences like withdrawal symptoms. Behavior cues have been found to be involved in the development of dependence to smoking. It has seen that behavior cues of sight of cigarettes pack or cigarette, the act of lighting contribute to repetitive behavior of smoking. The effect of modeling, imitation and identification on behavior can also lead to substance abuse disorders.

Psychodynamic Theory

According to Sigmund Freud's psychodynamic view addiction is a substitution for regressive infantile autoeroticism which was first pleasurable than turns into unpleasurable. In this gratification of pleasurable effect following the substance use, leads to guilt and loss of self-esteem. These feelings produce unbearable anxiety which in turn leads to repetition of the act in order to find relief.

According to infantile Abraham, alcoholism in males reduce their intense conflicts about homosexuality and that alcohol allows them to express these unconscious infantile in a way that is socially acceptable.

In the words of Wider and Kaplan use of substance is related to infantile of stress that the individuals can not achieve by his own psychic efforts.

The following defense mechanisms are frequently associated with the individual abusing substances:

- *Denial:* Here, the person denies the use of pattern, harmful effects, problems, lack of control over one's use and the need for external help in substance taking behaviors.
- *Rationalization:* The person provides logical explanation for the use of substance and its pattern.
- *Projection:* The person projects his substance use pattern and or related problem on some other person or source instead of being part of one's own behavior.

Sociocultural Factors

Society and one's culture plays an important role in addiction and dependence of substances. The availability of one or more substances, the cultural pattern of use and attitude and the legal control are important factors. In some cultures use of substances like alcohol, opium and tobacco are considered normal and even encouraged. Research studies have shown that the cultural tradition and permissiveness of alcohol use in Punjab has been associated with higher rates of alcohol use disorders.

DRUG DEPENDENCE AS A MEANS OF COPING

The Selye's general adaptation syndrome and proper choice of adaptation methods can be applied to the issues of substances, abuse and dependency. Drug use, abuse and dependency serve a purpose for the chemical/drug dependent person. There are legitimate reasons for the use of many drugs. Ethyl alcohol is a drug and a legal substance with approved recreational and social use. Many people drink alcoholic beverages without encountering problems. Some drugs, such as narcotics and sedative—hypnotics are controlled substances, and are used for medical purposes to alleviate physical pain and emotional suffering, when taken as prescription by doctor, these drugs maybe used to diminish stress without the serious adverse consequences of abuse and dependency.

For the person who abuses or is dependent on substance, the drugs have become a way of coping or adapting to any life's stressors. In other words, drugs are a way of life for this person.

The person may use drugs to relieve anxiety or unpleasant feelings of any kind, to experience and increase pleasant or 'high' sensations, to sustain a world of daydreams or an existence beyond the bounds of reality and to express or repress feelings of joy, love, anger, or hatredness. Drugs not only do things to people who take them, they also do things for people who take them. Thus, it is important to understand what these substances do for people to effect primary prevention of chemical dependence and to help people adapt to or cope with stress in a more effective, healthy manner.

Substance abuse and dependence cuts across all socioeconomic and cultural groups and all ages. The reasons for misuse of, abuse of, and dependence on drugs generally include an attempt to adapt to stress. Ironically, the process becomes a vicious cycle, because the method of adapting to life's stressors becomes another stressor and eventually a disease of dependency. There is no single etiological concept to explain the cause of substance related disorders. Biological, social, psychological and learning factors are considered to have a part in the cause. Although the cause is multifunctional using substances as a coping mechanism for stress must also be considered as a factor in the development of the disease process (Fig. 9.1).

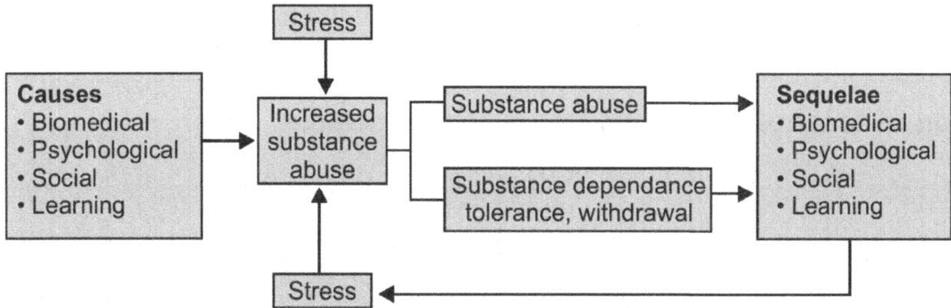

Fig. 9.1: A conceptual model of substances abuse

The use of drugs as a coping mechanism destroys or diminishes a person's ability to master life's concepts and events. Letting go of substance abuse as a method of adaptation and learning healthy methods of adaptation may result in successful recovery from drug dependence.

EPIDEMIOLOGICAL FACTS OF DRUG ABUSE

According to WHO's (2010) report:

- The harmful use of alcohol results in globally 2.5 million deaths each year.
- Around 3,20,000 young people between the age of 15–29 die from alcohol related causes, resulting in 9% of all deaths in that age group.

- At least 15.3 million people have drug use disorders.
- Injecting drug use reported in 148 countries, of which 120 report HIV infection.
- Recent estimate (2010), 155 to 250 million people or 3.5 to 5.7% of the world's population aged 15–64 use other psychoactive substances such as cannabis, amphetamines, cocaine, opioids and nonprescribed psychoactive prescription medication. Globally, cannabis is the most commonly used (129–190 million people) followed by amphetamine type stimulants then cocaine and opioids.
- WHO estimated that 0.7% of the global burden of disease in 2004 was due to cocaine and opioids use, with the social cost of illicit substance use being in the region of 2% of GDP in countries.

DYNAMICS OF SUBSTANCE ABUSE

Alcohol Abuse

Excess alcohol consumption is one of the major health problems around the world. On the other hand, it is associated with increased probability of death.

Nature of Alcohol

The substance commonly referred to as alcohol is ethyl alcohol (C_2H_5OH), also known as chemically as ethanol. It has pharmacological properties that produce mind and mood altering effects. It is a CNS depressant similar to barbiturates and ether. Chloral hydrate and paraldehyde are sedative hypnotic drugs derived from ethyl alcohol (Fig. 9.2).

Alcohol containing beverages include beer, wine, rum, and distilled spirits. The alcohol content of a beverage is expressed as proof, that is, the concentration of ethyl alcohol.

Alcohol often is erroneously considered a CNS stimulant. The reason for this misconception is that after drinking alcohol beverages, people may become more talkative or hyperactive, euphoric, self-confident or aggressive. This behavior has been attributed to the disinhibiting effect produced by a low dose.

Association of Alcohol and Other Drugs with Problems

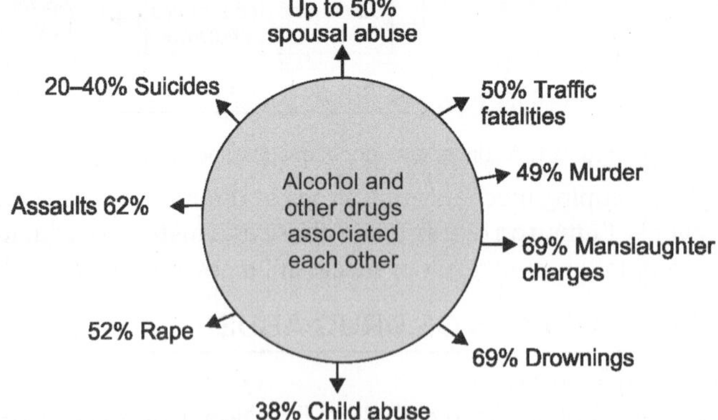

Fig. 9.2: Interlinks between alcohol and its effects (source: officer of substance abuse prevention 2001)

Alcohol Concentration in the Body

The physical and behavioral manifestations of the effects of alcohol on the CNS are related to the level of alcohol in the blood, the concentration of alcohol in the brain and other contributing factors. The blood level of alcohol is expressed in the number of milligrams of alcohol per milliliter of blood.

Blood alcohol level is determined by a laboratory blood test to measure the degree of alcohol intoxication. It maybe used in medicolegal procedures to rule out intoxication in a person who is comatose. The degree of intoxication also maybe measured by a breathalyzer.

Alcohol concentration in the blood depends on the rate of absorption, transportation to the CNS, redistribution to other parts of the body, metabolism and elimination. Alcohol is absorbed through the mouth, stomach and small intestine. It is absorbed unchanged into the blood and circulates throughout the body, including the brain. It also crosses the placenta into the fetal circulation. Intoxication occurs when the circulating alcohol interferes with the normal functioning of brain nerve cells.

The rate of absorption into the blood varies with the following factors:

- Substances in the beverage, such as the carbonation (CO_2) in Thums-up/Champagne, increase absorption.
- The rate of alcohol ingestion can affect the rate of absorption. Drinking alcoholic beverages slowly over a long period may slow absorption and allow for metabolism of alcohol by the liver. Because the body metabolizes alcohol at a steady rate, when a person drinks faster than the body can metabolize the alcohol, it accumulated in the blood.
- The rate of drinking may vary, but alcohol leaves the body at a fixed rate.
  - Oxidation, which occurs mainly in the liver, eliminates 90% of the alcohol absorbed by the body. The other 10% is eliminated unchanged through breath, sweat, urine and other body fluids. The healthy liver metabolizes approximately 1 Oz (30 ml) of alcohol per hour; the excess alcohol that the liver cannot metabolize continues to circulate in the blood. Food in the stomach slows absorption; whereas empty stomach increases absorption. The drinker's emotional state also affect absorption. For example, stress, fear, anger and fatigue may increase or decrease absorption. The drinker's body size also affects the concentration of the alcohol in the blood. A person's body chemistry and cultural influences may also alter the behavioral effects of alcohol.

Tolerance

Prolonged heavy drinking results in physical and behavioral tolerance. Physical tolerance or tissue adaptation, means that changes occur in the cells of the nervous system so that more drug is required to achieve the desired effects. When physical tolerance develops, the person may experience withdrawal or abstinence after cessation or syndrome after cessation or a decrease in alcohol consumption. Physical tolerance to alcohol never reaches the high doses of opiates. The behavioral tolerance to alcohol is manifested by the ability to mask the behavioral effects, for example, the acquired ability not to slur words, to walk straight and to function in ways that would not be possible in a nondependent person.

Blackout

Persistent heavy drinking frequently results in the chemically induced alcoholic blackout. During this period—the person appears to function normally while drinking but later is unable to remember what occurred. It may last a few hours or several hours.

Alcohol Induced Disorders

Intoxication

Intoxication occurs after drinking alcohol and is evidenced in behavior such as fighting, violence, impaired judgment, interference with social or occupational functioning or other maladaptive behavior. Physiological signs such as slurred speech, incoordination, unsteady gait, nystagmus and flushed face may accompany intoxication. Psychological signs also maybe observed, such as mood changes, irritability, talkativeness, etc.

Alcohol Withdrawal

Alcohol withdrawal or abstinence syndrome, occurs after reduction in or cessation of prolonged heavy drinking. A tremor of hand, tongue and eyelids may occur, as may nausea and vomiting, general malaise or weakness, autonomic nervous system hyperactivity (e.g. increased BP, pulse, HR), anxiety, a depressed or irritable mood, and orthostatic hypotension. Sleep disturbances, insomnia and nightmares may also be seen.

Alcohol Withdrawal Delirium/Delirium Tremens

Tremens is the most serious form of withdrawal syndrome. It occurs after cessation of or reduction in prolonged heavy drinking and can occur as long as one week after cessation of drinking symptoms include clouding of consciousness; inability to shift, focus and sustain attention to stimuli in the environment; misinterpretation, illusions or hallucinations, that are usually visual and vivid, incoherent speech; insomnia or daytime drowsiness; increased or decreased psychomotor activity; frequent agitation and increased blood pressure; sweating and temperature. Seizures may occur as a result of alcohol withdrawal. If untreated, this causes serious medical complications such as fluid and electrolyte imbalance, pneumonia and dehydration.

Alcoholic Hallucinosis

It occurs within 48 hours after cessation of or reduction in drinking. The symptoms are vivid and threatening, auditory hallucinations may develop but clouding of the consciousness does not occur. The person's response to the hallucinations is typically anxiety or fear. Auditory hallucinations are usually experienced as voices but maybe experienced as hissing or buzzing sounds.

Alcoholic Amnestic Disorder

The alcoholic amnestic disorder results from heavy, prolonged drinking and is thought to be related to poor nutritional intake. If the disorder is related to thiamine deficiency; it is known as Wernicke-Korsakoff syndrome. Amnesia consists of impairment in the ability to learn new information (short-term memory) and to recall remote information (long-term memory). Other neurological signs, such as neuropathy, unsteady gait or myopathy maybe present.

Alcoholic Dementia

Alcoholic dementia is associated with prolonged, chronic alcohol dependence. Signs of dementia include loss of intellectual ability that is severe enough to interfere with social or occupational functioning and impairment in memory, abstract thinking and judgment. The degree of impairment may range from mild to severe and may include permanent brain damage.

Medical Consequences

Heavy consumption of alcohol can adversely affect almost everybody system. Gastrointestinal problems occur as a result of the irritating effects of alcohol on the gastrointestinal tract, resulting in gastritis or ulcers. Acute or chronic pancreatitis may occur. Esophagitis may result from the direct toxic effect of alcohol on the esophageal mucosa; increased acid production in the stomach or frequent vomiting. Alcohol cardiomyopathy results from the direct toxic effects of the substance and malnutrition.

The liver is highly susceptible to the damaging effects of alcohol because it is the primary organ that metabolizes alcohol. Alcohol is toxic to the liver regardless of the person's nutritional status. Alcohol liver disease has been divided into three major types. In fatty liver, deposits of fats (triglycerides) build up in the normal liver cells. This condition is reversible. Alcoholic hepatisis is a more serious condition involving inflammation and necrosis of the liver cells. This condition is also reversible. Cirrhosis of liver is irreversible. In cirrhosis, the liver cells are destroyed and replaced by scar tissue. A high risk of cancer especially of the mouth, pharynx, esophagus, pancreas, cardia of the stomach and colon is also associated with alcoholism.

Sedative-Hypnotic Drugs

The barbiturates and other CNS depressants are called sedative—hypnotics and anxiolytics. The main difference between a sedative drug and a hypnotic drug is the degree of sedation produced compared with anxiolytics.

EFFECTS

The barbiturates and similarly acting drugs are capable of producing intoxication, withdrawal and physical and psychological dependence and tolerance. The route of administration maybe oral or parenteral (i.e. IV/IM). Basically, the organs with greater blood flow absorb the drug first. Most commonly used barbiturates are metabolized by the liver; some (e.g. phenobarbital) are not metabolized and are excreted unchanged by the kidneys. Because barbiturates cross the placental barrier, the fetus of a drug dependent mother may experience physical dependence. Physical withdrawal symptoms may occur in the infant up to seven days after delivery and may include high pitched cry, tremors, restlessness, disturbed sleep, increased reflex action, hyperphagia, diarrhea, vomiting and seizures.

Barbiturates and alcohol produce cross tolerance and when taken together, will increase absorption and produce addictive depression of the CNS. Because of this reason, people have taken barbiturate overdoses while intoxicated with alcohol, perhaps unaware of the additive effects of alcohol and the sedative hypnotics.

Pattern of Abuse

Barbiturates are frequently used by people who abuse or are dependent on drugs to relieve or counteract the effect of other drugs. For example, barbiturates maybe used to relieve symptoms of heroin withdrawal. The person maybe unaware that cross tolerance does not occur between opiates and barbiturates and may think that because tolerance to heroin is high, tolerance to barbiturates will be high also; as a result the person may unintentionally overdose on barbiturates. Heroin addicts may substitute barbiturates for heroin when heroin is unattainable and because there is no cross tolerance; may develop physical dependence on both drugs.

Barbiturates also maybe taken to relieve the anxiety related so flashbacks from lysergic acid diethylamide (LSD) abuse or to counteract the symptoms of anxiety, paranoia and depression due to excessive use of amphetamines.

Sedative-Hypnotic or Anxiolytic Induced Disorders

- *Intoxication:* It occurs after a recent ingestion of sedatives, hypnotics or anxiolytics. Signs and symptoms are similar to alcohol intoxication.
- *Withdrawal:* It occurs hours to several days after decrease in or cessation of prolonged heavy use of the barbiturate or similarly acting sedative-hypnotic agent. Signs and symptoms of withdrawal are similar to those of alcohol withdrawal. They do not necessarily follow a specific sequence and their severity depends on individual differences, doses and duration of use. Abrupt withdrawal from these drugs is not recommended; detoxification should be carried out in hospital settings.

Withdrawal Delirium

Withdrawal signs and symptoms from the barbiturates are the same as those of alcoholic withdrawal delirium and usually occur within one week after cessation or reduction of the drug. Some people experience delirium without seizures, some experiences seizures only, and some exhibit both. This condition is a medical emergency requiring immediate hospital interventions.

Amnestic Disorder

It occurs after prolonged heavy use of barbiturates or similarly acting sedative-hypnotics. Predominant signs and symptoms are impaired short-term memory (inability to learn new things) and long-term memory (inability to remember learned information).

Medical Consequences

Severe complications may result from intravenous barbiturate use. Inadvertently injecting the drug into subcutaneous tissue may cause cellulitis, in which subcutaneous tissue become swollen, inflamed and painful. Vascular complications occur if the drug is accidently injected into an artery; these may result in the loss of hand (paralysis) or fingers. The intravenous user may also suffer other medical complications from self-injections, particularly serum hepatitis,endocarditis, pneumonia, tetanus or malaria bacterial infection. They may have syphilis or malaria may result, as may allergic reactions to substances that may have been added to the drugs.

The Opiates

Opiates are narcotic drugs that relieve pain, often induce sleep and include drugs such as heroin, which has no medical use; codeine, which is used as a cough suppressant or pain medication and methadone, a synthetic narcotic that is a heroin substitute to help heroin addicts. Medicinal narcotics that are abused include paregoric, codeine-containing cough syrups, demerol, methadone and morphine.

Opiate abuse begins when client starts taking the medicine on their own wishes, more frequently than what physician has recommended. But opiate abuse is also seen as a street drug. It is more prevalent in those who use it as a recreational drug.

Effects

These are essentially CNS depressants, the opiates produce analgesia, mood changes and sedation; depress respirations and inhibit coughing. They are effective pain relief medications. The physiological actions of heroin are similar to morphine, but heroin is four or five times more potent than morphine. The body metabolizes heroin and morphine similarly. Heroin is converted into morphine, metabolized primarily in the liver with end products secreted through urine and bile. Tolerance to the opiates develops rapidly and physical dependence occurs a brief period of use.

Pattern of Abuse

Opiate abuser are of two classes: Street abuser and those who obtain opiates from health sources. The latter generally are an older, middle class, well-established group; the street abuse obtain opiates from illegal and in unethical manner.

The street abuser tends to be a young generation. The person begins using opiates occasionally but progresses to daily use and quickly develops dependence and tolerance. Frequently, there is a history of delinquent or antisocial behavior. The drugs illegal status brings legal problems. There is a high incidence of death in this group due to suicide, homicide, accidents and related health disorders; such as infections and tuberculosis. The mortality rate tends to 5 to 15 people per 1000 opiate users.

Medical abusers tend to be women from a middle class status or those with different pain disorders who misuse their prescribed drugs and often misuse other drugs as well. Two high-risk groups for this of abuse are of people with pain syndromes and health care workers, especially nurses, physicians and other health care providers. Opioid abuse and dependency is usually preceded by a period of poly drug use, which continues after opioid use is acquired.

Opioid-Induced Disorder

- *Intoxication*: Opiate intoxication is marked by papillary constriction, drowsiness, slurred speech, impaired attention or memory, euphoria, dysphoria, apathy and psychomotor retardation. Problems in social or occupational functioning and impaired judgment may result in maladaptive behavior.
- *Opioid withdrawal:* After reduction of opioid use, withdrawal symptoms may include tearing, runny nose, dilated pupils, gooseflesh (piloerection), sweating, diarrhea, yawning, mild hypertension, tachycardia, fever and insomnia. Accompanying symptoms maybe irritability, depression, restlessness, tremor, weakness, nausea, vomiting and muscle and joint pains. Duration of the withdrawal period depends on the specific drug.

Medical Consequences

Prolonged heavy opiate use often results in decreased motivation to engage in high quality life experiences, personal and social deterioration that usually involves problems with police and law agencies and family and interpersonal problems. Serious medical problems may result from drugs overdose, additives in the street drugs, poor nutrition and health and infection due to unsterile needles and equipment used in self-injection. Some common problems encounter are abscesses and infection of skin and muscle, tetanus, malaria, liver disease hepatitis, HIV, gastric ulcers, endocarditis, heart arrhythmias, anemia, infections of bones and joints, pneumonia, tuberculosis, lung abscess and kidney failure caused by infections of additives in street drug mixtures. Sexual function problems may occur secondary to low testosterone levels during chronic opiate use. In addition, serious emotional problems such as depression may result from opioid abuse.

Amphetamine and Cocaine: CNS Stimulants

Stimulants act directly on the CNS. The person taking stimulants becomes more talkative and active has increased sense of well-being; self-confidence and alertness. Stimulants are frequently used to decrease appetite, reduce fatigue and combat mild depression. A common stimulant is caffeine, an ingredient in coffee, tea and soft drinks.

Amphetamine is the prototype for this class of drug and other chemically related drugs with similar pharmacological properties. Cocaine is also a stimulant, classified as a narcotic and falls under PNDCACT.

Effects of Amphetamines and Similarly Acting Sympathomimetics

This category includes all substituted phenylethylamine structures, such as amphetamine and methamphetamine (or speed), substances with different chemical structures but amphetamine—like actions; and some substances used as diet pills. These substances maybe taken orally or intravenously. Tolerance develops within hours to days, and there is cross-tolerance to most stimulants.

Amphetamines (pep cells) are drugs that directly stimulate the central nervous system and create a feeling of alertness and self-confidence in the user. They are also referred by drug abusers as 'wake-up', 'speed', 'eye-openers', 'uppers', etc. Medically used in weight control measures (Dexedrine, Benzedrine); treatment of mild depression, fatigue, hyperkinesis or narcolepsy and local anesthetic.

A crystallized form of methamphetamine known as crystal, ice, glass or quartz (because it resembles transparent crystals). It can be taken orally, inhaled, injected or smoked. When smoked, the drug produces a high in few seconds; which may last up to 24 hours. It also have adverse effects including acute psychosis, severe paranoia, hallucinations and violent/aggressive behavior. These effects may last from a few days to weeks or even months. A person can quickly become addicted after using it just a few times.

Patterns of Use

Abusers of amphetamine generally can be classified into medical abusers and street abusers. Medical abusers may obtain these drugs to aid in weight loss or to treat fatigue and strain. Students may use them to help stay awake when studying for examinations; truck drivers may use them to stay awake during long distance driving. After the medication is discontinued, fatigues results and need for sleep leads to an increased dose, eventually leading to chronic use.

Street abusers use amphetamine or similar drugs to get high or achieve an altered state of consciousness. The drug maybe used alone or with other drugs.

Amphetamine and Sympathomimetics-Induced Disorders

- *Intoxication:* Physical symptoms of amphetamine intoxication include increased heart rate, and blood pressure, dilated pupils, perspiration, chills, nausea and vomiting. Other physical

symptoms include headaches, pallor, diarrhea and unclear speech. Psychological symptoms include psychomotor agitation, elation, grandiosity, delusions, auditory and visual hallucinations or a drug psychosis, talkativeness, loquacity and hypervigilance. People intoxicated with amphetamine display maladaptive behavior, such as fighting, violence, interference in social and occupational functioning and impaired judgment.
- *Delirium:* Symptoms of amphetamine delirium usually occur within one hour of oral intake or immediately after the intravenous injection and subside within six hours. Symptoms include hallucination (visual, tactile and olfactory), labile affect, violent and aggressive behavior.

Delusional Disorders

The prolonged, chronic use of moderate to high doses of amphetamine may result in a delusional disorder. Symptoms include persecutory delusions, ideas of reference, aggressiveness, hostility, anxiety and psychomotor agitation. The delusional person may experience distortion of body image or tactile hallucinations; such as feeling bugs crawling under skin. The delusional disorder may last for one week or of body image or tactile the delusional disorder may last for one week or longer, even for as long as one year.

Withdrawal

Amphetamine withdrawal follows prolonged use with abrupt cessation or reduction in use. Symptoms include dysphoric mood (e.g. Depression, irritability, anxiety), fatigue disturbed sleep and increased, dreaming. Dysphoric mood is the main symptom; if it is severe, agitation or suicidal ideation may occur. The sleep disturbance is related to an increase in rapid eye movement sleep and may persist for weeks. The withdrawal syndrome occurs within three days of cessation or reduction in the use of substance and speak in two or four days. Depression and irritability, however, may continue for months together.

Medical Complications

The overdose of amphetamine causes complications. Medical problems, such as tetanus, hepatitis, abscesses and infections may results due to self-injection of drugs. Cerebrovascular accident may result from strong contractions of blood vessels caused by stimulants. The increase in blood pressure may cause intracranial hemorrhage.

EFFECTS OF COCAINE

Cocaine is an alkaloid obtained from the coca plant (Erythroxylum coca). It is a white, odorless, fluffy powder that looks like snow, giving the substance one of its street names. It maybe taken by sniffing through the nose (snorting), where it is absorbed through the nasal mucus membranes. It can be absorbed from all mucous surfaces, including the gums, or mucous lining of the mouth, rectal and vaginal mucosa, and abrasions of the skin surface. All these routes are used to abuse.

Cocaine maybe injected intravenously, mixed in the same syringe with heroin or smoked. Because cocaine hydrochloride decomposes at high temperature, freebace is the term used globally when the cocaine alkaloid is freed from the hydrochloride salt. Some users have a kit to use.

Smoking cocaine is an efficient way of delivering the drug in a concentrated form to the brain. The alveoli of the lung offer a large area for absorption of the chemical substance. The appeal of smoking to users is the rapid circulation time from the lungs to the brain about 6 to 8 seconds—whereas circulation from arm to the brain takes about 16 seconds. It is metabolized by plasma enzymes and the liver and excreted in the urine.

Newer research findings shown that cocaine acts directly on the brain's pleasure centers, brain structures that, when stimulated, produce an intense desire to experience the pleasurable effects again and again. This causes changes in the brain activity and by allowing the neurotransmitter dopamine to remain active longer than normal, triggers an intense craving for more of the drug.

Cocaine Induced Disorders

- *Intoxication:* Cocaine intoxication is marked by maladaptive behavioral effects, such as fighting and impaired judgment and problems in occupational or social functioning. Physical and psychological symptoms occur within minutes to one hour of taking the drug. The psychological symptoms include an increased sense of well-being and confidence, increased awareness of sensory input, psychomotor agitation, elation, talkativeness, pacing and pressured speech, physical symptoms are increased heart rate, dilated pupils, increased BP, sweating, chills, nausea and vomiting. Cocaine use, especially by IV injection, causes a characteristic rush or feeling of increased self-confidence and well being. A severely intoxicated person may experience confusion, incoherent speech, anxiety, paranoid thoughts, headache and palpitations. Following the physical effects, the user is likely to feel anxious, tremulous, irritable, depressed and fatigued. In this stage, known as crashing stage, the user craves more cocaine for relief to these unpleasant symptoms. Recovery from intoxication occurs in 24 hours.
- *Delirium:* The symptoms of cocaine delirium usually occur within one hours of use (occurs immediately by IV use) and subside within 6–10 hours. Symptoms include labile affects, violent aggressive behavior, and tactile and olfactory hallucination.

Delusional Disorder

An organic delusional syndrome occurs soon after use of the drug. Symptoms include rapid development of persecutory delusions, distortion of body image and misperception of faces. Persecutory delusions may lead to aggressive or violent behavior; tactile hallucinations, such as the feeling of insects crawling under the skin, etc.

Cocaine Withdrawal

Cocaine withdrawal follows abrupt cessation or reduction in prolonged use. Symptoms include a dysphoric mood (e.g. depression, irritability, anxiety) along with fatigue psychomotor agitation, insomnia or hypersomnia. Paranoid and suicidal thoughts may occur; suicide is a major concern. Symptoms last for more than 24 hours after cessation of drug use.

Medical Consequences

Cocaine intoxication leads to many problems. Severe skin ulcerations may result because of digging out insects. Overdose can produce cardiac arrhythmias, convulsions and respiratory depression. Repeated heavy use by snorting the drug can abuse tissue ulcerations in the nasal septum. It can produce a paranoid psychosis which needs a longer treatment regime.

Hallucinogens/Psychomimetics

These drugs alter mood and perception. Ingestion of these drugs results in alterations in time and space perception, illusions, hallucinations, and delusions. These drugs produce 'bad trip'. The most potent and common hallucinogenic drug is LSD. Lysergic acid comes from ergot, a fungus that spoils grain. It was converted to LSD by a Swiss chemist in 1943. The odorless, colorless and tastelessness drug is classified as a hallucinogenic because it produces hallucinations.

The LSD trips start within one half hour after taking the drug and last for varying lengths of time. It is unknown how LSD acts on the nervous system, but is so powerful that only small doses 100 to 250 mg are needed for effects. The drug is liquid form is usually placed on a sugar cube: It has been also put on chewing gum, cookies and blotting paper. The side effects include flash backs and chromosomal damage, may result for LSD use.

Hallucinogen-Induced Disorder

Hallucinogen Hallucinosis

After drug ingestion, a hallucinogen hallucinosis may result. It is evidenced by perceptual changes, dilated pupils, increased heart rate, sweating, palpitations, blurred vision, tremors and incoordination. Also seen are maladaptive behavioral effects, such as severe anxiety or depression, fear of losing one's mind, ideas of reference, paranoid ideation, impaired judgment and interference with social and occupational functioning. The perceptual changes, the main feature of the hallucinogenesis, occur in a state of wakefulness and alertness and include subjective intensification of perceptions, depersonalization, illusions, hallucinations and synesthesias (e.g. seeing nose). The hallucinations are often visual and colorful and contain geometric forms and patterns. It begins within one hour after ingestion and lasts for several hours. Individual variations of the experience are related to the user's personality, the setting and the user's expectations. Euphoria is common. The person is usually aware that the changes in perception are due to the hallucinogen, although in some instances, the person fears loss of sanity and believes this will be a permanent state.

Hallucinogen Delusional Disorder

The use of hallucinogens may result in an organic delusional disorder that exists beyond the period of the direct effects of the substance, lasting longer than 24 hours after cessation of use. The perceptual changes of hallucinogen hallucinosis occur, but the individual believes that these misperceptions and thoughts are based on reality.

Hallucinogen Mood Disorder

An organic mood syndrome caused by hallucinogen ingestion may result in a disturbance in mood, often a depressed mood accompanied by feelings of guilt, fearfulness and restlessness. The person maybe talkative and unable to sleep. The disorder may last for a brief or a prolonged time and maybe difficult to differentiate from bipolar disorders.

Medical Consequences

Main symptoms include flashbacks, recurrences of hallucinations when the drug is no longer being used, may occur weeks or months after stoppage of drug use. People who have abused hallucination for a prolonged period are more likely to experience flashbacks. The episodes cause anxiety and the fear of going crazy. Physical dependence on hallucinogens does not develop. Tolerance develops and disappears quickly. Psychological dependence occurs in some people after chronic use. These people are known as acid heads, implying a personality change as a result of long-term hallucinogen use. The person becomes more passive and introspective and may lose the ability to concentrate. The research on these induced chromosome damage that produces congenial malformation. Medical problems are related to self-injury during periods of impaired judgment or delusions.

Cannabis

Cannabis is a generic term used to denote the several psychoactive preparations of the plant Cannabis Sativa. The major psychoactive constituent in cannabis is Delta tetra hydro cannabinol (DTHC). Compounds which are structurally similar to THC are referred to as cannabinoids the unpollinated female plants are called hashish. Cannabis oil (hashish oil) is a concentrate of cannabinoids obtained by solvent extraction of the crude plant material or of the resin.

Epidemiology

Cannabis is by far the most widely cultivated, trafficked and abused illicit drug. Half of an drug seizures are cannabis seizures. The geographical spread of those seizures is also global. According WHO (2010) report, about 147 million people, 2.5% of the world's population, consume cannabis compared with 0.2% consuming cocaine and 0.2% consuming opiates. In present, cannabis abuse has grown more rapidly than cocaine and opiate abuse.

Effects

Acute Heath Effects of Cannabis Use

The acute effects of cannabis use include the following:

- Cannabis impairment cognitive functioning which include the organization and integration of complex information involving various mechanisms of attention and memory processes. Including associative processes; free recall of previously learned items is often impaired.
- Cannabis impairs psychomotor performance in a wide variety of tasks, such as motor coordination, divided attention and operative tasks of many types. Human performance on complex machinery can be impaired for as long as 24 hours after smoking as little as 20 mg of THC in cannabis. There is increased risk of motor vehicle accidents.

Chronic Health Effects of Cannabis Use

- Selective impairment of cognitive functioning which include the organization and integration of complex information involving various mechanisms of attention and memory processes.
- Prolonged use may lead to greater impairment, which may not recover with cessation of use and which could affect daily life functions.
- The most predominant effects of cannabis are euphoria and altered level and consciousness without hallucinations. The drug can be smoked or eaten. The metabolities are excreted in feces and urine.
- Cannabis use can exacerbate schizophrenia in affected individuals.

- Epithelial injury of the trachea and major bronchi is caused by long-term cannabis smoking, airway injury, lung inflammation and impaired pulmonary defence against infection from persistent cannabis consumption over prolonged periods.
- Higher use can results in bronchitis and use during pregnancy may lead to postnatal risks of rare forms of cancer.

Cannabis Induced Disorders

- *Intoxication:* Cannabis intoxication is marked by increased heart rate, conjunctival injection (blood shot eyes), increased appetite, dry mouth, euphoria, subjective intensification of perceptions, sensation of slowed time and apathy. Maladaptive behavioral effects may include impaired judgment, interference with social or occupational functioning, panic attacks, suspiciousness, paranoid ideation or excessive anxiety.
- *Cannabis delusional disorder:* This delusional syndrome may occur with persecutory delusions during an episode of intoxication or immediately following use of cannabis. This disturbance does not usually last longer than 6 hours of cessation of use.
- *Medical consequences:* The smoke irritates the mucosa of lungs and causes acute or chronic bronchitis and sinusitis. Increased hear rate and decreased strength cardiac contractions invariably results. Research has indicated that chronic use can leads to impotency in men and causes malformation in neonates.

MANAGEMENT OF DRUG ABUSE: MEDICAL AND NURSING

Application of Nursing Process Model

Assessment

Medical assessment: The main objective of assessment is to ascertain the severity and extent of the problem as well as the client's biological, psychological and social resources. Identification of the problem and needs will help to provide therapeutic nursing and medical interventions. The interview for assessment should be therapeutic one.

- *Chief complaints:* These are the reason for admission. Here, the information getting from client maybe partially reliable. Collecting from client and his/her significant family members is crucial for further interventions. This provides an insight for attitude of the client and family member regarding disease process.
- *Present complaints:* Noting substance use pattern, complication related to use, abstinence attempted and treatment history will be collected. Before collecting information the nurse should be prepared with all baseline information regarding the client which will help her to establish a therapeutic relationship.
  - *Substance use pattern:* The nurse collects in depth information about the types, frequency, amount and duration of substances consumed by the client.
  - *Complication of substance use:* The complications of substance use include all complications arising in every sphere of one's life like physical, occupational, social, family as well as legal complications.
  - *Abstinence attempts:* Detail history of attempts of abstinence should be noted. It can be self-imposed of or treatment related. The nurse will note every attempt whether it is successful or unsuccessful with contributory factors.

- *Treatment history:* Includes detail information of treatment taken, complication of treatment if any and its outcomes and reason for relapse.

- *Past history:* It includes history of any long-term physical illnesses like tuberculosis, hypertension, HIV, syphilis, etc. these maybe related to prolong abuse.
- *Family history:* Family has an important role in causation as well as in its abstinence. So, in detail history should be collected towards its causes.
  - The family can have various factors which can lead to substance abuse like primary family dysfunction, marital disharmony, attitude and response of family members towards substance, impact of substance abuse on family, impulsive and pathogenic family, etc. This information will help to plan adequate treatment plan.
- *Personal history:* It will reflect contributory factors with an individual leading to substance abuse. A detail information regarding personal development, educational history, occupational history (especially influencing factor), peer relationship, marital relationship and psychosexual history should be noted down.
- *Premorbid personality:* Premorbid personality shows specific character traits, behavior pattern, suggestive of personality traits and their relationship with substance abuse. Detailed assessment should be made to ascertain whether antisocial behavior has occurred only during the period of substance abuse as a consequence of compulsive use or other dependence phenomena or it is a part of an overall pattern of antisocial traits.
- *Physical examination:*
  - Note physical deformities and physical complications and its effects of substances on body.
  - General appearance of the client shows signs of malnutrition, sign of liver disease, jaundice, palmer arrhythmia or pedal edema.
  - Abdomen may have epigastric tenderness, hepatomegaly and splenomegaly.
  - Cardiovascular system may indicate cardiac murmur and hypertension.
  - Respiratory system may show signs of bronchiolitis, emphysema and COPD.
  - Nervous system may show signs such as nystagmus and ataxia.
- *Mental status examination (MSE):* Assess for orientation, insight, level of consciousness, memory perception, mood and also for client's motivation for treatment. For the client with comorbid psychiatric illness, a detail mental status examination should be carried out.
- *Laboratory investigation:*

Two types of laboratory investigations are used in case of substance use disorders:

- Laboratory investigation for screening of substances.
- Laboratory investigation for assessment of physical health complications.
  - Laboratory investigation for screening of substances: Common tests used for screening are Gas Liquid Chromatography (GLC), Radio Immune Assay (RIA), and Thin Layer chromatography (TLC). Breath analyzer is the most common method to detect alcohol in exhaled air.
  - Laboratory investigation for assessment of physical health complication. Laboratory investigations for assessments of health complications include routine laboratory investigation like hemoglobin estimation, blood counts, urine examination, blood sugar, blood urea, X-ray, specific investigations like liver function test, lipid profile, test for HBsAg and HIV, ECG, CT scan etc.

Recognizing Emergency Conditions

Substance intoxication, overdose, severe alcohol and sedative hypnotic withdrawal, withdrawal delirium, withdrawal seizures and prolonged narcotic withdrawal maybe life threatening disorders that necessitate interruption of assessment for immediate intervention. The severity of withdrawal or abstinence syndrome depends on many factors such as type of drug consumption, extent of the additions, drug history, nutritional status of fluid and electrolyte balance.

- *Intoxication:* Almost all the drugs cause intoxication. If it is severe, symptoms include lethargy and stupor, and an overdose of the drug maybe a possibility. The intoxicated client may also demonstrate bizarre behavior, panic, fright, confusion or physical problems, such as vomiting and pain. The nursing interventions and treatment measureness for simple intoxication may consist of careful observation of symptoms, emotional support and protection from injury. Usually, intoxication resolves within a few hours.
- *Overdose:* Drug overdose maybe a severe medical problem needs critical care until the emergency situation is resolved. It occurs mostly with alcohol, sedative-hypnotics and narcotic drug use.

Withdrawal Syndrome

Various medications are given for detoxification purposes and relief of withdrawal symptoms. The nurse should be knowledge about the drug or drugs taken, dose, route of administration, reaction and possible effects and side effects, complication of the drugs. Generally, the following medications are used in withdrawal stage.

- The barbiturates are used primarily for barbiturate withdrawal.
- Anxiolytics, such as chlordiazepoxide (Librium or Diazepam Valium) are used for alcohol withdrawal disulfiram as antadict.
- Codeine, propoxyphene or other opiate drugs are given for relief of narcotic withdrawal symptoms; if these symptoms are severe, morphine or methadone maybe administered.
- Anticonvulsant drugs, particularly phenytoin are given for alcohol and sedative-hypnotic withdrawal seizures.
- Thiamine and multivitamin drugs are usually given in alcohol withdrawal treatment phase to prevent Wernicke-Korakoff syndrome.

Recognizing Behavioral Defenses

Defense or mental mechanisms are processes within the mind (i.e. intrapsychic processes) that are usually unconscious and that relieve the client's emotional conflict, stress and anxiety.

Denial

Denial is the most common defense used by clients. It is especially more seen in alcohol abuse and dependency. Denial is an unconscious process used to protect against intolerable feelings, thoughts, wishes, needs or external reality factors by blocking knowledge of these factors from conscious awareness. Coping mechanisms are used in normal ways to adapt to stressful or threatening situations, such as at the stage of grief in terminal illness. The use of defense mechanism becomes unhealthy when they are used haphazardly or inappropriately and when they interfere with healthy functioning. The person who abuses drugs often seem, unaware of the adverse bipsychosocial consequences of excessive drug use. Frequently, the abuse or dependency disorder develops gradually, and denial and other defense mechanisms protect the individual from acknowledging the fact that the disorder is developing. This is specially true to alcoholism. Although denial is found in almost all clients who abuse drugs, it is most predominant in alcoholics and allows alcoholics laterally to drink themselves to death.

People with alcohol abuse or dependence often cannot admit that alcohol is causing serious problems, so they continue drinking. One of the reasons for this denial in alcoholism is the blackouts that occur. The guilt feelings, the stigma attached to the behavior or disorder, and the possibility of rejection by others foster the development of denial. The family and care taker also contribute by denying that the drinking is a problem and by assuming care taking or enabling roles rather than allowing the person to experience the serious consequences of the drinking behavior.

Projection

It is an unconscious mechanism whereby that which is emotionally unacceptable to the self is rejected and attributed to other. Clients do not take responsibility for certain unacceptable behaviors and place their behavior outside of themselves, blaming others, places and things.

Rationalizing

This is also unconscious mechanism by which the client justifies, by seemingly believable means, feelings, behavior or motives that would otherwise be intolerable. For example, the client gives a reason for excessive use of a substance other than dependency. The drug use is not denied, an inaccurate, reasonable explanation is provided instead.

Diversion

The client may use certain tactics or techniques to change the subject to avoid the topic of abuse and dependency.

Minimizing

The abuser may admit to some drug or dependence but makes it seem like a minor problem.

Anger

The drug abuser may express anger or displeasure in response to the subject of drug abuse of dependency. This reaction tends to induce the nurse to change the subject, rather than confronting or dealing with the anger the discussion produces in the client.

The nurse practitioner recognizes that the denial process is a real phenomenon; that is, the client is not aware of the reality or extent of substance abuse or dependency disorder, because the initial experience with the use of the drug was enjoyable and although the pleasant aspects of the experiences have diminished and unfavorable consequences have developed; the search for recapturing the pleasure remains. The psychological compulsion to continue the drug use becomes very great that it becomes the prime priority in a dependent persons' life. What begins as a stress—relief or pleasure experience becomes the stressor. Denial helps drug—dependent client maintain some sense of self-worth and remove themselves from the harmful consequences of behavior. In the process, clients loose touch with reality of their situations.

Assessing Physical and Safety Needs

The physical needs of the client require constant assessment. The potential for infection is increased due to injuries, various medical consequences of the drugs and factors that may result from substance-induced organic mental disorders.

The potential for physical injury is a serious concern. Ensuring safety and protecting the client from harm must be primary focus. Substance-induced organic mental disorder present altered states of consciousness and impaired reality testing that will require vigilant assessment, through analysis and appropriate nursing interventions.

Sleep disturbances are common and conditions such as insomnia may result from withdrawal states, from the prolonged pattern of abuse or dependency or from personal or family stress. Also, nightmares and increased dreaming may occur. Nursing measures to assess and alleviate sleep disturbances are undertaken; sedative-hypnotics are usually discouraged because of the abuse disorder.

Assessment and intervention must be individualized to deal with the feelings of anxiety stemming from underlying conflicts and other issues related to substance abuse or dependency and cessation of use.

Depression or feelings of profound sadness are related to decreased self-esteem because of substance abuse behavior or its familial, social and legal consequences. These feelings require assessment and individualized treatment. Antidepressant medication maybe used in conjunction with other supportive measures. The potential for suicide is a priority consideration and requires appropriate interventions.

Noncompliance with treatment is manifested in many ways, indicating a lack of motivation for treatment. It maybe due to the denial syndrome and to a lack of understanding of the disorder. The nurse needs to be alert to these manifestations and help the client obtain insight into behavior.

Medication Management

The ultimate goal of treatment is to make the client achieve and maintain abstinence from substances and over time it should include the treatment for complications, improving social and psychological functioning and preventing relapse. So the treatment plan should be comprehensive viewing multi and interdisciplinary thought with family and social participation.

The treatment can be at different settings. The nonhospital settings are half way homes, rehabilitation centres, community clinics and specialized treatment units.

Goals

- *Immediate goal:* It includes treatment of intoxication and than detoxification, treatment of acute medical condition and crisis intervention.
- *Short-term goal:* It aims at treatment of comorbid and psychiatric disorder, maintenance of abstinence, vocational replacement and family reintegration.
- *Long-term goals:* It focuses on relapse prevention, psychosocial rehabilitation and improvement of quality of life inducing personnel empowerment.

Phases of Treatment

- *Pretreatment phase:* Preparation and acceptable on the part of the client about the problem and need for outside support.
- *The detoxification phase:* Usually, casts two to four weeks followed by active treatment phase.

- *Active treatment phase:* Usually, lasts three to twelve months or more and involve the choosing from many pharmacological and psychosocial modalities of treatment.
- *Post-treatment phase:* Usually, lasts for three to five years or even longer. In this phase family member and other social groups play a more active role to maintain abstinence and rehabilitation of the client.

Specific Management

Alcohol Withdrawal

In detoxification phase, the client is provided with benzodiazepines. These are useful in controlling alcohol withdrawal. Usually daily doses of 20–60 mg. of Diazepam or 40–120 mg of chlordiazepoxide are administered.

Clients with symptoms of Wernicke's syndrome or other signs of vitamin B deficiency (specially thiamine and nicotinic acid) are immediately treated with IV Thiamine HCL 100 mg twice in a day for first five days.

Treatment for Delirium Tremors

Delirium tremors are an psychiatric emergency. It develops in first five days of abstinence in about 5% of client. It typically begins 48–72 hours after the last drink and subsides within one to five days. It requires immediate hospitalization and IV administration of diazepam in doses of 10 mg every 20 minutes till client is sedated or signs symptoms of withdrawal decrease significantly. Supportive treatment comprises administration of thiamine, fluid and electrolyte correction, maintain safe and secure environment and monitoring vital signs.

OPIOID WITHDRAWAL

Management

The management of opioid withdrawal starts after estimation of amount of opioid consumed by the client in last 24 hours for estimation of dose of detoxification drugs. Usually, it is given in the range of dose is 1.2–3 mg of buprenorphine or 60–120 mg of methadone. Usually, these drugs are administered for 2–3 weeks and then tapered off by 5–25% daily.

- In accelerated detoxification low doses of naltrexone with clonidine are used.
- The client is reassured that these symptoms will disappear and should be kept motivated for further follow-up. Fluid and electrolyte correction if needed is done with management of other minor symptoms like administration of antidiarrheal agents, sleep inducing agents, etc.
- Aversion therapy is also used for opioid dependence. Here small dose of opium is administered by an emetic agent. This agent give rise to vomiting leading to conditioning of the client therapy decreasing the opium taking behavior.

SEDATIVE-HYPNOTIC WITHDRAWAL

Management

It is generally managed by gradual tapering off the substance of dependence. Client with mild to moderate dependence and those who are well motivated towards treatment out patient detoxification can be carried out by tapering of the drug. In severe cases, detoxification is carried out in inpatient setting by tapering off the drug at the rate of 10% daily. Withdrawal symptoms are managed by symptomatic management. After the detoxification stage, follow-up supportive treatment is essential to prevent relapse of the disease.

 NICOTINE WITHDRAWAL

Nicotine withdrawal is not so distressing, so it is treated with psychological therapies and with or without benzodiazepines for few weeks. Nowadays, chewing gum of nicotine content are available as an alternative consumption.

 CANNABIS WITHDRAWAL

Cannabis withdrawal includes supportive and symptomatic treatment. It requires hospitalization and administration of antipsychotics with family therapies.

 MULTIPLE SUBSTANCE WITHDRAWAL

Client with dependence of more than one substance requires specific medication for each category of the substance used. These clients require longer in patient treatment and detoxification period than those with single substance dependence.

Long-Term Treatment

The aim of long-term pharmacological treatment is to maintain abstinence after completion of detoxification phase. It helps to overcome expressed emotions of client to overcome psychosocial consequences.

 LONG-TERM TREATMENT FOR ALCOHOL DEPENDENCE

Mainly used drug is disulfiram (tetraelylthiuram disulfide).

Disulfiram Therapy

- Disulfiram was discovered in 1930 and most widely used.
- When alcohol is metabolized in body, it is converted into acetaldehyde then acetate and at last into carbon dioxide and water. When alcohol is ingested by the client who is on therapy, acetaldehyde cannot be converted into acetate in the presence of disulfiram therapy, acetaldehyde cannot be converted into acute in the ressence of disulfiram and hence leads to accumulation of acetaldehyde in blood and liver respectively. The accumulation results in disulfiram-ethanol reaction (DER) characterized by flushing, tachycardia, hypotension, tachypnea, headache, sweating, nausea, vomiting, giddiness and sense of impending doom as symptoms.
- Disulfiram-ethanol reaction occurs within 30 minutes of ingestion of alcohol and may subside after/within two hours of ingestion of alcohol. This occurrence of DER or any cognitive awareness of occurrence of DER prevents the drinking response. Prevention of drinking response helps in maintenance of abstinence and the client also gets an opportunity to control the behavior of drinking.
- It is administered after getting consent. The usual dose is 250 mg/day, however the dose can be increased to 500–750 mg/day in clients who fail to develop DER with the dose of 250 mg/day. It is generally given as single dose in the morning but a single bedtime may also be given.

Adverse Effects

The common adverse effects are drowsiness and gastric irritation while others are hepatotoxicity, neuropathy, skin reaction and psychosis.

Contraindications

It is contraindicated in clients with hepatic dysfunction, peripheral neuropathy, psychosis, first trimester of pregnancy and clients with cognitive deficits who cannot understand and remember the consequences of use of alcohol when on disulfiram.

Points to Remember During Therapy

- Disulfiram works well when it is given under supervision as it increases compliance. It can be done by any family member, preferably by spouse or significant family members.
- The therapy should be started only after proper explanation regarding use and precautions and about Disulfiram Ethanol Reaction (DER). Family member and the client should be educated about symptoms of DER and action required to be taken in case of DER.
- It should be explained that DER can occur with small doses of alcohol, so the client should avoid products containing alcohol such as shaving creams, antiemetics, etc.
- Disulfiram therapy should be started after Ethanol Challenge Test so that the client can experience DER in controlled condition.

Psychosocial Rehabilitation

Alcoholics Anonymous (AA)

This is an international movement which was founded in 1935 by Bill Wilson and Dr Bob Smith. It is a major self-help group or organization for the treatment of alcoholism. Both were alcoholics and wanted to quit alcohol. During this, they found that they could remain away from alcohol through mutual support. They accomplished it as peers who were able to share their common experiences, soon they were working with other alcoholics; who in turn worked with others. This movement grew remarkably and individually who had been treated unsuccessfully be professionals were able to maintain sobriety through helping one another.

Functioning of Alcoholic Anonymous Program

- AA members share their experience with anyone seeking help with a drinking problem; they give person-to-person service or 'sponsorship' to the alcoholic coming to AA from any source.
- The AA program, set forth in 12 steps, offers the alcoholic a way to develop a satisfying life without alcohol.
- AA program is discussed at AA group meetings. Open speaker meetings: open to alcoholics and nonalcoholics. At meeting, AA meeting 'tell their stories'. They describe their experience with alcohol, how they came to AA and how their lives have changed as a result of AA.
  - *Open discussion meetings:* One member speaks briefly about his or her drinking experience and then leads a discussion on AA recovery or any drinking related problem anyone brings up.

- *Closed discussion meetings:* Conducted just as open discussion are, but for alcoholic or prospective AA only.
- *Step meetings (usually closed):* Discussion of one of the twelve steps.
- AA members also take meetings into correctional and treatment facilities.
- AA members maybe asked to conduct the informational meetings about AA as a part of ASAP (Alcohol Safety Action Project) and DWI (driving while intoxicated) program. These meetings about AA are not regular AA group meetings.

Narcotic Anonymous (NA)

Narcotics anonymous is a nonprofit fellowship or society of men and women for when drugs had become a major problem. The recovery addicts who meet regularly to help each other stay clean. This is a program of complete abstinence from all drugs. There is only one requirement for membership, the desire to stop using.

NA's primary approach to recovery is its belief in the therapeutic value of one addict helping another. Members take part in NA meeting by talking about their experiences and recovery from drug addiction.

NA meetings are informally structured, held in space rented by the group and are led by members who take turns opening and closing the meeting. NA meetings and other services are funded entirely from donations by addict members and the sale of recovery literature. Financial contributions for non embers are not accepted. Most NA meetings are held regularly at the same time and place each week usually in a public place.

LONG-TERM TREATMENT FOR OPIATE DEPENDENCE

- It is based on use of substitution agents and antagonist agents.
- The commonly used agent is methadone. It will relieve the persistent narcotic substance craving without creating euphoria, sedation, impaired mental and physical performance and without modifying emotional reactions. Commonly it is administered orally 80–120 mg/day in a single dose. Adverse effects of methadone occur in early phase of treatment and are usually mile. These are constipation, seating, transient skin reaction, weight gain and water retention.
- Commonly used antagonist agent is naltrexone. Opioid antagonists are substance that bind to opioid receptors but do not produce morphine like effects. If the client who is on opioid antagonist take opioids he/she will not experience euphoric effects as the opioid receptors are already occupied and not available for opiate agonist.
- Naltrexone is available as 50 mg tablet. It is well absorbed from GI tract and after ingestion effective receptor blockade is obtained for 48–72 hours.
- There are three common regimens are seem in naltrexone administration. First is 50 mg daily, second is thrice a week (i.e. on Monday and Wednesday 100 mg and 150 mg on Friday), third is twice a week (i.e. 150 mg on Monday and 200 mg on Thursday) however daily dose is preferred.
- Naltrexone therapy should be started only after completion of detoxification phase. Common adverse effects of naltrexone are mild opiate withdrawal like symptoms and skin rashes.
- The only contraindication for this therapy is hepatic failure. So basic liver function tests are mandatory before starting this therapy.

- Recommended duration of this therapy is 6–12 months. Family members should be involved in treatment process to increase compliance and others, psychotherapeutic approaches should be used simultaneously.

Nursing Diagnosis

Because of the wide range of physical and emotional needs of clients with substance abuse disorders, many nursing diagnosis will be erupted. These are:
- Fluid volume deficit
- *Altered nutrition:* Less than body requirements
- Risk for injury
- Risk for infection
- Pain
- Ineffective airway clearance
- Impaired skin integrity
- Sleep pattern disturbance
- Constipation or diarrhea
- Self-care deficit.

Some diagnoses apply to the client's emotional state:
- Ineffective individual coping
- Ineffective family coping
- Hopelessness
- Self-esteem disturbance
- Altered role performance
- Personal identity disturbance
- Knowledge deficit
- Risk for violence
- Impaired social interaction
- Spiritual distress
- Sensory/perceptual alterations.
- Altered thought process
- *Altered family process:* Alcoholism
- Ineffective Denial

PLANNING

Developing therapeutic plans facilitate the client's participation in the treatment process and ultimate recovery. Individualized nursing assessment and intervention help the client to achieve the desired behavioral outcomes that will aid in the restoration of emotional and physical well-being. Ultimately, the recovery client strives for increased satisfaction in a way of life free from mood and mind—altering substances. Goal setting for clients who abuse or are dependent on substances includes the following elements.
- Provision for physical facilities
- Maintenance of emotional stability
- Minimal use of pathological defense mechanisms

- Understanding and acceptance of the substance abuse of depending disorders
- Developing hope for full recovery
- Resocialization and empowerment
- Development of alternative coping skills
- Improvement of motivation to continue treatment and prevention of noncompliance
- Involvement of family and significant member in treatment and in psychosocial rehabilitation.

For example:

- Disorientation and/or confusion related to alcohol withdrawal and environmental misinterpretation.
- *Nursing goals:* To make the client oriented to time/place/person. To make the client verbalize his feelings, needs and anxiety/fears.

Nursing interventions	Rationale
• Assess the level of consciousness.	• Alcohol is a CNS depressant, so disordination, confusion, slurred speech, muscle incardination are observed.
• Reorient the client to times place and person.	• The client is provided frequent explanation regarding situation, setting, person, time and so forth repetitively.
• Therapeutic communication in a simple, direct and concrete way. Do not try to discuss client's feelings. Plan for treatment or changes in lifestyle while the client is intoxicated or in severe withdrawal.	• The client can only respond to simple and direct statement. As he is in a state of intoxication, his ability to deal with abstract ideas are limited. Attempts to discuss emotions issues further confront the client.
• Provide nursing care with the help of others.	• Recognition of care giver promotes trust and sense of consistency which decreases fear and feelings of insecurity.
• Make the environment safe and therapeutic to the client.	• As the client is not having sense of reality and also may have suicidal ideation, his safety is top priority and therapeutic environment speeds up the recovery.

- *Nursing diagnosis:* Potential for injury to self or others related to aggressive behavior, suicidal ideation or environmental misinterpretation.
- *Nursing goal:* Protect the client from harming self and others.

Nursing interventions	Rationale
• Administer seizure precautions.	• Seizures can develop during intoxication and withdrawal. Precaution can minimize potential for injury.
• Assist the client in activities of daily living as needed.	• Prevent falls or any others accidents.
• Remove all potential hazardous articles from the reach of the client, provide environmental safety.	• Clients safety is a prime nursing priority.
• Administer medication as prescribed like benzodiazepines and others.	• Benzodiazepines maybe administered to decrease withdrawal as well as to calm the patient.

Substance Withdrawal

- Ineffective denial related to weak and underdeveloped ego evidenced by statement explaining no problem with drug use.
- *Nursing goal:* Client will accept the relation between complication and substance taking behavior.

Nursing interventions	Rationale
• Develop trust, convey an attitude of acceptance. Make sure that the client understands the consequences of his behavior.	• Unconditional acceptance promotes feelings of dignity and self-worth.
• Correct misconception of the client regarding his drug taking behavior like 'I only take to get rid of fatigue', 'nothing happens everybody drinks' by matter of fact and in nonjudgmental way.	• This will help to understand that this is the illnesses which requires treatment.
• Control client's behavior of rationalization or blaming others for substance taking behaviors. Confront the client in positive manner.	• Rationalizing and blaming others gives the client an excuse to continue his current behavior.
• Explain about the substance, dependence, tolerance and their effects on body.	• The first step in decreasing use of denial is for client to see the relationship between substance use and personal problem.
• Consistently redirect the client's focus to his own problem and to what he personally can do about them.	• This will facilitate client's acceptance of responsibility for his own behavior.

- Ineffective coping as evidenced by substance taking behavior (as a coping strategy).
- *Nursing goal:* Client will be able to understand and verbalize adequate coping strategies. Client will utilize coping strategies in a positive way.

Nursing interventions	Rationale
• Help the client to develop skill and defining problems, planning, problem solving approaches, implementing solutions and evaluating the process.	• Teaching problem solving process help the client to deal with the problem in a better way.
• Set limit on manipulative behaviors, administer consequences when limits are violated, confront the client and explain the reason for those behaviors.	• As client ego is weak he/she cannot delay the gratification and unable to set the limit. Client may tries to get the substances from various sources in the hospital.
• Help the client to verbalize and express his feelings in acceptable ways and provide positive reinforcement.	• It may help the client to resolve long unresolved issues and positive feedback encourages the client to continue to express feelings.
• Encourage the client to explore alternative ways of dealing with stress and difficult situations rather than restoring to substance use.	• The client may have minimal or no experience to deal stress without substance. Practice these techniques in day-to-day life. The client maybe learning these alternative methods for the first time.

- *Nursing diagnosis:* Imbalanced nutrition less than body requirement related to substance use rather than eating as evidenced by loss of weight, under nutrition/ malnutrition, weakness and lethargy.
- *Nursing goals*

Nursing interventions	Rationale
• Assess the level of malnutrition by assessing height, weight, skin color and body built.	• Assessment is required before starting interventions.
• In the beginning stage, parental support maybe needed.	• To correct fluid, electrolyte and some vitamin deficiencies.
• Collaborate with nutritionist/dietician for calorie requirement record input and output chart.	• It helps to decrease malnutrition.
• Provide foods that are not irritating the client and following the instructions provided by dietician regarding calorie intake.	• To avoid irritation to stomach adequate selection of food items help in adequate calorie intake.

Contd...

Contd...

Nursing interventions	Rationale
• Provide small frequent feeding of client's favorite foods.	• To ensure adequate intake of food.
• Meals should be supplemented by adequate multivitamin and minimal preparations.	• To achieve adequate nutritional needs.

Psychosocial Rehabilitation for Drug Abusers

Psychosocial interventions refers to non pharmacologic in nature designed to decrease symptom severity or distress, avoid frequent hospitalization, improve psychosocial functioning (e.g. Work and social relationships). Usually PSR involves teaching new skills and helping individuals take control over their lives; or modifying environments in which clients live to make them more therapeutic and conducive to helping them attain personal goals. It is an ongoing basis treatment modality.

Psychosocial rehabilitation for drug abuses include mainly different interventions. These include:

- The assertive community-case management
- Family interventions
- Supported employment
- Socials skills training and illness self-management
- Cognitive interventions (cognitive therapy and rehabilitation)
- Integrated treatment of substance use disorders
- Psychoeducation.

The overall objective of rehabilitation to bring back the abuser to his previous days. These are relatively long-term treatment modalities ranges from few months to years.

Nursing Management of Patients with Personality, Sexual and Eating Disorders

PERSONALITY DISORDERS

Introduction

Personality is a pattern of behavior, thought and emotion unique to an individual; and the ways they interact to help or hinder the adjustment of a person to other people and situations. It is very difficult to say normal and abnormal personalities. There are no hard demarcation between abnormal and normal personality.

A normal personality can be defined as the characteristic pattern of behavior and modes of thinking that determine a person's adjustment to environment. It includes factors such as intellectual abilities, attitudes, beliefs, moral values, emotional reactivity and motives acquired in the development process.

World Health Organization (WHO) defines 'abnormal personality as deeply ingrained maladaptive pattern of behavior, continuing throughout the most of adult life, although often becoming less obvious in middle or old age. The personality is abnormal either in the balance of its components; their qualities and expression or in its total aspects.

On a social response continuum behaviors ranges from adaptive behaviors to maladaptive ones. Adaptive behavior provides for mutually satisfying interactions. Maladaptive behaviors result in loneliness, suspiciousness and withdrawn behavior. These disorders occupy somewhere within the maladaptive range. The degree of maladaptiveness depends on the type of disorder and the severity of symptoms.

According to DSM–IVTR–personality disorders occur when personality traits become inflexible and maladaptive and cause significant functional impairment or subjective distress.

TYPES/CLASSIFICATION OF PERSONALITY DISORDERS

Personality disorders (PD) are classified into many types. According to United Kingdom's Psychiatric Association, these are grouped into three categories.

Suspicious	Emotional and impulsive	Anxious
Paranoid	Borderline	Avoidant
Schizoid	Histrionic	Dependent
Schizotypal	Narcissistic	Obsessive-compulsive
Antisocial		

Avoidant and dependent personality disorder are very similar, as are schizoid and schizotypal and histrionic and narcissist personality disorders.

The DSM-IVTR classified personality disorders as Axis II diagnosis, that fall into one of three clusters.

Cluster A: This cluster contains odd or eccentric personality disorders like Paranoid, Schizoid and schizotypal personality disorders.

- A person with one of these disorders is aloof and emotionally distant from others.
- The person's behaviors are considered strange or eccentric.
- The individuals with one of these disorders use following defense mechanisms: Projection: It involves attributing to another person thoughts or feelings of one's own that are unacceptable such as prejudice, excessive fault finding and paranoia.
- Fantasy is the creation of an imaginary life with which the clients deal with loneliness.
- Paranoia/ suspiciousness is thinking of being prosecuted or treated unfairly by others.
- Biologically persons with cluster 'A' personality disorders may have vulnerability to cognitive disorganization when stressed.

Cluster B: The dramatic, emotional and erratic group includes Antisocial, Borderline, Histrionic and Narcissistic personality disorders.

- A person with one of these disorders appears extremely ego centric with little ability to understand another's perspective.
- The person's behaviors are erratic and dramatic.
- Affected individual uses the following defense mechanisms.
  - *Dissociation:* It involves the forgetting of unpleasant feelings and association. It is unconscious splitting off some mental process and behavior from the normal or conscious awareness of individuals.
  - *Denial:* Such person refuses a thought, feeling or act as if he/she is unaware of doing so.
  - *Splitting:* Such person divides individuals into all good and bad and cannot experience an ambivalent relationship often seen in borderline personalities.
  - Acting out involves actual motor expression of a thought or feelings that is intolerable to the person.

Cluster C: The anxious and fearful group consists of avoidant, dependent, and obsessive compulsive personality disorders and those not otherwise classified.

- A person with one of these disorders appears overly anxious about various social and personal issues.
- The person tends to the unusually concerned with rules, procedures and acceptance by others.
- Affected individuals use the following defenses:
  - Isolation occurs when unacceptable feelings, act or idea is separated from the associated emotion. Individuals are orderly controlled and can speak of events of their lives without feelings.
  - Passive aggression occurs when resistance is indirect and often turned against the self. (e.g. Failing examination are aspect of passive aggression).
  - Hypochondriasis is often present in persons with personality disorders particularly in dependent passive aggressive individuals.
  - Biologically, these persons may have a tendency toward higher levels of cortical arousal and an increase in motor inhibition.

Etiology

There is no exact cause for personality disorders. The probable causes are the following:

Biological Theory

- *Genetics:* This theory emphasize that genetic predisposition to personality disorders exists,especially among people with a Cluster 'A' disorder or those with family history of alcoholism or other psychiatric conditions.
- A person with schizoid personality disorder, for example, is likely to have a family member who is schizophrenic.

Psychodynamic Theory

- Poor parenting during the first five years of life results in inadequate mastery of developmental issues and conflict centering on autonomy, separation—individuation, abandonment, dependency, control or authority, which can lead to development of personality disorders in adulthood.
- People who have a cold, indifferent and emotionally deficient childhood have a good chance of developing a personality disorders.

Environmental Theory

This is the surrounding the individual grew up in events that occurred and relationships with family members and others. It includes such things as the type of parenting the individual had, whether loving or abusive. This the 'nurture' part of the nature v/s nurture subsequent.

Sociocultural Theory

In some cultures, gender—specific child rearing practices may predispose, women to dependent personality disorder. Cultural norms influence the establishment of relationships: when casual friendships are not encouraged, lack of social mobility and lack of close family ties promote loneliness and involuntary isolation which in turn lead to personality disorders.

RISK FACTORS

Although the precise cause of personality disorders is not known, certain factors seem to increase the risk of developing or triggering personality disorders, including:

- A family history of personality disorders or other mental illness
- Low socioeconomic status
- Verbal, physical or sexual abuse during childhood
- Neglect during childhood
- An unstable or chaotic family life during childhood
- Being diagnosed with childhood conduct disorder
- Loss of parents through death or traumatic divorce during childhood.

Paranoid Personality Disorders

- More prevalent in males than females. The exact prevalence is very difficult to note because persons with this disorder seldom seek treatment and require hospitalization. They can lead their life with this disorders.

- DSM—IVTR defines paranoid personality disorder as 'a pervasive distrust and suspiciousness of others such as that their motives are interpreted as malevolent, beginning by early adulthood and present in a variety of contexts'.

Characteristics

- Distrust and suspicious of others
- Believing that others one trying to harm
- Emotional detachment
- Hostility
- Inability to find out the context of a given situation, so that person misperceives single acts or events within the situation
- Cold, aloof and overly serious affect
- Inability to express warmth and tenderness
- Use of projection as a primary defense mechanism.

Management

- Treated with antipsychotics and antidepressants.
- *Psychotherapy:*
  - Individual therapy
  - Cognitive behavior therapy
  - Dialectical behavioral therapy
  - Psychodynamic psychotherapy
  - Psychoeducation.
- Therapies that involve confrontation of feelings and alliances with others are not effective.

Nursing Diagnosis

- Altered growth and development related to unmet needs.
- Altered parenting related to lack of knowledge about the parenting role.
  - Risk for violence at others related to antisocial behavior
  - Fear related to being harmed by others.

Nursing Interventions

- Maintenance of an unambiguous environment.
- Classification of meanings, and conversations, situations and events.
- Develop and nurture trust in the nurse-client relationship.

SCHIZOID PERSONALITY DISORDER

Having a schizoid personality disorder means that you are not really interested in forming close relationship with other people. You feel that relationships interfere with your freedom and tend to cause problems. You prefer to be solitary and inward looking and choose to live your life without interference from others. Other people will see you as a loner. Few things in life give you pleasure and you may have little interest in sex or intimacy.

It is diagnosed in clients who display a lifelong pattern of social withdrawal. Their discomfort with human interaction, their introversion and their bland, constricted affect are notable. These are often seen as eccentric, isolated in nature.

The prevalence is not exactly established but it is thought that nearly 8% of the general population may have this disorder.

General ratio maybe 2:1 male to female.

Characteristics

- Lack of interest in social relationships.
- Limited range of emotional expression.
- Inability to pick up normal social cues.
- Appearing dull or indifferent to others.

Nursing Interventions

- Provide safety and calm environment.
- Allow the physical and emotional space needed by the client.
- Foster the development of basic social skills.

SCHIZOTYPAL PERSONALITY DISORDER

Individuals with this disorder are odd, eccentric, strange but do not meet the criteria for schizophrenia.

Characteristics

- Wearing peculiar dress, thinking, beliefs or behavior.
- Perceptual alterations, such as those affecting touch
- Discomfort in close relationships
- Eccentric behavior
- Magical thinking (belief that the person possesses special powers)
- Inability to form and maintain age—appropriate relationships
- Anxiety in social isolation
- Dysphoria
- Believing that messages are hidden for you in public speeches or displays.

Management

- Administration of antipsychotics
- Social skill development
- Intensive psychotherapy and counseling
- Steadfast determination to remain distant and aloof
- Emotionally restricted affect
- Use of intellectualization as a primary defense mechanism
- Men may not marry because they are unable to achieve intimacy
- Unable to express anger directly
- Maybe attached to animals
- Day dreaming.

Treatment

- *Drugs:* Antipsychotics and antidepressants.
- *Psychotherapy:* Individual psychotherapy and Group therapy.

- In group therapy settings, the clients with schizoid personality disorder maybe silent for long period; the client should be protected against aggressive attacks by group members. With time the group members become important to schizoid clients and may provide the only social contact in their isolated existence.

Nursing Diagnosis

- Diversional activity deficit related to unsustained social contact.
- Social isolation related to aloof and withdrawn behavior.
- Altered role performance related to eccentric behavior.
- Altered thought processes related to unrealistic ideas.
- Self-care deficit related to inability to take care of personal affairs.
- Sensory perceptual alteration related to self-centered feelings.

Nursing Interventions

- Institute safety precautions.
- Assist the client in developing basic social skills.
- Help the client with grooming and hygiene.

ANTISOCIAL PERSONALITY DISORDER

It is formerly called as sociopathic. Individuals with this disorder have difficulty in following societal rules and regulations.

Characteristics

- Consistent antisocial behavior (more common in males)
- Disregard for others
- Persistent lying or stealing
- Sustained history of irresponsibility and impulsiveness
- Lack of guilty feelings for one's destructive actions
- Repeatedly violating the rights of others
- Aggressive, often violent behaviors
- Anxiety and depressive symptoms
- Disregard for the safety of self or others
- Anger that result in hostile outbursts
- Use of rationalization and acting out as primary defense mechanisms.

Management

- Group therapy.
- Confrontation of inappropriate behaviors.

Possible Nursing Diagnosis

- Noncompliance with treatment related to the client's denial of problems.
- Risk for violence related to a disregarded for the feelings of others.
- Sexual dysfunction related to harmful relationships.
- Impaired social interactions related to a disregard for the feelings or property of others.

Nursing Intervention

- Provide stable and calm environment.
- Apply behavioral limits judiciously.
- Assist the client in taking responsibility for the consequences of actions.

BORDERLINE PERSONALITY DISORDER (BPD)

BPD may cause a number of problems in different areas of life. You may feel that you do not have a strong sense of who you really are, and others may describe you as very changeable. You will suffer from mood swings switching from one intense emotion to another very quickly, often with angry outbursts, and you may have brief episodes when you hear voices or see things that others cannot. You may end up doing things on impulses which you later regret. You may have episodes of harming yourself and think about taking your own life. You will probably also have a history of stormy or broken relationships and you will have a tendency to cling on to very damaging relationship, because you are terrified of being alone.

Characteristics

- Impulsiveness
- Emotional liability
- Unstable identity
- Self-mutilation
- Bouts of depression
- Anxiety
- Use of splitting, idealization, devaluation and projective identification as primary defense mechanisms.
- Harmful, unstable, intense relationships.

Management

- Group psychotherapy.
- Individual psychotherapy.
- Structured living under supervision.
- Treatment with antipsychotic medication.

Nursing Diagnosis

- Ineffective individual coping related to unmet dependency needs.
- Self-esteem disturbance related to feelings of worthlessness.
- Personal identify disturbance related to identity uncertainty.
- Risk for self-directed violence related to manipulative behavior.

Nursing Interventions

- Maintaining a structured, supportive and consistent environment.
- Counter the client's attempts to cause dissension among staff members.
- Adhere strictly to the treatment plan.
- Refuse to engage in third party conversation.

HISTRIONIC PERSONALITY DISORDERS

People with histrionic personality disorders are excitable, emotional and behave in a colorful, dramatic and extroverted fashion.

Characteristics

- Constantly seeking attention
- Excessively emotional
- Extreme sensitivity to other's approval
- Unstable mood
- Excessive concern with physical appearance
- Melodramatic, colorful, highly energetic personality
- Development of shallow relationships
- Seductive and self-centered nature
- Use of somatization and dissociation as defense mechanisms.

Management

- Psychoanalytically oriented psychotherapy will help in client with this disorder as they are unaware of their own feelings.
- Antidepressants and antianxiety drugs can be useful for depression, somatic complaints and anxiety.
  - Antipsychotic drugs are useful for derealization and illusion.

Nursing Diagnosis

- Self-esteem disturbance related to unsatisfactory personal relationships.
- Impaired social interaction related to seductive behavior.
- Risk for violence related to poor impulse control.

Nursing Interventions

- Reduce the client's anxiety about meeting needs for love and affection.
- Teach the client ways to delay needs for gratification.
- Assist the client in assuming a mature adult role.
- Assist the client in identifying feelings and in learning how to express them in a socially acceptable ways.

NARCISSISTIC PERSONALITY DISORDER

- Believing that you are better than others.
- Characterized by heightened sense of self-importance and grandiose feelings of uniqueness.

Symptoms

- Fantasizing about power, success and attractiveness.
- Exaggerating constant praise and admiration.

- Failing to recognize other people's emotions and feelings
- Lack of empathy
- Rage
- Depression
- Shame and humiliation.

Management

- Complicate to treat by drugs. Group therapy maybe useful.
- Lithium can be used to treat mood swings.

Nursing Diagnosis

- Self-esteem disturbance related to feelings of worthlessness/grandiose ideations.
- Altered role performance related to demands for attention.
- Defensive coping related to grandiosity.

Nursing Interventions

- Enhance the client's self-esteem and sense of self-worth.
- Assist the client in identifying feelings and in learning how to express them in a socially acceptable manner.
- Maintain a stable environment for the client and apply limit consistently.
  - These interventions tend to enhance the person's sense of safety.
  - This also can help reduce manipulative behaviors.

AVOIDANT PERSONALITY DISORDER

Individuals with avoidant personality disorder are sensitive to rejection and because of this they lead socially withdrawn life. This disorder is assumed to be equally seen in both genders.

Symptoms

- Hypersensitivity to criticism/rejection
- Feeling inadequate
- Social isolation
- Extreme shyness in social situations
- Timidity
- Anger
- Use of avoidance as a primary defense mechanism
- Anxiety and depression.

Treatment

- Assertive training
- Social skills training (SST)
- Relaxation exercises1
- *Group therapy:* Drugs to deal with anxiety and depression.

Nursing Diagnosis

- Social isolation related to persistent avoidance of interpersonal contact.
- Anxiety related to the possibility of making social mistakes.
- Powerlessness related to helpless lifestyle.
- Self-esteem disturbance related to feelings of being unable to deal with life's events.

General Nursing Interventions

- Enhance the client's ability to confront social situations.
- Role play events; then discuss what the client thoughts would happen.

DEPENDENT PERSONALITY DISORDER

Dependent personality disorder is characterized by a pervasive and excessive need to be taken care of that leads to submissive and changing behavior and fears of separation.

Sign and Symptoms

- Excessive dependent on others
- Submissiveness toward others
- A desire to be taken care of
- Tolerance of poor abusive treatment
- Urgent need to start a new relationship when one has ended
- Abdication of decision making to others
- Depression and anxiety
- Having feelings of low self-worth
- Avoid position of responsibility
- Inability to take risks.

Management

- Insight oriented psychotherapy
- Family therapy
- Assertiveness training
- Relaxation training
- Anxiolytics and antidepressants to deal with symptoms of anxiety and depression.

Nursing Diagnosis

- Impaired adjustment related to dependence on others
- Decisional conflict (delayed decision making) related to lack of experience in making choices without help
- Altered role performance related to fear of initiating actions.

General Nursing Interventions

- Enhance the client's ability to speak out and assume age appropriate responsibilities
- Give assignments that involve the client in risk taking behaviors.

OBSESSIVE-COMPULSIVE PERSONALITY DISORDERS

Characterized by emotional constriction, orderliness, stubbornness and indecisiveness. Most important symptoms are perfectionism and inflexibility.

Characteristics

- Preoccupation with orderliness and rules
- Perfectionism
- Desire to be in control of situations
- Inability to discard broken or worthless objects
- Inflexibility
- Either anger or emotional constriction
- Inefficiency caused by constant worry over doing things correctly.

Management

Investigations

- Physical examination
- Laboratory tests
- Psychological evaluation. MSE
  - Personality disorders are managed by multidisciplinary services.
  - Behavioral therapies.
  - Cognitive therapies.
  - Use of leisure activities.
  - Anti-depressants are useful to decrease obsessive compulsive symptoms if present.
  - Anxiolytics to decrease anxiety.
  - *Cognitive behavior therapy:* This combines the features of both cognitive and behavior therapies to help you identify unhealthy, negative belief and behaviors and replace them with healthy, positive ones.
  - *Dialectical behavior therapy:* It is a type of cognitive behavior therapy that teaches behavioral skills to help you tolerance stress, regulate emotions and improves relationship with others.
  - *Psychodynamic psychotherapy:* This therapy focuses on increasing the awareness of unconscious thoughts and behaviors developing new insights into motivation, and resolving conflict to live a happier life.
  - *Psychoeducation:* It teaches about illness, treatment options and coping strategies and problem solving skills.

Self-care Steps for Personality Disorders

- Stick to treatment plan
- Taking medications as directed
- Learning the condition
- Pay attention to warning signs
- Get active role
- Avoid drugs and alcohol
- Get routine medical care.

Coping Strategies for Personality Disorder Clients

- Simplify the life
- Write in a journal to express pain and hidden emotions
- Read reputable books
- Do not become isolated
- Taking care of yourself by eating a healthy diet and getting sufficient sleep
- Join a support group, like humor clubs, like minded
- Stay focused on your goals
- Learn relaxation and stress management
- Time your big decision.

Probable Nursing Diagnosis

- Sleep pattern disturbances related to preoccupation with obsessive compulsive behaviors
- Anxiety related to the need for perfection
- Altered heath maintenance related to difficulty in completing activities of daily living.

General Nursing Interventions

- Assist the client in becoming more flexible and in generating alternative solutions to life situations
- Confront invalid assumptions so that client can reassess a situation and develop a new perspective
- Teaching the art of maintaining peace and harmony
- Involving the client in art, music and dance therapies may help to express the inner feelings.

SEXUAL DISORDERS

Introduction

Human sexuality is a result of biological, chemical and psychosocial influences on a person. Sexuality can be expressed in many forms such as verbally, can be communicated in written form such as letters, poetry or songs and it can be expressed artistically. Behavioral expressions of sexuality include looking, touching, hand-holding, kissing and so forth. It can be expressed in various ways during the development of an intimate interpersonal relationship.

Sexuality Defined

Roper et al (1996) defines sexuality in terms of gender, personality, behavior, appearance, procreation and sexual intercourse.

The expression of sexuality maybe influenced by cultural, religious views, health status, physical attributes, age, environment or personal choice as a result of one's personality development. Sexuality has been defined as a desire or need for human contact, warmth or love. 'Normal' sexual behavior is generally described as a sexual act between consenting adults, lacking any type of force and performed in a private setting in the absence of unwilling observers. Abnormal sexual behavior would be considered as an act that does not meet the criteria of a definition.

Sexual Disorders

DSM-IVTR defines sexual disorders as disturbance in sexual desire and in the psychophysiological changes that characterize the sexual response cycle and cause marked distress and interpersonal difficulty.

DSM-IVTR classifies sexual disorders as follow:

- *Sexual desire disorders*
  - Hypo-active sexual desire disorder
  - Sexual aversion disorders.
- *Sexual arousal disorders*
  - Female sexual arousal disorder
  - Male sexual arousal disorder.
- *Orgasmic disorders*
  - Female orgasmic disorders
  - Male orgasmic disorders
  - Premature ejaculation.
- *Sexual pain disorder*
  - Dyspareunia (not due to general medical condition)
  - Vaginismus (not due to general medical condition).
- **Sexual disorders due to general medical condition**
  - Female hypoactive sexual desire disorder due to general medical condition
  - Male hypoactive sexual desire disorder due to general medical condition
  - Male erectile disorder due to general medical condition
  - Female dyspareunia due to general medical condition
  - Male dyspareunia due to general medical condition
  - Other female sexual dysfunction due to general medical condition
  - Other male sexual dysfunction due to general medical condition
  - Substance induced sexual dysfunction
  - Sexual dysfunction nos.
- *Paraphilias*
  - Exhibitionism
  - Fetishism
  - Frotteurism
  - Pedophilia
  - Sexual masochism
  - Transvestic fetishism
  - Voyeurism
  - Paraphilias nos.
- *Gender identity disorders*
  - In children
  - In adolescents or adults.
    - Gender identify disorder nos.
    - Sexual disorder nos.

Sexual Dysfunctions

Sexual dysfunction refers to a problem occurring during any phase of the sexual response cycle that prevents the individual or couple from experiencing satisfaction from the sexual activity. The sexual response cycle usually includes excitement, plateau, orgasm, and resolution. Desire and arousal are both part of the excitement phase of the sexual response.

SEXUAL DESIRE DISORDER

Hypoactive Sexual Desire Disorder

- It is defined as by persistent or recurrent deficiency or absence of sexual fantasies and desire for sexual activity which leads to marked distress or interpersonal difficulties.
- Sexual desire disorders or decreased libido characterized by a lack or absence for some period of time of sexual desire or libido for sexual activity or of sexual fantasies.
- The sexual aversion disorder is characterized by persistent or recurrent avoidance of all genital sexual contact with sexual partner which cause marked distress or interpersonal difficulties.
- An estimated 20% of the total population has hypoactive sexual desire disorder. These are more common in females than males.
- This can be because of unacceptable homosexual impulse, stressful life situations, anxiety, depression and abstinence from sex for a long time.
- The causes vary exactly, but the probable theory suggests that decrease in the production of normal estrogen in women or testosterone in both men and women. Other causes maybe aging, fatigue, pregnancy, medications (e.g. SSRI, antipsychotics, anxiolytics etc.)

SEXUAL AROUSAL DISORDERS

- Sexual arousal disorders were previously known as frigidity in women and impotence in men. Impotence is known as erectile disorder/dysfunction and frigidity as desire or arousal dysfunction.
- These are female sexual arousal disorder and male erectile disorders.
- Female sexual disorder is identified as a persistent or recurrent partial or complete failure to attain or maintain an erection until the completion of the lubrication and swelling response of sexual excitement until the completion of the sexual act, which cause marked distress or interpersonal difficulty.
- Male erectile disorder is defined as the recurrent and persistent partial or complete of the sexual act. This disturbance may cause marked distress or interpersonal difficulty. Primary erectile dysfunction refers to cases in which the male has never been able to have intercourse and secondary erectile dysfunction refers to cases in which the male has difficulty getting or maintaining an erection but has been able to have vaginal or anal intercourse at least once.
- These maybe caused by medical disorders, such as decreased blood flow or lack of vaginal lubrication and the nature of the relationships between the partners.

ORGASMIC DISORDERS

These are classified into:

- *Female orgasmic disorder:* It is defined as persistent or recurrent delay in, or absence of orgasm following a normal sexual excitement phase which leads to marked distress or interpersonal difficulty. This condition was earlier known as an orgasmia.

- *Male orgasmic disorder:* This disorder is defined as persistent or recurrent delay in or absence of orgasm, following a normal sexual excitement phase, which causes marked distress or interpersonal difficulty. The most common form of male orgasmic disorder is inability to experience orgasm although he can ejaculate from a partner's manual or oral stimulation.
- *Premature ejaculation:* It is characterized by persistent or recurrent ejaculation with minimal sexual stimulation before on or shorty after penetration and before the person wishes it, which cause marked distress or interpersonal difficulty. Diagnosis should be based on factors that affect duration of the excitement phase such as age, novelty of the sexual partner or situation and recent frequent of sexual activity.
  - The cause maybe strict religious background, viewing sex a sinful, drugs like antidepressants, nervous etc.

SEXUAL PAIN DISORDERS

- *Dyspareunia:* This disorder includes recurrent or persistent genital pain associated with sexual intercourse in either a male or female and which causes marked distress or interpersonal difficulty. It is not because of vaginismus, lack of lubrication, other general medical condition or physiological effects of substance use.
- *Vaginismus:* Vaginismus is characterized by recurrent or persistent involuntary spasm of the musculature of the outer third of the vagina that interferes with sexual intercourse and which causes marked distress or interpersonal difficulty.

SEXUAL DISORDERS DUE TO GENERAL MEDICAL CONDITION

These sexual disorders are due to a general medical condition is the presence of clinically significant sexual dysfunction that is judged to be exclusively due to the direct physiological effects of a general medical condition. These are dyspareunia, hypoactive sexual desire, male erectile disorder or other forms of sexual dysfunction (e.g. orgasmic disorder) and cause marked distress or interpersonal difficulty. There must be evidences from the history, physical examination or laboratory finding that the dysfunction is fully explained by the direct physiological effects of a general medical condition. These are not better accounted by other mental disorders such as depression.

- *Substance-induced sexual dysfunction:* The characteristic features of substance induced sexual dysfunction is a clinically significant sexual dysfunction that results in marked distress or interpersonal difficulty due to the direct effects of substance used (i.e. a drug of abuse, a medication or exposure to toxics). The drug of abuse can be evident from history, physical examination and laboratory findings.
- *Sexual dysfunction no other specified:* This category involves disorders which do not meet criteria for any sexual disorder.

PARAPHILIAS

The DSM-IVTR describes paraphilia as a disorder in which unusual or bizarre sexual acts or imagery are enacted to achieve sexual excitement. An example would be simulated bondage, in which pain is inflicted with materials such as leather belts, handcuffs and chains etc. Paraphiliac imagery is subclassified further as severe sexual sadism when the imagery involves a nonconsenting partner who is injured as a result of such activity. Sexual masochism describes the injury of self during imagery.

Paraphiliacs generally are not seen by mental health professionals unless their behavior has created a conflict with society. Nonconsenting partners may report such activity to police. Concerned neighbors may suspect that children are the object of sadistic sexual behavior and informs the police and other agencies.

The major types of paraphilias according to DSM-IVTR are exhibitiasm, frotteurism, pedophilia, sexual masochism, sexual sadism, voyeurism, transvestic fetishism and a separate category for otherwise paraplegias not specified.

These disorders are characterized by presence of recurrent (for more than 6 months) intense urge and fantasies involving unusual acts or activities. The individual either acts on the urges or is markedly distressed by them. These unusual acts and activities can be nonliving things, suffering and humiliation of self and/or sexual partner, children or nonconsenting persons.

Exhibitionism

Usually an adult male obtains sexual gratification from repeatedly exposing his genitals to unsuspecting strangers, usually women and children who are involuntary observes. He has a strong need to demonstrate masculinity and potency.

These behaviors are recurrent, intense, sexual urge, behavior or sexually arousing fantasies of at least 6 months duration involving the exposure of one's genitals to an unsuspecting stranger. Masturbation may occur during exhibitionism. Very common in males, but also seen in women which they expose their breasts and even their genitals.

Fetishism

Sexual contact with inanimate articles (fetishes) results in sexual gratification. Most often it is a piece of clothing or footwear. Parts of the body may also take on fetishistic significance. Its occurrence is almost exclusive with men who fear rejection by members of the opposite sex.

Frotteurism

Sexual excitement is achieved by touching and rubbing against a noncounseling person. Frottage is often involved in such activities in crowed places and he may use his hands to rub are unsuspecting victim the individuals with the disorders are extremely passive and isolated and frottage is the only sources of his gratification.

Sexual Sadism

The characteristic feature of this disorder is sexual arousal by physical and/or psychological humiliation; suffering or injury of the sexual partner. The method used can be retaining by tying, beating, burning, cutting, stabbing to rape, torture and even killing the individual.

Sexual Masochism

This is opposite to sexual sadism. Here, the person is sexually aroused by physical and/or psychological humiliation, suffering or injury inflicted oneself by others (usually sadists). Here masochistic activities maybe fantasized (being rape) and maybe performed alone (e.g. Self-inflicted pain) or with a partner (e.g. being restrained, spanked or beaten by the partner).

Voyeurism

It is characterized by recurrent preoccupation with fantasies and acts that involve observing people who are naked or are engaged in disrobing/grooming or even in sexual activity (peeping tom) followed by masturbation to orgasm usually occurring during or after the event.

Bestiality/Zoophilia

Sexual contact with animals serves as a preferred method to produce sexual excitement.

Necrophilia

Sexual arousal occurs while the person is using corpses to meet sexual needs.

Pedophilia

The use of prepubertal children is needed to achieve sexual gratification. It can be actual act or fantasy.

Telephone Scatologia

Sexual gratification is achieved by telephoning someone and making lewd or obscene remarks.

Transvestism

A heterosexual male achieves sexual gratification through wearing the clothing of a woman (cross dressing). It is a learned response due to encouragement by family members. As a child, the male person was considered more attractive when dressed up as a girl.

Characteristics of Paraphiliacs

A person may experience more than one paraphiliac disorder at the same time or may exhibit clinical symptoms of other psychiatric disorders (e.g. a personality disorder, or schizophrenia).

The associated symptoms or characteristics of persons with paraphilias include:

- Emotional immaturity
- Fear of a sexual relationship that could result in rejection.
- Shyness.
- The need to prove masculinity, demonstrated by the exhibitionist.
- The need to inflict pain on another to achieve sexual satisfaction (seen in sadistic behaviors).
- The need to endure pain to achieve sexual satisfaction.
- Low and poor self-concept.
- Depression.

Not all of these characteristic are present in each paraphilia. Theorists state that the way a paraphiliacs expresses himself or herself sexually affords a clue to the paraphiliac's self-concept. For example, the fetishist who has a very low self-concept chooses inanimate objects to satisfy sexual needs and therefore does not have to fear rejection by a partners.

Characteristics of Sexual Dysfunction

These may include frustration, depression, anxiety, guilt and a fear of failure in maintain a satisfying sexual relationship.

Treatment of Sexual Disorders

Medical treatment is individualized according to the type of disorder, underlying causative factors and presenting symptoms.

Medication

When a medication is the cause of the dysfunction, a change in the medication can help. Men and women with hormone deficiencies may benefit from hormone replacements, shots, pills or creams. For men, drugs like sildenafil (viagra) may help improve sexual function by increasing blood flow to the penis.

Sex Therapy

It counsels the couple to overcome sexual problems through therapeutic communication.

Behavioral Therapy

Behavioral therapy, group therapy and aversive therapy all focus on altering or managing unacceptable or undesirable behaviors. In aversive therapy, negative stimuli (e.g. anomeric or electric shock) are used to condition the person each time an undesirable sexual act occurs. The undesirable behavior decreases because the person wishes to avoid the punishment associated with the negative stimuli.

Environmental manipulation has proven effective in relieving anxiety and altering undesirable behavior. Incarceration maybe practicized legally to protect the public, especially children from being victimized. Hormonal therapy to reduce sex drive has been reported in research. Drugs such as Androcur, provera and depo provera used as adjunctive therapy to reduce incidents of cross dressing or transvestism.

Psychotherapy

Helps to relieve anxiety, fear or guilt that may have an impact on sexual function.

Mechanical Aids

Aids such as vacuum devices and penile implants may used to help men with erectile dysfunction.

Education and Communication

Education about sex and sexual behaviors and responses may help a man overcome his anxieties about sexual performance. Open communication and dialogue with partner helps to overcome many barriers to a healthy sex life.

Nursing Management

Primarily, nurses must examine feelings about their own sexuality before they are able to care for paraphiliacs who sexually act out or present symptoms of psychosocial disorders. Nurses are not immune to the development of psychosexual dysfunction. Feelings of disgust, contempt, anger or fear need to be identified and explored so that they do not interfere with the development of a therapeutic relationship. This is one of the reasons clients do better with a team approach rather than individual therapy. If the nurse is unable to be objective while providing care, the nurse should have another member of the health team care of the client. The quality of nursing care will depend on the nurses ability to be nonjudgmental and to understand the behavior of a client who is sexually acting out. The nurse needs to be supportive yet set limits, so that the client's behaviors is socially acceptable.

Nursing interventions for client who exhibit symptoms of sexual disorders also include planning nursing care to meet the basic human needs, providing a structured environment, providing protective care for the client, exploring methods to rechannel sexually unacceptable behavior, and participating in a variety of therapies, including behaviors therapy, aversive therapy, psychotherapy and psycho sex education. The nurse must also assume the role of client advocate to ensure the promotion of sexual health when the opportunity arises.

The common nursing diagnosis includes:
- Altered sexuality patterns
- Sexual dysfunction
- Self-esteem disturbance
- Body image disturbance
- Anxiety
- Fear and guilt.

EATING DISORDERS

Introduction

Eating disorders are mental illnesses that cause serious disturbances in a person's every day diet. It can manifest as eating extremely small amount of food or severely overeating. The condition may begin as just eating too little or too much but obsession with eating and food over takes over at the life of a person leading to severe changes. In addition to this, eating patterns are distress and concern about body weight or shape. These disorders frequently coexist with other mental illnesses such as depression, substance abuse and anxiety disorders.

ICD-10 Classification of Eating Disorders

The world Health Organization defines eating disorders under ICD-10, F 50. These are:
- F 50.0 Anorexia nervosa.
- F 50.1 Atypical anorexia nervosa.
- F 50.2 Bulimia nervosa.
- F 50.3 Atypical bulimia nervosa.
- F 50.4 Overeating associated with other psychological disturbances.
- F 50.5 Vomiting associated with other psychological disturbances.
- F 50.8 Other eating disorders.
- F 50.9 Eating disorder, unspecified.

Eating disorders when manifested at a young age can cause severe impairment in growth, development fertility and overall mental and social well-being. The addition, they also raise the risk of an early death. People with anorexia nervosa are 18 times more likely to die early compared with people of similar age in the general population.

Eating disorders can affect both men and women and are slightly more common among women. Often these disorders begin during adolescence or young adulthood but may also develop during childhood or later in life.

ANOREXIA NERVOSA

- Anorexia nervosa is characterized by an intense fear of being obese and a continued pursuit of becoming this.
- It is defined as refusal of eat with morbid fear of gaining weight. The individual is present with gross distortion of body image, preoccupation with food and refusal to eat.

Epidemiological Facts

- Mainly seen in young women. Most anorectics are teenaged girls or women who are generally bright achievers, males also suffer from this disorder.
- Age of onset is usually late adolescence, male 8 to 11 years of age, as while as women over age 30. It occurs 10 to 20 times more in females than males.
- According to statistics provided by Herzog.
  - Of all anorectics, 90 to 95% are female.
  - Of diagnosed anorectics, 10 to 20% die. Half of these deaths are due to suicide.
  - Anorexia occurs mainly in upper middle-class families however, victims maybe from any socioeconomic group.
  - Usually the youngest daughter of several children is afflicted.

Many factors contribute to the development of this disease include disturbed self-image, parent-child conflicts, past and present experiences resulting in feelings of dependency and helplessness; the adolescent's desire to return to the alleged comfort and safety of childhood, a stressful life situation, psychotic depression, or early manifestation of schizophrenia. Starvation is an attention getting device that permits the anorectic client full control of her body, allows her to remain in or revert to prepubertal state, and is considered manipulative behaviors.

The DSM-IVTR states that the anorectic has an intense fear of becoming obese although weight loss occurs. Even when emaciated, the person insists that she is fat, displaying a distortion of body image. A weight loss of at least 15% of the original body weights is seen, as well as the refusal to maintain at least minimal body weight for age and height. No known physical illness or disease is responsible for the weight loss.

Here, various methods are used to lose weight. These include induced vomiting, laxatives, enemas, diuretics, diet pills, excessive exercise, binging and purging, stimulant or refusal to eat. Deceitful behavior may prevail as the anorectic client disposes of food she is supposed to eat.

Other Factors of Causation

Family Influences

Negative influences within the family can trigger and maintain eating disorders. Poor parenting attitudes and behaviors maybe a primary cause. Poor parenting by both, mothers and fathers has been implicated in eating disorders. Often if one of the parents, especially the mothers, had a history of eating disorders, the child is likely to develop them. The research shows that parental criticism of weight can lead to binging and purging in young males.

History of drug addictions in the family and other emotional disorders also influences. These client's parents likely to have alcoholism or substance abuse than are those in the general populations.

Cultural Factors

Attitude to food in different cultures and often triggers one of the eating disorders. Media influences and pressures on being thin make eating disorders. Media showcasing anorexic young models sexually desirable, most clothes are designed and as displayed for thin bodies and eating junk food is also a cause for eating disorders.

Genetic Influences

Most of the eating disorders run in families. Anorexia is eight times more common in people who have relatives with the disorder. Twins also seem to have tendency to share specific eating disorders. Many research studies have linked chromosome 10 to eating disorders. Researchers suggest that genes may determine the interplay of neurotransmitters like serotonin, involved in well-being and appetite. They found certain proteins such as brain derived neurotrophic factors (BDNF). This has influence an individual's susceptibility to developing an eating disorders.

Hormonal Disturbances

Disturbances in thyroid hormone and HPA axis causes eating disorders. These are strongly linked to stress, well-being and appetite. Many of these chemical changes are certainly a result of malnutrition or other aspects of eating disorders.

Another important trigger is ghrelin, a hormone that increases the feelings of hunger and slows metabolism. Increased ghrelin is noted in clients with anorexia and bulimia. The HPA system is also responsible for the production of important reproductive hormones that are severely reduced in anorexics.

Psychological and Biological Factors

- Low self-esteem
- Feelings of inadequacy
- Feelings of lack of control in life
- Difficulty expressing emotions and feelings
- Personality types like obsessive, compulsive and sensitive avoidant are more at risk
- People with eating disorders tend to be perfectionist. They tend to have an unrealistic expectation of themselves and others
- Eating disorders maybe triggered to avoid sexuality.

Clinical Symptoms

- Severe dieting by restrictive dieting or binge-eating and purging
- Usually maintain caloric diaries and records of all they eat. Weigh and measures food
- Extreme weight loss
- Intense or irrational fear of weight gain
- Extreme weight loss
- Intense or irrational fear of weight gain

- Refusal to eat in front of others
- Ritualistic eating including cutting food into small pieces or avoiding certain foods
- Reactivity and hypersensitivity to cold
- Binge eating followed by self-induced vomiting
- They maybe hoarding of food
- Social withdrawal
- Clients may abuse laxatives and diuretics to loose weight and involve in ritualistic exercising, extensive cycling, walking, jogging and running
- Long periods without menstrual periods among women
- Delay in menses in young girls
- Hair loss from scalp
- Yellowish skin
- Swollen feet and hands.

Psychological Symptoms

- Confused, poor memory and judgment
- Conversations and projects revolving around food and weight loss
- Beliefs regarding thinners equating to happiness
- Anxiety, depressed, angry, stubborn or mood swings
- Incapability to adjust to changes of routines
- Severe fear of weight gain
- Refusal to believe anything is wrong and denial for need for help. Client may become sulky, angry or defensive when concern is expressed.

BULIMIA NERVOSA

Episodic binge eating with a rapid consumption of a large amount of food within two hours is classified as bulimia. The person is aware that the behavior is abnormal, fears the inability to stop eating voluntarily, is self-critical by may experience depression after each episode.

According to DSM-IVTR, it is recurrent episode of binge eating. A sense of lack of control over eating during the eating binges; self-induced vomiting; the misuse of laxatives or diuretics, fasting or excessive exercise to prevent weight gain and present self-evaluation unduly influenced by body shape and weight.

Incidence and Prevalence Rates

It is more prevalent than anorexia nervosa. More common in females than males. The onset is early in adulthood and male-female ratio is usually about 1:10.

CLINICAL SYMPTOMS

- Sudden episodes of eating large amount of food or buying large quantities that seem to disappear.
- Individuals with bulimia have an intense fear of getting obese and are very sensitive to weight gain because they lack impulse control.
- Binge eating stops when abdominal discomfort occurs.
- Eats in private and in a restrictive way.

- They are usually on high fat, high carbohydrate and high sugar "junk" foods.
- Behavioral problems like shoplifting, binge spending, alcohol or drug use and/or sexual promiscuity.
- Decline in work and school attendance.
- Perfectionist exercising.
- Dehydration.
- Chronic edema.
- Dental erosion.
- Chronic inflammation of esophagus, stomach and other organs.
- Electrolyte imbalance, leading to arrhythmias of the heart and metabolic alkalosis.
- Heart problems, irreversible congestive heart failure and death due to abuse of drugs.
- Chronic enlargement of the parotid gland.
- Irritable bowel syndrome or abnormal dilatation of the colon.

Etiology

Genetic Factors

Hereditary factors have a role in predisposition of bulimia.

Biological Factors

HPA dysfunction causes bulimia. Abnormality in serotonin, dopamine and norepinephrine regulation and increased cortical level in CSF. Presence of high level of endogenous opioids in the spinal fluid of the client with bulimia shows these chemicals may contribute do denial of anger.

Psychodynamic Factors

Psychodynamic theory suggests that deficits in ego development may predispose young children to anorexia. These clients typically lack sense of autonomy and selfhood. Many experience their bodies somehow under the control of their parents, so self-starvation maybe an effort to gain validation as a unique, independent and special person.

Social Factors

Family system theory suggests that anorexia nervosa is caused by intrafamilial conflicts and dysfunctional family. Families with eating disorders may exhibit high levels of hostility, chaos and isolation and low levels of nurturance and empathy. Conflict avoidance is the strong factors in the interpersonal dynamics of some families in which children develop eating disorders.

MANAGEMENT

- Treat the treatable cause with appropriate medications.
- *Psychotherapy:* Individual and group psychotherapy are useful.
- Behavior therapy.
- *Drugs:* Antihistamines and antiserotonin agents are used, e.g. Amitriptyline, pimozide, CPZ and fluoxetine can be given.

PICA

Persistent eating of non-nutritive substances such as clay, paint, plaster, ice or starch or the compulsive eating of one food is referred as Pica. Such behavior may occur between 1 and 2 years of age and may persist into adolescence or through adulthood. Possibly it is caused by mental retardation, neglect, poor supervision or mineral deficiency (e.g. Zinc, iron). Pica can present serious health consequences. This behavior must occur for at least one month to be diagnosed as pica.

According to DSM-5 to be diagnosed with Pica a person must display:

- Persistent eating of non-nutritive substances for a period of at least one month.
- The eating of non-nutritive substances is inappropriate to the development level of the individual.
- The eating behavior is not part a culturally supported or socially normative practice.
- If occurring in the presence of another mental disorder (e.g. Autistic disorder) or during a medical condition, e.g. pregnancy, it is severe enough to warrant independent clinical attention.

OBESITY

Individuals exhibiting clinical symptoms of obesity and coexisting diagnoses such as anxiety or depression are also treated in psychiatric setting. Such individuals frequently refer to themselves as bulimias who do not purge. They generally respond to and benefit from treatment modalities.

MANAGEMENT

- Comprehensive treatment plan with psychotherapeutic interventions.
- Correction of client's nutritional status like dehydration, starvation and electrolyte imbalances.
- Behavior group therapy is helpful in inducing weight gain, control over exercises and self-induced vomiting.
- Administration of drugs like antihistamines and antiserotonergics, e.g. Amitriptyline, pimozide, chropromazine and fluoxetine, etc.
- *Family therapy:* Changes in family unit will result in reduction of eating behaviors.

Nursing Management

Nursing Assessment

- The assessment of the client with eating disorders shows the presence of features of eating disorders.
- Family and peer group assessment provides understanding about the family dynamics and role of family in development of the disease.
- Collect the client's history of social, educational/occupational and medical details.

Nursing Priorities

- Reestablish adequate/appropriate nutritional intake
- Correct fluid and electrolyte imbalance
- Assist client to develop realistic body image/improve self-esteem
- Provide support/involve significant other, if available in treatment regimen

- Coordinate total treatment program with other health faculty.
- Provide health education information about disease, prognosis and treatment.

Discharge Goals

- Adequate nutrition and fluid intake maintenance.
- Maladaptive coping behaviors and stressor that precipitate anxiety recognized
- Implementation of adaptive coping strategies and techniques for anxiety reduction and self-control.
- Enhanced self-esteem.
- Understanding of disease process, prognosis and treatment regimen.
- Plan in place to meet the needs.

Nursing Diagnosis

Altered nutrition less than body requirements and fluid volume deficit related to refusal of food, self-inducing vomiting and abuse of laxatives/diuretics.

General Interventions

- Administration of the IV fluids to correct dehydration.
- Calculation of calorie requirement and inducing weight gain.
- Weigh the client daily and monitor it.
- Stay with the client during meals.
- Put restriction on client, that if he/she fails to eat, tube feeding will be initiated.
- Implement restriction in nonpunitive and matter of fact manner.

Nursing Diagnoses

Ineffective denial related to retarded ego development and fear of losing life.

Interventions

- Develop a trusting relationship, convey positive regard.
- Arguing or bargaining with the client should be avoided. Maintain therapeutic communication.
- Encourage the client to ventilate the feelings regarding his/her role in the family, dependence/independence; control, need of achievement and sexuality.
- Help the client to gain control over his/her problematic areas of life.

Nursing Diagnosis

Disturbed body image/low self-esteem related to altered perceptual input, dysfunctional family system and improper development of ego.

Nursing Interventions

- Help the client to develop a realistic perception of body image and relationship with food.
- Explain discrepancies between specific measurement of the client's body and client's perception.

- Promote feelings of independence within the environment through participation and independent decision-making.
- Encourage the client to accept his or her weakness as well as strength and provide positive feedback.
- Help the client realize that perfection is unrealistic and explore this need with him/her.
- Involve the client actively in family therapy with members.
- Educate family regarding the client illness and encourage active involvement of family in group therapy sessions.

Nursing Management of Childhood and Adolescent Disorders Including Mental Deficiency

INTRODUCTION

Throughout the history, childhood was considered a happy, joyous period of life. Children were not thought to suffer mental or emotional problems because they were spared the stresses of adults. Research conducted since 1970s, however, shows that children suffer from depression and manic depressive psychosis and anxiety disorders, illnesses once thought to be reserved for adults. From 3 to 6 million children suffer from clinical depression and are at high-risk for suicide, the third leading cause of death among young people. Every hour, 57 children and teenagers try to kill themselves, everyday 18 will succeed.

Classification

The DSM-IVTR classifies the disorders diagnosed in infancy, childhood or adolescence in the following category:

- Mental retardation
- Hearing disorders
- Motor skills disorders
- Communication disorders
- Pervasive developmental disorders
- Attention-deficit and disruptive behavior disorders
- Feeding and eating disorders of infancy or early childhood
- Tic disorders
- Elimination disorders
- Other disorders of infancy, childhood and adolescence.

The ICD–10 classifies childhood disorders under following sections:

- F90-F98: Behavioral and emotional disorders with onset usually occurring in childhood and adolescence.
- F90: Hyperkinetic disorders.
- F91: Conduct disorders.
- F92: Mixed disorders of conduct and emotions.
- F93: Emotional disorders with onset specific to childhood.
- F94: Disorders of social functioning with onset specific to childhood adolescence.
- F95: Tic disorders
- F96: Other behavior and emotional disorders with onset usually occurring in childhood and adolescence.
- F99: Unspecified mental disorders.

INTELLECTUAL DISABILITY/MENTAL RETARDATION

Mental retardation is a term that was once commonly used to describe someone who learns and develops more slowly than other kids. But, nowadays it is not used as much anymore because it hurts people's feelings and emotions. Instead, the terms like 'intellectual disability' or 'developmental delay' are used. These clients have trouble learning and functioning in everyday life. But these can be learned. It can be mild (smaller) or major (bigger). The bigger the disability the more trouble someone will have in learning and becoming an independent person.

Incidence

It is estimated to be about 2–3%. It is not a disease rather it is the result of a pathological process in the brain characterized by limitations in intellectual and adaptive function.

Definition

According to Mayo, intellectual disability (ID), once called mental retardation, is characterized by below average intelligence or mental ability and a lack of skills necessary for day-to-day living. People with intellectual disabilities can learn new skills, but they learn them more slowly. There are varying degrees of intellectual disability, from mild to profound.

Mental retardation is a disorder, characterized by significantly subaverage general intellectual functioning, associated with significant impairment in adaptive behavior including thinking, learning social and occupational functioning, which manifests during the development period before 18 years of age. The 'General intellectual functioning' means result of a standardized intelligence test, significantly subaverage includes two standard deviation below the mean (behavior below the mean usually IQ below 70). 'Adaptive behavior' is the person's ability to meet the responsibilities of social, personal, occupational and interpersonal areas of life according to his or her age and sociocultural and educational background.

Measurement of IQ

$$\text{IQ (Intelligence Quotient)} = \frac{\text{Mental Age}}{\text{Chronological Age}} \times 100$$

Mental retardation (MR) is defined by American Association on Mental Retardation (AAMR) as referring to substantial limitations in present functioning, characterized by subaverage intellectual functioning existing concurrently with related limitations in two or more applicable adaptive skill areas. The adaptive skill areas are communication, self-care, home living, social skills, communication use, self-direction, health and safety, functional academics, leisure and work. Mental retardation manifests before age 18.

Etiology of MR

Intellectual disabilities occur because the brain gets injured or a problem presents the brain from developing normally.

Antenatal Causes

- Deficiency of folic acid and iron during pregnancy of mother.
- Viral infection to mother during first trimester (TORCH, HIV).

- Exposure of pregnant mother to radiations.
- Consumption of intoxicants like lead, thalidomide, etc.
- Placental dysfunctions.
- Endocrine disorders like hypothyroidism.

Intranatal Causes

- Birth asphyxia
- Preeclampsia
- Prolonged or difficult labor
- Instrumental delivery
- Birth injuries (head injury, bleeding, IVH).

Postnatal Causes

- Cranial injury (accident and battered baby).
- Infections such as meningitis and encephalitis whooping cough, drug, use, malnutrition, measles.
- Kernicterus

Genetic Causes

Associated with chromosomal anomalies like Down's syndrome, Doris syndrome, Klinefelter's syndrome, Fragile-X-syndrome, Trisomy X, Turner's syndrome.

Metabolic Disorders

- Disease of protein metabolism like phenylketonuria, maple syrup disease, hartnup disease, homocystinuria.
- Disorders of fat metabolism like Taysach's disease, Gaucher's, disease, Niemann- pick's disease.
- Disorders of carbohydrate metabolism like galactosemias, gargoylism.
- Disorders of purine metabolism like Lesch-Nyhan syndrome.
- Disorders of mucopolysaccharides like Hurler's syndrome, Hunter's syndrome.
- Miscellaneous disorders like Wilson's disease, Toni-Fanconi syndrome.

Diseases of Brain

- Tuberous sclerosis
- Epilepsy
- Neuron fibromatosis

Cranial Malformations

- Microcephaly
- Anencephaly
- Hydrocephaly

Psychiatric Disorders

- Autism
- Rett's syndrome

- Childhood onset schizophrenia
- Asperger's syndrome

Classification of MR

According to IQ level, MR is classified into 4 categories.

1. *Mild Mental Retardation (51–70):* This is very common type of MR accounting for 85–90% cases. Children with IQ 51–70, fall in this category. During infancy, mild mental retardation often remains unnoticed. During later life, the caregiver may note developmental delay in language, social development and motor skills. During schooling, these children may face problems in reading and arithmetics. With the help of special education, these children can progress up to 6th grade of school. This group is referred as 'educable' in adulthood. In adulthood, mild mentally retarded people may live independently.
2. *Moderate Mental Retardation (35–50):* About 10% of mentally retarded have moderate mental retardation. IQ ranges between 36–50. Moderately mentally retarded children display delays in motor development and speech. Often they drop out of school 2nd grade. These group can be 'trained' to support themselves by performing semiskilled or unskilled work, under constant supervision. So, this group is termed as 'trainable'. During adolescence, these people can work in supervised occupational settings.
3. *Severe Mental Retardation:* About 4% of mentally retarded children fall in this group. The IQ varies in between 21–35. It is often recognized early in life, due to delayed or poor motor development and absent or markedly delayed speech and other communication skills. Later in life, these children can be given elementary training in personal health care and they can be taught to speak. At the most, they can perform simple tasks under close supervision. This group was earlier known as 'dependent'.
4. *Profound Mental Retardation:* This section of retardation accounts for 1–2% of all mentally retarded. Their IQ is below 20. Physical defects associated with retardation are more associated in these children.

   The achievement of developmental milestones is delayed. These children often need complete medical and nursing care of 'life support' under a carefully planned and structured environment like rehabilitation institutions.

Disorders Associated with MR

The following disorders are more frequently seen in mentally retardation children. These are:

- *Physical Defects:*
  - Sensory disorder (found in 20–25% of cases)
    - Defect in hearing and vision.
    - Motor defects like spasticity, ataxia, athetosis, and epilepsy, heart alert problems.

Psychiatric Disorders

- Schizophrenia
- Depression
- Neurosis
- Personality disorders

- Organic psychiatric disorders like dementia
- Autism and overactivity syndrome
- Behavior disorders like mannerisms, head banging and hyperkinetic syndrome.

Clinical Manifestations

There are many different signs of intellectual disability among children. Signs may appear during infancy or they may not be noticeable until a child reaches the school age. It often depends on the severity of the disability. Some of the most common signs of intellectual disability are:

- Rolling over, sitting up, crawling or walking late.
- Having trouble in speech/delayed developmental milestones in speech and hearing.
- Difficulty remembering things.
- Slow to master things, like toilet training, dressing and feeding himself or herself.
- Inability to connect actions with consequences.
- Behavior disorders such as explosive tantrums.
- Difficulty with problem-solving or logical thinking.
- Aggression, dependency, impulsivity, passivity, self-injury, stubbornness, low self-esteem and low frustration tolerance. Also associated with psychotic and attention deficit symptoms. Sometimes shortness in stature and malformation of facial elements.
- Failure to meet intellectual developmental milestones.
- Lack of enthusiasm and curiosity.

Diagnosis of MR

MR is diagnosed on the following basis:

- Physical examination and history.
- Mental status examination.
- Developmental assessment including IQ score.
- Tests used for intellectual and adaptive functioning are:
  - Denver developmental screening test-II.
  - Stanford-Binet intelligence scale.
  - Wechsler intelligence scale.

If IQ is below 70 on Stanford binet test it is classified as 'mentally retarded'.
The following are the possible referral characteristics of tests:

Intellectual

- Subaverage intellectual functioning, performs poorly on verbal and nonverbal intelligence tests.
- Difficulty applying abstract processes, such as conceptualization, generalization, transfer.
- Limited intellectual functioning in area such as memory, imagination and creativity.

Academic

- Subaverage learning performance in basic academic skills.
- Experiences difficulty in activities requiring reading and listening comprehension, such as following complex directions, gaining insight into problem situations and generalizing from rules and principles.

- Oral communication skills generally exceed written communication skills.
- Limited in incidental learning acquired through experience.

Behavior

- Lacks age appropriate skills.
- Difficulty in comprehending social situations.
- Low frustration tolerance.
- May exhibit poor self-concept.
- Seeks approval therefore easily influenced.

Communication

- Below average for age in language skills.
- Display limited vocabulary.
- Delayed speech and language.
- Displays articulation disorders.
- Limited written communication skills.
- Slow processing of questions often resulting in delayed responses.

Physical

- Physical development generally proceeds at a slow rate.
- May manifest caulis or chronic health problems.

MANAGEMENT

There is no exact cause of MR so it needs multidisciplinary approach. Prevention plays more important role than cure.

Primary Prevention

It includes action taken to identify and reduce the incidences of mental retardation. It involves strategies of heath promotion and specific protection.

Health Promotion

- Safe antenatal care.
- Empowering socioeconomic status.
- Educating public about misconceptions about mentally reacted individuals.
- Family and genetic counseling.
- Innovative techniques to improve the curative aspects of retardation.

Specific Protection

- Immunization to prenatal, natal and postnatal mothers and child.
- Safe natal and postnatal care.
- Avoiding high-risk pregnancy and its consequences.
- Avoiding first degree consanguineous marriages.
- Prompt management of prematurity and neonatal medical conditions.

Secondary Prevention

It involves early diagnosis and case finding, followed by medical intervention to limit the disability.

Early Detection and Treatment

- It includes early detection and treatment of preventable disorders which may lead to mental retardation like phenylketonuria, maple syrup urine disease, and hypothyroidism.
- Early detection and treatment of sensory motor and behavioral handicaps.
- Early treatment of correctable disorder, e.g. infection, skill configuration anosmatic (surgery is performed).
- Early recognition of presence of intellectual abilities. A delay in diagnosis may cause unfortunate delay rehabilitation.

Tertiary Prevention

The aim is to limit disability and promote rehabilitation.

Disability Limitation

It includes:

- Treatment of physical and psychoneurological problems.
- Institutional care of severe or profound mental retardation.
- Education in special school, if educable.
- Vocational training if trainable.
- Regular physiotherapy to improve physical abilities.

Psychosocial Rehabilitation

Rehabilitation in vocational, physical and social areas is the cornerstone of management of intellectual disability children. It depends on client's intelligence level and his capacities.

Nurse Role in Institutionalized Intellectual Disability Clients

Persons with intellectual disability maybe educable or trainable or require custodial or institutional care. Such clients may have dual diagnosis of mental retardation and mental illness, as well as a physical disability or limitation.

The psychiatric nurse working in an institutional setting is challenged to provide environmental stimulation as well as to meet the needs of the child emotionally and physically because persons with mental disability do not always communicate physical symptoms. Helping the child to master the activities of daily living may be a slow process involving multiple therapies including behavior therapy. Protective care may be utmost necessary. If the client is epileptic prone to acting out behavior, disoriented or masochistic (head banging or biting self). The administration and monitoring of anticonvulsants and psychotropic drugs is also the responsibility of the nurse.

Education of the family is an important factor not to be overlooked because many clients who are mentally retarded attend an institution during the week but go home for weekend or on holidays. Others attend a day hospital, special school or sheltered workshop and return home at night as well as weekends. The nurse is the client's advocate, both in the institutional setting and when relating to the family. Identifying the family's ability to cope and continue with the therapy at home setting is important to promote progress as well as to minimize the stress that can occur when changing environments.

Community Psychiatric Nursing Care

Community care includes care provided by the general public and by health professionals for the intellectual disability clients in the community.

Tasks of the Psychiatric Community Nurse are:

- Coordination of services for the mentally retarded.
- Psychoeducation of public and professionals.
- Counseling and support
- Training and psychosocial rehabilitation of the disabled for community living.
- Placement in the community and supervision.

The above care would be rendered through a multidisciplinary health professionals which include a psychologist, doctor, psychiatric social worker, occupational therapist, physiotherapist, teacher and NGOs.

The overall nursing tasks and interventions at community include:

- Acceptance by the community.
- Promotion of normalization.
- Mobilization of the community.
- Prevention of mental retardation.
- Involvement in psychosocial rehabilitation.

The management of mental retardation is a joint venture between the client and health care team, requiring very hard work and patience.

The possible nursing care plan includes:

Nursing need	Objective	Interventions	Evaluation
• Prevention of mental retardation	• To reduce the number of people with intellectual disability.	• If there is a history mental retardation, provide genetic counseling.	• Mental retardation is prevention and fetal outcomes are improved.
		• During the antenatal period provide proper care to the mother like nutritious diet, prevention from infections, prevention from unnecessary exposure to radiations, abstenence from alcohol, smoking and abstenence drugs.	
		• Help the mother go through easy labor and prevent any trauma to the neonate.	
		• Encourage the mother for abortion, if the fetus has major congenital anomalies.	

Contd...

Contd...

Nursing need	Objective	Interventions	Evaluation
		• Protect the infant from any type of infections.	
		• Educate the mother about signs of early detection of mental retardation like delayed milestones.	
• Assessment of degree of mental retardation	• To help the couple know about degree of mental disability in the child and plan for the care of the child accordingly.	• Assess the milestones according to the child's age, teacher and mother also.	• Parents are able to identify the needs of the child and are provided are accordingly.
		• Refer the couple for child guidance clinics to treatment, counseling and follow-up.	
		• Assess the IQ of the child to determine the degree of mental disability.	
		• Educate parents about care of the newborn and elder children.	
		• Provide valid health information to empower their intellectuality.	
• Acceptance of the child with disability	• To help the couple in accepting the child with his/her deficits and treat him as other children of family members.	• Help the couple to ventilate their feelings and listen to the parents with a supportive attitude.	• The parents are able to accept the child with his strengths and weakness.
		• Encourage the parents to maintain a safe environment at home and care for the child at home.	
		• Explain the couple, the causes and empower them to overcome shame and guilt.	
		• Provide love and affection health care.	
• Impaired communication	• To help the child express his feelings and communicate well.	• The children with MR have poor communication ability. So, teach the couple to use simple words while communicating with child.	• Communication skills of the child improves.
		• Educate to impart rewards and positive reinforcement for successful acts.	
		• Teach new words/phrases day by day.	
• Impaired attention and concentration	• To improve the child's attention and communication span.	• The child should be given one simple command or activity at a time.	• The child's attention and concentration spar interview to some extent.

Contd...

Contd...

Nursing need	Objective	Interventions	Evaluation
		• Encourage the child to practice same activity till he/she learns to do.	
		• Remove the distraction in the environment while the child is practicing the activity.	
• Self-care deficit	• To help the child be as independent as possible in performing ADL	• Demonstrate and teach simple activities of daily living to the child like toothbrushing, combing, tongue cleaning, etc.	• The child is able to perform those activities of daily living that are with in its capacity of doing.
		• Teach the child patiently and in simple manner.	
		• Demonstrate each activity daily till the child learns it.	
		• Provide positive reinforcement to motivate the child.	
		• Demonstrate buttoning and unbuttoning of clothes.	
		• Provide the child with clothes having big holes and buttons.	
		• Teach the child how to eat and drink.	
		• Teach the child to chew the food slowly and properly.	
		• Provide special utensils like big spoon with long handle and special cup so that the child can grasp them properly.	
• Safety and health care needs	• To protect the child from diseases and accidents.	• Teach the parents that these children are prone to infections and accidents, so they must be careful.	• Child remains healthy and safe.
		• Treat any infection promptly.	
		• The child may have hearing and visual defects so, counsel to get hearing aids or spectacles for use.	
		• Keep sharp and harmful objects away from the child to avoid accidental injury to the child	
		• Teach the child what is hot and dangerous by letting him feel it once.	
		• Maintain calm and safe environment at home/setting.	

Contd...

Contd...

Nursing need	Objective	Interventions	Evaluation
• Rehabilitation needs	• To help the child learn productive activities and become more independent.	• Help the parents identify the strength and interest of the child.	• Productivity level of the child is improved and gain maximum independence.
		• Tell the parents to send the child to day care center and half-way homes or other available facilities.	
		• The child should be put in sheltered workshops where he can be supervised constantly and taught productive activities.	

LEARNING DISORDERS

Introduction

Parents are often worried when their child has learning problems in school. There are varied reasons for school failure, but a common one is learning disability. Children with learning disabilities can have intelligence in the normal but the specific learning disability may make tutors and parents concerned about their general intelligence, often, these children may try very hard to follow instructions, concentrate and 'be good' at home and in school. Yet, despite this effort, he or she is not mastering school tasks and falls behind. These affect at least 1 in 10 children.

After 1990s more research has done gradually related learning disabilities specially reading, written expression and mathematics. The DSM-IV-TR states that learning disorders are diagnosed when the child's academic achievement in reading, writing is substantially below that would be expected for age, schooling and intellectual ability. Learning problems must significantly interfere with achievement at school or the performance or activities of daily life that require reading, mathematics or writing skills.

Definitions

The term 'learning disorders' is used by DSM–IV-TR to refer to a group of disorders that are characterized by learning problems resulting in an individual's measured academic achievement falling substantially below the level expected for given the person's chronological age, educational level and intellectual ability.

Learning disability means a disorder in one or more of the basic psychological processes involved in understanding or in using language, spoken or written which may manifest itself as an imperfect ability to listen, think, speak, reading, spell, reason out, or doing mathematical problems.

Learning disabilities vary from person to person. One person with learning disabilities may not have the same kind of learning problems as another person with learning disabilities. One person may have trouble of reading and writing. Another person with learning disabilities may have problems with understanding with maths. Still another person may have trouble in each of these areas, as well as with understanding what people are saying.

Epidemiological Facts

These are more commonly seen in children and adolescents. About 2–10% of the population and than man 10% school children have significant academic difficulties. Learning disabilities are reported four times more common in males than females. Reading disorders constitute the greatest proportion of children identified with learning disabilities, probably 80–90%.

Types of Learning Disorders

There are three major types of learning disorders:
1. Reading disorder.
2. Mathematics disorder.
3. Disorder of written expression.

Common Signs of Learning Disorders

In addition to the problems associated with the specific type of learning disorder, many children also suffer from:
- Low self-esteem.
- Socialization problems.
- Increased dropout from school.
- Absenteeism
- These disorders maybe associated with conduct disorder, ADD and ADHD, and depressive disorders. Learning disabilities are associated with brain dysfunctions that affect a number of basic skills. Perhaps the most fundamental in sensory-perceptual ability—the capacity to take in and process information through the senses. Difficulties involving vision, hearing and touch will have an adverse effect on learning. Although learning is usually considered a mental, rather than a physical pursuit, it involves motor skills, and it can also be impaired by problems with motor development. Other basic skills fundamental to learning include memory, attention and language abilities.

Reading Disorder

It is also known as Dyslexia. According to DSM–IV-TR–Reading disorder is reading achievement below the expected level for a child's age, education and intelligence with the impairment interfering significantly with academic success or the daily activities that involve reading.

Causes

No single cause has been identified. The possible causes are:
- *Genetic causes:* Frequently seen in family members.
- *Neurological causes:* Most likely cause appears to be disorder of brain maturation or brain dysfunction.

Social Factors

- Frequent changes of school, illiterate family background and poor school environment.
- Malnutrition.

Clinical Features

- Dyslexia is related to deficits in processing the basic sounds that make-up language, a skill that is referred to as phonological processing that result in difficulty with decoding or being able to 'sound out' words, although higher order cognitive skills of thinking, reasoning, and understanding concepts are intact even advanced.

- Difficulty in developing an awareness that spoken and written words are made-up of phonemes (smaller segments representing individual sounds), e.g. p-q, b-d.
- Difficulty with role memorization and rapid word retrieval.
- May highlight nonessential information and omit important information.
- Inability to quickly find the correct word is often misinterpreted as the person being slow or dimwitted.
- Have strong receptive vocabulary, syntactic and grammar skills, but have difficulty retrieving words on demand due to the inability to use phonemic properties.
- Confusion regarding word sounds leads to slip of tongue, e.g. intrepid for interrupted.
- Long pauses, use fillers (um) and use of nonspecific filler, e.g. 'That thing', 'this was'.
- The sentences they themselves use maybe fragmented or poorly constructed. The child may find it difficult to draw inference from a story read aloud.

Pathogenesis

The concordance rate of reading disorder in monozygotic twins is 80% whereas it is 50% in dizygotic twins. If one family member is affected, the ratio for other members is much higher than that in general population.

Early warning signs of reading disorder in children by end of kindergarten are:

- Delay in developing speech
- Difficulties with articulation or pronunciation
- Takes little enjoyment in hearing and repeating nursery rhymes
- Difficulty with rhyming
- Difficulty naming all uppercase and lower case letters
- Difficulty naming all words

Early warning signs of reading disorder in children by 1st grade:

- Difficulty segmenting words and grouping them by their initial, ending and middle phonemes
- Difficulty naming letters and sounds
- Difficulty counting number of sounds in small words
- Expressive language seems to lag behind receptive language.

Assessment

- Wechsler intelligence scale for children (WLSC).
- Stanford-Binet test for intelligence.
- Detailed developmental history.
- Asking child to name capital and lower case letters and identifying corresponding sounds.
- Interviewing parents.
- Gray oral reading test (GORT).
- Compressive test for phonologic processing (CTOPP).

Management

It is a coordinated effort of physician, parents, mental health professionals and educationists based on child's age, overall health condition and medical history.

- *Remedial Teaching:* It involves following steps:
  - Mastery of simple phonetic units.
  - Blending of these units into words or resentences.
  - Make use of different senses:
    - Early exposure to oral reading, writing and drawing.
    - Practice reading from different kinds of books.
    - Practice using multisensory structured language instruction.
    - Allow extra time for them to complete their assignment.
- *Parental counseling*
  - Parents are helped to accept the child as he is.
  - Provide practice in reading at home and listen to their reading and give correction constructively.
- *Counseling and psychotherapy of child*
  - Positive reinforcement provided immediately and contingently can accelerate the reading skills.
  - Allowing child to plan own program.
  - Help with the emotional issues that rise from struggling to overcome academic difficulties.

MATHEMATICS DISORDER

Introduction

Mathematics disorder is a learning disability that is characterized by difficulties with calculation, with understanding math concepts, and with applying math skills when solving functional word problems. Some children with the disorder struggle with the mechanical operations of math, such as basic calculations. Others have trouble understanding the language used in math. Children may struggle with all areas of mathematics or have difficulty with only one aspect of math functioning. In addition, the severity may vary given the child's other areas of strength and weakness. Mathematics disorder is not related to IQ, and children with the disorder might do well in subjects requiring logic instead of formulas. Some children struggle to visualize and understand spatial relationships that might be required in geometry or in using a number line. Some children struggle with multistep problems that require sequencing. Children who have difficulty with memory retrieval may have difficulty recalling basic math facts.

Definitions

Mathematics disorders, formerly called developmental arithmetic disorders, developmental acalculia, or dyscalculia, is a learning disorder in which a person's mathematical ability is substantially below the level normally expected based on his or her age; intelligence, life experiences educational background and physical impairments. This ability affects the ability to do calculations as well as the ability to understand word problems and mathematical concept.

Mathematics disorder involves difficulties recognizing numbers and symbols, memorizing facts, grasping various aspects of mathematical reasoning to solve problems or performing computation.

DSM-IV-TR defines mathematics achievement below the expected level of the child age, education and intelligence with impairment interfering significantly with academic achievement, daily activities and activities requiring mathematical skills.

Mathematical disorder was first described as developmental disorder in 1937. These disorders includes the following:

- Difficulty reading and writing numbers.
- Difficulty aligning numbers in order to do calculations.
- Inability to perform calculations.
- Inability to comprehend word problems.

ETIOLOGY

The causes of mathematical disorder are not well understood, different manifestations may have different causes:

- Genetic causes maybe incorporated.
- Abnormality in cerebral hemisphere. Research finding in adults has suggested that calculation involves the inferior prefrontal cortex in the left hemisphere as well as the angular gyrus.
- Environmental factors may also be involved.

CLINICAL FEATURES

Mathematics disorders symptoms can be grouped under the following headings.

Language Symptoms

- Difficulty in understanding and naming mathematical terms, operations and concepts.
- Difficulty in decoding written problems into mathematical symbols.
- Understanding concepts used in mathematical problems like more or less than, first and last, before and after.

Perceptual Symptoms

- Difficulty in recognizing and reading numerical symbols or arithmetic signs and symbols.
- Clustering objects into groups.
- Aligning strings of numbers during calculation.
- Ordering strings of numbers.
- Mathematical symptoms.
- Difficulty in performing basic mathematical operations and in memorizing numerical facts.
- Difficulty in following sequences of mathematical steps.
- Difficulty in counting objects.
- Difficulty in learning multiplication tables.

Attentional Symptoms

Inaccurate copying of numbers.

- Omitting digits, decimals or symbols when writing.
- Forgets to add in carried numbers.
- Fails to notice arithmetic signs.

Other than these, children also face these symptoms:

- Problem counting.
- Difficulty memorizing multiplication tables.
- Inability to group the difference between such operation as on addition and subtraction.

- Poor computation skills, many errors in simple arithmetics.
- Slowness in performing calculations.
- Difficulty arranging numbers in order (from smallest to largest).
- Inability to grasp information on graphs.
- Difficulty copying numbers or problems.
- Inability to graph the concept of place value.
- Inability to align two or three digit numbers to do calculations.
- Difficulty understanding word problems.
- Inability to understand mathematical symbols.

Diagnosis

It is not usually diagnosed before a child is in the second or third grade because of the variability with which children acquire mathematical fluency. Many bright children manage to get through fourth or fifth grade level in mathematics by using memorization and calculation tricks.

Treatment

- Specific individual educational plan to improve basic mathematical skills and concepts.
- Perceptual skill training: It focuses on skills like matching, sorting and arranging objects.
  - Teaching new concept with concrete objects like pencil, sticks, blocks, etc. then move to abstract ideas.
  - Cognitive developmental teaching: In this procedure, teacher facilitate learning through areas of cognitive strength in the child.
    - Use of graph paper for students who have difficulty in organizing on plain paper.
    - Encourage them to ask doubts.
  - Help in student to understand his abilities and weaknesses.
  - Some specific measures or techniques that can be used are:
    - Providing demonstration, modeling and feedback.
    - Increasing fluency.
    - Using concrete/abstract teaching sequence.
    - Setting goals.
    - Combining demonstration with permanent model.
    - Teaching strategies for computation and problem-solving.
    - Using computerized instructions.

Prognosis

Progress in overcoming mathematics disorder depends on the specific type of difficulties that the child has with mathematics; the learning resources available and the child's determination to work overcoming the disorder. If it prolongs, may develop low self-esteem and psychosocial problems.

DISORDER OF WRITTEN LANGUAGE

Disorder of written expression, formerly called developmental expressive writing disorder, is a learning disability in which a person's ability to communicate in writing is substantially below the level normally expected based on the individual's age, intelligence, life experiences, educational background or physical impairments. This disability affects both the physical reproduction of letters and words and the organization of thoughts and ideas in written compositions.

Definition

Disorder of written expression is significant impairment in written communication that is not attributable to low intelligence, visual or hearing defect, neurological disorder or lack of adequate instruction.

Written expression related to basic skills such as handwriting and spelling as well as executive functions such as planning, self-monitoring, organizing and perspective speaking.

Types of Written Disorders

- Inability to form letters and numbers correctly, also called dysgraphia.
- Inability to write words spontaneously or from dictation.
- Inability to organize into meaningful thoughts.
- Disorders of written expression usually appears in conjunction with other reading or language disabilities, making it hard to separate manifestations of the disability related only to written expression. Delays in attention, visual-motor integration, visual processing and expressive language may also contribute to writing disorders.

Causes/Etiology

The causes of disorder of written expression are unknown. Different manifestations of the disorder may have varied causes. For example, people who cannot form letters correctly on the page (dysgraphia) may have delays in hand-eye coordination and difficulties in concentrating. People who are unable to write words from memory or dictation appear to have deficits in their visual memory. They cannot remember what the words look like. People who produce legible script but cannot organize their thoughts and views on paper may be suffering from cognitive-processing problems.

The possible causes are genetic, biological, psychosocial and environmental including instructional variables.

CLINICAL FEATURES

- Poor or illegible handwriting.
- Poorly formed letters or numbers.
- Excessive spelling errors.
- Excessive grammar errors.
- Sentences that lack logical cohesion.
- Paragraphs and stories that are missing elements that do not make sense or lack logical transitions.
- Deficit writing skills that significantly impact academic achievement for daily life.

Spelling Errors

The most common is phonetic or grammatical error in which misspelling resemble the way the word sounds.

Example:

- Misspelling resemble the way the word sound
  - Fotograph for photograph.
  - CAIM for CAME.
- Misspelling resemble a pronunciation or slurring of word.
  - Offen for often
- Morphological errors.

Example:

- Laughted for laughed.
- Segmental errors.
  - A way for away.
- Reversals: God for dog
- Spelling error: Bitting for biting.

Grammatical Errors

- Word omissions, incorrect verb and pronoun usage and incorrect word endings.
- Written sentences maybe incomplete:
  - Punctuation and capitulation.
  - Excessively poor handwriting.
  - Letter forms are not decodable.
  - Rotations or invasions of letters.
  - Mixture of printing and cursive writing.
  - Inappropriate mixture of appear case letters and lower case letters.
- Poor organization of paragraphs.
  - Poor story composition like settings, character, theme, etc.
  - Poor cohesion, e.g. abrupt ending, transition that are not smooth in nature)

Demographies

Several research studies have estimated that between 3 and 5% of children/students have disorder of written expression. These are associated with other learning disorders. Deficits in written work maybe attributed to a reading, language, or attention disorders, limited educational background or lack of fluency in the language of instruction. Disorders of written language expression unassociated with any other learning disability is rare.

Diagnostic Criteria

There is no specific test to diagnose these disorders. These are normally diagnosed before the age eight because of the variability with which children acquire writing skills. Mostly diagnosed in the fourth or fifth grade.

The following tests maybe useful for diagnosis:

a. DEWS: (Diagnostic Evaluation of Writing Skills).
b. TEWL: (Test of Early Written Language).
c. Test of Adolescent Language.

Management

- *Remediation therapy:* Practicing the written material more and more.
- Consistently using a basic framework of planning, writing and revision.

- Encourage proper grip and posture for writing.
- Be positive and patient, encourage practice and praise efforts.
- Allow extra time for writing.
- Counseling and psychotherapy to the child and parents are helpful.
- Treat the treating causes well in advance.
- Holistic management.

Prognosis

Those who have this disorder may develop low self-esteem and social problems related to their lack of academic achievement. Later in life they maybe more likely to dropout of school and find employment is more difficult.

PERVASIVE DEVELOPMENTAL DISORDER

The pervasive developmental disorder (PDD), refers to a group of conditions that involve delays in the development of many basic skills most notably the ability to socialize with others, to communicate and to use imagination. Children with PDD are confused in their thinking and generally have problems understanding the world around him/her.

In more than two-third of children with PDD, there is evidence of atypical development before the child is one year old. In others, there is evidence of regression in speech, language and communication during the next six months and within two and half years for most children with PDD except those with childhood disintegrative disorders.

Conditions included in PDD are:

- Autism (autistic disorder).
- Asperger's disorder.
- Childhood disintegrative disorder.
- Rett's syndrome.
- Pervasive development disorder not otherwise specified (PDDNOS).

SYMPTOMS OF PERVASIVE DEVELOPMENT DISORDER

The use of the word 'pervasive' to describe these illnesses is really mean 'to be present throughout'.

General Symptoms

- Difficulty with verbal communication, including problems, using and understanding language.
- Difficulty with nonverbal communication, such as gestures and facial expressions.
- Difficulty with social interaction including, relating to people and to his/her surroundings.
- Repetitive body movement or pattern of behaviors, such as hand flapping, spinning head banging.
- Changing response to sound.

Autistic Disorder (Autism)

Kanner (1943) described features which is designated as early infantile autism, with an onset before 30 months of age through certain modifications were suggested over the years.

The following features are present in autism:
- Profound general failure of development of social relationships.
- These children did not want to be picked up, their eye to eye gaze will be different and they landed to turn away resulting in failure of maternal bonding and creating new friendships.
- A marked retardation in acquiring language or even loss of already acquired language with impaired comprehension, echolalia, pronominal reversal.
- A tendency for ritualistic and compulsive behavior was more or less the rule with a tendency for rigidity and wanting of sameness of the environment to be maintained.
- Stereotyped, repetitive movements of the hands and fingers are typical with tendency for posturing.
- A short attention span with difficulty of maintaining the concentration in a particular direction.
- A tendency to inflict self-injury and enjoy the situation.
- A delay in acquiring standee and bowel control.
- IQ testing showed mental retardation in 75% cases through it that may not always be actual.

Incidence

The incidence rate is 10 per 10000 children (Bryson, 1988). The male–female ratio for autistic disorder was 3:1 as found by Gillberg.

Diagnostic Scales

- Autistic diagnostic interview revised for parents (Lord, 1994).
- Interview for social and communication disorders for parents (Wing, 1999).
- Childhood autism rating scale (william, 1995).
- Autism diagnostic observation schedule (Lord, 2000).

Etiology

Psychosocial Hypothesis

According to Kanner, he called initially autism as inborn disturbance, emotionally rigid, detached and obsessive parents who raised their child in an atmosphere lacking emotional warmth led to autistic child's 'emotional refrigeration'. The autistic child was traumatized by the unconscious hostility of a negative mother who did not truly want her child leading to autistic withdrawal.

Biological Theories

Congenital Rubella and untreated phenylketonuria could be associated with the syndrome. It is now thought that it is a behavioral syndrome that can be caused or influenced by diverse conditions that adversely affect the control nervous system.

Genetic Causes

It may influence or contribute to the development of autism.

Perinatal Factors

Prenatal, perinatal and neonatal complications, bleeding after the first trimester of pregnancy, fetal distress, maternal use of medication during pregnancy, delayed cry, respiratory distress and neonatal anemia may contribute in causation of autism.

Neurochemical Hypothesis

In one-third of autistic children increased levels of serotonin in the blood was reported primarily in 1961. Dopamine hyperdopaminergic functioning of the cells might explain the hyperactivity and stereotype seen in autism.

Viral Infections

- Congenital Rubella
- Cytomegalovirus infection
- Herpes simplex encephalitis
- Winter influenza infection.

Sign and Symptoms

It is characterized by withdrawal of the child into self and into a fantasy world of him or her own. The child has markedly abnormal or impaired social communication and interaction. The following features are observed:

- Absence of social smile.
- Lack of eye to eye contact.
- Solitary play.
- Nonattachment with loved parents and absence of separation anxiety.
- Inability to make friends.
- Absence of fear in presence of danger.
- Impaired language and communication.
  - Lack of response to voice or sounds.
  - Absence of communication sounds like babbling during infancy.
  - Absent or delayed speech.
  - Impaired abstract thinking.
  - Abnormal speech content and pattern like echolalia, preservation, poor articulation, etc.
- Abnormalities in behavior.
  - Mannerism
  - Stereotyped behavior like head-banging, body-spinning, rocking, clapping, hand-flicking, etc.
  - Ritualistic and compulsive acts.
  - Attachment to nonliving things/objects.

Mental Retardation

- Less than 25% of autistic children have an IQ of more than 70. Most of them have moderate to profound mental retardation. About 70% of these children lead dependent lives.
- Other features:
  - Epilepsy is very common.
  - Exceptional calculating ability or musical ability maybe present.

Treatment Modalities

The goal of treatment of children with autistic disorder is to reduce behavioral symptoms and to promote learning and development, particularly the acquisition of language skills. The goal is achieved through a comprehensive and highly individualized treatment program of which special education and language therapy are essential components. The treatment consists of three modes that maybe used together.

Behavior Therapy

It includes positive reinforcements to teach self-care skills, speech therapy and or sign language teaching and behavioral techniques to encourage interpersonal interactions.

Psychotherapy

Parental counseling and supportive therapy are useful in allaying parental anxiety.

Pharmacotherapy

Drug treatment is used for the treatment of autism and associated epilepsy. Fenfluramine is helpful in increasing brain serotonin levels.

Antipsychotic

It was hypothesized that the stereotype and hyperactivity seen in autism children were a function of increased dopaminergic activity that was the rationale for the use of antipsychotics which block dopamine receptors in autism children. In individually regulated dose of 0.25 to 4.0 mg/day or from 0.016 to 0.217 mg/kg/day; the high potency antipsychotic Haloperidol proved to be more effective which decreases dopamine levels in brain and thus decreases hyperactivity and abnormal behavioral symptoms.

Naltrexone

It is an opioid antagonist reduced stereotype, withdrawal and increased language production in autistic children. It can be given 0.5 to 1.0 mg/kg/day. The adverse effects are drowsiness, nausea and vomiting which are mild and transient.

Clonidine

- Clonidine reduced noradrenergic activity can be used which decreases stereotype behavior, hyperactivity and temper.
- Antiepileptic drugs are used for generalized seizures.
- Education plans should be individualized for each child and should take into account not only the child's shortcomings but also strengths that the tutor may capitalize to facilitate the acquisition of new skills.

RETT'S DISORDER

Rett's syndrome is a rare, serve, 'girls only' form of autism. It is usually diagnosed in the first two years of life. It is an autism spectrum disorder that affects girls almost exclusively, occurs between 6–8 months of age. It is seen only about one in 10000 to 15000 girls.

The Rett's syndrome diagnostic criteria work group agreed on the following criteria for diagnosis of Rett's disorder.

- An initial period of normal development including normal perinatal head circumference.

- Between 5 months to 4 years of age, there is deceleration of head growth followed by loss of hand skills and appearance of stereotype hand wringing movements.
- Social skills and receptive language also deteriorate at 2 or 3 years of age.
- Ataxia and apraxia become prominent and gait becomes broad and jerky with stiff legs and side-to-side swaying.
- Breathing dysfunction maybe severe.

Epidemiological Data

- 1:10000 to 1:15000 in females.
- Annual mortality rate is 1:2%.
- 100% concordance in monozygotic twins.
- It occurs in females and is X-linked dominant mutation with lethality in homozygous males.
- Mutations in gene MECP 2 (methyl- cpG – binding protein).

Symptoms

- Loss of speech and motor control.
- Functional hand use replaced by compulsive hand movements.
- Disordered digestive and breathing problems.
- Orthopedic abnormalities including scoliosis and fragile bones.
- Disrupted sleep patterns.
- Extreme excessive anxiety.
- Seizures.
- Impaired cardiac and circulatory function.
- Parkinsonian tremor.

Management

No specific treatments supportive measures are applied. Children may benefit from special education. Physical therapy maybe introduced. Drugs maybe administered to decrease stereotype movements and wetting of hands with saliva. Haloperidol maybe tried.

CHILDHOOD DEGENERATIVE DISORDER

Thomas Heller, an Austrian educator, first described childhood disintegrative disorder in 1908. It is a complex disorder that affects many different areas of the child's development. He described it as infantile dementia, that also known as Haller's disorder.

Causes

The cause of childhood disintegrative disorder is unknown. Research findings shown that, abnormalities of different neurotransmitters in brain, changes in EEG and also associated with seizures.

Characteristics (Research based)

- A child after 2–4 years of normal development regressed in social, communicative and adaptive skills.

- The condition maybe associated with metachromatic leukodystrophy and schilder's disease but no specific neuropathological process was identified.
- A number of children development seizures in the proportion of 7:3 when compared to autism.
- The mean age of onset was 36 months (ranges 24–70 month).
- These children often had IQ less than 40.

Diagnosis

To be diagnosed with CDD, a child must show loss or regression in at least two of the areas listed below. Usually regression occurs in more than two areas.
These are:

- Receptive language skills (language understanding).
- Expressive language skills (spoken language).
- Social or self-help skills.
- Play with peers.
- Motor skills
- Bowel and bladder control.

Treatment

- Educational interventions.
- Behavior therapy.
- Guidance and counseling to parents and child.
- Support group therapy.

ASPERGER'S DISORDER

Asperger's syndrome, also called Asperger's disorder, is a type of pervasive development disorder (PDD). This involves delays in the development of many basic skills most notably the ability to socialize with others, to communicate and to use imagination. Children with Asperger's syndrome typically function better than autism. In addition, children with this disorder, generally have normal intelligence and near-normal language development, although they may develop problems communicating as they get older.

- Asperger described the following characteristics of this disorder.
- High functioning and autism spectrum disorder symptoms.
- Normal language development as young children but facial expression, prosody and social gestures and interactions are minimal.
- Intuitive knowledge of how to approach others.
- If highly intelligent interested in one or two subjects like astronomy geology.
- Ability to use knowledge quite successfully despite their very inceptive, social skills and quite successful in earning a living.
- In spite of normal language development' presence of delayed milestones and clumsiness but no significant delays in cognitive development of age appropriate self-help skills and adequate behavior.

 CLINICAL MANIFESTATIONS

The symptoms of Asperser's syndrome may vary and can range from mild to severe. Common symptoms include:

- Problems with social networking: Difficulty in interacting with others and often are awkward in social situations. They show difficulty in initiating and maintain conversation.
- Eccentric or repetitive behaviors.
- Unusual preoccupations or rituals.
- Communication difficulties.
- Limited range of interest.
- Coordination problems.
- Exceptionally skilled or talented, e.g. music/maths.

Diagnosis

- Physical and neurological examination.
- X-ray of brain and lab investigations.
- Mental status examination.

Management

- Special education.
- Behavior modification.
- Occupational/speech/physical therapy.
- Social skills training.
- *Medication:* Treated for anxiety, depression and other associated symptoms.

 ATYPICAL AUTISM

It is the term to designate persons with pervasive developmental disorders where symptoms developed after 30 years of age or who showed atypical or subthreshold symptoms. Many attempts have been made to distinguish the different entities contributing to PDD especially those by Ghaziuddin (1994) but without any convincing differentiation.

Autism Spectrum Disorder

This considers autism as a spectrum ranging from severe to mild. Piver considered the spectrum model as a means of understanding those individuals including their relations who were autistic with significant impairments in social knowledge and pragmatic communication and whose behavior, interests and activities were socially nonfunctional but the symptoms were not severe enough to meet the criteria for autism. The diagnosis of autism spectrum disorder is also a means to avoid differentiation that is often confusion and difficult in nature.

 HABIT DISORDERS

Introduction

Habit disorders also known as nervous habits. It refers to persistent, largely involuntary patterns of dyscontrol of motor functions in children. Commonly these disorders include bedwetting, soiling, nail biting, thumbsucking, overeating, sleepwalking, tics and stuttering. Since, these habits have been repeated frequently so often in the past, and are so overlearned, they are notoriously resistant to change. They tend to be automatic reactions that the child has little control over. According to Sigmund Freud, he tells many of us are unconscious about our habits, often we perform habits without realizing that we are doing them, e.g. nail biting.

Common Etiology of Habit Disorders

Some psychologists suggest that they offer a release of nervous tension or anxiety and are pleasant or satisfying to some instinctual impulse. Other behaviorists assume that habits are learned and can be unlearned in a systematic way. Still others assert that habits are often a symptom of an underlying conflict which must be treated before the habit will disappear. Most likely the cause includes combination of different factors.

THUMBSUCKING

We know that many babies and young children calm themselves by sucking their thumbs. While most children stop on their own, some children continue till the age of 4 or 5 years. Thumbsucking is normal in babies. A natural instinct leads some babies to suck their thumbs during their first few months of life. They may also suck on their fingers, hands or some other items also.

It is a tendency that occurs when the child is able to raise his fingers to his mouth. It acts like a substitute at the breast or bottle, while the oral habits seem to soothe the infant in all types of stress. It cannot be considered as a psychological problem unless it causes harm.

Definition

It is defined as non-nutritive sucking of fingers or thumb.

Age of Occurrence

Thumb sucking is common in oral stage (0–1 year) as babies have a natural urge to suck. This usually decreases after the age of 6 months. Many babies continue to suck their thumb to soothe themselves. Most children stop thumbsucking by 3–6 years.

ETIOLOGY

Babies have a natural urge to suck that usually decreases after the age of 6–12 months. However, many babies continue to suck their thumbs to soothe themselves much longer. Eventually, it will become a habit in babies and young children who use it to comfort themselves. Most common, they are sucking thumbs when they feel hungry, afraid, restless, quiet, sleepy or bored. The fact is that about 70 to 90% of infants suck their thumbs. Most of these children gradually stop on their own between ages three and six, but if that does not happen, it became habit disorders. The other possible causes are:

Parental Causes

- Over protection by parents.
- Neglect by parents.
- Overstrictness of parents.
- Disharmony between parents.

Causes Related to School

- Excessive strictness by teachers.
- Excessive punitive attitude of teachers.
- Excessive competition.
- Separation from parents and siblings.

Other Causes

- Loneliness and boredom.
- Tiredness.
- Frustration and anxiety.
- Separation from parents.

Problems Caused by Thumbsucking

Thumbsucking in children younger than four years is not a problem; but if it continues up to 5 or above, it indicates presence of an emotional cause.

Prolonged thumbsucking may lead to dental problems like maligned teeth or sometimes malformation of the upper palate of mouth. The child may also develop speech problems like mispronouncing 'T' and alphabet 'D' lisping, thrusting out the tongue while talking. A child with this type of problem needs to be evaluated by a physician.

Management

Thumbsucking treatment involves many approaches. It can be managed at home by setting rules and providing distractions by care providers. Many have opinion that ignoring thumbsucking in children as most children stop it on their own. However, following points are also considered.

Do's

- Divert the child's attention. Engage children in play.
- The hands and fingers of the child should be kept busy.
- Offer praise and rewards to the child for not sucking thumbs.
- Distract the child when he/she feels bored.
- Put gloves on child's hands or wrap the thumb with a cloth or bandage.
- A nontoxic bitter tasting substance can be opted on child's thumb so that he may not suck it.
- Take help of elder children for explanation.
- Encourage the child to socialize utmost.
- If the child is sucking thumb due to anxiety or distress, address the causes of discomfort. Talk to the child and reassure him/her.

Do Not's

- Do not punish/beat the child.
- Do not tie child's thumbs and fingers.
- Do not nag, scold the child.
- Do not leave the child repeatedly cold, wet or hungry.

Therapies

- Behavioral therapy.
- Substitution therapy: Behavioral therapy is combined with tapping fingers together quietly. It works best when all are used.

Hypnotherapy

It is very effective tool to help reduce symptoms and to uncover issues that maybe causing thumbsucking.

 NAIL BITING/ONYCHOPHAGIA

Onychophagia or nail biting is a common oral compulsive habit in children as well as adults. It is just a way of coping with stress or comforting self.

Nail biting is a body focused repetitive behavior that results in the destruction of one's own finger nails and often the skin around the nails.

Incidence

Several research studies have shown that approximately 28 to 33% of children aged 7–10 are biting their nails, as well as the 44% of adolescents, 19 to 29% of young adults and 5% of older adults. It is very common in boys. Stereotypic movements are common even in infants and toddlers.

Causes

Nail biting can be caused by:

- Sensory deprivation (blindness/deafness).
- Drug use (cocaine, amphetamines).
- Brain disease (seizures, infection)
- Major psychiatric disorders (anxiety disorder, OCD, autism).
- Mental retardation.
- Out of curiosity or boredom.
- Lack of confidence.
- Poor time management strategies.
- Poor management of leisure activities.
- Tiredness.
- Constant nagging.
- Fear.
- According to Freud: It is a symptom of oral fixation.

Symptoms

- Extremely short finger nails.
- Paronychia (infection around nail).
- Oral herpes.
- Damaged dentition.

- Apical root resorption.
- Fractures to incisors.
- Gingivitis.
- Warts around the nail bud.

Management

- *Medications:* Same as used for OCD–antidepressants (SSRIS).
- *Natural remedies:* Vit B inositol which seems to reduce the urge to pull or pick.
- *Psychotherapy:* Cognitive behavior therapy has been used to treat nail biting and mental disorders. The techniques used are the following.

Habit Reversal Training (HRT)

It is a four step process which teaches the person with how to relax; how to breathe and feel centered and to perform muscle response exercises. It also includes self-monitoring and stimulus control and social support.

Self-monitoring

- It is simply making the nail biter more aware of their behaviors. As the behavior can often be unconscious, awareness can be improved by simply keeping a log of picking behaviors. The act of recording the behavior also interrupt the process and reduce the picking.
- *Stimulus control (SC):* It is a behavioral treatment used for sufferers to identify and eliminate, avoid or change the environmental factors, moods or circumstances that trigger nail biting. The goal is to consciously control these triggers to create new learned connections between the urges and alternative, nondestructive behaviors. For example, if nail biting usually occurs while alone, the person will be encouraged to spend time more with others. If nail biting occurs at home while reading, then the person maybe asked to wear gloves during this time.

Competing Response

It is a technique designed to give the person an alternative to nail biting. This include toys, knitting, beading or other activities to keep the hands busy, chewing gum, tooth picks and other orally oriented behaviors maybe also used to satisfy the urge to chew.

Hypnotherapy

Helps to cope with anxious situations and stress triggers in a constructive way.

Alternative Methods

- Coating the nails with a bad-tasting nail polish.
- Wearing a rubber band on wrist: Having friends and family members snap it, when they see nail biting.

HEAD BANGING

Head banging exemplifies a stereotypic movement disorder that can result in functional impairment. According to DSM-IV-TR the male to female ratio is 3:1.

Head banging begins during infancy between 6 and 12 months of age. Infants strike their heads with a definite rhythmic and monotonus continuity against the crib or another hard surface. They seem to be absorbed in the activity which may persist until they become exhausted and fall asleep. The head banging is often transitory but sometimes persists into middle childhood. It is a component of temper tantrum differs from stereotypic head banging and ceases after the tantrum and their secondary gains have been controlled.

TIC DISORDER AND TOURETTE SYNDROME

Definition

Tic disorders are characterized by the persistent presence of tics, which are abrupt, repetitive in voluntary movements and sounds that have been described as caricatures of normal physical acts.

Meaning

Tics are sudden nonrhythmic behaviors that are either motor (related to movements) or vocal, e.g. knee bends, lip smacking, tongue thrusting, grimacing, eye blinking, throat clearing and so on. These are seen in transient tic disorder, chronic vocal or motor tic disorder and Tourette's disorder. Tourette's syndrome is characterized classically by convulsive muscular jerking and explosive utterances. Coprolalia (absence utterances) and copropraxia (absence gestures) do occur but not as frequent as used to be thought. Associated psychiatric problems are very common and include social and relationship difficulties, obsessive-compulsive behaviors, impulsiveness, distractibility and inattentiveness maybe associated with Tourette syndrome.

Types of Tics

Tics can be of the following types:

- *Simple:* Using only a few muscles or simple words.
- *Simple motor tics:* These are simple brief meaningless movements like eye blinking, facial grimacing, head jerks or shoulder shrugs. They usually last less than one second.
- *Simple phonetics:* These are meaningless sounds or noises like throat clearing, coughing sniffing, barking or hissing.

Complex Tics

These involve using many muscle groups or full words and sentences:

- *Complex motor tics:* These tics involve slower, longer, and more purposeful movements like sustained looks, facial gestures, biting, banging, sustained or twisting around or absence gestures.
- Complex phonic tics include syllabus, words, phrases and statements like 'shut up' or 'yes, you have done it'. The child's speech maybe abnormal with unusual tones, rhythms and accent.

Age of Onset

The age of onset of tic disorders is 2–15 years. In 75 to 80% cases of Tourette's disorder, the symptoms appear by the age of 11 years. Transient tic disorder occurs in approximately 4–24% of school children. Tourette's disorder is 3–4 times more common in boys than girls.

Etiology

In earlier times, emotional factors were considered as cause of tics, but now the search for causes focus on biological, chemical and environmental factors. There appear to be both functional and structural-abnormalities in brains of people with tic disorders. It is postulated that abnormal neurotransmitters contribute to this disorder. Researchers have also found changes within brain especially basal ganglia and anterior cingulate cortex.

- *Genetics:* A genetic basis to Tourette's syndrome has been confirmed and the exact nature of inheritance remains unclear. Both single gene and polygenic effect have been suggested.
- *Neurologic:* Recent brain imaging studies suggest a loss of the normal symmetry of the basal ganglia and a trend towards smaller left metabolic lateral ventricles. PET scanning has shown metabolic and perfusion abnormalities in the basal ganglia and frontotemporal area.
- *Neurochemical:* Abnormal dopamine metabolism is suggested by the beneficial effect of dopamine antagonists like haloperidol and pimozide.
- *Familial, environmental and other stress factors:* Undue parental or school pressures may aggravate problems. The child's bizarre behavior may itself be the cause of severe family disturbances.
- *Individual psychopathology:* There is no clear evidence that repressed aggressive or sexual urges underlie these disorders. In severe cases individual psychopathology occurs secondarily to the problem.
- *Medications:* In some cases, tic disorders appear to be caused or worsened by recreational drugs like psychomotor stimulants such as methylphenidate, pemoline, amphetamines and cocaine. In smaller cases, antihistamines, TCA's, antiepileptic medications and opioids also worsens the effects.
- Some forms of tic maybe triggered by environment. A cough that began during an upper respiratory infection may also begin as limitations of normally occurring events, such as mimicking a dog barking.

CLINICAL MANIFESTATIONS

Chronic motor or vocal tics or vocal tic disorder is characterized by either motor tics or vocal tics, but not both.

The tics occur many times a day nearly everyday, or intermittently for a period of more than one year. During this time, the client is never without symptoms for more than three consecutive months. The severity of the symptoms and functional impairment is usually much less than three consecutive months. The severity of the symptoms and functional impairment is usually much less than for clients with Tourette's disorder.

For a diagnosis of Tourette's disorder, a client must have experienced both multiple motor and one or more vocal tics at sometime during the illness, though they do not have to occur at the same time. The tics occur many times a day, usually in bouts, nearly everyday or intermittently for a period of more than one year. The client is never symptom free for more than three months at a time.

Children and adolescents with Tourette's disorder frequently experience, additional problems including aggressiveness, self-harming behaviors, emotional immaturity, social additional problems including aggressiveness, self-harming behavior, emotional immaturity, social withdrawal, physical complaints, conduct disorders, affective disorders, anxiety, panic attacks, stuttering, sleep disorders, migraine headaches and inappropriate sexual behaviors.

Treatment

A holistic client approach is recommended for the treatment of tic disorders. A multidisciplinary team should work together with the affected child's parents and teachers, to make a comprehensive treatment plan. Treatment should include the following:

- Educating the client and family about the course of disorder in a reassuring way.
- Completion of necessary diagnostic tests including self-reports by child and parents.
- Comprehensive assessment including the child's cognitive abilities, perception, motor skills, behavior and adaptive functioning should be done from the child, parents and if possible by teaching staff. Check for any emotional or behavioral problems or developmental delays. Physical examination is usually negative. Interviewing the child may exaggerate the movements because of anxiety. Observe parents reactions to tics. Differential diagnosis include other dyskinesias including the athetoid and choreiform.
- Including the athetoid and chores form movements seen in cerebral Palsy and Huntington's and Sydenham's Choreas.
- *Medications:* Medications are used to reduce severity of the tics. Pharmacotherapy is most effective when it is combined with other therapeutic approaches.
  - *Haloperidol:* Haloperidol is the drug of choice. The dosage is 0.05 to 0.075 mg/kg/day in two or three divided doses. Children should be monitored carefully as they may develop adverse effects.
  - *Pimozide:* It is useful where haloperidol is not effective or where it produces severe adverse effects. The close is 1 mg twice daily and can be increased up to 3–5 mg/day.
  - *Clonidine:* It is useful in severe cases with associated hyperactivity. Doses should be low in the range of 0.025 to 0.5 mg/day in single or divided doses.
  - *TCA and SSRIs:* They can be used occasionally especially when there are features of depression and OCD.
- *Cognitive behavior therapy:* The client is asked to deliberately perform tic movement for specified period of time interspersed with brief periods of rest.
- Contingency management is another behavioral treatment. It is based on positive reinforcement, usually administered by parents. Children are praised and rewarded for not performing tics and replacing them with alternative behaviors.
- Habit reversal is most commonly used technique, which when combined with relaxation exercises, awareness training and contingency management shows 64–100% success rate.

Nursing Management

- *Nursing diagnosis:* Risk for self-directed or violence directed towards others related to low tolerance for frustration.
- *Nursing objective:* Client will not harm self or others.

Nursing interventions	Rationale
• Observe client's behaviors frequently through routine activities and interactions. Become aware of behaviors that indicate rise in agitation.	• Stress commonly increases tic behavior. Recognition of behaviors help to intervene before violence occurs.
• Monitor for self-destructive behavior and impulses a staff member can stay with the client.	• Client's safety is primary.
• Redirect violent behaviors with physical outlets for frustrations.	• Excess energy is released through physical activities and a feeling of relaxation is induced.

- *Nursing Diagnosis:* Impaired social interaction related to impulsiveness and aggressive behavior.
- *Nursing objective:* Client will be able to interact with staff and peers.

Nursing interventions	Rationale
• Develop a trusting relationship with the client. Convey acceptance of the person.	• Unconditional acceptance increases feelings of self-worth.
• Discuss with the client the behaviors that are acceptable and those are not. Describe in manner the consequences of unacceptable behaviors.	• Aversion reinforcement can alter miserable behaviors.

- *Nursing diagnosis:* Low self-esteem related to shame associated with tic behaviors.
- *Nursing objective:* Client will verbalize positive aspects about self not associated with tics.

Nursing interventions	Rationale
• Convey unconditional acceptance and positive regard.	• Communication of client as a worth while human being may increase self-esteem.
• Set limit on manipulative behaviors. Take cautions not to reinforce manipulation behavior by providing desired attention.	• Aversive consequences may work to decrease or extinguish unacceptable behaviors.
• Help client understand that he/she uses manipulation to try to increase own self-esteem.	• When a client feels better about self, the need to manipulate others will diminish.
• If client chooses to suppress tics in the presence of others provide a specified tic time during which he/she vents tics, feelings and behaviors (alone or with others).	• Allows for release of tics and assists in sense of self-control and management of symptoms.

Preventive Measures/Alternate Therapies

- Many theorists postulated that dietary changes and nutritional supplements are used to prevent and manage symptoms of tic disorders. Some suggested that hidden food and chemical allergies or nutritional deficiencies may influence the development and maintenance of tic disorders. Recommendations include eating organic food and avoiding pesticides: taking antioxidants increasing the intake of folic acid and the 'B' vitamins eating foods high in zinc and magnesium; eliminating caffeine and avoiding artificial sweetness colors and dyes.
- Prevention of maternal emotional stress during pregnancy and severe nausea and vomiting during first trimester of pregnancy may affect tic severity.
- Stress Management Techniques.

ELIMINATION DISORDERS

Disorders of elimination include mainly encopresis and enuresis. These disorders are considered only when a child is chronologically and developmentally beyond the point at which it is expected that these functions can be mastered. Bowel and bladder control develops gradually overtime. Toilet training is affected by many factors such as child's intellectual capacity and social maturity, cultural determinants and the psychological interactions between child and parents. The normal sequence of developing control over bowel and bladder functions is the development of nocturnal fecal continence, diurnal control and nocturnal bladder control.

ENURESIS

Definition

Enuresis or bedwetting is a disorder of involuntary micturition in children who are beyond the age, when normal bladder control is acquired. Bladder control is normally mastered by the age of 2.5–3 years. If it is not acquired beyond 4–5 years of age, it is considered as abnormal. When bedwetting occurs repeatedly it is known as 'Enuresis'.

Types of Enuresis

It is divided into three categories

1. *Primary nocturnal enuresis:* It refers to children who have never been successfully trained to control urination. There maybe delay in maturation of sphincter control.
   It is very common in children. It occurs three times more frequently in boys and often disappears without intervention. The actual cause of night time wetting is not known, but it is believed that a developmental delay in the sleep-wake mechanism or bladder capacity of the child maybe a cause.
2. Day time (diurnal) wetting is less common. It is usually seen in shy, timid children or those with ADHDs. Day time wetting occurs usually between boys and girls. An estimated children of 60 to 80% wet the bed at night.
3. Secondary enuresis develops when a bladder trained child becomes incontinent. Usually it follow a stressful event, such as the birth of a sibling or a divorce. Both diurnal and secondary enuresis are associated with high levels of emotional stress, anxiety and mental health problems.

Etiology of Enuresis

- *Inappropriate toilet training:* The age at which toilet training is started has an important impact on child. If toilet training is started very early, produces stress in the child.
- *Neurological developmental delay:* This is the most common cause of bedwetting. There is delayed development in the ability to stay dry. Bedwetting maybe due to delay in nervous system's ability to process feeling of a full bladder.
- *Genetics:* Bedwetting has a strong genetic link. Children, whose parents were not wetting bed, have only 15% of incidence of bedwetting. When one or both parents were bedwetters, the rates jump to 44 and 77% respectively. Genetic research forecasted that bedwetting is associated with genes on chromosome 13 and 12q.
- *Emotional factors:* Emotional and psychological disturbances due to death in family, sexual abuse, extreme bullying, severe punishment or scolding, jealousy feeling or sibling rivalry and feeling of being rejected create internal tension in the child which may lead to secondary enuresis.
- *Organic causes:* Enuresis may occur due to anatomical defects of urinary tract and bladder, diabetes insipidus, urinary tract infection, etc.

Management

For management of bedwetting, it is essential to assess the home conditions of the child, his/her socioeconomic status and family conditions. Explore the child and parent's relationship. Child's relationship with playmates, teachers and siblings is also noted for evaluation.

- Reassure the child and parents.
- Try to build the child's self-confidence.
- Parents should be explained about the possible contributing factors for bedwetting.
- The child should not be given any liquids like tea or milk after late evening.
- The child should be habitually made to pass urine before going to sleep.
- The parents should arouse the child after 2–3 hours of sleep and persuade him/her to walk unaided to the toilet to empty bladder.
- The child is trained to hold the urine for longer time. This maybe practiced by making the child drink large quantity of water during day and persuading him to delay emptying bladder as long as possible.
- Bedwetting alarms Physicians frequently suggest bedwetting alarms, which produce a loud noise notice when they sense moisture. This can help the child to wake at sensation of full bladder.
- *Medications:* Used in very resistant cases like tricyclic antidepressants, etc. amitriptyline, imipramine, and nortriptyline are given orally, at night for 2 months. Desmopressin, which is a synthetic replacement for antidiuretic hormone (ADH) is also prescribed as it reduces urine production during sleep.

ENCOPRESIS

Encopresis is fecal incontinence in a child over 4 year of age with no physical abnormalities. It is defined as 'the repeated, usually voluntary, passage of feces in inappropriate places (Clark 1995). In other terms, it is known as paradoxical diarrhea is involuntary fecal soiling in children who are past the age of toilet training.

Incidence

As each child achieves bowel control at his or her own rate, physician do not consider stool soiling to be a medical condition unless the child is at least four years old. The estimated prevalence of encopresis in 4 years old children is between 1–3%. It affects boys four times more than girls and is rarely seen in adolescence.

Causes

It is rarely caused by any congenital defect. In majority of cases it develops as a result of chronic constipation. In most children, the problem begins with painful passage of hard constipated stool. Over the time, child becomes reluctant to pass stool or holds stool to avoid pain. This 'holding in' of stool becomes a habit. As more and more stool collects in child's colon, the colon goes on stretching and finally the child loses the natural urge to pass stool. Eventually, the partly formed stool from high up in the intestine, leaks around the large intestine.

Collection of hard stool at the bottom of rectum and then leaks out of the anus. As time passes, more and more stool leaks and then the child starts passing entire stool in his or her panties.

Management

The management of encopresis focuses on the following principle:

- Empty the colon of stool.
- Establish regular, soft and painless bowel movement.

- Promote regular bowel habits.
- Behavior therapy for modification of child's behavior.

A combination of medical and behavioral therapy works best in evacuation of hard stool from the colon. Evacuation can be accomplished in the following manner:

- Administer an enema or series of enemas, as it creates pressure within the rectum and gives the child an urge to pass stool.
- Suppositories and laxatives can also be used to promote bowel evacuation.
- Establish a regular toilet routine. The child should be made to sit in toilet for 5–10 minutes after breakfast and again after dinner everyday.
- Behavioral techniques: Offer age appropriate positive reinforcement for developing regular toilet habits.
- *Training:* Children may respond to teaching about appropriate use of muscles to defecate. Children are taught how to use their abdominal, pelvic and anal sphincter muscles which they have so often used to retain stool.
- The duration of treatment varies from child to child. Treatment should continue, until the child has developed regular and reliable bowel habits. This usually needs several months of time.

FEEDING AND EATING DISORDERS

Introduction

Feeding and eating disorder in infancy or early childhood includes persistent symptoms of inadequate food intake, recurrent regurgitation and rechewing of food or repeated ingestion of non-nutritive substances. The DSM-IVTR includes three distinct disorders feeding and eating disorders in this age group: Pica, rumination disorder and feeding disorder of infancy or early childhood.

PICA

Introduction

- The word 'PICA' is presumed to be derived from the word 'Magpie' is a scavenger bird that picks up whatever it sees.
- The DSM-IVTR described Pica as persistent eating of non-nutritive substances such as clay or chalk for at least 1 month of duration. The behavior must be developmentally inappropriate, not culturally accepted and sufficiently severe to attract clinical attention. In general, pica is the persistent eating of substances such as dirt or paint that have no nutritional value.

Incidence

Pica appears much more frequently in younger children than adults. It also occurs in persons who are mentally retarded (15%). It appears to affect both genders equally.

Types

The subtypes of pica are characterized by the substances eaten, for example:

Amylophagia: Consumption of starch.
Coprophagy: Consumption of animal feces.
Geophagy: Consumption of soil, clay or chalk powder.

Hyalophagia: Consumption of glass.
Pagophagia: Pathological consumption of ice.
Trichophagia: Consumption of hair or wool.
Urophagia: Consumption of urine.
This type of pattern should last for at least 1 month to be diagnosed as pica.

Causes/Etiology

Many research theories have been put forward to explain the cause of pica but none has been globally accepted. A higher expected incidence of pica looks to occur in the relatives of persons with the symptoms.

Nutritional deficiencies have been postulated as cause of pica. At particular circumstances craving for nonedible substances have been produced by dietary insufficiencies, e.g. craving for dirt and ice are associated with iron and zinc deficiencies.

During teething, the infants want to bite something hard and accordingly they tend to eat paint and varnish from their cradles, toys and even form walls. It can also serve as a means to get attention. Separation anxiety also acts as contributory factors.

Pica is more common in poorly nourished, neglected and badly supervised children. It tends to occur more commonly in those belonging to lower socioeconomic status.

Theories related to psychological deprivation, and subsequent ingestion of nonedible substances have suggested that pica is a compensatory mechanism to satisfy oral needs. The children who exhibit pica have either had an over satisfactory oral phase of psychosexual development or deficient one. Stressors such as maternal deprivation family issues, parental neglect, pregnancy, poverty and a disorganized family structure are strongly linked to pica.

Treatment

Pica maybe managed by combination of psychosocial, environmental, dietary and family guidance care approach. For pica that appears to be of psychotic etiology, therapy and medications such as SSRIs have been used successfully. Other treatment techniques are as follows:

- Presentation of attention, food or toys not contingent on pica being attempted.
- Discrimination training between edible and nonedible items.
- Detect nutritional deficiencies and treat them, e.g. anemia, hypoglycemia, etc.
- Make meal times pleasant.
- Meet the emotional needs of the child.
- Do not ignore and leave the child alone.
- Keep the child busy, as boredom may give him time for eating nonedible substances.
- Mild aversion therapy and negative reinforcement techniques maybe used sometimes.
- Positive reinforcement, modeling, behavioral shaping and overcorrection treatment are the other choice.

Complications of Pica

Eating certain items such as paint, mud, clay can contain lead or other toxic substances and consuming them can lead to poisoning, increasing the child's risk of complications including learning disabilities and brain damage.

ANOREXIA NERVOSA

Eating Disorders

An eating disorder is an ongoing disturbance in behaviors associated with the ingestion of food. The most common eating disorders are anorexia nervosa and bulimia. Although, obesity is not classified yet, it is now alarming the society as it presents more than 30% of our population (Fig. 11.1)

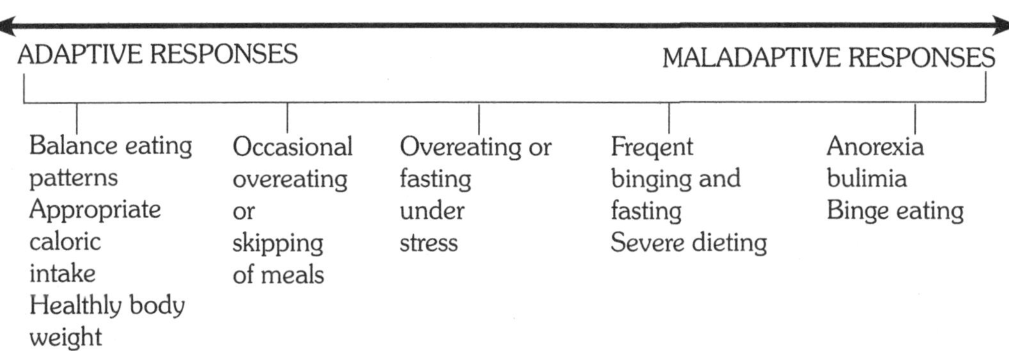

Fig. 11.1: Continuum of eating regulation responses (redrawn from Stuart GW, 1995)

Anorexia Nervosa

Definition and Meaning

Anorexia nervosa is characterized by voluntary refusal to eat, significant weight loss, an intense fear of becoming overweight and a pronounced disturbance of body image. The individual with anorexia nervosa may restrict food intake or engage in binge eating followed by self-induced vomiting or misuse of laxatives.

It is a condition that is seen mainly in young women, has become increasingly prevalent. Usually these are bright achievers, males also suffer from this disorder. It is characterized by an aversion to food, it may result in death owing to serious malnutrition.

The onset of anorexia nervosa is typically in mid to late adolescence (14–18 years) and rarely is after 40 years of age. Its onset is associated with stressful life events. It is seen in about 5% of adolescent females and 5–10% of all males. It usually starts by the age of 10–19 years.

Causes/Etiology

The exact etiology of anorexia nervosa is not clear. Several theories offer insight into the nature of disorder.

- Biological theory suggests that anorexic individuals suffer a disturbance in levels of neurotransmitters in brain.
- Psychodynamic theory suggests that deficits in ego development may predispose young children to anorexia.
- Family system theory views that anorexia nervosa is caused by intrafamilial conflicts and dysfunctional family.

Some other factors that may contribute to the development of this disorder include disturbed self-image, parent-child conflicts, past and present experiences resulting in feelings of dependency and helplessness, the adolescent's desire to return to the alleged comfort and safety of childhood, a stressful life situation, psychotic depression or early manifestation of schizophrenia. Starvation is an attention-getting device that permits the anorectic client full control of her body, allows her to remain in or revert to a prepubertal state, and is considered manipulative behavior.

CLINICAL FEATURES

- Extreme weight loss.
- Intense or irrational fear of weight gain.
- Distorted body image, weight or shape.
- Other physical manifestations like amenorrhea for up to 3 months, hypothermia, muscle wasting, cardiac dysrhythmias, hypotension, dry skin, brittle nails and cold intolerance.

Three main key features of anorexia nervosa are:

1. Refusal to maintain a healthy body weight.
2. An intense fear of gaining weight.
3. A distorted body image.

The DSM-IVTR states that the anorectic has an intense fear of becoming obese although weight loss occurs. Even when emaciated, the person insists that he/she is fat, displaying a distortion of body image. A weight loss of at least 15% of the original body weight is seen, as well as the refusal to maintain at least minimal body weight for age and height. No known physical illness or disease is responsible for the weight loss.

Various methods are used to lose weight. They include induced vomiting, laxatives, enemas, diuretics, diet pills, excessive exercise, binging and purging, stimulants for refusal to eat. Deceitful behavior may prevail as the anorectic client disposes of food as she is supposed to eat.

Types of Anorexia Nervosa

There are two ways of anorexia. In the restricting types of anorexia, weight loss is achieved by restricting calories (following drastic diets, fasting and excessive exercising). In the purging type of anorexia, weight loss is achieved by vomiting or using laxatives and diuretics.

Major Risk Factors for Anorexia Nervosa

- Body dissatisfaction.
- Strict dieting.
- Low self-esteem.
- Difficulty expressing feelings.
- Perfectionism.
- Troubled family relationships.
- History of physical or sexual abuse.
- Family history of eating disorders.

Management

The initial goal of management is overall improvement of body weight, normalization of eating patterns and restoration of physical health by weight gain. These goals cannot be attained unless the disordered thinking is corrected because the real issue is not with food but issues like poor self-esteem, need for perfection, and myth of slimming and dieting. So the client requires holistic interventions which include:

- Nutritional counseling by dietician and psychologist.
- Individual therapy to correct distortions and deficits in psychological thinking.
- Family therapy to correct disturbed patterns of interaction in family.
- Antidepressants and SSRIs maybe tried to be effective.
- Enhance self-esteem and self-worth of the individual so that he/she learns to like self, learns to trust and develop an identity beyond their thin body.
- Cognitive analytic therapy (CAT): This therapy combines psychodynamic with behavioral factors and focuses on interpersonal transference issues of the client.

Nursing Management

- Cognitive and behavioral therapy to positive and negative reinforcement, focus is on client's responsibility to gain weight.
  - Privileges are gained with weight gain.
  - Privileges are lost with weight loss.
- Increase self-esteem by acceptance and nonjudgmental approach so the client will realize that they do not need to artificial perfection as they believe what thinness provides. Assist so find other positive qualities about self.
- Health education about the disorder. The more information they receive that validates their problem, the less likely they will deny it.
- Monitor weight three times a week but weigh the patient facing away form the weighing machine to help them reduce their focus on weight. Makes sure the client is not hiding heavy objects under clothing.
- As soon as the ideal weight is gained allow the client to regulate his or her own progression and program.
- High protein and high carbohydrate diet, serve foods, the client prefer in small frequent feedings. NGT if the client refuses to eat.
- Limit setting to avoid manipulative behavior:
  - Restrict use of bathroom for 2 hours after eating.
  - Accompany to the bathroom to ensure that they will not self-induce vomiting.
  - Stay with client during meals.
  - Do not accept excuses to leave eating area.
- Help the client identify and express feelings. Avoid being judgmental. People with eating disorders are thought to be afraid of expressing strong emotions; they express their feelings unconsciously by vomiting, starvation and purging.
- Help the patient to identify and express other bodily concerns such as hair style, clothing, typically anorectic people have little bodily awareness other than a distorted perception of their size.
- Identify the clients nonweight related interests. This could help reduce anxiety, become creative outlet for energy, raise self-esteem and divert attention from eating and weight.

- Avoid being confrontational and engaging in long discussions or explanations about food or body.
- Ignore manipulative behaviors.
- Refer and involve self-help groups.

BULIMIA NERVOSA

Introduction

Bulimia nervosa is opposite to anorexia nervosa. Just as emotional factors contribute to refusal of food they also contribute to overeating. Food seems to be a source of satisfaction, security, love and relief also.

Definitions

- Bulimia nervosa/Purge disorder is disorder characterized by alternating dieting, binging and purging through vomiting, enema and laxatives.
- Bulimia nervosa is a disorder of binge eating, where the individual consumes large amount of food with lack of control followed by various compensatory behaviors like self-imposed vomiting to control weight.
- Episodic binge eating with a rapid consumption of a large amount of food in two hours is classified as bulimia. The person is aware that the behavior is abnormal, fears the inability to stop eating voluntarily, is self-critical and may experience depression after each episode.
  - According to DSM-IVTR the person with bulimia nervosa consumes high calories, easily ingested food, eats inconspicuously and terminates binging or gorging by self-induced vomiting, going to sleep or engaging in social functions and activities. The person may stop eating because of abdominal pain.
  - The person may stop eating because of abdominal pain, repeated attempts are made to lose weight by fasting or dieting; by abusing laxatives, enemas or diuretics, by self-induced vomiting or by abusing over the counter weight control drugs. Weight fluctuation is observed during the owing to alternating dieting or fasting and binging.

Incidence and Causes

Incidence of bulimia nervosa is higher than anorexia nervosa. Bulimia occurs in about 1–15% females with lower rates in males. The disorder is seen in age group of 15–30 years, with peak incidence at about 18–19 years of age. It is usually found in individuals involved in sports or careers that require low body weight (like models, dancers, wrestling, etc.), those who have been sexually abused and who have a family history of depression, substance abuse and eating disorders.

The onset of bulimia nervosa occurs in adolescence or early adult life. Many adolescents feel insecure about their physical shape and size in a society that places value on external appearance and nurturing. Parents and family members also play a great deal of influence during the development of the adolescent's self-concept and perceptions of the world.

Certain traits are found among individuals who view themselves as unlovable, inadequate and unworthy. The desire to please becomes very powerful as the adolescent strives to be perfect, thin, loved and accepted. The psychiatric implications are significant because approximately

50% of clients with bulimia nervosa also experience depression and require antidepressant medications. Substance abuse is commonly seen. Bulimia nervosa may develop into a chronic disorder and occur intermittently over several years.

CLINICAL FEATURES

- Individuals with bulimia have an intense fear of getting fat and are very sensitive to weight gain because they lack impulse control.
- Binge eating stops when abdominal discomfort occurs.
- After binge eating, the adolescents feel out of control, depressed, guilty and anxious.
- Self-induced vomiting and misuse of laxatives and diuretics is also observed, due to which the person loses the ability to experience hunger and satiety.
- Fasting or excessive exercise as compensatory behaviors to prevent weight gain.

Common Complications Related to Manner of Purging

- Chronic inflammation of the living of the esophagus due to induced vomiting, acidic gastric secretions irritates esophageal mucosa.
  - Rupture of the esophagus and stomach.
  - Electrolytic imbalance or abnormalities, leading to arrhythmias of the heart and metabolic alkalosis.
  - Dilation of the stomach.
  - Chronic enlargement of the parotid gland.
  - Rectal prolapse or abscess.
  - Dental erosion.
  - Chronic edema.
  - Fungal infection of vagina and rectum.

Management

- Behavior modification is used to control binge eating and then induced vomiting.
- Cognitive therapy maybe opted, as bulimic individuals have distorted thoughts and beliefs related to food, weight, body image and self-concept. Cognitive therapy helps in developing a sense of self, perception of one's body and enhancing self-esteem and self-concept.
- Dietary counseling maybe tried out.
- SSRI drugs have been shown effective in reducing the urge to binge and in treating depression.

Nursing Management

Nursing Diagnosis

- Alterations in health maintenance.
- *Altered nutrition:* Less than body requirements.
- *Altered nutrition:* More than body requirements.
- Anxiety
- Body image disturbance.
- Ineffective family coping compromised.
- Ineffective individual coping.
- Self-esteem disturbance.

Nursing Interventions

- Client with bulimia are aware of their problems as they want to be helped because they feel helpless and unable to control themselves during episode of binging. But because of their intense desire to please and need to conform, they may resort to manipulative acts and may provide half-truths. During assessment to gain trust and acceptance of health worker, creates an atmosphere of trust. Accept person as worthwhile individual. If they know that no rejection or punishment is forthcoming, they disclose their problem, they will be more open and honest.
- Develop strength to cope with problems. Encourage patient to discuss positive qualities about themselves to increase self-esteem.
- Help client identify feelings and situations associated with or that triggers binge eating.
  - Assist to explore alternative and positive ways of coping.
  - Encourage making a journal of incident and feelings before, during and after a binge episode.
  - Make a contract with the client to approach the nurse when they feel the urge to binge so that feelings and alternate ways of coping can be explored.
- Encourage adhering to meal and snack schedule of diet. This decreases the incidence of binging, which is often precipitated by starvation and fasting.
- Encourage participating in group activities with other persons having the same eating disorder to gain additional support.
- For young adolescent living at home, encourage family therapy to correct and modify dysfunctional family patterns.
- Cognitive behavioral therapy is the ideal therapy to help the bulimic understand the problem and explore appropriate behaviors.
- Practice positive reinforcement, modeling, behavioral shaping and overcorrection treatment may also be used.

OBESITY

According to Diagnostic and Statistical Manual of Mental Disorders (DSM-IVTR), obesity is not listed as a mental health disorder because it has not been established that obesity is consistently associated with mental health or behavioral problems. However, obesity is linked to many physical and psychological problems including socioenvironmental; that cause distress for most overweight individuals.

Obesity is defined as an excess of body weight. Clients are classified as mildly obese (20 to 40% above normal weight), moderately obese (41 to 100% above normal weight) and severely (morbidly) obese (over 100% above normal weight). Concern with being overweight is common in modern global societies in which the luxury of chronic overeating and underexercising is available. Nowadays, India is also facing this menace.

Obesity is the result of too many calories consumed or not enough calories burned. Although, the eating pattern of obese individuals do not pose an immediate threat, being chronically overweight can eventually result in severe physical and emotional problems. Today, much money and time is spent on the pursuit of losing weight throughout the world.

The causes of obesity are many and complex. Changes in neurochemicals also a contributory factor. Heredity appears to play a major role in the development of obesity. The children of obese parents tend to be overweight themselves. Obese persons have larger fat cells in their bodies. Lack of sufficient exercise also contributes greatly to obesity.

Faulty eating behaviors appear to begin in childhood. Many overweight persons once relied on food to numb the emotional discomforts of growing up. Throughout childhood they learned to cope by eating, which helped to relieve the emotional distresses of life. This pattern of lessening emotional pain by eating is called compulsive overeating. In time, food becomes like a drug, with a 'fix' that temporarily lessens psychological discomforts of an ever-growing for more food.

As the individual continues to find comfort in food, he/she grows physically more obese and becomes less attractive to others. This behavior serves only to increase feelings of worthlessness, an the person begins to replace social relationships with the comforts of food. Compulsive overeating can become a lonely way of life.

CLINICAL PRESENTATION

The first sign of obesity are seen early in life. An estimate maybe made by comparing one's height and weight to a standardized chart, e.g. IAP, obesity scale, ICMR obesity chart. Usually children who are 20% over normal for their height and weight should undergo further evaluation, including height and weight history of the child, parents and siblings, as well as eating habits, appetite and hunger patterns and physical activity.

As overweight children grow and mature, they begin to sense society's disapproval of their obesity. Youngsters may begin to diet and exercise or react by continuing to find comfort in food. Dieting and other weight loss methods soon become a way of life for many overweight people at a young age.

During adolescence, weight becomes an important part of a newly forming body image. Teens may discard against parental pressure to lose weight or become unwilling to control their caloric intake. They may resort to unhealthy methods, such as prolonged-fasting or purging, to gain some control over their weight. Not infrequently they will ignore their obesity and continue to eat as though a problem does not exist.

The cycle of ' I am not attractive, so I shall eat because it makes me feel better becomes ingrained as a way of coping in childhood and early adolescence. Many overweight individuals become more obese as they grow older. Eventually, the numerous chronic health problems associated with moderate or severe obesity begin to appear. These problems increase anxiety and further encourage the individual to seek the comfort that food has so frequently brought in the past. The cycle continues and problems grow. Obesity is managed by exercises, counseling and in extreme conditions bariatric surgery can be performed.

ATTENTION DEFICIT HYPERACTIVE DISORDERS (ADHD)

Attention deficit hyperactivity disorder (ADHD) is one of the most common childhood disorder and can continue through adolescence and adulthood.

ADHD is a behavioral disorder that is characterized by hyperactivity, impulsiveness, inattention or a combination of these behaviors that are more frequent and severe than would be expected for the age. It is usually not diagnosed before the age of four and is more common in boys than girls.

ADHD characteristics include a short attention span, impulsivity and distractibility.

TYPES OF ADHD

- *Predominantly hyperactive-impulsive type of ADHD.*
  - It is characterized by the presence of symptoms of hyperactivity.
  - Impulsivity at least 6 months.
- *Predominantly inattentive-types of ADHD.*
  - Characterized by the presence of symptoms of inattention and absence of or less symptoms of hyperactivity for at least 6 months.
- *Combined hyperactive-impulsive and inattentive type of ADHD.*
  - Most children and adolescents have this type of ADHD. In this type both symptoms of inattention and hyperactivity are present for at least 6 months.

Causes/Etiology

Researchers are not sure what causes ADHD, although many research studies suggest that genes play a large role. Like any other illnesses, ADHD probably results from a combination of factors and are studying now brain injuries, nutrition, drugs and social environment might contribute to ADHD.

Genetics

Heredity factors appear to be involved in the development of ADHD. Research have shown that parents who had symptoms of hyperactivity in their own childhood had hyperactive children.

Biochemical Theories

According to biochemical theories, ADHD may be caused by low levels of dopamine and norepinephrine in the brain.

Prenatal Causes

Prenatal factors involved are complications and problems in pregnancy, difficult deliveries, maternal smoking and drug abuse, and exposure to toxins during pregnancy.

Environmental Factors

Exposure to environment maybe considered as a causative factor in the development of ADHD.

Food Additives

Recent British researchers linked a possible cause with consumption of certain food additives like artificial colors or preservatives and an increase in activity.

Sugar

Research postulated that refined sugar causes ADHD and makes symptoms more worse.

Psychosocial Factors

These include maternal illness, pathological families, paternal criminality, low socioeconomic status, disruption of bonding in the first 3 years of life and infant malnutrition.

SIGNS AND SYMPTOMS

There are three different categories of ADHD symptoms:

1. Inattention
2. Hyperactivity
3. Impulsivity

Inattention may not become apparent until a child enters the challenging environment of school. In adults, symptoms of inattention may manifest in work or in social situations.

A person with ADHD may have some or all of the following symptoms:

- Difficulty paying attention to details and tendency to make careless mistakes in school or other activities, producing work that is often messy and careless.
- Easily distracted by irrelevant stimuli and frequently interrupting ongoing tasks to attend to trivial noises or events that are usually ignored by others.
- Inability to sustain attention on tasks or activities.
- Difficulty finishing school work or paperwork or performing tasks that require concentration.
- Frequent shifts from one uncompleted activity to another.
- Procrastination.
- Disorganized work habits.
- Forgetfulness in daily activities (e.g. missing appointments, forgetting to bring lunch).
- Failure to complete tasks such as homework or household chores.
- Frequent shifts in conversation, not listening to others, not keeping one's mind on conversation and not following details or rules of activities in social situations.
- *Hyperactivity:* Symptoms maybe apparent in very young preschoolers and are nearly always present before the age of seven. Symptoms include:
  - Fidgeting, squirming when seated.
  - Getting up frequently to walk or run around.
  - Running or climbing excessively when it is inappropriate (in teens, this may appear as restlessness).
  - Always being 'on the go'.
  - Often talking excessively.
- Hyperactivity may vary with age and developmental stage.
- Toddlers and preschooler's with ADHD tend to be constantly in motion, jumping on furniture and having difficulty participating in sedentary group activities for instance. They may have trouble listening to a story or poem.
- Schoolage children display similar behaviors but with less frequency. They are unable to remain seated, squirm a lot, fidget or talk excessively.

Impulsivity symptoms include:

- Impatience.
- Difficulty delaying responses.
- Blurting out answers before questions have been completed.
- Difficulty awaiting one's turn.
- Frequently interrupting or intruding on other to the point of causing problems in social or work situations.
- Initiating conversations at inappropriate times.

Impulsivity may lead to Impulsivity such a knocking over objects or banging into people. Children with ADHD may also engage in potentially dangerous activities without considering the consequences for instance, they may jump or climb to precarious positions.

Many of these symptoms occur from time to time in normal youngsters. However, in children with ADHD they occur frequently at home and at school or when visiting with friends. They also interfere with the child's ability to function as other children of the same age or developmental level.

ADHD is diagnosed only when children consistently display some or all of the above behaviors in at least two settings, such as at home and in school for at least six months.

Long-term Prognosis with ADHD

- Some children with ADHD approximately 20 to 30% develop learning problems that may not improve with ADHD treatment. Hyperactive behavior may be associated with the development of other disruptive behaviors.
- As they grow older, may experience periods of anxiety or depression.
- Several of the symptoms of ADHD may get work as the demands at school or home increase they include:
  - Difficulty following instruction.
  - Being unable to get organized either at home or at school.
  - Fidgeting especially with the hands and feet.
  - Talking too much.
  - Failing to finish project, including chores and homework.
  - Not paying attention to and responding to details.
  - Getting poor grades in school.
  - Being isolated from peers due to poor grades and secondary depression.

Diagnosis

Children mature at different rates and have different personalities, temperaments and energy levels. Most children get distracted, act impulsively and struggle to concentrate at one time or another sometimes. These normal factors maybe mistakes for ADHD. ADHD symptoms appear early in life, often between the age of 3 and 6 or 7 and because symptoms vary form person to person, the disorder can be hard to diagnose. Parents may first notice that their child loses interest in things sooner than other children or seems constantly 'out of control'. Often teachers notice the symptoms first, when a child has trouble following rules, or frequently 'spaces out' in the classroom or on the playground.

Some children with ADHD also have other illnesses or conditions such as learning disability, oppositional defiant disorder, conduct disorder, anxiety and depression, bipolar disorder, Tourette's syndrome, etc. ADHD also may coexist with a sleep disorder, bedwetting, substance abuse or other disorder illnesses.

Treatment

The treatment of ADHD focus on reducing the symptoms of ADHD and improving functioning. The treatment include medication, various types of psychotherapy, education or training or a combination of these.

Treatments can retrieve many of the disorder's symptoms but there is no cure with treatment, most people with ADHD, can be successful in school lead productive lives.

Pharmacological Treatment

CNS stimulants are prescribed to these children. It actually has a calming effect in children to treat ADHD.

Commonly used stimulants are dextroamphetamine with doses of 2.5 mg/day to 40 mg/day. Methylphenidate 5 mg/day to 60 mg/day and pemoline 37.5 mg/day to 112.5 mg/day. These drugs acts on reticular activating system causing stimulation of inhibitory influences on the cerebral cortex, thus decreasing hyperactivity and/or destructivity. Other drugs are used:

- Bupropion 3 mg/kg/day
- Imipramine 1 mg/kg/day to 2.5 mg/kg/day.

Behavior Therapy

Counseling and supportive psychotherapy can also helps

- *Parenting skills training:* It helps parents learn how to use a system of rewards and consequences to change a child's behavior. Parents are taught to give immediate and positive feedback for behaviors they want to encourage. In some cases, the use of 'time-outs' may be used when the child's behavior gets out of control. In a time-out, the child is removed from the upsetting situations and sits alone for a time to calm down.

Parents are also encouraged to share a pleasant or relaxing activity with the child, to notice and point out what the child does well, and to praise the child's strength and abilities. They may also learn to structure situation in more positive ways. For example, they may restrict the number of playmates to one or two, so that their child does not become overstimulated or if the child has trouble completing tables, parents can help child divide large tasks into smaller, more manageable steps. Also, parents may benefit from learning stress, management techniques to increase their own ability to deal with frustration, so that they can respond calmly to their child's behavior.

Sometimes the whole family may need therapy. Therapists can help family members find better ways to handle disruptive behaviors and to encourage behaviors changes. Finally, support groups help parents and families connect with others who have similar problems and concerns. Groups often meet regularly to share frustration and successes, to exchange information about recommended by specialists and strategies and talk to specialists.

Cognitive Behavior Therapy

Cognitive behavior therapy helps the child to control their thought and in turn their behavior.

Social Skills Training

Here the child is taught important social skills like having a conversation or playing cooperatively with colleagues and other playmates.

Anger Management

The child is taught how to recognize the signs of growing frustration and taught coping skills designed to manage anger and aggression. Relaxation techniques and stress management skills are also taught to them.

Encouragement

Many children with behavior disorders experience repeated failures at school and in their interaction with others. Encouraging the child to excel in their particular talents like sports/ gardening/painting can help to build and rebuild self-esteem.

Nursing Management

Nursing Interventions

The nurse may participate in assessing and therapies to provide nursing interventions in a hospital setting. Rules for establishing a therapeutic relationship with a child are:

- Accept a child or adolescent as an equal when able, keeping in mind the person's age.
- Do not be baby like, or use substandard language. Listen to the emotions expressed and encourage verbalization of feelings.
- Do not force yourself on the patients or push him or her to confide in you.
- Accept the person but discerns any undesirable behavior. Each behavior needs to be evaluated to decide the appropriate approach.
- Be a good role model.

Another suggestion is to watch one's body language or nonverbal communication. Children and adolescents are quite observant of what adults say and how they can communicate feelings both verbally and nonverbally. They should know that adults have good and bad days that can affect their interpersonal relationships especially in the area of communication.

Other aspects of nursing interventions include:

- Helping the child to master developmental tasks to overcome regressive slow or impaired developmental behavior.
- Establishing a method of communication with persons who have difficulty communicating, such as the withdrawn, disoriented, mute, hostile, preoccupied or autistic child.
- Identifying stimuli that might foster abusive, destructive or otherwise negative behavior and
- Allowing time for the person to respond to therapeutic interventions.
  - Nurses should be aware of their own reaction to client's behaviors. If unable to handle feelings or behaviors, they should seek assistance from peers or supervisory personnel. They also should respect the child's spatial territory and not invade her or his privacy. Therapeutic touch is used only after exploring the person's feelings about being touched (e.g. a battered or abused child).
  - Psychiatric nurse may plan activities appropriate for the child's development level and age. They should consider the child's energy level and need to calm down after an activity.
  - The main nursing management for an ADHD child is to change the environment so that the child is able to alter or improve his or her reaction to the environment. Environmental stimuli are kept at a minimum while the child is medicated with CNS stimulants that have a paradoxical effect that prevents flooding of the cerebral cortex by impulses. The role of nurse is to identify, reduce or eliminate such stimuli as well as to administer the medication. The nurse may also work with the family or teachers to plan a firm, consistent, predictable environment. Limits and standards must be set while employing behavior therapy. The symptoms generally subside at puberty.

CONDUCT DISORDERS

Conduct disorder is a childhood behavior disorder, characterized by aggressive and destructive activities that cause disruptions in the child's natural environments such as home, school, playground, church/temple or the neighborhood. The main iconic feature of conduct disorder is the repetitive and persistent pattern of behaviors that violate societal norms and the civil rights of other people. Earlier it was called as juvenile delinquency.

Definition

According to DSM-IVTR conduct disorder is a repetitive and persistent pattern of behavior in which the basic rights of others or major age appropriate societal norms or rules are violated.

Common Conduct Disorders in Children

- Lying
- Stealing
- Fire setting
- Constant disobedience
- Truancy from school
- Running away from home
- Sexual problems
- Gambling
- Drug abuse.

Other forms of conduct disorders that are not so commonly seen are assault, robbery, rape, homicide, burglary, theft, forgery, fraud, trading stolen goods and property, vandalism, prostitution, boot-legging and smuggling.

Aggression may Include

- Bullying
- Fighting
- Weapon use
- Cruel to people and animals
- Stealing with confrontation
- Forced sex

Destruction of Property may Include

- Fire setting
- Other property destruction
- Vandalism

Deceitfulness/Theft

- Breaking in (house, car/jeep)
- Lying
- Stealing

Serious Rule Violations

- Staying out late (before 13)
- Frequent truancy (before 13)
- Running away overnight.

The specific behavior used to produce a diagnosis of conduct disorder fall into four groups:

1. Aggressive conduct that causes or threatens physical harm to other people or animals.
2. Nonaggressive behavior that causes property loss or damage, deceitfulness or theft and serious violations of rules, deceitfulness or theft, and serious property violations of rules. Severity is classified as mild, moderate or severe, depending on the number of problems exhibited and their impact on other people.
3. The negative consequences of conduct disorder, particularly childhood onset, may include illicit drug use, dropping out of school, violent behavior, severe family conflict and frequent delinquent acts.
4. The financial costs of crime and correction of repeated juvenile offenses by youth with conduct disorders are extensive and enormous. The social costs include citizen's fear of such behavior, loss of a sense of safety, and disruptions in school that interfere organizational climate. The costs to the child and his/her family are enormous in terms of the emotional and other resources needed to address the consequences of conduct disorders.

Etiology

There is no known exact cause for conduct disorder. The frustrating behavior of youngsters with conduct disorder frequently leads to blaming and other unproductive activities. Children who are 'acting out' do not inspire sympathy or the benefit of the doubt. They are often ostracized by other children. Parents of such children are often blamed as poor disciplinarians or bad parents. As a result, parents of children with conduct disorder maybe reluctant to engage with schools or other authorities. At the same time, there is a strong correlation between children diagnosed with conduct disorder and a significant level of family dysfunction, poor parenting practices, an overemphasis on coercion and hostile communication patterns, verbal and physical aggression and a history of maltreatment.

Genetics

Genetic vulnerability is a newer concept. The XXY syndrome and conduct disorder is far from probable. Criminality and antisocial behavior has been reported in clients of Klinefelter's syndrome (XXY) by Brown (1962) and Frossman (1966). Eysenck (1970) felt that neurotic extroverts had a special predisposition to delinquency while Hoghughi and Forest (1970) applying this theory to school boys, failed to confirm this hypothesis. It has now been realized that both behavioral as well as physical characteristics may have a genetic predisposition. The dermatographic and buccal smear studies of juvenile delinquents carried out by Agarwal Sethi and Gupta (1978) reported the following findings:

- Incidence of tented arch on index finger was higher.
- Incidence of ulnar loop on ring finger was significantly higher.
- No differences in position of axial tri radii in both hands.

- Frequency of open patterns in thenar area was lower.
- No differences were seen in palmar crease.

Body Build

The XXY syndrome is associated with maleness and muscularity and these traits generally belong to the psychopathic group. Sheldon (1949) postulated that the children of mesomorphic group were represented more in group of juvenile delinquents. Stott (1976) inferred that certain parental factors affected the behavior patterns and body build of these children. Lombroso (1986) stated that criminals had some typical features like short stature, particular shape of skull, longer lower jaws, flat nose, scanty beard and low sensitivity to pain. This was replicated by Goring (1913). Hooton (1939) stated that the primary cause of crime was biological inferiority.

Gender

The number of boys compared to girls is very large. Schwartz (1949) put the ratio at 12:1. Maller (1949) in New York stated that 93% of delinquents were boys. After 1935, the girls showed an increase and each year showed a rise in number of girls. The researchers conducted a study at Mumbai and put male-female ratio at 7:3. Murthy, Ghosh and Verma (1974) analyzed the children of a child guidance clinic and conferred the ratio at 10:1.

Age

Delinquency usually starts with the onset of puberty. In India, it occurs as early as 12 years and increases after 12. The upsurge of sex at the time of puberty contributes largely to delinquency. Aggressive and antisocial behavior is seen between 4–6 years of age in boys.

Intelligence

Delinquency has been associated with both superior intelligence as well as borderline mental retardation.

Family Background

Fergusson (1952) found that delinquents generally belong from poor families, where the number of children was large and parents were unable to attend to the individual needs of children. Also single child shows less delinquency than middle or youngest one.

EEG Studies

The EEG has helped far and wide in many disorders, but with regard to delinquency there has been little to look for. Loomis (1965) did a detailed study of EEGs of delinquents, but failed to show that it differed from that of nondelinquents.

Personality Testing

Abrahamsen (1960) mentioned that behavior problems might be a direct expression of repressed desires that might be result of an ego that had become maladjusted because of the conflicting forces excreted on it by id and superego. Somasundram and Ponnudurai (1980) used the Jesness Inventory while studying juvenile delinquency in girls and found it very useful to distinguish between delinquent and normal girls, on the subtests of social maladjustment, immaturity, autism, alienation, aggression and the antisocial index. On personality testing the delinquents show characteristics traits of egocentricity, antisocial attitude, antisocial tendencies, hyperactivity, fear, epileptoid features and social maladjustment.

CLINICAL MANIFESTATIONS

The DSM-IVTR indicates that for conduct disorder to be diagnosed, the patient has repeatedly violated rules, age appropriate social norms and the rights of others for a period of at least twelve months. This is shown by three or more of the following behaviors, with at least one having taken place in the previous six months; aggression to people or animals, property destruction, lying or theft and serious rule violations.

Aggression to people or animals includes:
- Engaging in frequent bullying or threatening.
- Often starting fights.
- Using a weapon that could cause serious injury (gun, knife, club, broken glass).
- Showing physical cruelty to people.
- Showing cruelty to animals.
- Engaging in theft with confrontation (armed robbery, extortion, mugging, purse snatching).
- Forcing sex upon someone.

Property destruction includes:
- Deliberately setting fires to cause serious damage.
- Deliberately destroying the property of others by means other than fire setting.

Lying or theft includes:
- Breaking into building, car or house belonging to someone else.
- Frequently lying or breaking promises for gain or to avoid obligations (called 'conning')
- Stealing valuables without confrontation (burglary, forgery, shop lifting).

Serious rule violation include:
- Beginning before age 13, frequently staying out at night against parent's wishes.
- Running away from parents overnight twice or more once if for an extended period.
- Engaging in frequent traunancy beginning before the age 13.
- Mild severity would mean there are few problems with conduct beyond those needed to make a diagnosis and all of the problems cause little harm to the people. Moderate severity means the number and effect of the conduct problems is between the extremes of mild and severe. Severe is indicated if there are many more conduct symptoms than are needed to make diagnosis (more than three in the previous twelve months or more than one in the previous six months) or the behaviors cause other people considerable harm.

Treatment/Management

Conduct disorders need multimodal approach. It is very difficult to decide, whether conduct disordered should be put in an institution or not.
- *Preventive aspects*
- *Corrective therapy:* These include:
  - Protective therapy, which not only extends to custodial care, but also to probation or parole.
- *Punitive therapy:* To bring about certain changes in the personality and behavior of the delinquent.

- *Rehabilitative therapy:* Helps to lead a normal life.
- *Family therapy:* Here, parents learn to apply behavioral principles effectively, how to play with their children, and how to teach and coach the child to use new skills.
- *Medication management:* These are useful in aggression. Tranqualizers in adequate dose should be administered. Chlorpromazine 25–50 kg, three times a day is the ideal choice. Also haloperidol can be given orally in dose of 1.5–10 mg, three times a day. In case of severe uncontrolled aggression, IV/IM can be administered.

OTHER PROBLEMS OF ADOLESCENTS

Sexual Problems: Inappropriate Sexual Activity

Ideally, the adolescent is supposed to wait until a certain age when economic independence has been achieved and marriage and subsequent monogamous, heterosexual activities are condoned. In this age group, stimulation for sexual activity is generally strong.

Sexual behavior can be the cause of many teenage problems. Adolescents tend to use their sexuality to sublimate other needs such as love and security; personal anxiety about sexual adequacy and peer pressure.

Some may involve sexual activity for experimentation and joy leading to risk for HIV infection and other sexually transmitted diseases. Substance use and improper health information may increase the risk potential of adolescents because they are more likely to have unplanned sexual activity.

Stress and Its Related Disorders

The adolescent is subjected to pressure from many sources. Many of his/her difficulties are caused by culture, and society in which they live. They feel that he/she does not belong, that he/she is different, that others view him with suspiciousness and hostility.

Depression and Suicide

Depression is more prevalent due to more stressor, or abstract thinking, rumination and personal fable. The symptoms increase during adolescence, then decrease in adulthood.

Adolescents may develop feeling of helplessness, hopelessness and worthlessness leading them to develop depression and suicidal ideation and attempts. Between the age of 11 and 15 years, the rate of depression in girls rises rapidly, while slightly low in boys. Girls think and worry more than boys.

Suicide is the fourth leading cause of death among children age between 10–14 years and third leading cause of death among youth age between 15–24 years. One of most common causes of adolescent's suicide is lack or loss of a meaningful relationship. Parent-adolescents relationship can play an important role in prevention. The nurse who is serving with an adolescent having suicidal ideation idea tan should make it clear that this behavior is not confidential and that parents will be counseled. Family involvement is essential to avoid angry, hostile and hopeless feelings.

Insecurity and Anxiety are Caused by Thwarting

The adolescent faces great deal of insecurity in his relations with others and particularly with adults. The society hopes and expects that he/she should behave like an adult but not too much like an adult. The adolescent is also eager to play adult behavior but he/she does not know whether he/she has gone too far enough. The state of affairs causes a sense of insecurity and anxiety. Anxiety is caused by the fact that the adolescent is living at two kinds of societies—teenage society and adult society. The behavior that satisfies one irritates the other therefore, all these causes tension in adolescents.

Runaways

The number of adolescents who runaway or are forced to run from their homes and become homeless is growing nowadays. Many adolescents leave their home because of dysfunctional or abusive family, sexual harassment and poverty. Runaways result from conflicting thoughts and feelings of depression and independence. This can result in panic that motivates running away to prove autonomy and self-image to escape painful circumstances of life. Often adolescents become involved in dangerous, unlawful, unethical activities after running away from homes. Most of them may involve in drug abuse.

Violence and Criminal Offences

Violence and aggressive behavior is a human impulse that must be channeled constructively by a learned process that occurs within a supportive loving relationship. Under favorable condition a child learns the healthy expression of aggression by involvement in activities that result in pleasure and active problem-solving attempts. Under unfavorable conditions aggression can result in destructive activities that are harmful to self and others. Sometimes, these activities can lead to adolescents involving in criminal offences. Most adolescents involving in violent activities have experienced frustration and had violent role model during their childhood. Adolescents who have committed extreme acts of violence is homicide are often from families in which violence is condoned in some form. These adolescents may have experienced physical or sexual abuse or they may have witnessed violence between their parents. Violent adolescents may have the history of dangerous assaults on family members and pets, drug abuse, poor school performance and a history of fighting and violence. In severely violent adolescents, violent behavior maybe followed by calmness and lack of sorrow and guilt.

Unwed Motherhood

Pregnancy in adolescents is a complicated issue. It can be of various origins. It can occur accidentally after sexual exploration, unawareness about contraceptive methods and sometimes pregnancy is an effort to escape a difficult family situation or to force the parents to accept and agree to a marriage. Pregnancy in unmarried adolescents may also be associated with sexual promiscuity. Sometimes pregnancy occurs within close caring relationship. Decision-making and involving abortion, continue with pregnancy and marriage are difficult issues. Attitudes and laws play an important role in it. Marriage, abortion and continue with pregnancy are various alternatives which can be taken into consideration. The adolescent girls should make her decision with the help and support of her parents, the family members, the nurse and others involved health care professionals.

Substance Use

Substance use and abuse are significant problem of youth in every country and culture. It carries serious consequences among adolescents causing 50% of the deaths in younger age of 15–24

years. Drugs and alcohol abuse is one of the risk taking behaviors among adolescents. These are capable of providing pleasure by giving relaxation and prolonged heightened sensation. These drug consumption also contribute to assaults and rapes by adolescents. Alcohol is the most commonly used and abused substances by youth. Most of youngers of higher secondary report some taste of alcohol. Higher levels of adolescent alcohol use are associated with the three most frequent forms of mortality among adolescent accidental deaths, homicides and suicides. Nearly 75% of automobile accidents involve the use of alcohol and other drugs.
Adolescents often report a wish for closeness that is expressed by sharing a drug experience with colleagues and near and dear ones.

Drug users can experience an illusion of closeness, a sharing attitude because of drug use. The drug consuming behavior can be an expression of rebelliousness with support of a peer towards authority of parents and teachers as well as a way of obtaining gratification. Repeated and regular use of drugs for recreational purposes can lead to problems of anxiety and depression. Some adolescents use substances to decrease their anxiety especially when socializing. Use of tobacco is another substance very much consumed nowadays. Smoking usually starts in 6th to 9th grades and addiction typically occurs before the age of 20 years. Tobacco can be the first drug, adolescents use before expanding the experimentation to other substances. It has also been noted that smoking teens tend to fight more, carry weapons and engage in high-risk sexual behaviors.

MOOD DISORDERS IN ADOLESCENTS

Mood disorders in adolescents appear in children of all ages and gender. It is increasingly diagnosed and treated with multimodal therapies. Depressive disorders and bipolar I are generally episodic and onset maybe insidious, comorbidity is also common in children.

Mood disorders in preschool age are extremely rare (0.3% in community and 0.9% in clinical area). In hospitalized children and adolescents about 20% of children and 40% adolescents are tend to be depressed. In adolescents dysthymic disorder is less common than major depressive disorder. The prevalence rate is about 3.3% for dysthymic disorder and 5% for depressive disorder. The lifetime rate of bipolar I disorder is 0.6% in community. Depression is seen more in boys than girls among school age people.
Major depressive episode is characterized by insidious onset and may occur after hyperactivity.

- Depressed or irritable mood, loss of interest or pleasure
- Anhedonia, failure to meet expected weight gains and loss of appetite.
- Daily insomnia or hypersomnia, psychomotor agitation or retardation, sudden or gradual marked lowering of mood and daily fatigue or loss of energy. Retardation of movement, speech, agitation and pressure of speech.
- Thoughts of unworthiness, guilt, hopelessness about future, desire of death and suicidal behavior.
- Delusions and hallucinations are usually absent.

Bipolar I disorder is characterized by elevated, expansive or irritable mood that lasts for one week or any duration. The usual symptoms include-decreased need for sleep, pressure of speech, racing of thoughts, distractibility, increase in goal directed activities and excessive involvement in pleasureable activities. Delusions and hallucinations of adolescents may involve grandiose notions about their power, worth, knowledge, family and relationships. Persecutory delusions and flight of ideas are very common. Gross impairment in reality testing in adolescents having mania.

SCHIZOPHRENIA

Childhood schizophrenia affects an estimated one in 40000 children under the age of 13. During early teen years, the rate of onset of schizophrenia in the general population is enhancing and the peak rates of onset lie between the ages of 15 and 30 years.

In males the onset of schizophrenia is at the younger side of this range, while onset in females is usually at the older side of end.

A child or adolescent with schizophrenia may experience severe deterioration in the ability to function in social, personal and regular daily activities. Signs and symptoms include typical psychotic features like hallucinations, delusions, disorganized thinking, grossly disorganized irrational behavior, physical immobility, excessive mobility with no purpose, absent or inappropriate emotional expression, little verbal communication with other people (withdrawal) and absence of future plans.

Psychosocial and Personal Problems

The adolescent is faced with many emotional/psychosocial problems. He/she does things which, he later regrets. He/she wishes he were more popular but he finds himself ignored, isolated and rejected. He worries about little things but he cannot find answers to them. He wants to improve his prestige and position but fails.

He needs to develop self-confidence but he is not given ample opportunities. He is easily hurt. He is not sure of himself. He hesitates to assume responsibilities. In short, he remains in a continual tense psychological/emotional state which risks for psychiatric problems. Adolescence has therefore, been regarded as the period of stress and strain.

Management

When working with the adolescent's knowledge of normal adolescent's development is necessary to differentiate between age-expected behavior and maladaptive responses. When dealing with the adolescents it is recommended to have direct contact with the adolescents. By seeking direct contact with the adolescents' the psychiatric nurse aligns with the client's independent and mature aspects. Family session can also play an important role in thorough assessment, understanding family interactions and establishing family support.

PSYCHOEDUCATION

The psychiatric/mental heath nurse is in an excellent position to educate the client, the parents and in whole as community. Adolescents maybe interested in information regarding what activities are healthy and unhealthy, including facts regarding exercise, nutrition, dealing with anger, sexuality, conflicts, frustration resolutions and where they can access help and support. Basic health education can be provided in such areas as drug abuse, sex and contraception, suicide prevention/crime prevention and promotion of mental health. The nurse can also provide information regarding healthy emotional functioning including coping with stress, anxiety and morbidity.

The nurse can play an important role in educating the teachers and parents regarding normal adolescent's development, dealing with adolescents and dealing with problematic adolescents. Encouraging independence and decreasing power struggle can produce a positive change in adolescent's relationship with adults and their feelings about themselves.

Family Therapy

The psychiatric nurse needs to assess the level of family functioning and determine how to best interact with the help of family towards adolescents. Family therapy is particularly useful when disturbed family interaction is interfering with adolescent's development.

Group Therapy

It addresses adolescent's need for peer support. Conflicts with authority can be better detected by peers rather than adults, so involving adolescents in group therapy is particularly helpful for adolescents. Group therapy can be used effectively to teach adolescents the skills of relating and dealing with others and development of positive and meaningful attitude.

Individual Therapy

Individual therapy is provided by a trained therapist specialist psychiatric nurse. It is helpful with adolescents requiring help. Once the decision of individual therapy is made, a pact between the nurse and the adolescents is established and a therapeutic relationship is initiated.

Pharmacological Management

Various treatment options are used to manage complex problems of adolescent's psychological problems. Care should be taken while administrating drugs to adolescents. The use of SSRIs is preferred over TCAs because of their lower adverse effects profile and safety in overdose. The use of benzodiazepines is generally not recommended. Lithium is well tolerated by adolescents in the treatment of mania, aggression and conduct disorders. Antipsychotics are the standard treatment for psychiatric symptoms in adolescents. Use of psychological therapies and alternative therapies is very useful in treatment of adolescents looking into holistically.

Nursing Management of Organic Brain Disorders

INTRODUCTION

Organic brain disorders/syndrome is an umbrella term used to include a wide range of impaired mental functions due to cerebral damage or insult often called brain damage syndrome. Any brain damage may occur with no obvious mental changes, most clients with neurological signs of cerebral damage would show minor psychosocial deficit and the mental changes may continue even after the physical signs have disappeared.

These maybe acute, subacute or chronic. the common features include:

a. *Learning disorder:* That is speech, hearing.
b. *Motor disorder:* Over activity in coordination, involuntary movements.
c. *Emotional disorders:* Mood swings, impulsive behavior, catastrophic reactions, antisocial behavior and
d. *Cognitive disorders:* Poor memory, poor concentration, specific defects due to local lesions.

Definitions

- Organic brain disorders are the group of disorders resulting from identifiable cause in brain occurring due to general medical condition or a substance or a combination of these factors thus giving rise to psychosocial disturbances.
- Organic brain syndrome (OBS) is a general term for decrease in mental function that are not caused by a psychiatric disorder. Reduced mental function could include:
  - Problems with memory.
  - Difficulties understanding language.
  - Changes in behavior.
  - Trouble in performing daily activities.

Incidence and Prevalence

The exact incidence and prevalence of organic brain disorders are difficult to calculate. They are much seen among hospitalized inpatient such as medical, psychiatric and at out patients' clinics. It is believed to affect at least 10 to 30% of all causes.

Classification

Diagnostic and Statistical Manual of Mental Disorders: Fourth Edition (DSM-IV) uses the term Delirium. Dementia and the amnestic disorders (characterized by the primary symptoms common to all, i.e. impairment in cognition, in memory, language and attention) replacing the old terminology organic mental disorders.

Classification According to DSM-IV

- **Delirium**
  - Delirium due to a general medical condition.
  - Substance induced Delirium.
  - Delirium due to multiple etiologies.
  - Delirium not otherwise classified.
- **Dementia**
  - Dementia of the Alzheimer's type.
  - Dementia due to other general medical conditions.
  - Dementia due to HIV disease.
  - Dementia due to head trauma.
  - Dementia due to Parkinson's disease.
  - Dementia due to Huntington's disease.
  - Dementia due to Pick's disease.
  - Dementia due to other general medical conditions.
  - Substance induced persisting dementia.
  - Dementia due to multiple etiologies.
  - Dementia not otherwise specified.
- **Amnestic disorders**
  - Amnestic disorders due to general medical condition.
  - Substance induced persisting amnestic disorder.
  - Amnestic disorder not otherwise specified.
  - Cognitive disorder not otherwise specified.

ICD-10 Classification

- **F 00–F 09**: Organic, including symptoms, mental disorders.
- **F 00**: Dementia in Alzheimer's disease.
- **F 01**: Vascular dementia.
- **F 02**: Dementia in other disease classified elsewhere.
- **F 03**: Unspecified dementia.
- **F 04**: Organic amnestic syndrome, not induced by alcohol and other psychoactive substance.
- **F 05**: Delirium, not induced by alcohol and other psychoactive substances.
- **F 06**: Other mental disorders due to brain damage and dysfunction and to physical disease.
- **F 07**: Personality and behavioral disorders due to brain disease, damage and dysfunction.
- **F 08–F 09**: Unspecified organic or symptomatic mental disorder.

CLINICAL TYPES OF ORGANIC MENTAL DISORDERS

Delirium

According to Beresin (2008), the incidence of delirium among clients in medical and surgical departments of general hospitals was reported to be 12 to 17%. The incidence in elderly clients was more reported.

It is a very common organic disorders in medical and surgical units. It is presumed as everyone's psychosis, meaning anybody and everybody can develop this syndrome. It is the state of mental confusion and excitement characterized by disorientation in time and place/ person usually associated with different hallucinations and illusions.

Epidemiological Facts

Delirium is generally developed in clients admitted in general hospital, it is estimated that about 5–15% of clients in medical and surgical units develops delirium. It is also usually observed in Alzheimer's disease when a severe infection or other medical condition is superimposed on the pre-existing condition. It is also estimated that in elderly above 65 years of age, the prevalence rate ranges from 30–50%. Delirium can also be the first sign or only indicator of illness ranging from pneumonia, hypoglycemia to myocardial infarction. Failure to recognize delirium can lead to significant mortality and morbidity.

Causes

DSM-IV has described following types of delirium on the basis of etiology, although they share the same symptomatology.

- Delirium due to general medical condition.
  - This type of delirium develops when delirium symptoms are the result of any medical abnormality which can be evidenced by history, laboratory examination or physical examination.
  - These conditions can be:
  - Systemic infection that can be acute and chronic.
  - *Metabolic causes,* e.g. hypoxia, hypoglycemia, water and electrolyte imbalance, metabolic acidosis or alkalosis.
  - Nutritional deficiencies like thiamine deficiency and folic acid deficiency.
  - Postoperative state.
  - Hypertensive Encephalopathy.
  - Intracranial causes like epilepsy, head injury migraine, etc.

Substance Induced Delirium

Substance induced delirium is due to the adverse effects of medication, ingestion or withdrawal of substances or toxin poisoning. This type of delirium may result due to drugs like anesthetics, auticonvulsants corticosteroids, immunosuppressive drugs, lithium carbonate, antipsychotic medications and cardiovascular medications. Toxins can be insecticides, carbon monoxide, volatile substances such as inhalants and fuels.

Substance Intoxication Delirium

Delirium develops after taking high doses of substances like opiates, cocaine, alcohol and hallucinogens.

Substance Withdrawal Delirium

Withdrawal delirium develops when the client reduces or stops taking substances suddenly which he/she was taking in higher doses like opioids, opiates or sedative drugs.

Delirium Due to Multiple Etiologies

This category is characterized when more than one etiology is involved in developing symptoms of delirium.

Clinical Features/symptoms

The signs and symptoms of delirium appear over a short period of time, from a few hours to a few days. They often fluctuate throughout the day, so a person may have periods of no symptoms. Primary signs and symptoms include the following.

Reduced Awareness of the Environment: This may result in:

- An inability to stay focused on a topic or to change topics
- Wandering attention
- Getting stuck on an idea rather than responding to questions or conversation
- Being easily distracted by unimportant things
- Being withdrawal with little or no activity or little response to the environment.

Clouding of Consciousness

In delirium impairment can range from mild dulling of awareness to coma with characteristic worsening at night, with fatigue and decreased environmental stimulation. The client has reduced ability to direct, focus, sustain and shift attention. Diurnal variation and sun down effect is severe enough that worsening of symptoms occur in evening and night.

Cognitive impairment: Poor thinking skills.

A client with delirium may have difficulty in understanding his/her surroundings and hence, experiences difficulty in goal directed behavior. Memory thinking and perception are affected markedly.

- *Memory:* Poor memory, particularly of recent events. Impairment in memory is commonly observed. The client may have difficulty in recalling immediate and recent memory (the client tries to overcome this with the help of confabulation) but remote memory is relatively intact. Disorientation of time is very common but disordenation of place and person may also take place gradually.
- *Perception:* Marked perceptual disturbances are seen in delirium. Hallucination and illusions both can be observed. Hallucinations are more prominent and common in younger clients than elderly and these are found in clients with alcohol or other substance induced delirium (substance withdrawal), visual hallucinations are more common and can be simple sound or light to group of people and whole scenes. Auditory hallucinations if present are usually accompanied by visual hallucinations.
- *Thinking:* In delirium, thought process impairment are obvious. This process becomes fragmented and disjoined: later on speech and thought disorders like slurring of speech, incoherence, dysarthria and delusion may develop.

Changes in Psychomotor Functions

- The disturbances in psychomotor behavior presents in two forms—hyperactive behavior and hypoactive behavior. Hyperactivity is characterized by purposeless, repetitive and stereotyped activities. Sometimes hyperactivity may occur as a result of hallucination or delusions.
- In hypoactivity, motor behavior decreases considerably as impairment in consciousness is increase.

- These behaviors are also accompanied by emotional disturbances like apathy, depression, irritability, euphoria, anxiety or fear and wandering tendency.
- Disturbed sleep habits.
- Extreme emotions, such as fear, anxiety, angel or depression.

Diagnostic Evaluation

Diagnosis of delirium can be done on the basis of:
- Complete and detailed history
- Bedside physical examination of the client
- Mental status examination
- Laboratory investigation
- Physical and neurological examination.

MANAGEMENT

The primary goal of treatment for delirium is to address any underlying causes or triggers–by stopping use of a particular medication, e.g. or treating an infection. Treatment then focuses on creating the best environment for healing the body and calming the brain.

Nursing Therapeutics/Supportive Care

It aims to prevent complications by protecting the airway, providing fluids and nutrition, assisting with movement, treating pain, addressing incontinence and keeping people with delirium oriented to surroundings.
The nursing actions include:
- Clocks and calenders to help a person stay oriented
- A calm, comfortable environment that includes familiar objects from home
- Regular verbal reminders of current location, time, place and event
- Involvement of family members
- Avoidance of change in surrounding and caregivers
- Uninterrupted periods of sleep at nights with low levels of noise and minimal light
- Open blinds during the day to promote daytime alertness and a regular sleep-wake cycle
- Avoidance of physical restraints and bladder tubes
- Adequate nutrition and fluids
- Use of adequate light, music, massage, yogic and relaxation techniques to ease agitation
- Provide opportunities to get out of bed, walk, and perform self-care activities
- Provision of eye glasses, hearing aids and other adaptive equipments as needed.

COMPLICATIONS

Delirium may last only a few hours or as long as several weeks or months. If factors contributing to delirium are addressed, the recovery time is often shorter. The degree of recovery depends mainly on the health and mental status before the onset of delirium. People with dementia, e.g. may experience a significant overall decline in memory and thinking skills. People in better health are more likely to recover fully. People with other serious, chronic or terminal illness may not regain the levels of thinking skills or functioning that they had before the onset of delirium. Delirium in seriously ill people is also more likely to lead to general decline in health, poor recovery from surgery, need for more prolonged institutionalized care and enhanced risk of death.

Preventive Aspects of Delirium

The most successful approach to preventing delirium is to target risk factors that might trigger an episode. Hospital environments present a special challenge—frequent room changes, invasive procedures, loud noises, poor lighting and lack of natural light can worsen confusion.

The following strategies help prevent or reduce the severity of delirium in hospitalized clients:

- Provide adequate fluids.
- Provide stimulating activities and familiar objects.
- Encourage the use of eye glasses and hearing aids, if applicable.
- Use simple and regular communication about people, current place and time and events.
- Provide mobility and range-of-motion exercises.
- Reduce noise and avoid sleep interruptions.
- Provide appropriate pain management and offer indigenous/nondrug treatment for sleep problems and stress.

DEMENTIA

Introduction

Dementia is a general term for a decline in mental ability severe enough to interfere with daily life. It is not a specific disease. It is an overall term that denotes and describes a wide range of symptoms associated with a decline in memory or other thinking skills severe enough to reduce a person's ability to perform everyday activities.

Dementia Defined

Dementia is a complex disorder of all mental processes with progressive deterioration of a previous normal intellectual functions secondary to brain damage or disease. It is essentially subacute a chronic or primary and secondary.

Epidemiological Facts

The average prevalence of dementia is about 3 to 5%. The prevalence of dementia increases with age. It is estimated that prevalence of dementia below age 60 is 0.1% to 15 and 20 % by the age of 80 years. The incidence of dementia will become epidemic as our demographic and social trends are changing with the increase in elderly population.

Signs and Symptoms

Dementia is characterized by deterioration in intellectual or cognitive ability of the individual with impaired personal, social and occupational functioning. Impaired cognitive function are memory, abstract thinking, problem-solving ability and learning new material. In addition to these, there is profound change in personality with errors in judgments, lack of personal care, defective control of emotions and impulse control.

Memory Impairments

- Memory impairments are common and early in dementia. Usually recent memory is impaired than remote memory. This impairment in memory will lead to faulty orientation and difficulty in registration of events.
- Intellectual abilities are grossly impaired. The client's ability of reasoning, abstract thinking, and generalization is lost. Preservation and delusions maybe seen at chronic stage.

Personality Changes

The demented client presents with emotional lability (marked variation in emotional expression). There is decreased drive and enthusiasm leading to lack of interest in day-to-day activities. When client is encountered with new learning and new task which is beyond his/her intellectual ability, client may into sudden rage, anxiety and depression. As disease progresses the client becomes very self-centered, withdraws himself/herself from the environment with lack of concern and feeling for others. Inability to carry-out day-to-day activities and inflexibility in thinking and behavior is also observed.

Other Features

Anxiety and depression, inability to carry-out complex tasks may lead to violent emotional responses in the clients known as Catastrophic Reaction. Hallucinations and delusions may-be found in 20 to 40% of demented clients. Clients with vascular dementia may also have neurological symptoms such as headaches, dizziness, faintness, lethargy, dysarthria and dysphagia. People with dementias may have problems with short-term memory, keeping track of a purse or wallet, paying bills, planning and preparing meals remembering appointments or traveling out of the neighborhood. Many dementia are progressive, i.e. start out slowly and gradually get worse.

Diagnostic Criteria

Symptoms of dementia can vary greatly, at least two of the following core mental functions must be significantly impaired to be considered dementia.

- Memory loss or alterations
- Communication and language
- Ability to focus and pay attention
- Reasoning and judgment
- Visual perception.

Etiology

DSM-IV differentiates between disorders of dementia by their etiology, although they share more common symptoms presentation. Types of dementia according to DSM-IV are:

- Dementia of the Alzheimer's type.
- Dementia due to other general medical conditions
- Dementia due to HIV disease
- Dementia due to head trauma
- Dementia due to Alzheimer's type disease
- Dementia due to Alzheimer's type disease
- Dementia due to Pick's disease
- Dementia due to other general medical condition
- Substance induced persisting dementia
- Dementia due to multiple etiologies
- Dementia not otherwise specified.

Among the various types of dementia, dementia of Alzheimer's type and vascular dementia accounts 75% of clinical features.

Common causes of dementia are:

Degenerative diseases of central nervous system: Dementia is caused by damage to brain cells. This damage interferes with the ability of brain cells to communicate with each other. When brain cells cannot communicate normally, thinking, behavior and feelings can be affected. The brain has many distinct regions, each of which is responsible for different functions. When cells in a particular region are damaged, that region cannot carry-out its functions normally. Different types of dementia are associated with particular types of brain cells damage in particular regions of the brain. For example, in Alzheimer's disease, high levels of certain proteins inside and outside brain cells make it hard for brain cells to stay healthy and to communicate with each other. The brain region, i.e. the hippocampus is the center of learning and memory in the brain, and the brain cells in this region are often the first to be damaged. This is the reason, to get memory loss on the earliest symptoms of Alzheimer's disease.

- Senile dementia
- Huntington's disease
- Multiple sclerosis
- Pick's disease
- Wilson's disease
- Parkinson's disease

- *Vascular causes*:
  - Vascular dementia
  - Subarachnoid hemorrhage
  - Carotid antery occlusive disease
- *Metabolic disorders*:
  - Renal insufficiency
  - Hepatic insufficiency
  - Dialysis dementia
  - Cushing's syndrome
  - Hypothyroidism and hyperthyroidism
  - Pulmonary insufficiency
  - Cushing's syndrome
  - Parathyroid disease
- *Infections*:
  - Meningitis
  - Acquired Immune Deficiency Syndrome (AIDS)
  - Encephalitis
  - Multifocal leukoencephalopathy
- Epilepsy
- Head injury
- *Nutritional disorders*:
  - Wernicke-Korsakoff's syndrome (Thiamine deficiency)
  - Vitamin B_{12} deficiency.
  - Pellagra
- *Hypoxia:*
  - Congestive cardiac failure
  - Secondary to cardiac arrest

  - Postcarbon dioxide poisoning
  - Postanesthetic hypoxia.
- *Toxins:*
  - Alcoholic dementia
  - Heavy metal poisoning (lead, mercury, arsenic, etc.)
  - Sedative-hypnotic intoxication.
- *Other causes:*
  - Electric shock injury
  - Heat/cold stroke.

Dementia of Alzheimer's Type

Alois Alzheimer first described in 1907. It occurs in people over the age of 60. The time frame of the disease varies from person to person, however, the average length of the disease is from 7–20 years. Damage to the brain begins 10 to 20 years before signs and symptoms of Alzheimer's are visible.

STATISTICAL DATA

A study by John Hopkin's Bloomberg School (2009) of Health reports 26 million people worldwide suffer from Alzheimer's. These numbers are expected to rise dramatically. The study reports 106 million people will suffer from the condition by 2050. This is one in 85 persons worldwide. Current 5.1 million people in the US are diagnosed with Alzheimer's. These numbers will rise to 16 million by 2050. According to a CBS news report, Hispanics and African–Americans are at a higher risk of being diagnosed with Alzheimer's syndrome. The Alzheimer's Association reports African–Americans are twice more likely to be diagnosed than whites and Hispanics 1.5 times more likely.

Causes

According to National Institute of Aging, several changes occur in the brains of persons with Alzheimer's. The characteristics are plaques, which are microscopic deposits between the neurons consisting of insoluble proteins, neuron fragments and other protein materials. Tangles or clumps of a protein called tan protein, are also present inside the neurons. Tangles represent a breakdown in the infrastructure of neurons. The plaques and tangles lead to a loss of connection between neurons and cell death. It is also associated with all of the neuronal degradation is inflammation of the brain tissue.

The exact mechanism is unknown and the final diagnosis is made on the basis of neuropathological examination of the brain by CT scan/MRI; which reveal a degenerative pathology of the brain including atrophy, widened cortical sulci and enlarged cerebral ventricles. Microscopic examination shows senile plaques, neuronal loss and ventricles of the neuron in the brain. In the client with Alzheimer's disease, the activity of acetylcholine and norepinephrine is dramatically reduces. Aluminium toxicity is also considered as one of the causes of Alzheimer's disease as high levels of aluminum is found in the brain of the client with Alzheimer's disease. Genetic factors are also presumed to play role in occurrence of Alzheimer's because of 40% of client suffers from Alzhemer's disease have a positive family history of dementia.

RISK FACTORS

The new research suggests a positive association between excess belly fat, type II diabetes and cognitive decline. Having a gene associated with late-onset, Alzheimer's also increases the risk. Other risk factors include genetics, diabetes, Down syndrome, mild cognitive impairment, head injury, low levels of formal education, menopause in women, history of clinical depression, strokes, high cholesterol, high bold pressure, stress, inadequate exercising of the brain and body and obesity.

Without assistance and disorientation are signs of stage II Alzheimer's disease. During this stage, the client might begin to have trouble comprehending spoken or read words and he could have difficulty speaking. Depression and irritation are common as a result of the realization that self-care is becoming less likely. The symptoms from disease, I however, they are markedly worse. Generally, this stage of Alzheimer's disease lasts two to ten years.

Stage: III Terminal/Severe

A client with severe Alzheimer's disease, also known as stage III, usually requires around the clock care. On top of the symptoms from prior stages, the client also might sleep more. However, this sleep is often disturbed and the client may grunt and groan while sleeping. Loss of bodily functions, including swallowing, as well as bladder and bowel control, is likely in this stage. Because of the inability to move on her own, a client might experience skin infections and respiratory problems. The client might begin to have seizures. This is the stage of Alzheimer's usually associated with the inability to recognize loved ones and friends. This final stage of Alzheimer's disease is caused by severe damage to the brain and typically lasts one to three years.

Stages of Alzheimer's Disease/Psychopathology

Brain Cell Changes

Alzheimer's disease in thought to be caused by changes in brain cells. There are two ways in which brain cells are affected: tangles and plaques. Tangles, which may lead to neuron death, occur when tan proteins in the brain that are normally straight become twisted. Plaques occur when beta-amyloid proteins, which are normally harmless, begin to interfere with brain cell communication causing neuron dysfunction and/or neuron death.

Stage I/Mild/Onset

Mild Alzheimer's disease, which is classified as stage I, occurs when symptoms are mild. These symptoms include minor memory loss and minor mood swings. Irrational thinking, getting lost and trouble communicating are also signs of this phase. A client with stage 1, Alzheimer's might place things in odd places and begin to perform poorly on daily tasks, including work tasks. This stage of the disease usually lasts two to four years. Memory loss is important landmark of disease progression. It is also marked by anxiety, confusion and depressive symptoms. Personality changes are more evident.

Stage II/Moderate

As the damage to the brain worsens, the client moves to stage II. A client in this stage of Alzheimer's disease might be able to distinguish past events from present events. Inability to perform complicated tasks without assistance stage III.

FORMS OF ALZHEIMER'S DISEASE

Familial Alzheimer's Disease (FAD)

A small percentage of people with Alzheimer's disease (<5%) have familial. Alzheimer's disease or FAD (formerly known as 'early onset Alzheimer's disease). At some point in their family history genes mutated and developed the abnormal characteristics that cause FAD. These inherited genes have a powerful influence. If one parent has FAD, each child has a 50% chance of inheriting the disease, and with two parents with FAD, 75% of their children will go onto develop Alzheimer's disease in adulthood. These inherited genes differentiate FAD from the more common sporadic form of Alzheimer's disease, but the disease itself is nearly identical. The risk increases further if both parents have the disease. So aside from the FAD- related genes, there are other Alzheimer's disease related genetic factors shared by family members.

Sporadic Alzheimer's Disease

The sporadic form of Alzheimer's disease (earlier called 'late onset Alzheimer's disease') was formerly assumed to have no family linkages. Now we know that a person with a direct relative (parent or sibling) with Alzheimer's disease has a three times greater chance of developing the disease than someone who does not.

Warning Signs of Alzheimer's Disease

Alzheimer's disease is a progressive, degenerative disease of the brain. Symptoms include loss of memory, difficulty with day-to-day tasks and changes in mood and behavior. People may think these symptoms are part of normal aging but they are not. If you notice any of these symptoms or changes in abilities or behavior, it is important to consult a doctor. The changes maybe due to other conditions such as depression, drug interactions or an infection.

- Memory loss that affects day-to-day activities
- Difficulty in performing familiar tasks
- Problems with language
- Disorientation in time and space
- Impaired judgment
- Problems with abstract thinking
- Misplacing things
- Changes in mood and behavior
- Changes in personality
- Loss of initiative.

Diagnostic Evaluation

The process of diagnosis involves the following procedures:

- Thorough history taking and recording
- Mental status examination
- Physical and neurological examination
- Laboratory tests like:
  - Detailed blood test
  - Thyroid tests

- X-ray
- EEG
- CT and MRI of brain.

Treatment

Pharmacological Treatment

Cholinesterase Inhibitors

These help to preserve the ability of damaged nerve endings to transmit messages from one nerve cells to another. These are:

- Aricept (Donepezil)
- Rivastigmine (exelon)
- Reminys.

These drug are considered for people whose symptoms are early to middle stage and Aricept has been scientifically proved for treatment of early, middle and late stage Alzheimer's disease.

Memantine Hydrochloride

Neurotransmitters send messages across the space between nerve cells. As Alzheimer's disease progresses the neurotransmitter glutamate leaks out of nerve cells and is reabsorbed at levels that are toxic to the cell.

Memantine hydrochloride, known by the trade name Ebixa(R), works by blocking the reabsorption of glutamate into nerve cells. It is the first drug therapy approved for individuals whose symptoms are middle to late stage. Ongoing research indicates that there maybe greater benefit to using cholinesterase inhibitors and memantine hydrochloride together.

Aricept

Used to treat moderate, mild or severe one. It help clients with their mental and thought processes. Side effects include cramps, lack of appetite, insomnia, constipation, drowsiness, headaches, depression, blurred vision, frequent urination, dizziness, weakness and pain.

Razadyne: (generic-galantamine) maybe used in mild and moderate Alzheimer's disease treatment. Galantamine slows the breakdown of acetylcholine in the brain. This chemical is broken down by Alzheimer's. It helps the brain work. In order for galantamine to function, it must be used early in treatment because farther along there may not be enough acetylcholine left to allow it to have an effect. Side effects of galantamine include dry mouth, confusion, breathing difficulties, chest pain, cramps, mood changes, irregular heartbeat, rapid heartbeat, convulsions and skin wrinkling.

Rivastigmine

Rivastigmine, commonly marketed as Exelon, is a cholinesterase inhibitor that treats Alzheimer's disease. It increases acetylcholine so that memory and thinking improve. The side effects include stomach pain, weight loss, constipation, diarrhea, confusion, and dizziness. In some instances, rivastigmine leads to trouble falling asleep and lack of energy. A few of Rivastigmine's serious effects include fainting, bloody vomit, depression, seizures, aggression and painful urination.

Nutritional Supplements

Nutritional supplements include Phosphatidyl Serine, trimethylglycine, antioxidant supplements, acetyl-carnitine, fish oil are helpful in reducing symptoms.

Nonpharmacological Management

- *Behavior therapy:* These therapeutic approaches use a combination of basic behavioral and cognitive sessions, and are being increasingly used in combination with drugs.
- Other therapies like music therapy, aroma therapy, pet therapy and massage is used as in holistic thought.

Other Types of Dementias

Vascular Dementia

It is the second most common cause of dementia caused by brain damage from cerebrovascular or cardiovascular problems (strokes) or other problems that inhibit vascular function, symptoms are similar to Alzheimer's but personality and emotions affected only late in the disease.

Lewy Body Dementias

It is common and progressive where cells in the brain's cortex die and other contain abnormal structures (lewy bodies); symptoms overlap with Alzheimer's disease but also include hallucinations, shuffling gait and flexed posture with symptoms that may vary daily.

Frontotemporal Dementias

It is linked to degeneration of nerve cells in the frontal and temporal brain lobes and some evidence for a genetic factor. Commonly seen in 40 to 65 of ages. The symptoms include alterations in judgment, social behavior such as stealing, neglecting responsibilities, increased appetite, compulsive behavior and eventual motor skills problems and memory loss.

HIV-associated Dementia

It is due to infection of the brain with HIV virus symptoms include impaired memory, apathy, social withdrawal and concentration problems.

Huntington's Disease

It is a heredity disorder caused by a faulty gene and children of a person with the disorder have a 50% chance of getting the disease, symptoms begin in 30 to 40 years of old people with personality changes such as anxiety, depression and progress to show psychotic behavior, severe dementia and chorea—involuntary jerks, arrhythmic movements of the body.

Dementia Pugilistica

Also known as Boxer's syndrome. It occurs due to traumatic injury (often repeatedly) to the brain; symptoms commonly are dementia and parkinsonism.

Corticobasal Degeneration

It is a progressive nerve cell loss in multiple areas of the brain; symptoms begin at about age 60 on one side of the body and include poor coordination and rigidity with associated visual-spatial problems that can progress to memory loss, hesitant speech and dysphagia.

Creutzfeldt-Jakob Disease

It is a very rare disease that related to a gene mutation that causes rapid degenerative and fatal brain disease in people usually over 60 years old; personality changes and reduced coordination develop, rapidly followed by impaired judgment and vision and many clients develop a coma before they die.

Secondary Dementia

These dementias occur in patients with other disorders of movement such as Parkinson's disease or multiple sclerosis and maybe because of multiple etiology.

Nursing Care Management

The general principle of management of confusion state is the same except that early diagnosis and establishment of the underlying cause is the key to proper management. In all cases, sympathetic, gentle handling is the best approach to a frightened, potentially violent and aggressive client. The primary nursing aim lies in the confinement in a separate well-lit-room with minimum distraction and external stimuli. The attending nursing person should be a familiar good companion or a regular constant nurse because changing faces and surroundings increases the tendency to misinterpretations and illusion. The secondary nursing aim is to attend to the cerebral hypoxia if any by drugs like aminothymidine, ephedrine, etc. The third nursing aim is the question of hydration by oxygen administration and adequate respiratory ventilation by fluid intake by mouth or glucose intravenously with vitamin supplement like Vitamin B complex and ascorbic acid, preferably high potency parentrovite intravenously twice daily in glucose drip of 5% dextrose in normal saline depending on the diagnosis. Haldol (haloperidol) drops in the same drip can be a safe and effective combination. The fourth aim should be that sedation-barbiturates should be avoided as they are cerebral depressants and can potentiate the effect of alcohol and increase the cerebral hypoxia. A safe sedative is oral chloral hydrate, paraldehyde or chlorpromazine. In severe excitement, chlorpromazine intramuscular may help the client to settle down with the minimum physical restraint.

Nursing Care Assessment

Nursing assessment of client with delirium, dementia and amnestic disorders is difficult when we rely much on the client regarding information. So, the mental health nurse collects data from other sources like family members, friends and other members of health team. A mental health nurse can also take the help of various laboratory findings and cognitive tools to gather data regarding clients.

When interviewing the client or administering an assessment test, a positive physical and psychological climate is must as the client have cognitive impairments. Certain points should be kept in mind. The room should be free from distractions, quite dim lighted and away from noise of any activity. The nurse should speak therapeutically in direct and in simple manner, establish eye contact and sit in front of the client. If any printed material is provided to the client, it should be in large letters, heavy type and easily read. Adequate time should be allotted to the client to answer, attitude of the nurse should be nonjudgmental, friendly and nonthreatening. From the client the psychiatric nurse should collect the following information:

Physical Manifestations

Nutritional status: Client should be assessed for signs of malnutrition, weight loss/gain due to change in eating habits, skin color, eye color and weight should be observed. The client from these disorders often develops dehydration so it should be noted correctly.

Gait changes are also noted in clients. These can be secondary to vision problems, middle ear infection/disturbances, pain from osteoarthritis or an injury and or can be due to neuropathy resulting from vascular and diabetic problems. Feeling of cold even in warm climate is also a common problem depending upon level of activities and amount of body fat.

Incontinence first of urine and in later stages fecal maybe present in all these clients. Many causes can lead to bladder and fecal incontinence among them. Muscle weakness/loss of muscle control, chronic use of laxatives/abuse, lack of exercise or diet, low fiber intake in diet, adverse effects of drug and cognitive deficits, etc. are also present.

Emotional Manifestations

Emotional manifestations should be assessed before administration of any psychotic medication, by doing MSE and other cognitive assessment tools.

Secondary depression can be the commonest condition in the client with dementias or Alzheimer's disease. Psychological assessment with Zung or Beck Depression Scale can be useful. Observe for suicidal ideation, guilt feelings and delusions.

Disorientation is also very common in delusion, dementia and in other amnestic disorders. Client should be assessed for orientation towards time, place and person.

Determination of client's ability to carry-out activities of daily living and degree of independence should be observed because these things help in retaining client's self-esteem and engaging in worthwhile activities. Behavior related to emotional conditions are:

- Pacing, wandering, may show anxiety symptoms
- Decreased or inappropriate socialization may indicate apathy
- Refusal to eat, bath, groom may indicate depression
- Hoarding, scanning nature, accusations and alterness may indicate paranoia
- Reversal of sleep-wake cycle
- Falls/accidents show disorientation to surroundings
- Delusions, hallucinations and suspiciousness
- Inappropriate toilet activities
- Inappropriate sexual behavior
- Inappropriate social and communicative behavior
- Inappropriate eating.

Assess and note the differences between delirium and dementia.

Characteristics	Delirium	Dementia
• Onset	• Rapid (hours to days)	• Very gradual in years.
• Course	• Usually recover if cause is known and treated	• Chronic and slow (usually protected)
• Level of consciousness	• Fluctuates from hyperalert to difficult to arouse	• Usually normal
• Orientation	• Client is disoriented and confused	• Usually normal
• Affect	• Fluctuating	• Labile, apathy in later stage
• Attention	• Always impaired	• Maybe intact
• Behavior	• Agitated, restless, may wander	• Client maybe apathetic
• Speech	• Rapid or space, inherent	• Rapid or space, maybe repetitive
• Memory	• Impaired specially for recent and immediate facts and figures • Immediate recall and retention normal	• Remote memory is impaired in later stages.
• Content of thought	• Incoherent, confused deluded and stereotyped	• Disorganized, deluded and paranoid
• Perception	• Prencence of illusions and hallucinations	• Hallucinations maybe seen.
• Judgment	• Poor	• Poor, socially inappropriate behavior
• Insight	• Maybe present in lucid periods	• Absent
• Other characteristic	• Asterisks and multifocal myoclonus	• Catastrophic reaction and preservation

- *Nursing diagnosis:* Disturbed thought processes related to cerebral degeneration leading to inability to process and synthesize information as evidenced by recent memory loss, descreased ability to analyze reason and form judgment.
- *Nursing goal:* The client uses his/her intellect and judgment to the best of his/her ability.

Nursing intervention	Rationable
• Develop a positive stimulating therapeutic activities program.	• Cognitive stimulating in deficit areas and positive reinforcement will promote self-esteem and encourage the client to attain the highest functional level possible.
• Assess the environment, activities and frequently orient the client and collaborate with other staff to: – Use simple clothes, colors, foods and activities – Use multiple sensory cues, especially auditory, visual and tactile senses to indicate choices – Speak always slowly, in a low voice with the use of simple sentences.	• All these interventions help in maintaining orientation. Simple choices give control back to client and aid client in memory and recognition.
• Develop simple calenders with daily routines and easy to read clock. Notes and large bold signs are useful as reminders. Encourage family members to repeat frequently their names and relationships often in conversations.	• Adverse effects of medication may induce or deteriorate thought processes.
• Monitor for adverse effects of medications.	• The use of multiple, varied sensory cues stimulate be of sensory memory.
• Formulate daily periods of reminiscence using old photos. Incidence and specifically designed books.	

- *Nursing diagnosis:* Self-care deficient related to perceptual and cognitive alterations secondary to neuronal damage in the brain as evidenced by inability to carry-out activities of daily living.
- *Nursing goal:* The client will accomplish activities of daily living to the best of his/her ability and unfulfilled neds will be net by health care providers.

Nursing interventions	Rationale
• Assess and monitor client's physical mobility, provide safe and structured environment.	• Understanding the client's ability to carry-out activities of daily living help in planning the interventions.
– After identifying deficit areas, provide assistance as needed. Motivate for independent actions if possible. – Provide safe, simple and consistent schedule for performing activities of daily livings. Avoid frequent changes in schedule. – Provide plenty of time in performing activities of daily living. – Provide guidance and support for independent action. Employ positive reinforcement after successful completion of task. – Simplify dressing choices and stack clothes in order to avoid too many buttons, tight, belts, buckles and use elastic, loose clothing.	
• Always carry-out ongoing assessment for client's ability, safety, his/her nutritional status and needs and medication effects and need for communication.	• Clients, safety and security are nursing priorities actions.

- *Nursing diagnosis:* Risk for injury related to inability to recognize and identify dangers in the environment.
- *Nursing goal:* Client will be protected from injuries, fall and trauma.

Nursing interventions	Rationale
• The following interventions will help to protect the client from injuries and trauma: – Provide room to the client near to the nurse's station and observe frequently. – Provide assistance in mobility/ambulation. – Store only frequently used things near the client with easy access. – Use limited furniture and other items in room which accommodate client's with disability. – Bedrails should be up when client is in the bed. – Do not give any hazardous item to the client like match box, cigarettes. Allow client to smoke only when someone is present with the client. – Keep a dim light at night. – Frequently orient the client with time, person and place. – Restraints can be applied if the client is aggressive or hyperactive to ensure safety and security. – If client has wandering tendency provide adequate safe area to wander.	• All these interventions help to ensure client safety.

- *Nursing diagnosis:* Altered nutrition less than body requirement related to loss of appetite, forgetfullness.
- *Nursing goal:* Client's nutritional level will be adequately maintained and recorded.

Nursing interventions	Rationale
• Observe the client's pattern of food and fluid intake. Record input and output and daily weight.	• These client may not be aware of meeting his/her physical needs.
• Provide foods that are easily chewed, fruit juices with additional supplements of vitamins and minerals and high protein diet.	• As client is not interested in eating highly nutritional foods that require little efforts to eat can be effective.
• Client should be served with foods according to his/her tastes and likes.	• It encourages eating.
• If client is overeating, limit access to food and kitchen, schedule meals and snacks, serve limited carbohydrates.	• The client should consume balance and healthy diet.
• Observe and record client's pattern of bowel movement. Provide enough fiber diet and also increase fluid intake.	• These client may become severely constipated.
• Provide plenty of time to eat and maintain record of diet.	• Due to many physical problems eating may become a slow process like loss of teeth.

Psychoeducation

- The client and family members should be provided information on the nature of illness which includes possible causes, signs and symptoms and probable treatment options.
- The management of the illness can be explained further with ways to ensure client safety, maintaining orientation and touch with the reality, providing assistance in activities of daily living, nutritional requirement and modification required, difficult behavior of the client and its management, medicine administration and their adverse effects.
- The family member can be taught about general health measures to deal with client with organic disorders and ways to ventilate feelings and reduce stress.
- Family members are to be advocated about various organizations which help like self-help group (SHGs), day care centers, home health care, centers with domestic care facilities and other available socioeconomic resources. Psychiatric nurse should help to link the client to the community psychiatric nurses for daily follow-up.

Psychiatric Emergencies and Crisis Intervention

INTRODUCTION

The treatment of psychiatric clients has undergone dramatic changes in managed care area. Managed care, changes in health care delivery systems and decreasing access to mental health services are increasing the prevalence of psychiatric emergencies.

Psychiatric emergency is an acute disturbance of behavior, thought or mood of a client, which if untreated may lead to harm, either to the individual or to others in the environment. Thus, the definition of a psychiatric emergency differs from other medical emergencies in that the danger of harm to the society is also taken into account. Emergencies maybe classified as major, where there is a danger to life to the client or to others in his environment or minor where there is no threat to life but causes severe incapacitation.

Psychiatric Emergency Defined

The following conditions parallel for psychiatric emergency:

- Danger of harm to self or others.
- Level of functioning and capacity for self care.
- Severity of psychiatric symptoms.
- Ability to comply with treatment measures.
- Comorbid psychiatric and physical disorders.
- Quality and availability of support systems.
- Client and family preferences.
- Available resources.

Psychiatric emergencies are mostly dealt in emergency/casualty department of hospital but these can be encountered in any routine psychiatric setting. Psychiatric emergencies do not mean that the client is suffering only from psychiatric disorders but they may superadded due to medical condition or condition unrelated to medical field like disaster, rape/assault and violence. In initial assessment the emergency department of hospital after receiving client should quickly assess the client's condition and evaluate the nature of the condition and implement care according to seriousness of the situation.

Staff of emergency department should have basic understanding and knowledge as well as training of handling psychiatric emergency. Essential psychiatric medicine to deal with psychiatric emergencies should be available in an emergency area. Hospital security should be adequate to control violent and dangerous clients.

History and clinical finding should be recorded in clinical file clearly. Client's condition and plan of management should be explained clearly to the person(s) accompanying the client. It is observed that client is not kept for longer times in emergency department. A psychiatric evaluation is modified and specific to save time in decision making. If possible old health records of the client are retrieved particularly in cases in which little information is obtained.

Features indicating a possibility of medical illness:

- Old age.
- Memory impairment.
- Acute onset.
- Catatonic state
- Disorientation/confusion.
- Drug overdose.
- Neurological symptoms like unconsciousness, seizures, head injury and visual problems.

General Guidelines for Management of Psychiatric Emergencies

- Make personal and health-staff safety a priority.
- Realize that violence can occur anywhere.
- Position yourself between the client and exit.
- Gather/collect in depth information as possible from the client, including history of violence and legal problems.
- Maintain calm and quit environment.
- Handle emergencies tactically and with patience.
- Staff should be trained for management.
- Deal with the situation in a family manner.

Common Psychiatric Emergencies

Major Psychiatric Emergencies

- Suicidal attempts
- Agitation/aggression/and violent attacks.

Minor Emergencies

- Grief reaction
- Disaster
- Rape/assault
- Crisis.

Medial Emergencies in Psychiatry

- Delirium due to life threatening condition
- Neuroleptic malignant syndrome
- Serotonin syndrome
- Drug overdose
- Overdose with withdrawal from common drugs abuse substance
- Environmental problems

- Personality disorders
- Sundowning syndrome
- Pisa syndrome
- Acute psychosis
- The patient who has stopped eating
- Catatonia
- Acute mania
- Adjustment disorders
- Catastrophic reactions.

Suicide

Suicide is the action of intentionally taking one's own life. Globally it is considered as an immoral act committed by the sinful or insane. It has historically served as a solution to life's great obstacles or disappointments.

Epidemiological Aspects of Suicide

Suicide rate in India was 11.2 per 100000 in 2002. The rates vary across with states such as Kerala having the highest suicide rate of 30.8 per lakh in 2002. Suicide rates in Army, Airforce and Naval personnel were 0.04, 0.11 and 0.12 per thousands respectively.

Rates are higher in urban areas than rural community. Studies of completed suicides shown that 90–94% of the clients are mentally ill while committing the act. Depressive disorder accounts for nearly half the number of clients committing suicide followed by alcohol abuse (34%) and schizophernia (13%). The suicide risk is highest for primary psychiatric disorder and least for organic disorders with substance use disorders falling in between. Indian research studies show that most people attempting suicide are in the age group of 15–30 years and are predicted to increase further in the forthcoming years. Suicide is very common in the unmarried individuals. Rates are also high in the unemployed and in those who are suffering from chronic or terminal medical illness. More men than women commit suicide though more women attempt it.

Continuum of Behavioral Responses Towards Suicide

Suicide (sui means self, cide means murder or deliberate self harm) can be defined as the intentional taking of one's own life in a culturally non-endorsed manner. Attempted suicide (parasuicide, pseudosuicide) is defined as any act of self-harm or damage carried out with the apparent intention of self destruction however half-hearted, vague and ineffective.

According to Maslow's hierarchy theory, safety and security are fundamental requirements of life. Individuals behave in many ways to secure these basic needs. Some individuals respond with behaviors that promote growth, whereas others begin a journey to self destruction (Fig. 13.1). Adaptive behaviors result in a greater understanding and acceptance of oneself; but nonadaptive self-protective responses, if not changed, can eventually read to subtle or overt self-harm.

Self-destructive behaviors may taken two forms: direct and indirect way. Direct-self destructive behaviors relate to any form of active suicide behavior, such as threats, gestures or attempts to intentionally end one's life. Here, the individual is aware of and intends to achieve the desired outcome; death. Although the person may waver between wanting to live and need to die, the behaviors communicate an active wish to end the suffering of the present.

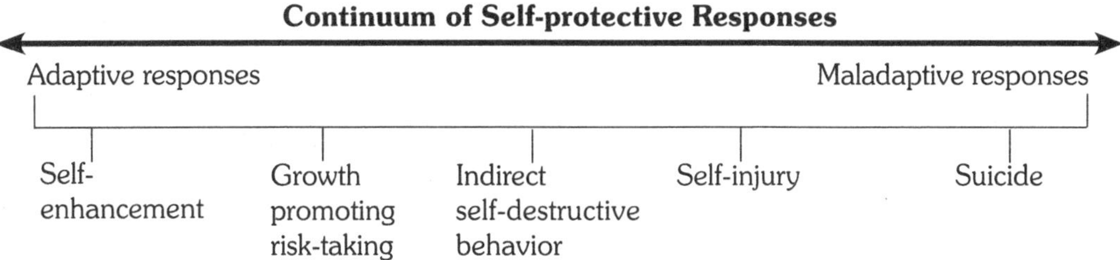

Fig. 13.1: Continuum of self-protective responses

Many people, however, engage in indirect self-destructive behaviors, which are the more subtle responses to self-protection. Indirect self-destructive behaviors are described as any behaviors or actions that may result in harm or death to the individual's well-being. In this case, people have no actual intention of ending their lives. They may be unaware of the potential harm when engaging in these activities and deny the possibility of danger even when confronted. Examples of indirect self-destructive behaviors include substance abuse, riding bike/vehicles overspeed, engaging in dangerous activities and an unwillingness to change negative thoughts and actions.

As the continuum of self-protective responses moves toward maladaptive behaviors, indirect self-destructive behaviors progress to active attempts to injure oneself. Self-injuries reaffirm to individuals that they are still alive. Pain serves as a reminder of their connection with the body and its physical world.

The last and ultimate maladaptive self-protective response is suicide; the ending of one's own life. Suicide is a complex and emotional issue, but it is one with which most nurses must cope.

Myths About Suicide

Many misconceptions and half-truths are existing about suicide in society. Although, suicide was found at the beginning of evolution, education has provided little effort to change the mindsets. Today, many false ideas about suicide still exist. Table 13.1 shows cases the myths and highlights facts to more accurately reflect the nature of suicide.

Table 13.1: Myths and facts about suicide.

Myth	Fact
• People who talk about it will not commit suicide. One does not need to take a suicide threat seriously.	• Most people communicate their intent, verbally in writing, through art, with behaviors.
• A failed suicide attempt is manipulative behavior.	• Manipulation is usually not a factor in suicide.
• People who are really serious about suicide give no clues.	• Many people communicate warnings of their wish by such things as tidying up their affairs, giving away possessions and being occupied with death.
• It is harmful to discuss the subject of suicide with clients.	• Most suicidal persons need acceptance and emotional support: discussing the topic demonstrates interest and concern.
• Only psychotic or depressed people commit suicide.	• Depression is a very high risk factor for suicide, but not all suicidal persons are depressed. Mental illness is a high risk factor for suicide.
• Suicide occurs only in the lower socioeconomic group, the poor.	• Although poverty is a risk factor, suicide occurs in all strata of classes.

Contd...

Contd...

Myth	Fact
• Young children never commit suicide.	• Suicidal behavior is the leading cause of psychiatric hospitalization for young children. It can occur in children as young as teen.
• When people show signs of improved mood, the threat of suicide is over.	• Depressed people often show improved moods, attitude and behaviors before their deaths because the decision to commit suicide has been made.

Causes and Impact of Suicide on Society

Over more than 1000 suicides occur throughout the world everyday. In India, 150- 200 people commit suicide everyday. The average prevalence of suicide varies and is about 10 per lakh of population. The ratio of attempted suicide to suicide is 8–10:1.

Cultural Factors

No one knows exactly why a person chooses suicide, but many cultural, social and individual factors have an influence. The laws, customs, beliefs, values and norms of a culture usually include a view of suicides.

Social Factors

Inability to meet basic needs such as food, shelter, social support are the main contributors for suicide. Nowadays, easily accessibility of weapons also a cause.

The chronic and incurable disease like cancer, HIV/AIDS, has positive influence on suicide. The philosophy of these clients, the 'death with dignity' has also influenced to choose time and place for suicide. This form of suicide is called 'rational suicide'; because the choice to end one's life was made from a sound mind, freely and rationally.

Characteristics of Suicide

Suicide is an act of individual meaning. The actual reasons for choosing such a final course of action will probably never be known to anyone but the individual. However, it is likely that more than one motive drives a person for such activity.

In the physical dimension, thoughts of suicide produce many of the same biochemical changes in the body as depression. Often suicidal persons will not eat, drink or rest enough to maintain required energy levels. Recent research studies have suggested a link between low serum cholesterol levels and suicide attempts in men. The results of one study found that 'among men' those with low cholesterol were about twice as likely to have made medically serious suicide attempts (Golier and others, 1998).

One's method of choice for committing suicide differs by gender. Men usually prefer on firearms, hanging or drowning and also by jumping from higher places; whereas women prefer drugs/pills or to inhale carbon monoxide.

The emotional dimension of functioning for the suicidal person is filled with feelings of ambivalence, guilt, anger, aggression, helplessness and hopelessness. Ambivalence is a state in which an individual experiences conflicting feelings, attitudes, or drives. For the suicidal person, the struggle is between self-preservation (life) and self-destruction (death). Often, suicidal individuals treat or attempt suicide and then seek out treatment, behaviorally acting out their feelings of ambivalence.

Anger and aggression are turned inward in suicidal persons. Fears of being abandoned or rejected add to the dynamics. Many persons who feel trapped in frustrating dependant relationships commonly react with rage that becomes-directed and harmful.

Guilt can also become to suicide. Suicidal individuals shoulder the guilt of the world. They feel sinful and carry around the belief that they must have done something very wrong to deserve their misfortunes. Often personal guilt is exaggerated until the only way to make up for one's transgressions is to offer the final sacrifice-the self.

For the suicidal person, the emotional inspect of psyche is marked by overwhelming feelings of helplessness and hopelessness. Nothing the person tries to do works out the way it was expected.

The self becomes unable to function emotionally. Life becomes bleak and hopeless as its meaning and purpose slips from the suicidal person's control. Self-esteem will be very very low.

The intellectual dimension, the intense emotional suffering of a suicidal person leads to distorted thinking and self-defeating thoughts. The self becomes devalued, worth little. Everything becomes depressing, which leads individuals to a negative and pessimistic view of the future. One's internal aspect of self-talk becomes self-defeating; which soon becomes reflected in negative behaviors. Thinking is self-centered rather than oriented toward solving problems.

The social dimension of functioning includes the suicidal person's views of others. Many suicidal individuals depend on the feedback of others to frequently reaffirm their self-worth. Self-esteem is very low in suicidal people. Their feelings of inferiority, of being less than others, interfere with social relationships and lead to the isolation and loneliness that often accompanies suicide.

In the area of spiritual dimension, suicidal individuals grapple with the cultural, religious and ethical dilemmas associated with bringing about one's own demise. Many people respond by blaming other people, their society or their religious practices. Others 'make their peace' with the spiritual sides of themselves and experience a spiritual calm and serenity before committing suicide. Some people believe they will be reunited with loved ones in a new life after leaving this reality.

Theories of Suicide

Because suicide is an end result, it is difficult to understand all the factors that led up to one's decision to end his/her life. The study of the nature of suicide is called suicidology. Several theories attempt to explain the causes of suicidal behavior.

The psychoanalytical theory states that all humans have the instinct for life and death within them. Suicidal persons experience much ambivalence between wanting to live and wanting to die. Anger turns inward, and when stressful life events activate their death wish, suicide becomes an option.

Sociological theory looks at the relationship between the number of suicides and the social conditions of an area. These theorists believe that suicide rates are affected by group support (or the lack of it); social changes, regulations, religion, legal sanctions or limitations and philosophical beliefs. In short, the sociological theories consider the impact of social factors on the occurrence of suicide.

According to interpersonal theory by H.S. Sullivan, suicide is viewed as the outcome of a failure to work with or resolve interpersonal conflicts.

The biological theory, suggests that alterations in neurotransmitters, their imbalance causes people to have difficulty regulating their moods; specially irregularities of serotonin.

Risk Factors for Suicide

- Abuse, neglect, exploitation.
- Accident prone.
- Academic stress, school/college problems.
- Chronic illness, disability, HIV/AIDS, terminal illness.
- Dysfunctional family relationships.
- Family/self history of anxiety, depression, previous suicide attempts or other mental health problems.
- Inadequate childbearing practices.
- Loss of parent or significant family member.
- Low socioeconomic status, poverty, homelessness.
- Male, unmarried, divorce, unemployed.
- Member of certain fanatic religious groups.
- Negative outlook for future.
- Parental/self history of alcoholism, substance abuse or previous suicide attempts.
- Profession/occupation: Policeman, fireman, air traffic controller, physician, psychiatrist, college student.
- Social/Isolation, lack of social support.
- Stressful or unhappy personal relationships, peer pressure.

Therapeutic Management of Suicidal Client

Thoughts about suicide can be described on several levels. Suicidal ideation is described as thoughts or fantasies that are expressed but have no definite intent. Ideas may be expressed directly or symbolically. Suicidal threats are verbal or written expressions of the intent to take one's life, but they are without actions. As the seriousness increases, suicidal gestures may be observed. These are suicidal actions that result in little or no injury but communicate a message of suicidal purpose. Suicidal attempts are serious self directed actions that are intended to do harm or end life. Parasuicidal behaviors are unsuccessful attempts and gestures associated with a low likelihood of success. The last level is completed suicide, the successful attempt to end one's life. Motivation for the successful suicide may be conscious or unconscious.

Preventive Aspects of Suicide

Prevention is the most important nursing action for clients who may be suicidal. Preventing a suicide from occurring means saving a life. Prevention requires a knowledge of the dynamics of suicide and the ability to recognize the potential for suicidal actions in every client and an individual. Applying nursing process is an excellent method for working with clients who may be considering suicide.

Assessment of Suicidal Potential

Nowadays, suicide is becoming so prevalent. It is important for nurses to evaluate every clients for its potential. To achieve this, assess the risk factors for the age of the client. Then ask the client directly if he/she has any thoughts relating to suicide. Asking clients will not encourage them to take any suicidal actions. On the contrary, it gives them permission to discuss their inner feelings and attitudes.

Questions to Ask a Client for the Potential for Suicide

- What has been the most difficult moment for you in the recent past?
- Have things been so bad that you have thought about escaping? If so, How? Describe it.
- Are there times when death seems like an attractive option to you ?
- Have you thought of harming yourself ?
- Have you thought about killing yourself ?
- If you were to harm yourself, how you carry out?
- Do you have access to the items you would need to carryout you plan? (This includes, pistol, gun, medicine a rope, etc).
- Have you thought about or attempted to harm yourself in the past?
- What has kept you from harming yourself thus far?
- What might keep you from harming yourself in the near future?

(From Lueckenotte AG: Gerontological Nursing St. Lowis. 1996, Mosby).

The most important question to ask is 'do you think you can control your behavior and refrain from acting on your thoughts or impulses?' If the answer is negative, then hospitalization may be required for the client's safety and protection. Not every question may be appropriate for every client, but a serious of questions like these will usually bring out expressions of suicidal thoughts if they are present.

Suicidal intentions can exist with any medical or psychiatric diagnosis. Clients who are depressed must be carefully monitored for expressions of hopelessness. Table 13.2 lists, the basic components of a suicide assessment. When used as part of a nursing history, it will yield valuable information about the client's suicidal intentions (if any) along with numerous clues to help understand the unique individual of the client.

Table 13.2: Suicide assessment

Assessment	Description
• Suicide ideation (thoughts)	• Client talks about wanting to be dead, imagines AIDS or other serious illness, seems gloomy, brooding.
• History of suicide attempts	• Client has tried to end own life before, there may be history of suicide in family.
• Present suicide plan	• The more detained a suicide plan, the more likely it will be carried out.
• Availability of items to carry out plan	• What guns, rifles, knives or ropes, other weapons are available ? How difficult is to obtain such items ?
• Substance use or abuse	• Suicide rates are higher in people who abuse alcohol or other drugs.
• Level of despair	• Ask about the future; when despair is high, hope is at a low level.
• Ability to control own behavior	• Inpatient hospitalization is indicated for individuals who are unable to control their suicidal impulses.

Nursing diagnoses for suicidal persons are based on each client's identified problems and needs. Commonly identified diagnoses include anxiety, impaired adjustment, ineffective coping, denial, body image disturbance, dysfunctional grieving, spiritual distress, risk for self-directed violence, loneliness and powerlessness.

Nursing Interventions for Suicidal Clients

The first and foremost priority for the care of suicidal clients is protection from harm. If the client is actively attempting suicide, he/she must be physically prevented from doing so. If the risks are so high that a serious attempt may be made, then suicidal precautions are carried out.

One of the most important therapeutic interventions with suicidal persons is to establish a support. Many suicidal people are alone and most have little or no self-esteem. The majority of individuals are distressed and experiencing emotional reactions, but they will usually agree to make a no-self harm contract or agreement with their nurse not to engage in self-destructive behaviors.

Establishing a therapeutic relationship with a healthcare provider is important for clients. The focused communications and concerned actions of nurses encourage suicidal individuals to feel self with the encouragement and advocacy of their nurses, many suicidal clients are able to develop more effective strategies for living more satisfying lives.

Nursing Interventions: Suicide Precautions

Definitions

Reducing risk of self-inflicted harm for a client in crisis or severe depression.

Activities

- Determine whether client has specific suicide plan identified.
- Encourage the person to make a verbal no suicide contract.
- Determine history of suicide attempts.
- Protect client from harming self.
- Place client in least restrictive environment that allows for necessary level of observation.
- Demonstrate concern about client's welfare.
- Refrain from negatively criticizing.
- Remove dangerous items from the environment.
- Place client in room with protective window coverings, as appropriate.
- Observe closely during suicidal crisis.
- Educate client and significant others in signs, symptoms and basic physiology of depression.
- Instruct family that suicidal risk increases for severely depressed clients as they begin to feel better.
- Facilitate discussion of factors or events that precipitated the suicidal thoughts.
- Involve client in outdoor activities, as appropriately.
- Provide counseling whereas applicable.
- Instruct family on possible warning signs and symptoms.
- Refer to higher centers for further management.

AGITATED AND VIOLENT CLIENTS

Violence is a danger often faced in emergency or casualty setting. The risk of violence is especially high in those societies where there is easier access to firearms and alcohol/drug abuse. The use of alcohol also predisposes to violence. Specific psychiatric and medical disorders have also been associated with violent behavior. Certain characteristics predict an assault in the ward/emergency departments. Unemployed young (< 40 years) men with low socioeconomic status, past history of violence and who are usually noncomplaint with treatment, present with violent behavior in psychiatric settings. A threat to assault should' always be taken seriously. Signs predicting an impending assault are anger, demanding immediate attention, loud voice, excitement, staring eyes, flared nostrils, flushed face, hands clenched or gripping, possessing weapons, pushing furniture, uncooperativeness and suspiciousness, slamming objects and sudden movements.

Etiology of Violence

Biological Theory

- *Neurotrasmitters:* Serotonin metabolism appears to be involved. Its metabolite 5-HIAA has lower level in the CSF of offenders who kill with unusual cruelty.
- *Chromosomal abnormalities:* XXY, sex chromosomal abnormality is thought to involve in crime.
- *Alcohol and Other Drugs:* These is a positive link between violent behavior and drugs like consumption of alcohol, amphetamines, cocaine, phencyclidine and sedative-hypnotics.

Psychosocial Factors

- A history of child abuse.
- Easy accessibility to weapons like guns, pistol, etc.
- Crowding and temperature of discomfort.
- Poverty, marital disharmony, unemployment, caste discrimination, etc.

Social Learning Theory

It states that aggressive and violent behaviors are learned through role modeling, others in the environment. Aggression is believed to be a learned behavior based on the values, attitudes and actions of role models within the individual's environment.

Anthropological Theory

Anthropological theory explains violence and aggression as the result of cultural, social organizations or sexual differences. Because some cultures encourage the use of aggressive behaviors, their citizens learn to interact and cope aggressively. In other cultures, equality and harmony are stressed. Male and female roles are less defined in cooperative cultures than they are in cultures with hierarchies or degrees or power.

According to Dr. Sherry Turkle, cyber psychologist between that computer networks will change the way people think about themselves and their role in society. The fear is 'that young people will succumb to the temptation to leave 'real life' behind for the ever-so-much more controllable realm of cyber space' (Technology Review, 2006). As more people become member of the computer network society, the number of 'real', ' face to face interaction descreases. The lack of supportive relationships has been linked to many negative–even pathological consequences, including mental illness (net-addiction), crime and suicide'. It appears that social relationships are more important in preventing aggression and violence than other strategies.

Protection against Violence and Assault

Strategies recommended for protection against an assault are described in the following table and drugs used for controlling aggression nonspecific tranqualizers may be administered to first calm the client under control before an assessment can be carried out. Emergency staff should be familiar with the administration of these drugs which should readily be available. If the client is willing , drugs may be administered, orally, otherwise parenterally. Mostly Haloperidol 10 mg IM can be given at intervals of every half hour to a maximum 60 mg. Lorazepam 2 mg up to a maximum 10 mg is equally effective as haloperidol. It is especially useful where alcohol withdrawal is suspected. Once the client under control, assessment and mental status examination should be carried out.

Verbal assault	Physical assault
• Answer all questions politely, softly, simple manner and honestly. • Be empathic and calm. • Keep hands visible. • Keep the door always half often. • Stay at least an arm's length away from the client. • Stay to the side of the client. • Use non threatening body language. • Use reflective statements rather than judgmental ones.	• Call for help, if possible press the panic button to summon help. • Deflect a kick with your legs. • Deflect punches with you hands. • Try to escape as early as possible. • Face the person sideways. • If bitter do not pull away the bitter part, instead force the bitter part to the mouth and nose of the bitter to block his respiration. • If choked, tuck you chin to the chest to maintain the airway. • If the client grabs your hair, use your hands to control the hands of the client.

Psychiatric Disorders Associated with Violent Behavior

- Schizophrenia especially paranoid.
- Mania.
- Paranoid psychosis.
- Personality disorder–Antisocial.
- Alcohol intoxication or withdrawal.
- Multisubstance intoxication with cocaine, amphetamines, anabolic steroids, phencyclidine.
- Substance withdrawal.
- Post-traumatic stress disorder.
- Dementia.
- Learning disorders.

Medical Disorders Associated with Violent Behavior

- Neurologic illnesses:
  - Brain infections such as encephalitis, meningoencephalitis.
  - Head injury with intracerebral, subarachnoid or subdural.
  - Hematoma.
  - Cerebral infarction.
  - Seizure disorders (interictal, postictal or temporal lobe epilepsy).
  - Hepatic encephalopathy.
  - Huntigton's chorea.
  - Parkinson's disease due to levodopa toxicity.
  - Wilson's disease.

- Endocrinopathies:
  - Thyrotoxicosis
  - Hyperthyroidism
  - Cushing's syndrome
  - Hyperparathyroidism
- Metabolic disorders:
  - Hypoglycemia
  - Hypoxia
  - Electrolyte imbalance
  - Hypocholesterolemia
- Infections:
  - AIDS
  - Syphilis
  - Tuberculosis
- Vitamin deficiencies:
  - Folic acid
  - Niacin
  - Pyridoxine
  - Vit B_{12}
- Temperature disturbances
  - Hyperthermia
  - Hypothermia.

Prevention of Assault on Health Workers

The casualty department should have adequate security staff. Access to examination rooms and treatment areas should be limited. All consulting and examination rooms should have at least two exists. Similarly all rooms should have a call button, which can be pressed in an emergency so that all available staff can rush to the aid of the medical person being assaulted. All suspicious clients should be watched and reported in detail for future crisis. Medical personnel should also be careful not to provide an assault by being always polite and respectful, calm avoiding prolonged eye contact with potentially violent clients, giving clear instructions, remaining at a safe distance unless unavoidable, keeping clear exists, removing all articles in client's room which could be used for assault. All cases of assault must be investigated and discussed among the staff and the administration and lessons drawn for future.

NURSING INTERVENTIONS FOR VIOLENT/ HYPERACTIVE/AGITATED CLIENT

Nursing interventions	Rationale
1. Establish and maintain physical health and safety. • Provide adequate nutrition; offer snacks and fluids between meals. • Promote rest and sleep: If necessary administer sedatives.	Hyperactivity may become a physical concern because client who does not eat, drink or sleep may suffer complete exhaustion.

Contd...

Contd...

Nursing interventions	Rationale
• Keep the client in a quiet area for periods of time during the days to prevent and reduce overactive behavior. • Encourage personal hygiene. • Assess the client for suicidal, homicidal or elopement behavior and intervene accordingly. • Observe for adverse effects of medications: maintain hydration and adequate fluid intake. • If client is displaying acting out behavior, physical restraint or sedation may be administered when client calms down, an opportunity is provided for ventilation of feelings and thoughts.	These clients are over stimulating and are processing massive stimulation from the environment; removal to a nonstimulating environment reduces over activity. Increases self-esteem. Client's safety is a nursing priority. Moderate or severe anxiety may lead to threatening behavior or destructivenes of property and people. In this stage, physical control or restraints or chemical restraints maybe necessary to protect client and others.
2 Safeguard against destructive behavior. • Observe for mood or behavioral changes such as increasing irritability, demanding or increasing physical activity. • Provide for diversion and physical activities which channelize energy and decrease anxiety. • Assign same staff member to the client to assess and provide ego control. • Maintain a safe physical distance. • Set limit on client's behavior. • Give the client expectations that the behavior can be controlled. • De-escalate the client's behavior by using direct, simple quite comments and avoiding lengthy conversations. • Take the client to quiet area.	Acting out behavior may be prevented by assessing the behavior and intervening early. In early stages, expecting the client to control behavior providing diversion, encouraging the release of anxiety with physical activity or talking it out will de-escalate the behavior of the anxiety or overactivity is moderate or severe then limit setting is crucial.
3. Orient client to reality • Orient client to reality situation in every moment; protect client from stressful situations, provide protective environment and assure client's safety. • Recognize the client's feelings and reflect these back. • Encourage expression of anger, depression and guilt. Discuss the situation that precipitate these feelings. • Assess the signs which indicate that the client is becoming depressed.	The client may experience flight of ideas, loosening of association and unrealistic grandiose ideas which put client in an unsafe position and provide distance from other clients. Depression often followed a hyperactive period and is devastating to the client.
4. Establish discharge planning with the client. • Educate the client and significant others about early signs and symptoms of an over active episode. • Establish follow-up treatment • Educate the client and family regarding the purpose, dosage, closage, adverse effects and special precautions of medication. • Discuss and formulate discharge plans with the client.	Overactive clients often have recurrent episodes because they like the feelings of euphoria and stop talking their medication especially lithium salts. If the client is educate about the illness. The effects of medication and the importance of regular testing for lithium blood level. Active involvement in planning increase the client's chances for follow through.

DELIRIUM

Delirium is a transitional change in consciousness. It is managed with environmental manipulation to help orient the client (e.g. Leaving a light on at night, frequent orientation to time, place and person) and with drugs. Drugs should be prescribed only after the underlying disorder has been diagnosed or the process of determining the diagnosis has been initiated.

Haloperidol in low doses (0.5 to 2 mg) is frequently administered. Lorazepam 0.5 to 2 mg can reduce agitation and is preferable when substance withdrawal is the cause. Anticholinergic drugs (e.g. tropine) should be administered with caution in delirious client's especially the elderly, because anticholinergic toxicity like atropine psychosis can occur.

SUBSTANCE INTOXICATION AND WITHDRAWAL

- It may occur with a psychiatric disorder or as a primary presenting complaint. Alcohol, cocaine and phencyclidine are the substances that most commonly lead to violent behavior. Clients should be placed under observation in a secure room away from the stimulation.
- Physical restraints or sedation may be necessary for violent clients. Lorazepam 2 to 4 mg stat or diazepam 10 to 20 mg stat is recommended to treat agitation.
- Withdrawal from barbiturates, other sedatives and hypnotics (including benzodiazepines) and alcohol are similar clinically. When symptoms are very severe, treatment in a hospital is safest and is mandatory if the client is febrile (>38.30 c or 1010f) ; cannot hold down fluids to prevent dehydration or has a severe underlying physical disorder. Alcohol withdrawal can be life-threatening situation and seizures can also be expected to occur.
- Delirium tremens, a withdrawal syndrome that appears within 7 days of withdrawal (usually within 24 to 72 hours) is a medical emergency and should be treated in an intensive care units.
- Management is usually with high doses of benzodiazepines parenteral thiamine and maintenance of fluid and electrolyte balance.

OVERDOSE OF PRESCRIBED PSYCHOACTIVE DRUGS

It can also pose a threat to life apart from causing intoxication. Hence, the client should be jointly managed by a physician and a psychiatrist. If the client has taken a toxic dose and is awake, treatment consists of inducing emesis followed by administering activated charcoal. Overdose with tricyclic antidepressant or carbamazepine requires cardiac monitoring. Overdose of barbiturates or benzodiazepines and alcohol may cause respiratory arrest. Antipsychotic drugs, at therapeutic as well as toxic levels can cause acute extrapyramidal adverse effects including dystonia, oculogyric crisis, torticollis and akinesia.

Akinesia is a common adverse effect of high potency antipsychotics, when severe, it is accompanied by extreme anxiety or terror. Acute onset of oculogyric or orofacial dystonia in an otherwise healthy person may suggest purposeful or inadvertent ingestion of an antipsychotic. Immediate relief maybe provided with a parenteral antihistaminic such as promethazine 25 mg administered intramuscularly.

NEUROLEPTIC MALIGNANT SYNDROME (NMS)

NMS is a medical emergency and is best managed in the acute medical units. It may present differently and more subtly in elderly patient. It is a hypermetabolic reaction to dopamine antagonists, primarily antipsychotic drugs such as phenothiazines and butyrophenones. It usually occurs early in treatment and rarely during maintenance period. It develops in up to 3% of clients started on antipsychotics. Risk is increased in agitated male clients who have received large and rapidly increased doses. No genetic component is apparent. Its pathophysiologic basis is believed to be blockage of central dopamine receptors. The characteristic signs are muscle rigidity, high fever, an elevated CPK and respiratory and metabolic acidosis, myoglobinuria and leucocytosis. Mortality rates are between 10 to 20% treatment includes cessation of antipsychotic drugs.

Supportive care and aggressive treatment of myoglobinuria, fever and acidosis. The dopamine agonist bromocriptine 2.5 to 20 mg twice a day or Dantrolene up to 10 mg/kg IV and 4 hourly may be used as a muscle relaxant.

SEROTONIN SYNDROME

The serotonin syndrome is caused by drug-induced excess of intrasynaptic 5-hydroxy tryptaline. The clinical manifestations are mediated by the action of 5- hydroxytryptamine on various subtypes of serotonin receptors. Treatment includes administration of chlorpromazine and cyproheptadine.

VICTIMS OF DISASTERS

Victims of disasters are those people who have survived a sudden and unexpected natural calamity that is much more beyond human control like earthquakes, floods, riots, terrorism, natural and manmade disasters and cloud bursting and tsunami. Others victims can be relatives of survivors and rescue workers. The victims present with anger, frustration, guilt, numbness, confusion as well as flash backs.

Management

- Treatment of underlying physical problem.
- Crisis intervention.
- Ventilate victim's feelings, emotions by nursing therapies.
- Group therapy.
- Drugs like benzodiazepines to reduce anxiety and induce sleep can be given.
- Referral services.

RAPE AND REHABILITATION

Rape is defined as the penetration of the anus or vagina by a penis, finger or object or the penetration of the mouth by a penis. If a person is forced to penetrate someone in the anus, mouth or vagina with their penis, also regarded as rape (Polaschek, Ward and Hudson, 1997). The most commonly cited motives for rape are those of power, anger and sex.

Blaming, a victim for being raped is a form of 'secondary victimization', where victims can be made to feel guilt or shame because they are further victimized by negative feedback about their conduct. It has a number of profound consequences on victim and as well as society.

RAPE MYTHS

There are a number of rape myths which operate within a range of professional and everyday contexts.

- Women precipitate rape by their behavior or appearance.
- Rape is not damaging because, after all, it is only sex.
- Real rape victims have signs of injury to prove it because you cannot be raped against your will.
- Women often lie about rape because they are malicious and deceitful.
- Real rapists are psychopathic individuals.

Management

- Medical examination and treatment; if needed surgery.
- Inform police.
- Be supportive, reassuring and nonjudgmental.
- Educate the client about availability of medical, legal services.
- Referral to the Social group and SHG/NGOs, etc.
- Medications such on benzodiazepines to reduce anxiety and to induce sleep.

GRIEF

Grief and mourning are inseparable in life. Both these terms are used interchangeably, each has a separate meaning. Grief is the set of emotional reactions that accompany a loss. Mourning is the process of working through or resolving one's grief and bereavement is the emotional and behavioral state of thoughts, feelings and activities that follow a loss. The period of grief and mourning after a loss can be intense and painful. Feeling of loss, grief and mourning are deeply personal and each of us has our own way of coping with these emotions.

The experience of coping with a significant loss is called the grieving process. It involves a serious of events or situations. Grieving is a process, a method for resolving losses and a way of healing or recuperating.

Grief is a normal reaction to loss. It affects family, friends and relatives of the grieving person and colors the interactions and communications of those related to the loss. It serves several purposes. First, it allows individual to work through the feelings of anger, helplessness and emotions that result from the loss. Second, it offers a socially acceptable avenue for receiving physical and emotional support.

Grieving Process/Stages

According to Kubler–Ross (1969): It involves the following steps.

Denial and Isolation

- The first reaction to learning of terminal illness or death of a cherished loved one is to deny the reality of the situation. It is a normal reaction to rationalize overwhelming emotions. It is a defense mechanism that buffers the immediate shock. We block out the words and hide from the real facts. This is a temporary response that carries us through the first wave of pain.

Anger

- As the masking effects of denial and isolation begin to wear, reality and its pain reemerge. We are not ready. The intense emotion is deflected from our vulnerable core, redirected and expressed instead as anger. The anger may be aimed at inanimate objects, complete strangers, friends or family. Anger may be directed at our dying or deceased loved one.
  - Rationally, we know the person is not to be blamed. Emotionally, however, we may resent the person for causing us pain or for leaving us. We feel guilt for being angry and this makes us more angry.
  - Remember, grieving is a personal process that has no limit, nor one 'right' way to do it.

Bargaining Stage

- The normal reaction to feelings of helplessness and vulnerability is often a need to regain control:
  - If only we had sought medical attention sooner.
  - If only we got a second opinion from another doctor.
  - If only we had tried to be a better person toward them.

    Secretly, we may make a deal with God or our high power is an attempt to postpone the unexitable. This is a weaker line of defense to protect us from the painful reality.

Depression

Two types of depression are associated with mourning. The first one is a reaction to practical implications relating to the loss. Sadness and regret predominate this type of depression. We worry about the costs and burial. We worry that in our grief, we have spent less time with others that depend on us. This phase may be eased by simple classification and reassurance. We may need a bit of helpful cooperation and a few kind of words. The second type of depression is more subtle and in a sense. Perhaps more private in nature. It is our quite preparation to separate and to bid our loved one farewell. Sometimes all we really need is a hug.

Acceptance

Reaching this stage of mourning is a gift not afforded to everyone. Death may be sudden and unexpected or we may never see beyond our anger or denial. It is not necessarily a mark of bravery to resist the inevitable and to deny ourselves the opportunity to make our peace. This phase is marked by withdrawal and calm. This is not a period of happiness and must be distinguished from depression.

Loved ones that are terminally ill or aging appear to go through a final period of withdrawal. This is by no means a suggestion that they are aware of their own impending death or such, only that physical decline may be sufficient to produce a similar response. Their behavior implies that it is natural to reach a stage at which social interaction is limited. The dignity and grace shown by our dying loved ones may well be their last gift to us.

Coping with loss is ultimately a deeply personal and singular experience – nobody can help you go through it more easily or understand all the emotions that you are going through. But others can be there for you and help comfort you through this process. The best way you can do is to allow yourself to feel the grief as it comes over you. Resisting it only prolong the natural process of healing.

Unresolved Grief

When the grieving process is prolonged or impairs functioning overtime, mental health problems can result. Unresolved grief, dysfunctional grief, and complicated bereavement are terms to be used describe unhealthy or ineffective grief reactions. Although everyone who experiences a great loss grieves, people who are suffering from unresolved grief are unable to shift are unable to shift their attention from their loss to the realities of everyday life. They become so preoccupied with the loss that they are unable to function effectively.

There are two types of dysfunctional (unresolved) grief; bereavement related depression and complicated grief. Both are associated with expressions of distress about the loss, changes in eating, sleeping patterns, talking and changes and in activity levels. With bereavement-related depression, the griever feels the loss so intensely that feelings of despair and worthlessness overwhelm everything else in life. Everyday is a gray fog with no light as one looks toward the future. Life becomes a burden, and each new day is faced with remorse. This attitude overshadows all else, and the griever experiences changes in eating, sleeping and activity levels, angry, hostile moods and an inability to concentrate or complete work tasks. To complicate matters, individuals often become more and more socially isolated and react with hostility and anger when friends or relatives express concern. This type of grief commonly leads to the despair of suicide.

'Bereavement, related depression responds well to treatment when it is recognized and interventions begun early'. A combination of psychotherapy and medicine has been effective, but emotional and social support are always important factors.

Complicated grief is 'a persistent yearning for a deceased person that often occurs without the signs of depression'. Although the symptoms appear to be those of normal grieving they are associated with impaired psychological functioning and disturbances of mood, sleep and self esteem. The griever becomes preoccupied with the loss and may idealize and search for the lost person or object, relieve past experience and yearn fro the past. Because life in the present is not as desirable as past memories, the individual may become of others and socially isolated.

Treatment for unresolved grief depends on the presence of depressive symptoms. A psychotherapeutic and psychopharmacological approach treats depression, whereas grief is helped by emotional support and a responsive ear. Support groups, self help groups/NGOs and opportunities for social interactions add to the effectiveness of treatment in most cases.

The therapeutic nursing interventions for both types of unresolved grief involving listening, providing emotional support, and referring to appropriate resources. Psychiatric nurses are often the first to identify the signs and symptoms of dysfunctional grieving because of their focus on client's activities of daily living. Therapeutic listening helps in understanding the needs of the grieving individual. It also offers an opportunity to provide emotional support and comfort. Sometimes, when grievers are encouraged to verbalize their feelings, the real healing begins. Nurses are also instrumental in referring their clients to the therapists, support group, and educational opportunities that assist in effectively working through the grieving process.

Acute Mania

Acute mania is also one of the psychiatric emergency. The stressors can stimulate for manic symptoms. Acute mania can be treated with antidepressants/mood stabilizers like lithium, carbamazepine, lamotrigine, gabapentin or valporic acid.

Adjustment Disorders

The client comes with symptoms of agitation, tearful depressed, anxious or even psychotic. This can be dealt with reassurance, spending more time with the client, frequent orientation and with mild tranquilizers.

Catatonia

It is rarely a true emergency. Clients can come with symptoms of fever, uncertain etiology, tachycardia hypotension, hyperaphea, etc. Neuroleptic symptoms are also associated with catatonia.

Catatonia can be diagnosed if the client has three primary or two primary plus two secondary signs/symptoms.

- *Primary Signs/Symptoms*
  - Immobility
  - Mutism
  - Withdrawal
- *Secondary Signs/Symptoms*
  - Staring
  - Rigidity
  - Posturing
  - Waxy flexibility
  - Echo phenomena
  - Stereotype
  - Verbigeration (stereotypic verbalization)
- *Treatment includes ECT and drugs.*

The client who has stopped eating

Sudden stoppage of eating may trigger an emergency. The underlying cause maybe, the client will be suffering from apathetic syndrome depression/schizophrenia. This can be treated with antidepressants, ECT, diet therapy and by multiple psychotherapeutic interventions.

Pisa Syndrome

Also called as dystonic syndrome, first described by Ekbom (Germany) in 1972 as a side effect of neuroleptic treatment.

Criteria of diagnosis

- Tonic flexion of the trunk to oneside or also seen as a learning backward as well–patients unable to stand straight.
- Accompanied by a slight truncal rotation.
- Remarkable indifference to a grossly abnormal posture.
- Current neuroleptic or antidepressant treatment.
  - The very effective treatment is to reduce or discontinuing the medication causing the syndrome. Anticholinergics may be administered.

Sundowning Syndrome

Clients with demeting disorders often become more confused in the late afternoon or evening 'when the sun goes down'. Some feel that this is caused by the diurnal variation in blood melatonin levels or a special sensitivity of the suprachiasmatic nucleus. Clients with this syndrome usually become increasingly disoriented and exhibit agitated and/or aggressive behavior as daylight wanes. Often, the abnormal behavior associated with this syndrome continue into the night and usually cause massive disruption in the client's life as well as in the lives of those caring for the client.

Both pharmacological and non-pharmacological strategies are used to manage these clients. Low doses of neuroleptics or trazodone given just before the onset of this syndrome and then midway through the cycle has been identified. For example, for the client who starts showing symptoms at 4:00 pm, a dose of trazodone at 3:00–3:30 pm can help attenuate the severity of the syndrome; another dose given between 7:30–8:00 pm can relieve the client of further distress and help insure that both the client and his/her caregiver get rest at night. Trazodone dosing usually starts at 25 mg at each of the two times and is slowly increased until the correct dose for the client is found. A useful alternative is risperidone, oral concentrate, starting at 0.25mg and a slow upward titration of the dose if necessary is administered.

Crisis

A 'crisis' has been defined as–an acute disruption of psychological homeostasis in which one's usual coping mechanisms fail and there exists evidence of distress and functional impairment. The subjective reaction to a stressful life experience that comprises the individuals, stability and ability to cope or function.

Crisis is also defined as a state of disequilibrium resulting from the interaction of an event with the individual or family coping mechanism which are inadequate to meet the demands of the situation combined with the individual's or family's perception of the meaning of the event.

Largerquist defined crisis' as a sudden event in one's life that disturbs homeostasis, during which usual coping mechanisms cannot resolve the problem'.

The main cause of a crisis is an intensely stressful traumatic or hazardous event, but two other conditions are also necessary (1) the individual's perception of the event as the cause of considerable upset and/or disruption; and (2) the individual's inability to resolve the disruption by previously used coping mechanisms. It also refers to 'an upset in the steady state'. It often has five components; a hazardous or traumatic event, a vulnerable or unbalanced state, a precipitating factor, an active crisis state based on the person's perception, and the resolution of the crisis (Roberts, 2005).

Crisis may influence life in different ways. As a consequences of crisis experience, the individual may go down to a lower or less healthy level of functioning than what was before the crisis or he may resume the same level of functioning by repressing the crisis because the challenge of crisis sometimes can bring out new strengths, skills and coping skills; so crisis can act in both ways, it can have positive or negative impact on one's life.

Factors that influence the outcome of crisis are as follows:

- The individual problems solving experience.
- How the individual views the problem?
- The amount of help or hindrances shown by significant others in his life.
  - Maladaptive crisis resolution increases the probability that the individual will unsuccessfully resolve crisis in the future.

Types of Crisis

- Developmental or maturational crisis
- Situational crisis
- Adventitious crisis
- Crisis due to psychopathology.

Developmental/Maturational Crisis

As human being grows he/she passes through many different stages of development. The transmission between these stages can be emotionally disturbing period to any individual, e.g. child's first separation from home to attend school, a girl who attains puberty, etc.

A maturational crisis may occur during any of the transitional periods in normal growth and developmental period. Because each stage of development is dependent on previous stage, the inability to master the tasks of previous stage disturbs one's growth and development in subsequent stages of life.

In each stage of development, a person needs nurturance from others to work through the task of that stage. When adequate social support from family and relatives, friends is available, the individual is able to channel his increased anxiety and resultant energy into constructive work which leads to feelings of accomplishment.

Situational Crisis

It is a response to traumatic events that usually sudden and unavoidable. When the stressful event threatens the physical, emotional and social integrity of the individual, crisis may develop. The threat or loss of individual role viewed as necessary to maintain self image will usually lead to a crisis state, e.g. Loss of a good job, loss of life partner, diagnosis of terminal illness, etc.

The most common response to loss or deprivation is depression. The difficulty in dealing with situational crisis is compounded if it occurs at the same time when the individual is struggling with a developmental crisis.

Adventitious Crisis

- It is the result of epidemic or natural/manmade disaster and usually occurs at a large scale, for example, Cloud bursting, earthquakes, tsunami, floods, hurricanes, etc.

Crisis due to Psychopathology

Crisis develops due to maladaptive response of individual due to psychopathology. Examples of psychopathology that can precipitate crisis include borderline personality, severe neurosis or schizophrenia etc.

PHASES OF CRISIS

Experts of crisis theory have explained various stages of crisis for theoretical purposes. All individual's need not go through each stages of crisis. The phases are:

- *Phase of denial:* This is the phase which occurs soon after the incident or immediately after the individual receives the message of incident. The victim shows disability and unacceptance of the incident or change usually , within few hours the individual acknowledges the reality.
- *Phase of increased pension:* As the reality is acknowledged, the victim experiences anxiety. He/she tries to function but many show depression or over activity. Most often the increased

tension acts as a motivating factor and the individual keeps himself busy with the activities and even overactive and efficient, e.g. the individual who efficiently carries out the funeral arrangement of a close relative.

- *Phase of disorganization:* This is the stage when the individual experiences real anxiety and feels that he cannot go any longer. This is due to the flood of anxiety. The individual may fall apart and experience the loss badly, for example, when crisis is related to loss of loved one, the victim was able to keep himself busy and when funeral is over, the last relative also leaves; then the victim really starts to feel the loss and loneliness when there is nobody to support and share feelings with him/her.
- *Attempt to reorganize:* The affected individual tries to recognize his/her life inspite of the loss. He/she resumes his/her duties and gradually progresses into permanent adjustment. This is where the previous coping mechanisms become useful.
- *Phase of attempt to escape from the problem:* The victim is lying to make an attempt to escape the reality. In this attempt, he/she blames others for what had happened. The individual uses a great deal of projection. Blaming and getting upset at others complicates the situation because it destroys the support of other people. With the help and support of understanding people the victim may soon move into local reorganization.
- *Phase of general reorganization:* The individual learns to adapt to the new situation. The victim's life is organized according to the loss in consideration and new circumstances. A woman after her husband's death often may go through above mentioned stage and normally within 4–6 weeks starts accepting the loss. She will start getting busy looking after family affairs and establishing contact with people.
- *Paradigm of balancing factors:* Aguilera (1986) illustrates a paradigm of balancing factors that determine whether a crisis occurs as the result of a stressful event. These factors, which can affect a return to equilibrium, are:
  - Realistic perception of an event;
  - Adequate situational support and;
  - Adequate coping mechanisms to help resolve a problem.

A realistic perception occurs when a person is able to distinguish the relationship between an event and feelings of stress. For example, a 45-year-old executive recognizes the fact that his company is on the verge of bankruptcy because of inefficient projected financial planning by the board of trustees. He does not place the blame on himself and view himself as a failure, although he realizes the seriousness of the situation and feels stressed. His perception rather than the actual event will determine his reaction to the situation.

The executive may discuss the situation with a financial consultant, a lawyer or the firm's accountant. Such persons available in the climate are considered to be situational supports because they reflect appraisals of one's intrinsic and extrinsic values. Support by these people may prevent a state of disequilibrium and crisis from occurring. The less readily available emotional or environmental support systems (i.e. family or friends) are, the more overwhelming or hazardous with the person defining the event, thus increasing vulnerability to crisis.

Coping mechanisms are those methods which one usually employs to cope with anxiety or stress and reduce tension in difficult situations. They may be conscious or unconscious revealing themselves in behavioral outcomes such as denial, intellectualization, productive worrying, grieving, crying, aggression, regression, withdrawal, or repression. The executive may cope by burying himself in his work, calling an emergency meeting of the board of trustees to discuss the situation or withdrawing from the situation. Coping mechanisms are used during early developmental stages and if found effective in maintaining emotional stability, will become a part of one's lifestyle in dealing with daily stress. The person who met development tasks and achieved a level of personal maturity generally will adapt more readily in a crisis. Additional factors that may influence the developmental of a crisis include the physical and emotional status of a person, previous experience with similar situations and cultural influences.

CRISIS INTERVENTION

'Crisis intervention is an active but temporary entry into the life situation of an individual, a family or a group during a period of stress' (Mitchell and Resnick 1991). It is an attempt to resolve an immediate crisis when a person's goals are obstructed and usual problem-solving methods fail. The client is called on to be active in all steps of the crisis intervention process, including clarifying the problem, verbalizing feelings, identifying goals and options for reaching goals and deeding on a plan.

Crisis intervention can occur in a variety of settings, for example, the home, community, emergency settings, industrial clinics, classroom, intensive care unit or psychiatric unit. The generic approach focuses on a particular kind of crisis with direct encouragement of adaptive behavior, general support, environmental manipulation and anticipatory guidance. The individual approach stresses the present, shows little or no concern for the developmental past and places an emphasis on the immediate causes of disequilibrium. It can be used as secondary or tertiary prevention and can be effective in preventing future crisis.

The goals of crisis intervention are:

- To decrease emotional stress and protect the crisis victim from additional stress.
- To assist the victim in organizing and mobilizing resources or support systems to meet unique needs and reach a solution for the particular situation or circumstance that precipitated the crisis. It is hoped that this action will prevent hospitalization, reduce the risk of chronic maladaptation and promote adaptive family dynamics.
- To return the crisis victim to a precrisis or higher level of functioning.

Robert's Seven-Stage Crisis Intervention Model

In conceptualizing the process of crisis intervention, Roberts 2005 has identified seven critical stages through which clients typically pass on the road to crisis stabilization, resolution and mastery (Fig. 13.2). These stages, listed below, are essential, sequential and sometimes overlapping in the process of crisis intervention.

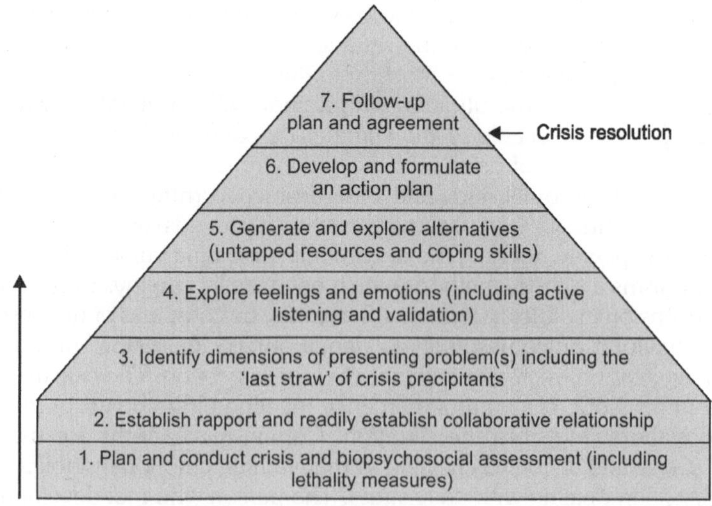

Fig. 13.2: Robert's seven-stage crisis intervention model

1. Plan and conduct a thorough biopsychosocial and lethality or imminent danger assessment;
2. Make psychological contact and rapidly establish the collaborative relationship.
3. Identify the major problems, includings crisis precipitants.
4. Encourage an exploration of feeling and emotions.
5. Generate and explore alternatives and new coping strategies.
6. Restore functioning through implementation of an action plan.
7. Plan follow-up and booster sessions.

- *Stage 1:* Psychosocial and Lethality Assessment
  - It should cover the client's environmental supports and stressors, medical needs and medications, current use of drugs and alcohol and internal and external coping methods and resources (Eaton and Ertl 2000).
  - Assessing lethality, first and foremost, involves ascertaining whether the client has actually initiated attempt, such as ingesting a poison or overdose of medication. If no attempt, assessment for 'potential, for self harm will be under taken.
- *Stage 2:* Rapidly Establish Rapport
  - Rapport is facilitated by the presence of counselor-offered conditions such as genuineness, respect and acceptance of the client (Roberts, 2005). Maintain good eye contact, nonjudgemental attitude, creativity, flexibility, positive mental attitude, reinforcing small gains and resilience.
- *Stage 3:* Identify the Major Problems or Crisis Precipitants: Crisis intervention focuses on the client's current problems which are often the one that precipitated the crisis.
- *Stage 4:* Deal with Feelings and Emotions.
  - By active listening, ventilate and express feelings, to vent and heal, and explain.
- *Stage 5:* Generate and Explore Alternatives:
  - This is a difficult stage to accomplish in crisis intervention. Clients, usually lack the equanimity to study the big picture and tend to doggedly cling to familiar ways of coping even when they are backfiring. However, if stage IV has been achieved, the client in crisis has probably worked out enough feelings to re-establish some emotional balance. Now, clinician and client can begin to put options on other table, like no-suicide contract or brief hospitalization for ensuring the client's safety; or discuss alternatives for finding temporary housing or consider the pros and cons of various programs for treating drug dependency. It is important to keep in mind that these alternatives are better when they are generated collaboratively and when the alternatives selected are 'owned' by the client.
- *Stage 6:* Implement an action plan: In this stage, strategies become integrated into an empowering treatment plan or coordinated interventions. These strategies are:
  - Maintaining safe and secure climate.
  - Negotiating safety.
  - Future linkage.
  - Decreasing anxiety and sleep loss.
  - Decreasing isolation.
  - Hospitalization.
- *Stage 7:* Follow up.
  - Crisis workers should plan for a follow-up contact with the client after the initial intervention to ensure that the crisis is on its way to be resolved and to evaluate the postcrisis status of the client. This postcrisis evaluation of the client can include:

- Physical condition of the client (e.g. sleeping, nutrition, diet, hygiene).
- Cognitive mastery of the precipitating event (does the client have a better understanding of what happened and why it happened ?).
- An assessment of overall functioning including, social, spiritual, employment and academic.
- Satisfaction and progress with ongoing treatment (e.g. financial counseling).
- Any current stressors and how those are being handled.
- Need for possible referrals (e.g. legal, housing, medical).

Follow-up can also include the scheduling of a 'booster' session in about a month after the crisis intervention has been terminated. Treatment gains and potential problems can be discussed at the booster session.

Nursing Perceptives

Merely, Messicle and Aguilera have identified four phases of crisis intervention:

- Assessment of the individual and problem.
- Planning the therapeutic intervention.
- Implementing the intervention.
- Evaluation of crisis/resolution and anticipatory planning.

Assessment of the Individual Client and Problem

- Assessment is carried to rectify the strength and limitations of the victim.
- Primarily the nurse must determine whether the person is really in crisis or it is perceived one.
- Assess for the precipitating situation like loss, and grief.

The Client's Feelings

The psychiatric nurse asks the client to describe the feelings he/she is experiencing by accepting client's feelings without judgment. The nurse assists him/her and accept his/her own feelings. It is important for the nurse to understand the client both cognitively and emotionally.

Assessment of the problem involves three areas of consideration.

- Client's perception of the problem.
- Situational support.
- Client's coping skills.

Client's Perception of the Problem

The nurse must explore the client's perception of the crisis precipitating event and identify the factors which are affecting the client's ability to solve the problem.

Ask the following questions:

- Why did you come for help today?
- What effect is this problem having on others around you?
- How do you see that this is affecting your future?
- What do you see as the solution of the problem?

- The nurse assesses how realistically or unrealistically the client perceives the problem and what factors are influencing the client's perception. An important factor which can influence perception is where the client starts in terms of the developmental cycle.

Situational Support or Support System

After determining the client's perception of event, the nurse focuses on who will be available to be supportive to the client. Significant individuals from client's life should be involved to maximize the effectiveness of intervention.
The use of question like:

- Who supports the client?
- With whom the client lives?
- With whom he/she interacts?
- On whom the client trusts more?
- How is her/his social network?

Client's Coping Skills

Coping skills involve the ways in which individual behaves when confronted with a problem that cannot be solved. Coping skills are very individual so the client must be asked the following:

- Has anything like this event happened before?
- What have you done to deal with anxiety, tension or depression?
- Have you tried the something this time?
- Has it worked out?
- Whatelse do you think might work?
- Is the person still continuing her/his occupation, academics or other roles?
- Are the significant others also affected?
- Are they also upset?
- The nurse then determines whether the client's coping mechanisms are adaptive or maladaptive. The nurse also assesses the degree to which the individual is affected by the client.

As assessment of the person in crisis is not complete without asking him/her about any plans regarding self-harm or blaming himself/herself. Many people will not volunteer this information, but when asked will really speak out the suicidal thoughts. If the client has ever attempted suicide or has decided how, when and where will kill himself/herself; the client needs protection. The suicidal client should not be left alone and needs an experienced therapist.

From the above assessment the nurse should know what is the nature of client's feelings, his/her perception of the precipitating event, how he/she copes with stress and what are his suicidal potentials?

Planning Nursing Therapeutic Interventions

Crisis intervention is a structured, objective problem-solving approach. To ensure the success of the plan the client must be involved in planning solution to the problem so that he/she can be provided with opportunity to grow and develop more constructive coping skills for future use.

Successful planning depends upon in-depth assessment and diagnosis of the client's level of functioning and his dependence needs. Together the client and the nurse define a time frame and goals for resolution of the crisis. Often in planning it is helpful for interviewer to outline the problem and available resources. The crisis must be identified whether it is self-related, family-related or a combination of these, e.g. a young couple experiencing normal stress of first time parenthood which can be converted into situational crisis after the birth of a retarded child.

Goal Setting for the Client in Crisis

The major goal is to establishing client's equilibrium for this, following points can be taken into consideration.

- Establishing a working relationship.
- Identification of client's specific problems.
- Reduction of the client's distorted perception of the problem.
- Improvement of client's self-esteem.
- Decreasing client's anxiety.
- Promotion of involvement of family and friends.
- Reinforcement of healthy coping mechanisms.
- Validation of client's ability to solve his/her problem.

Implementation of the Interventions

- In this phase the intervention can take place on many levels with the use of variety of techniques.
- Shields has described four specific level of crisis intervention which represent a hierarchy from the most superficial to the most in-depth.
- Environmental manipulation
- General approach
- Generic approach
- Individual approach.

Environmental Approach

It includes those interventions which directly change the client's physical or interpersonal support for the purpose of providing situational support or removing stress, e.g. a client who is having difficulty coping with children may temporarily send children to their grandmother's home. By this technique, some stress can be reduced. Similarly a client having difficulty on his/her job may take leave of a week, so he/she can be removed temporarily from that stress. Like this, involving the client in group therapy or family therapy also provides environmental manipulation for the purpose of providing support.

General Approach

It includes those interventions which provide the client with the feeling that the nurse is on his/her side and will be a helping person. The nurse's demonstration of therapeutic element of warm acceptance, empathy and caring with her reassurance results in this type of support.

Generic Approach

In this type of crisis intervention, emphasis is based on reaching high-risk individuals in great numbers in as short time as possible. It applies a specific method to all those individuals faced who similar type of crisis. The intervention then is set to ensure that the course of crisis intervention results in an adaptive resolution.

Individual Approach

It is a type of crisis intervention that is analogous to the model of diagnosis and client with a specific problem is a specific client. In this approach, the nurse needs to have a thorough understanding of the client's psychodynamics that led to the present crisis and most consequently use the intervention to aid the particular client to achieve an adaptive resolution of the crisis. This type of intervention is effective in combined crisis of situational and maturational type. The individual approach is also useful when symptoms include strong components of homicide and suicidal ideas. The individual approach is aided by the use of some techniques of crisis intervention that are as follows:

- **Abreaction:** This is a process similar to ventilation. The only difference is that the degree of emotional release is much greater here. The client might burst out sobbing while recounting his experiences. Usually abreaction is encouraged in crisis intervention. The nurse facilitates it by asking the client how he/she feels about his/her situation, recent events and significant people involved in his/her crisis. The nurse asks open ended questions and reflects the client's words back to him/her so that the client will further, ventilate his/her feelings. It is better to help him/her focus on thinking through the consequences of carrying out the act rather than encouraging free expression of the anger feelings.
- **Classification:** Classification is used when nurse encourages the client to express mere clearly the relationship for certain events in his/her life or the nurse herself/himself may point out possible relationships. Clarification enables the person to gain a better intellectual understanding of her/his feelings and how they led to the development of crisis.
- **Suggestion:** Suggestion is a process of influencing an individual so that he/she accepts an idea or belief. In crisis intervention the nurse influences the client to see her/him as a confident, calm, hopeful and empathetic leader.
- **Reinforcement of behavior:** This is reinforcing useful and adaptive behaviors of the client by the nurse. The nurse strengthens positive responses made by the client by agreeing with or complementing those responses.
- **Raising self-esteem:** This is important because the client in crisis feels helpless and may be overwhelmed with worthlessness. The nurse does this by communicating to the client that he/she can participate actively in finding solution to his problems.
- **Evaluation of crisis/resolution of the crisis and anticipatory planning:** To evaluate the crisis intervention, a reassessment is done to determine if the interventions were successful and the objective which was framed has been achieved. During this phase the nurse and the client summarizes what has occurred during the intervention. The nurse will also determine whether further follow–up or referral is needed or crisis is resolved.

STRESS: ADAPTATION AND COUNSELING

- In modern times, stress is a universal phenomena. Now, the psychiatric medicine fraternity are more concerned on this topic. It is most researched in the field of psychology and applied sciences. Hense, Selye (1956) defined stress in two different ways: one view states that stress

as the rate of wear and tear within the body: the other describes stress as the state manifested by a specific syndrome which consists of all the non-specifically induced changes within a biological system.
- Burgers (1997) defines stress in two different ways.
  - Stress is a stimulus that upsets an individual's balance or homeostasis and
  - Stress is an individual's response to a stressful stimulus.
- Stress maybe defined as a real or perceived threat to the physiological or psychological and/or behavioral response. It is a bodily or mental tension resulting from factors that tend to alter the existing equilibrium. Stress maybe negative or positive. It involves a stressors and a stress response.
- According to stress appraisal theory (1984), stress is a particular relationship between a person and the enviorment that is appraised by the person as taxing or exceeding his/her resources and endangering his/her well being.

STRESSORS

Stressors are the stimuli proceeding or precipitating a change. It maybe internal (fear, guilt) or external (trauma, environment) (Fig. 13.3).

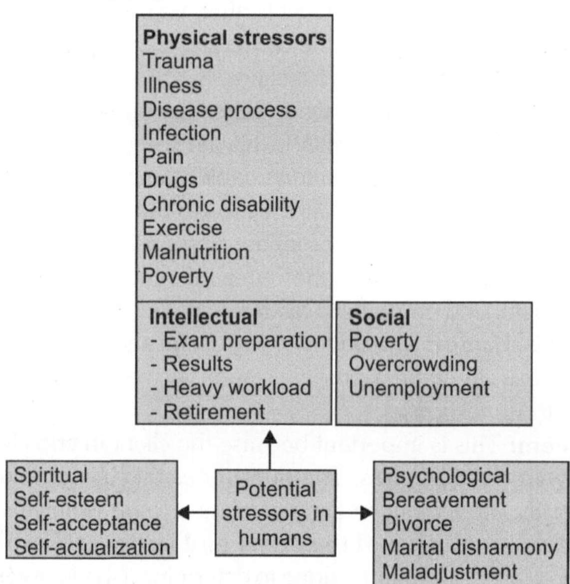

Fig.13.3: Potential stressors in humans

Stress Response

It is the compensatory reaction, the body makes to the disturbances caused by the stressors.

Types of Stress

- *Positive Stress/Eustress:* The stress that occurs from good hectic sources like marriages, celebrations, birth of a baby, conference, winning the lottery, etc.

- *Negative Stress/Distress:* It results from bad sources like difficult work environment, overwhelming sights and sounds, threat of personal injury, etc.
  - Results of Positive Stress:
    - Enables success and concentration.
    - Enhances performance.
    - Energized for further motion.
  - Results of Negative Stress:
    - Loss of motivation.
    - Reduced effectiveness.
    - Problems in physical, psychosocial domains.

THEORIES/MODELS OF STRESS

James-Lange: Theory of Emotion

In 1984–85, William James and Carl Lange proposed a correlation of stress and emotions. They proposed that emotions do not immediately succeed the perception of the stressor or the stressful event; they become present after the body's response to the stress. For example, when you see a barking dog, the heart rate increases, breath begins faster, then the eyes become wide open. According to theorists, the feeling of fear or any other emotion only begins after you experience these bodily changes. It means that the emotional behavior is not possible to occur unless it is connected to one's brain.

Cannon-Bard: The Emergency Theory

This theory is quite the opposite of Jame's and Lange's theory. According to Walter Cannon, emotion in response to stress can actually occur even when the bodily changes are not present. Cannon proposed that the visceral or internal physiological response of one's body is more slowly recognized by the brain as compared with its function to release emotional response.

Philip Bard expanded Cannon's theory by postulating that a lower brainstem structure, the 'thalamus' is important in the production of emotional responses. According to Bard, the emotional response is released first, and then sent as signals by the thalamus to the brain cortex for the interpretation alongside with the sending of signals to the sympathetic nervous system or SNS to begin the physiologic response to stress. Therefore, this theory argues that emotional response to stress is not a product of the physiologic response, rather they occur simultaneously.

The Schachater-Singer Theory

Stanley Schachater and Lerome Singer postulated that the appropriate identification of the emotion requires both cognitive activity and emotional arousal in order to experience an emotion. According to them, we become aware of the reason believed the emotional response and when we the reason is not obvious, we start to look for environmental clues for the proper interpretation of the emotion to occur.

Theory of Stress—General Adaptation Syndrome (GAS)

General adaptation syndrome (GAS) theory was propagated by Hans Selye (1907–1982). He was a Hungarian endocrinologist, first to give a scientific explanation to biological stress.

He explained, stress model based on physiology and psychobiology as general adaptation syndrome (GAS). According to Selye, he states that an event that threatens an organism's well-being (a stressor) leads to a three-stage bodily response.

- **Stage 1:** Alarm reaction.
- **Stage 2:** Resistance stage.
- **Stage 3:** Exhaustion stage.

Stage 1: Alarm Reaction/Phase

The alarm reaction is a typical fight-or-flight reaction, which is an immediate, short-term life-preserving sympathetic nervous system response to a stressor. The perception of a stressor triggers release of corticotrophin hormone releasing factor (CRF) which influences the hypothalamus to produce other hormones that initiate a cascade of physiological response. These responses include dilatation of pupils, increased cardiac rate, strength and output, increased blood flow to brain, heart and skeletal muscles, tension headache and pain leading to dilatation of bronchi with increased muscle tone, increased cellular metabolism, breakdown of fat to form free fatty acids that can be used by muscles; synthesis of more glucose from glycerol; increased ADH and aldosterone production, retention of salt and water by kidneys in order to boost blood volume and breakdown of glycogen in order to make more glucose.

Stage 2: The Resistance Phase

It is an adaptation stage that occurs due to continued exposure to the stressor or threat and is the body's way of adapting to the instability caused by the stressors. Neuroendocrine responses such as adrenocortical responses facilitate changes that enable the body to fight for self-preservation. This involves anabolic reactions and mobilization of all the body's resources. It is likely that the variables of psychosocial resources, optimism are part of this resistance or adaptation phase and help to define the individual differences in the ability to cope with stress.

Stage 3: Exhaustion Phase

It results from long-term continued exposure to stressors from both the internal and the external environments coupled with inadequate adaptive mechanisms. It is in this phase when resources are depleted that irreversible damage to tissues or to the individual occurs and this is sometimes followed by illness and death. For example, a person with a continued job stress may experience long-term stress, which can give birth to hypertension and may even to heart diseases.

The Unified Stress Model

The totality of the disruption to the individual's homeostasis and the response by the individual has inherent properties of a unified stress model (Fig. 13.4). It encompasses not only the potential stressors in human existence as stimuli but also the coping mechanisms within the individual, issues of perception, aspects of laws of control and adaptation. The following chart views this unified stress model whereby both the short and long-term effects of stress are observed. In this unified model any of the five dimensions of the individual (physical, emotional, intellectual, social and spiritual) have potential to or can generate a situation or event (the stimulus) that can be perceived by the brain as a stressor, and in addition the nature of the mind-body response to the stressor, coping mechanisms inherent in the individual and how the individual adapts are all shown. It is observed that adaptation is a continuation of the initial autonomic nervous system, endocrine, muscle and other organ responses. Adequate coping mechanisms to the activating stimulus lead to quick adaptation and a restoration of homeostasis. However, inadequate coping measures lead to lack of or breakdown in adaptation and a cycle of chronic stress with the possibility of development of mental illness.

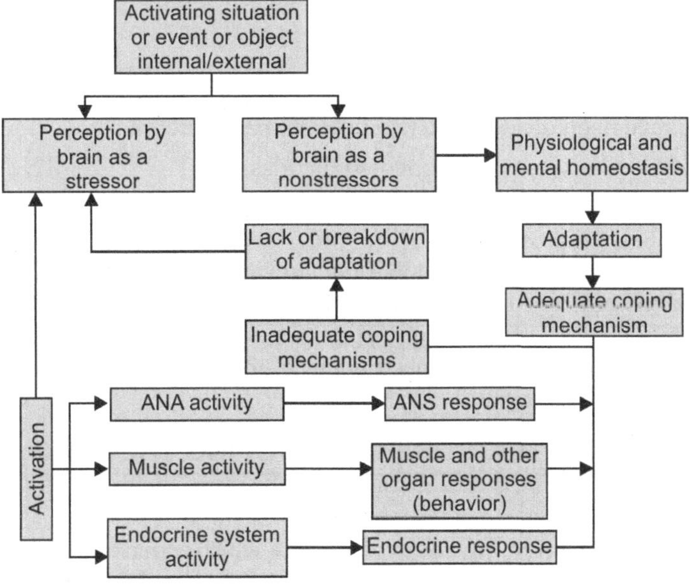

Fig.13.4: The unified stress model.

ADAPTATION/COPING

The Concept of Coping

Stress requires not only bodily adaptation, but also adaptation at the mental level. The organisms resist change and react to external challenges by mounting responses that maintain their equilibrium. There are equivalents at many levels. At the cellular level, maintaining homeostasis is the role of the immune system, at the organ level the endocrine and the limbic systems are involved, at the psychological, while at the social level, norms, philosophy, values and social sanctions maintain order.

Coping is expanding conscious effort to master, reduce or tolerate stress. It is defined as ongoing cognitive and behavioral efforts to manage specific external and internal demands that are appraised as taxing or exceeding the resources of the person (Lazarus, 1993).

It may also be defined as thoughts or actions designed to resolve or mitigate a problematic situation. Coping is not a fixed attribute, but is the dynamic capacity to apply suitable methods to control, avoid appraisal prevent distress. It is also a process that involves appraisal and reaction; we do not use identical responses in every situation. Coping refers to the management of responses; not mastery over stimuli. It normally refers to managing unusual demands that tax, even exceed, a person's resources; we do not generally speak of coping with making our bed or brushing our teeth.

Theories of Coping

Basically, coping refers to an individual's attempt to tolerate or minimize the effect of the stress. Whether it is the stressor or the experience of stress itself. Coping theories can be classified according to orientation or focus (trait-oriented or state-oriented) and approach (macroanalytic or microanalytic).

Classification of Coping Theories

Coping theories have been divided into two different parameters:

1. Trait-oriented theories versus state-oriented theories.
2. Microanalytic approach versus macroanalytic approach.

The trait-oriented theories focus on the early recognition of a person's resources and tendencies related to coping while the state-oriented theories emphasizes the actual coping of an individual and the outcome of his application of coping methods or strategies.

On the other hand, the microanalytic approach studies a wide variety of specific and concrete coping strategies; while the macroanalytic approach concentrates on fundamental and abstract coping methodologies.

MACROANALYTIC, TRAIT ORIENTED COPING THEORIES

Repression-Sensitization

This theory states that there is a bipolar dimension in which a person copes with the stress in only one of two opposite poles repression or sensitization. People who tend to be repressors cope with the stress by means of denying or minimizing its existence. They use the avoidance coping mechanism such that they are unable to realize the potential negative outcomes of the stressful experience. In contrast to this, sensitizers tend to react to stress with rumination, excessive worrying and obsessive search for information on stress-related cues.

Monitoring and Blunting

According to Miller, monitoring and blunting is a construct that is based on the repression-sensitization theory due to the similarity in their nature as cognitive informational styles. However, this construct, particularly blunting, explains the impact of uncontrollable stressful cues which can be reduced by the individual through the use of cognitive avoidance (e.g. denial, reinterpretation, distraction).

Under controllable stress, monitoring is said to be a more effective coping strategy, as it includes seeking information related to the stressor.

Model of Coping Modes (MCM)

This model originates from the monitoring blunting construct, and is also related to the repression sensitization conception, but expands concepts of vigilance and cognitive avoidance with an underpinning of cognitive motivational approach. It emphasizes that a person is stimulated to avert the situation and perceive the stressor in an ambiguous manner in the presence of the stressor.

Macroanalytic, State-Oriented Theories

The defense mechanism construct by Sigmund Freud in 1926 is one of the few macroanalytic, state-orientad theories of coping. A number of defense mechanisms were basically related to intellectualization and repression, the two basic forms that were emphasized by Freud in 1936.

Richard Lazarus and Susan-Folkman proposed yet another theory of coping in a macroanalytic approach. Concentrating on the coping strategies that are focused on emotion or on the problem itself, as well as the function related to them.

While the theory of Lazarus and Folkman proposed theory of coping in a macroanalytic approach, where in Lazarus et al was able to specify coping strategies and classify them into eight groups. These include self-controlling, confrontative coping, seeking social support, distancing, escape-avoidance, accepting responsibility, positive appraisal and planful problem-solving.

Defense mechanisms/coping mechanisms, are the unconscious (mostly) strategies used to deal with stress and as the term suggests involve defensive coping. They are different from conscious coping strategies. Coping can be adaptive or maladaptive. Maladaptive coping may appear to remove the stress. But it is not effective in long run duration. For example, those who consume drugs/withdraw from the social climate is maladaptive coping.

Types of Coping Strategies

Appraisal-focused Strategies

These occur when the person modifies the way he/she thinks (e.g. using positive appraisal or reframing a situation to see it in a positive way).

Problem-focused Coping

It is aimed at changing or eliminating the source of the stress (e.g. Learning new skills to manage the problem, seeking information or seeking social support).

Emotion-focused Strategies

These are directed at managing or reducing emotional distress (e.g. releasing pent-up emotions or watching TV excessively)/computer gaming, etc, so as to distract oneself from the problem.

- Coping is a process rather than an event. An individual may alternate between several of the above coping strategies in order to cope with a stressful event.
- Task-oriented or direct coping focuses on the immediate problem and aims to change an uncomfortable situation. They maybe categorized as follows:
  - Attack (confrontation): In confrontation all efforts are aimed at removing the obstacles to the goal. This could mean learning a new skill or putting in more effort.
  - Withdrawal: Sometimes, withdrawal is the only way of coping with stress and escaping from stress which cannot be overcome. Although this can shut the door to other options, it may, at times, be sensible and help people to move on in life situations.
  - Compromise: This could mean accepting substitute goals or settling for something slightly different from their original plan.

STRESS MANAGEMENT

Strategy 1: Avoid Unnecessary Stress

Not all stress can be avoided and it is not healthy to avoid a situation that needs to be addressed. Learn how to say 'no'—know your limits and stick to them. Whether in personal/professional life, refuse to accept added responsibilities. Taking on more can surefire for stress.

- Avoid people who stress you out.
- Take control of your environment.
- Avoid hot-button topics—such as politics, etc.
- Pen down your to do list.

Strategy 2: Stress Management

Alter the situation if you cannot avoid a stressful situation, try to alter it. Figure out what you can do to change things so the problem does not present itself in near future. Often, this involves changing the way you communicate and operate in daily life situation.

- Express your feelings instead of bottling them up.
- Be willing to compromise.
- Be more assertive.
- Manage your time better.

Stress Management Strategy 3: Adapt to the Stressor

If you cannot change the stressor, change yourself. You can adapt to stressful situations and regain your sense of control by changing the expectation and attitude.

- Reframe the problems.
- Looking at the big picture.
- Adjust your standards.
- Focus on positive things.

Stress Management Strategy 4: Accept the Things You cannot Change

Some sources of stress are unavoidable. You cannot prevent or change stressors such as the death of a loved one, a serious illness, or a national economic recession. In such cases, the best way to cope with stress is to accept things as they are. Acceptance maybe difficult, but in the long run, it is easier than railing against a situation you cannot change.

- Do not try to control the uncontrollable.
- Look for the upside.
- Share your feelings.
- Learn to forgive.

Stress Management Strategy 5: Make Time for Fun and Relaxation

Beyond a take-charge approach and a positive attitude, you can reduce stress in your life by nurturing yourself. If you regularly make time for fun and relaxation, you will be in a better place to handle life's stressors when they inevitably occur.

Healthy Ways to Relax and Recharge

- Walking.
- Spend time in nature.

- Call a good friend.
- Sweat out tension with a good work out.
- Write in your diary.
- Take a long bath.
- Light scented candles.
- Savor a warm up of coffee or tea.
- Play with a pet.
- Work in garden.
- Get a massage.
- Curl up with a good book.
- Listen to music.
- Watch a comedy.
- Connect with others.
- Do something you enjoy everyday.
- Keep your sense of humor.

Stress Management Strategy 6: Adopt a Healthy Lifestyle

You can increase your resistance to stress by strengthening your physical health.

- Exercise regularly.
- Eat a healthy diet.
- Reduce caffeine and sugar.
- Avoid alcohol, cigarettes and drugs.
- Get enough sleep.

Nursing Implications of Stress and Coping

Psychiatric nursing/nursing involves activities and interpersonal relationship that are often stressful. Carrying for clients who are experiencing high levels of anxiety can be stressed provoking. Some of the job/work related stressed that a nurse may experience are:

- Dealing with violence and drug addicts.
- Dealing with death and dying.
- Low job control.
- Heavy work pressure.
- Night shifts.
- Low socio-economic support.
- Frequent shifts of duty roaster.
- Dealing with uncooperative family member and clients.
- Uncertainty about client's treatment.

In addition, nursing being mostly female dominated, stresses resulting from the combined responsibilities of work, marriage and children are commonly observed. Nurses working with psychiatric clients are subjected to additional stressors as they experience a sort of violence at work. Intensive care nurses face stresses due to an increase in the number of critically ill clients and the introduction of highly sophisticated technologies in the intensive care environment.

Compassion fatigue and burnout are common among nurses. Compassion fatigue occurs when one cannot rescue or save an individual from harm. This results in 'frustration' a sense of loss of control, increased willful efforts and diminishing morale (Valent, 2002). Cross cultural research shows that nurses cope with workplace stressors by using effective problem-solving techniques, self-control, seeking social support and positive reappraisal.

COUNSELING

Counseling is 'a relationship in which one person endeavours to help another to understand and solve his adjustment problems' (English and English, 1958). In 1959, Patterson defines counseling as the process involving the interpersonal relationship between a therapist and one or more clients, by which the former employs psychological methods based on systematic knowledge of the human personality in attempting to improve the mental health of the latter. According to Patterson, counseling is not about providing information though information maybe given in counseling. It is also not giving advice, suggestions or recommendations.

Goals and Outcomes

- Counseling leads to change in one or more of the following areas-behavior, beliefs and level of emotional distress. Change in behavior is usually noticed first, since it is overt and observable.
- Counseling enhances an individual's ability to cope with life situations. For example, counseling can help people with terminal illness learn to accept suffering and appreciate the care and concern shown by family members, instead of cursing their fate and avoiding people.
- Counseling can improve a client's self-concept and make him/her feel more worthy.
- The purpose of counseling is to provide conditions which will help the client make independent decisions and become autonomous.
- Counseling leads to the resolution of problems of an emotional or interpersonal nature.
- Counseling helps individual clarify values for the future.
- An important goal of counseling is achieving positive mental health.

PRINCIPLES OF COUNSELING

- Counseling is a helping relationship that is usually carried out in a face to face situation. Two conditions are necessary for a relationship to be labelled as counseling. First, the client should have a problem, and second, the counselor should be skilled in working with such problems.
- It is directed at self-realization and self-direction.
- It is important for counsellors to recognize and understand a client's unique qualities. They must have genuine respect for clients and accept them as they are.
- It is necessary to allow clients to express their feelings without condemning or criticizing them. Only when the counselors are sensitive to the client's feelings, can they understand their meaning and respond to them accurately.
- The principle of confidentiality is very important in a counseling relationship. It is the right of a client to expect that what he reveals will not be disclosed to anyone.
- The client's freedom to make independent decisions must be encouraged. This will promote responsibility on the part of the client to make the necessary changes.
- A counselor does not have the right to impose his values on the client. Counselors must work within the framework of the basic value systems in a given society.
- The physical setting should be taken care of. Counseling has to be done in a private and relatively informal setting.
- Acceptance of the client as he/she is.

- Purposeful therapeutic working relationship.
- Nonjudgmentally.
- Immediacy.
- Lead.
- Advice.
- Classification.

PROCESS OF COUNSELING

Counseling is a process and involves certain steps towards the goal.

- *Identification of the problem:* The counselor and client must establish contact and the client's problems have to be identified.
- *In-depth exploration:* The counselor helps the client reach a clearer understanding of his problem and life situation.
- *Selecting goals and action plans:* A new sense of direction is formulated which enables the client to identify specific goals for change and action plans to implement the selected goals.
- Implementing and evaluating the action plan.
  It is possible to reach these steps only if good therapeutic rapport and trust have been established. As the client tries out his action plans, the counselor supports him and evaluates the effectiveness of newly-acquired behaviors or attitudes.

Counselor Skills

Egan (1986) identifies three stages of counseling relationship, which can be simplified as exploring, understanding and acting. Burnard has divided these skills into two categories namely: listening and attending skills and counseling intervention skills.

Active Listening

Listening is the most important skill a service provider must possess. Total attention should be paid to what is being said, observe nonverbal messages; the client is sending and encourage the client to talk by nodding the head and saying 'go on'. Some of the counseling behaviors which represent active listening skill are:

- Good eye contact.
- Head nodding are relevant places.
  - Saying (hummmmm).
  - Telling 'go on'.
- Not rushing the client during pauses while the client maybe finding words to express oneself.
- Not interrupting when the client is talking.
- Ask questions to facilitate conversation.

Reflecting

Questions and feelings are referred back to the client so that they maybe recognized and accepted and the client may recognize that his or her point of view has value. It is a good technique to use when the client asks the nurse for advice.

For example:

- *Client:* ' What do you think I should do about my wife's drinking problem?'
- *Nurse:* 'What do you think you should do?.'

- *Client:* ' My sister would not help a bit toward my mother's care. I have to do it all.'
- *Nurse:* ' You feel angry when she does not help.'

Focusing

- Taking notice of a single idea or even a single word.
  - *Example:* Like you and I discuss together.

Offering General Leads

- Offer the client encouragement to continue, e.g. yes I see, go on...

Summarizing and Paraphrasing

The main idea of what the client has said is repeated in his or her own words to check whether it has been correctly understood. This indicates to the client that the provider has been following and understanding what has been said by the client.
For example:
- *Client:* 'I cannot study, my mind keeps wondering.'
- *Nurse:* 'You have difficulty concentrating.'
- *Client:* 'I cannot take that new job. What if I cannot do it?'
- *Nurse:* 'You are afraid you will fail in this new position.'

Empathy

In empathizing with a client, the health personnel leaves aside her/his own frame of reference, and for the time being adopts the frame of reference of the client and then appreciated how the client experiences the events in his/her world. For empathy to have are impact, it is essential that the health personnel must communicate or reflect back to the client that the client's feelings are being understood and his/her emotional state is important. The client must feel understand. Empathy maybe communicated verbally, non–verbally or by a mixture of both.

Observations

Verbalizing what is observed or perceived. This encourages the client to recognize specific behavior and compare perceptions with the nurse.
- **Example**: Nurse – ' You appear tense today'
  - ' I notice you are pacing a lot. You seem uncomfortable when you........'

Analyzing Each Option with the Client

- The information given should include possible adverse reactions /failures and ways to tackle them.
- For example: To adopt the family planning method by eligible couples.
- The client must be actively involved in this process of checking out the gains and cost involved in implementation of his/her decision.

Reassurance

It can be used to relieve fears, boost self-confidence and promote hope (but to promote to client's hopes unreasonably by providing false reassurance or to intervene prematurely before the client has explained his situation fully should be avoided).

Explanation: (Interpretative Comments)

The therapist encourages the provision of explanation of such diverse matters as the nature of client's symptoms, the choice of treatment and the likely outcome.

Guidance and Suggestion

This involves the provision of direct and indirect advice. The client is taught how and when to ask for help. Advice maybe necessary with regard to particular problems, such as optimal ways of relating to particular difficult relative or handling a job interview or to general issues such as making contact with members of opposite gender.

Ventilation

The value of ventilation of feeling within psychotherapies is well accepted. It is useful for clients to be able to express emotions such as anger, frustration and despair openly.

Psychodynamic Life Narrative

This technique can be used as a supportive interpretation. The narrative is a formulation of the client's difficulties (crisis) as the inevitable product of previous life experiences. It serves to give or accepting his/her own emotional responses as justifiable and inevitable and to strengthen the client's alliance with the therapist.

Nontherapeutic Communication Techniques in Counseling

- Giving reassurance indicates to the client that there is no cause for anxiety, thereby devaluing the client's feelings.
- Rejecting/refusing to consider or showing contempt for the client's ideas or behavior. The client discontinues interaction with the nurse for fear of further rejection.
- Agree or disagree indicating according with or opposition to the client's ideas or opinions.
- Giving advice and telling the client what do or how to behave implies that the nurse knows what is best and the client is incapable of self-direction.
- Probing and pushing the client for answers to the issues which the client does not wish to discuss.
- Defending/attempting to protect someone.
- Using denial–when the nurse denies that a problem exists. He or she blocks discussion with the client.

GOOD COUNSELLOR

G – Good technical knowledge.
O – Obtains appropriate information from client.
O – Objectivity.
D – Demonstrates professionalism.
C – Confidentiality.
O – Observant.
U – Unbiased.
N – Nonjudgment.
S – Sensitive to the needs of the clients.

E – Empathetic.
L – Listen effectively.
L – Lets the client make decision.
O – Open minded.
R – Respects the rights of client.

Qualities of Counselor

- *Interpersonal relationship:* Friendly–nature gets along with others, fairness, sincerity, patience, tactful, attentive listener, ability to maintain confidentiality, tolerance power, openness and empathy.
- *Personal adjustment:* Shows mature behavior, maintains emotional stability, able to accept criticism, shows self-respect, self-confidence, aware about one's limitations, flexibility and adaptability.
- *Educational background:* He/she will have masters degree in the essential area of guidance program and ability to work with people.
- *Health and personal appearance:* Pleasing voice and appearance, poise and neatness, freedom from annoying mannerisms.
- *Leadership:* Ability to stimulate and lead others.
- *Philosophy of life:* Good character, wholesome, positive philosophy of life, civic sense, faith in human value and human nature.
- *Professional dedication:* He/she shows loyalty, has strong sense of professional ethics and professional growth.
- *Faith:* It is in the spiritual quality and a high sense of morality.

Types of Counseling

- **Individual Counseling:** This is carried out one-to-one counseling. It occurs between a professionally trained counselor and a client (counselee). It provides an opportunity to explore and understand one's personal problems.
- **Group Counseling:** It is a powerful tool for growth and self-awareness. Groups usually include six to eight people, who meet and discuss what is concerning them. These maybe issues like coping with grief, managing eating disorders, coping with substance abuse, etc....... These interactions provide an opportunity to increase self-understanding and learn more about the ways to interact and cope with such issues.

Online Counseling

Online counseling involves providing professional help through the internet media. Through email, video conferencing or by chatting through webcam. The advantages are convenience and privacy, but non-verbal signs are missing.

Special Areas of Counseling

Areas of counseling	Issues/problem encountered
• College/school counseling	Problems related to academic achievement, personal/social development so that students become well adjusted.
• Career counseling	To help clients make the right carrier decision and to provide help with job search and interview preparation.
• Work place counseling	Preventive and intervention services to combat work related stressor training workshops and enhancing personal and group effectiveness.

Contd...

Contd...

Areas of counseling	Issues/problem encountered
• Grief and bereavement counseling	To help people cope with grief and mourning following loss or death of loved ones, so that they can continue to carry on with life and accept the loss.
• Counseling the terminally	Providing support and helping client with terminal illness find meaning In their life and to help them deal with feeling of isolation.
• Rehabilitation counseling	Helping people to adjust the after-effects of injury or disease, helping those who have medical problem that require lifestyle changes and assisting individual with disability to achieve independent living.
• Trauma or crisis	Psychological first aid used in public health setting. Disease sites, suicide violence and robberies, to restore equilibrium to their biopsychosocial functioning and to minimize the potential for psychological trauma.
• Premarital counseling	Introducing communication, conflict, resolution, problem-solving and understanding their strength and weakness.
• Marital counseling	It helps couples to discover the strengths in their relationship and find out the causes of conflict and helps them towards improvement.
• Addition counseling	It helps enhance a client's motivation for change and includes teaching coping and problem-solving skills.

PSYCHODYNAMIC COUNSELING

This is based on the idea that past experiences have a bearing on experiences and feelings in the present and that important relationship, perhaps from early childhood, maybe replayed with other people later in life. It translates the principles and insights of psychoanalysis and psychoanalytic psychotherapy into once-a week format.

Here, the counselor usually aims to be as neutral as possible, giving little information about him or herself, making it more likely that important relationships (past and present) will be reflected in the relationship between the client and the counselor. This relationship is therefore an important source of insight for both and helps the clients to "work through" their difficulties. Developing a trusting and reliable relationship with the counselor is essential.

CLIENT-CENTERED OR PERSON-CENTERED COUNSELING

This is based on the principle that the counselor provides three 'core conditions' (or essential attributes) that are, in themselves, therapeutic. These are:

- Empathy (the ability to imagine oneself in another person's position).
- Unconditional positive regard (warm, positive feelings, regardless of the person's behavior)
- Congruence (honesty and openness)
  - Here also, counselor uses the relationship with the client as a means of healing and change.

TRANSPERSONAL COUNSELING

This is an integrative and holistic approach that utilizes creative imagination. It assumes a spiritual dimension to life and human nature. It also presupposes the interconnectedness of all beings with a higher spiritual power, and specifically addresses, the bridge between the two.

Transpersonal counseling emphasizes personal empowerment. It takes account of the client's past experiences, but also looks to the future and what is likely to unfold for them, the challenges they may face and the qualities that need to emerge in them to meet those challenges. Its basic belief is that whatever the hardships of human experience, the core essence or soul, remains undamaged.

TRANSACTIONAL ANALYSIS COUNSELING (TAC)

Transactional analysis counseling emphasizes people's personal responsibility for their feelings, thoughts and behavior. It believes people can change, if they actively decide to replace their usual patterns of behavior with new ones.

Here, the counselor offer:

- 'Permission' (for new messages about yourself and the world)
- 'Protection' (when changing behavior and thoughts feel risky)
- 'Potency' (to deliver what he or she promised)

Planning the goals of the counseling is part of the process. The focus is on uncovering the 'life scripts, (life plans) that reflect the messages the client was given as a child. The counseling teaches the client to identify in which of the following modes he or she is operating; at any given time:

- The 'child' (replaying their childhood)
- The 'parent' (copied from parents or parent figures)
- The 'adult' (appropriate to the present situation)

EXISTENTIAL COUNSELING

This helps people to clarify, think about and understand life, so that they can live it well. It encourages them to focus on the basic assumptions they make about it, and about themselves, so they can come to terms with life as it is. It allows them to make sense of their existence.

The counseling focuses the client on how much already they take change in their life, and not on what they are doing wrong. At the same time, it takes note of any real limitations, so that they can make choices based on a true view of the options available.

Personal Construct Counseling

Personal construct counseling is based on the idea that nobody can know absolute truth. Instead, each person constructs their idea of the truth from their own experiences, and this affects the way they see the world. The problem is that people get stuck with a view of things that prevents them from living life to the full, because they cannot find any alternative ways and seeing things.

Personal construct counseling helps people to look at different ways of behaving that may be useful in changing the way they see and view the world.

Gestalt Counseling

This is a more directive type of counseling, focusing on Gestalten (pattern of thought, feeling and activity). It encourages people to have an active awareness of their present situation, and also incorporates communication that goes beyond words. A key part of gestalt counseling is the dramatization or acting out, of important conflicts in a person's life. This could involve using two or more chairs, for instance, so that they can physically take up different positions to represent different aspects of themselves.

RATIONAL-EMOTIONAL BEHAVIORAL COUNSELING (REBC)

This takes the view that people have two main goals in life; to stay alive and to be happy. It aims to remove the obstacles that people place in their own way, and also to achieve a healthy balance between short-term and long-term goals.

Cognitive Behavioral Counseling

This is another directive model, concerned with the way people's beliefs about themselves shape how they interpret experiences. The objective is to change self-defeating or irrational beliefs and behavior by altering negative ways of thinking.

Clients learn to monitor their emotional upsets and what triggers them, to identify self-defeating thoughts, to see the connections between their beliefs, feelings and behavior, to look at the evidence for and against these thoughts and beliefs and to think in a way that is more realistic and less negative.

Here, the counselor usually gives the client tables or homework to do between sessions. This could mean recording thoughts and feelings or doing something that tests out a basic assumption about themselves. This might mean, for instance, going to the shops when their fear is that they may panic.

Brief Solution Focused Counseling Therapy

It is a structured therapy, usually carried out over one to five sessions. Unlike most other talking therapies, therapist and client usually spend little time on details and causes of the problem. The client is helped to define their own goals in the briefest time possible. It helps the client to recognize their own strengths, resources and abilities. To focus on what is getting better and to build on this.

Interpersonal Counseling Therapy (IPCT)

It is a semistructured therapy which examines how problems in relationships contribute to emotional difficulties such as depression and vice-versa. It primarily focuses on working and improving relationship with the aim of bringing about change, leading to improvements in mood, or other troubling symptoms.

Dialectical Behavior Counseling/Therapy

It is an outgrowth of cognitive behavior therapy and adapted to suit the specific needs of people with borderline personality disorder, etc.

Psychosynthesis

It is a holistic approach to self-realization and the development of potential. It includes creative approaches such as artwork, metaphor and imagery, visualization, therapeutic writing, etc.

Integrative Counseling

It combines ideas from more than one theoretical approach (usually includes person-centered and psychodynamic and others, drawing on elements of each as appropriate for the client/ issues.

Process-Oriented Counseling

- It is developed by A. Mindell. It emphasis on awareness over specific interventions. Process work counseling developed by Arnold Mindell, has roots in Jungian psychology and Taoism. Its methods reflect a dedication to accurately following the way of nature, while bringing awareness into the patterns structuring our lives; including those parts normally unseen, unappreciated, disturbing or marginalized bringing awareness into this interaction, a surprising, wisdom emerges and a creative way forward in even the most difficult situations.

Merits of Counseling

Counseling helps in many ways. These are:
- To learn new skills and better ways to cope.
- To understand the reality or real problem experiencing.
- To learn new ways of looking at what is happening.
- To solve problems and make decisions.
- To learn about strengths and how to use them.

ROLE OF NURSE

Nowadays, an increasing number of people find themselves using counseling skills, especially in the health/mental health profession. Developing counseling skills means learning how to be a better listener and how to communicate therapeutically and more effectively. Psychiatric nurses often find themselves in situations which require in-depth listening and responding skills. For example, in helping people come out from depression, disability and helping families cope with bereavement or chronic incurable diseases.

In the case of clients with dementia, nurses should support the caregivers and family by listening therapeutically. Palliative care clients have various needs like resolving unfinished business, the need to grieve and live the best they can until their end. Psychiatric nurses are having a big role by responding authentically.

Hospitalization causes a lot of stress and anxiety for most clients. Nurses can retrieve insecurities of client, especially depressed, and encourage them to become as independent as their condition permits, so that their sense of helplessness can be alleviated.

Nurses working in psychosocial rehabilitation centre have a strong role to play in counseling and mental health promotion. They spend a great deal of time in problem-solving with the clients and support them in their attempts at making lifestyle changes. There is also a great deal of scope to use counseling skills to promote mental health in community specially in drug dependence and other psychiatric disorders.

Legal Issues in Mental Health Nursing

Nursing as a profession is influenced in each country by legal acts referred to as the Nurse Practice Act. The practice of psychiatric nursing heavily demands an in-depth knowledge of the law, particularly involves the rights of mentally ill and the delivery of quality of care. History provides questionable practices in delivering nursing care such as the loss of individual rights. To overcome these, today's psychiatric nurses should know the legal and ethical context of care because; they are accountable for quality of care.

Legislation is an important component in the implementation of mental health care. Legislation is an expression of society with regard to the way it views and cares for mentally ill individuals.

THE INDIAN LUNACY ACT (1912)

Indian Lunacy Act (1912) is derived from English Lunacy Act; 1890 and it contains eight chapters. Act 4 of Indian Lunacy Act (ILA), 1912, replaced Act 36 of the Indian Lunatic Asylums Act 1958. It was enacted to govern reception, dentition and care of lunatics and their property and to consolidate and amend the laws relating to lunacy. The act was divided into four parts and eight chapters consisting of 100 sections. The enactment of Indian Lunacy Act of 1912 was followed by opening of many new mental hospitals, an improvement in the general conditions of hospitals and, an increase in awareness regarding the prevailing situation of mentally ill in such hospitals. It consists of the following.

PART I Preliminary:

- *Chapter I:* It contains preliminary information and definitions such as a asylum, cost of maintenance, district court, criminal lunatic, India Maintenance lunatic, magistrate, medical officer, medical practitioner, reception order, prescribed, relative and rule.

PART II

- *Chapter II:* Chapter second reception care and treatment of lunatics. It described about: first reception of person in asylum, reception order on petition, dentition of lunatic, order powers and duties of police, dentition of alleged lunatic, authority for reception, reception after inquisition.
- *Chapter III:* It describes the procedure to be followed for administering care, treatment and discharge. It includes appointment of visitors, monthly inspection, temporary release, removal, proof of insanity, powers of courts, management and administration of property, etc. Here,

the term 'parole' refers to the permission given to patients to perform certain rituals or attend certain family functions. During the parole, the patient can leave the hospital anytime and can be brought back forcefully if he does not return within a maximum period of 90 days.

Part III

- Chapter IV: It deals with proceeding of lunacy in presidency town.
- Chapter V: It deals with proceeding of lunacy outside presidency towns.

Part IV: Miscellaneous

- *Chapter VI:* Establishment of asylums.
- It deals with licensure of asylums, admission and discharge, cost maintenance, etc.
- *Chapter VII:* It deals with expenses of lunatics.
- *Chapter VIII:* This chapter focuses on rules to be imposed by the state government regarding care of lunatics.

Drawbacks:

- No definite guidelines for penalties or maintenance of hospital.
- No role of human rights.
- In 1950, a committee was appointed by Indian Psychiatry Society to prepare a draft of Indian Mental Health Act and sent to Government of India 1986, the Indian Mental Health Act was formulated after passed by Rajya Sabha.

LAWS RELATED TO PSYCHIATRIC DISORDER

MENTAL HEALTH ACT 1987

The enactment of the Mental Health Act, 1987 is a landmark in the mental care delivery in India. It is not simply a cosmetic improvement over the outdated Indian Lunacy Act, 1912 but represents the conclusion of lengthy presentation by the Indian Psychiatric Society to the Government of India. This act came into force in April 1993, as per the government of Indian order, even though it is still in liberation in some states.

The Mental Health Act is 'an act to consolidate and amend the law relating to the treatment and care of the mentally ill persons, to make better provisions with respect to their property and for matters connected with or incidental thereto'.

The Mental Health Act has the Following Objectives

- To regulate admission to psychiatric hospitals or psychiatric nursing homes of mentally ill persons who do not have sufficient understanding to seek treatment on a voluntary basis, to protect the rights of such persons while being detained.
- To protect society from the presence of mentally ill person who have become a danger or nuisance to others.
- To protect citizens from being detained in psychiatric hospitals or psychiatric nursing home without sufficient cause.
- To regulate responsibility for maintenance charges of mentally ill persons who are admitted to psychiatric hospitals or psychiatric nursing homes.

- To provide facilities for establishing guardianship or custody of mentally ill person who are incapable of managing their own affairs.
- To provide for the establishment of Central Authority and State Authorities for mental health services.
- To regulate the powers of the Government for establishing licensing and controlling psychiatric hospitals and psychiatric nursing homes for mentally ill person.
- To provide for legal aid to mentally ill person at state expense in certain cases. The Government of India has constituted Central Mental Health Authority. Before implementing the mental health act in the states, the states have to take action regarding the following:
  - To establish a State Mental Health Authority.
  - To spell out guidelines for establishment of private psychiatric hospitals and nursing homes.
  - Formation of a Board of Visitors.

In the Mental Health Act, 1987, a modest attempt has also been made to bring mental illnesses at par with physical illness, thus reducing the stigma attached to mental illnesses. The Mental Health Act has modified certain terms and definitions. The Act uses the term mentally ill person instead of lunatic, mentally ill person, instead of criminal lunatic. Other new terms are psychiatric hospital instead of lunatic asylum, psychiatric nursing home and psychiatrist. New terminology and definitions are provided in chapter 1. The Mental Health Act has 10 chapters in total, consisting of 100 sections.

Chapter: I

It contains Preliminary part and Definitions.

- *Mentally ill person:* A person who is in need of treatment by reason of any mental disorder other than mental retardation.
- *Mentally ill prisoner:* A mentally ill person for whose detention in or removal to, a psychiatric hospital, psychiatric nursing home, jail or other place of safe custody, an order referred to in section 30 has been made.

Chapter: II

It deals with establishment of mental health authorities at the center and at state levels. These authorities will regulate and coordinate mental health services under Central and State governments, respectively.

Chapter: III

It lays down the guidelines for establishment and maintenance of psychiatric hospitals and nursing homes. Also, there is a provision for a licensing authority who will process application for licenses. No private psychiatric hospital or nursing homes will be to allowed to function without at a valid license, which has to be renewed every five years. There is also a provision for an inspecting officer who will inspect the psychiatric hospitals and nursing homes to prevent any irregularities.

Chapter: IV

It deals with the procedures of admission and detention in psychiatric hospital or nursing homes. In addition to the five methods allowed by the Indian Lunacy Act-1912, one more method was included (Fig. 14.1).

Types of Admission

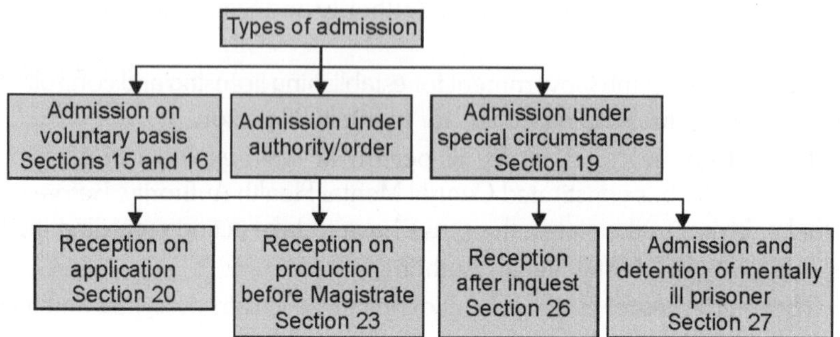

Fig 14.1: Admission and sections

Admission on Voluntary Basis

Any person who considers himself to be mentally ill and wishes to be admitted to a psychiatric hospital may apply to the medical officer in-charge; if he is a minor, the guardian can make this application on his behalf.

The medical officer should make inquiry within 24 hours and should admit the patient if he opines that treatment is required. The voluntary patient thus admitted is now bound to abide by the rules made by the institution.

Admission Under Special Circumstances

Any mentally ill who is unwilling for admission on a voluntary basis maybe admitted and kept as an inpatient in a psychiatric hospital/nursing home. For such purpose an application should be made out on his/her behalf by a relative or a friend of the mentally ill person, provided the medical officer deems fit for it. The clients who admitted under this section cannot be admitted for a period more than ninety days.

Admission Under Reception Order

On Application

Only a relative not other than husband, wife, guardian or a friend can make out an application for the admission of a mentally ill client. Such an application should be made out to the magistrate in black and white supported by two medical certificates, one of them issued by a gazetted medical officer. However, no person being a minor or one who has not seen the mentally ill client in the last 14 days can make such an application. The patient may now be admitted after the magistrate obtains consent from the medical officer in-charge of the mental inpatient treatment to more than six month by making such an application to the magistrate (Fig. 14.2).

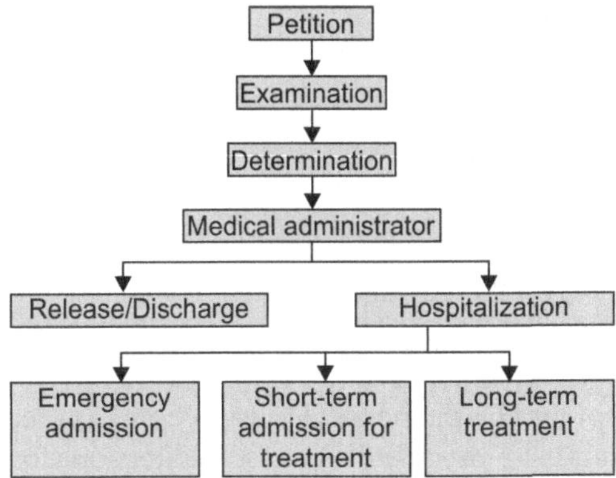

Fig 14.2: Admission procedure

On Production Before the Magistrate

Mentally ill patients, exhibiting violent behavior, creating obscene scenes and dangerous to the society can be detained by the police officer and produced in court within 24 hours of such detention, support by two medical certificates, subsequent to which the magistrate issues a reception order.

Admission in Emergency Conditions

If the psychiatric patient is in danger and the medical officer in-charge thinks such type of clients maybe admitted then within 72 hours, the client should be produced before magistrate or the magistrate is asked to come to the psychiatric hospital and get examined and pass a reception order.

Temporary Treatment Order

It is an order issued by the magistrate in cases where the risk is perceived to the patient's life or to that of others. If the medical officer in-charge feels it necessary to bring legal authorities into the picture he can do so by applying to the magistrate. Alternatively the relatives can get the magistrate to issue an order for treatment. In such case a single medical certificate is required which is valid for 6 months.

Admission of Mentally Ill Prisoners

A mentally ill prisoner maybe admitted into a mental hospital on the order of the presiding officer or by court.

Miscellaneous Admission

A mentally ill patient can be admitted either on humanitarian grounds (for examples, street wanderers) order from the magistrate pending report from medical officer.

Chapter V

This chapter deals mainly with the procedure to be followed for the discharge of mentally ill persons from a mental hospital under varied different circumstances (Fig. 14.3).

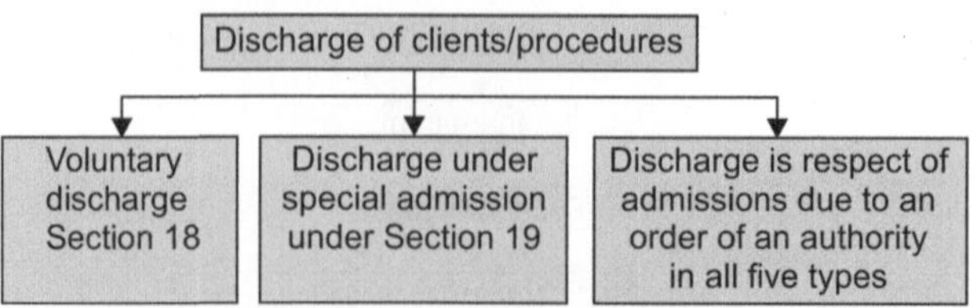

Fig 14.3: Discharge of clients/procedures

Discharge of a Patient Admitted on Voluntary Basis

Medical officer-in-charge of psychiatric hospital/nursing home on recommendations from two medical practitioners preferably a psychiatric, can issue directions for discharge of the patient.

Discharge of a Patient Admitted Under Special Circumstances

A relative or a friend can apply to the medical officer for care and custody of the patient. The relatives are required furnish a bond with or without sureties, along with an undertaking that the mentally ill person shall be prevented from causing injury to self or others.

Discharge of a Patient Admitted on Reception Order

An applicant who feels that the patient has recovered from illness may make an application for discharge to the magistrate. A certificate should contain such as application from medical officer-in-charge of the psychiatric hospital/nursing home. If the magistrate deems fit he may issue an order for discharge.

Discharge of a Patient Admitted by Police

In such cases where the police officer detain the mentally ill people in hospital, he maybe discharged after the family member agree in writing to take proper care, and the medical officer-in-charge opines that he is fit to be discharged.

Discharge of Mentally Ill Prisoner

The hospital authorities have to report every 6 months about the person's state of mind to the authority, which had ordered detention. As soon as they find that the person is fit to stand the trial, they have to inform and report about the same to the authority concerned. The person is then handed over to the prison officer for further legal action.

Leave of Absence (Section 45)

On application by a relative or others to the medical officer-in-charge and a bond duly signed stating that the patient will be taken proper care of and prevented from injuring self or others, leave of absence maybe granted (maximum two months).

Chapter: VI

This chapter deals with the judicial inquisition regarding alleged mentally ill person possessing property custody of their person and management of their property. If the court feels that the alleged mentally ill person is incapable of looking after both himself and his property an order can be issued for the appointment of a guardian. If however, it is felt that the person is only incapable of looking after his property but can look after himself a manager can be appointed.

Chapter: VII

It deals with the liability to meet the cost of maintenance of mentally ill persons detained in psychiatric hospitals or nursing homes. Under section 78 when a mentally ill patient is detained as an in patient and does not have property to bear the cost of treatment, in such cases his/her expenses shall be borne by the respective government of state.

Chapter: VIII

It is aimed at the protection of human rights of mentally ill persons. It provides that under section 81:

- No mentally ill person shall be subjected during treatment to any indignity (whether physical or mental) or cruelty.
- No mentally ill person under treatment shall be used for the purpose of research unless:
- Such research is direct benefit to him.
- A consent has been obtained in writing from the person (if a voluntary patient) or from the guardian/relative (if admitted involuntarily).
- No letters or communications sent by or to a mentally ill person shall be intercepted detained or destroyed.

Chapter: IX

It deals with procedures to be followed for the establishment and maintenance of psychiatric hospital/nursing homes and the penalties, which can be relatively severe and explicit, for contravening them. The article 6 (1) of the Mental Health Act prohibits the running of a home without license and article 11 (1b) views the licensing authority can revoke the license of the maintenance of the home is being carried-out in a manner detrimental to the moral, mental or physical well-being of the inpatients.

Chapter: X

This chapter deals with classification pertaining to certain procedures to be followed by the medical officer-in-charge of the psychiatric hospital/nursing home.

MERITS/POSITIVE QUALITIES OF THE NEW ACT

- The admission procedure are simplified to some extent
- The two new provisions of the often Mental Health Act in admission procedure are:
  - Admission of minor (below the age 18) by the parents/guardian.
  - Admission under special circumstance (maximum 90 days).
- It incorporates the latest scientific knowledge and psychosocial concepts.
- An attempt is made to reduce stigma to look similar to physical illness.
- The word 'treatability' is the essential criterion of treatment.
- MHA is not applicable to untreatable conditions like mental retardation and dementia.
- Formation of mental health authorities provide opportunities for better monitoring and management of services.
- Psychiatric patients admitted in general hospitals or nursing homes are spared.
- Out patient services are mandatory in psychiatric hospital or nursing homes.
- Admission and discharge procedures are simplified and easier.
- Efforts are kept to safe guard human rights.
- Provision for separate hospitals for children, addicts and psychopaths.
- Stringent punishment has been provided for those who subject the mentally ill to physical and mental indignity within hospitals.

Drawbacks/Critique of Act

- The notion of a care in the community has not been addressed in the current legislation. No effort has been made to provide after care services for the discharged client. There seem to be no thinking over the alternative to hospital care.
- Psychiatrists, running private psychiatric nursing home are facing too many medicolegal problems, difficulties and interference in the administration with regard to:
  - Getting and renewing licenses.
  - Board of visitor's control over their nursing home.
  - Constituting a medical board for their today hospital procedures like issuing certificates for admission to and discharge and leave absence, etc.
- Patients examined by psychiatrists and admitted in a psychiatric nursing home should not be compelled to undergo further examination by medical and or nonmedical visitors. It goes against the fundamental rights of a citizen or his family and such an exposure of any responsible citizen or his family and disclosure of his psychiatric illness to the knowledge of the public may amount to indignity and cruelty.
- Improper implication of the term consent and competence.
- Does an involuntary admission (e.g. admission through a reception order) necessarily imply competence? Can drugs and ECT can be administered without any informed consent? What is their statutory criteria for competence?

RIGHTS OF MENTALLY ILL CLIENTS AND NURSES' RESPONSIBILITY

Chapter VIII of Mental Health Act 1987 contains a very detail novel and explicit provision of protection of human rights. It is based on the philosophy that 'every human body and mind has an integrity which is inviolable. Every human being has certain irreducible barest minimum needs such as right to air, potable water, food, clothing, health, medical care and treatment, clean and hygienic conditions for living accommodation, environmental sanitation, personal hygiene and so on. Deprivation of any one of these amounts to violence to the person.

Universal Declaration of Human Rights (UDHR) in Article 24(1) explicitly mentions that 'Every one has the right to a standard of living adequate for the health and well-being of himself and his family, including food, clothing, housing and medical care and necessary social services'. Article of 5 or UDHR states no one shall be subjected to torture or to cruel, inhuman or degrading treatment or punishment. Article 66(1) of Persons With Disability Act states, the appropriate government and the local authorities shall within the limits of their economic capacity and development undertake or cause to be undertaken rehabilitation of all persons with disabilities. Mental illness is also recognized as disability according to section 2 of the Person With Disability (PWD) Act, 1995.

Psychiatric clients are often the least capable of protecting their own rights. It is therefore one of the responsibilities of the nurse to guide the clients and relatives in matters related to their rights and protect the client from any mistreatment.

Rights of Psychiatric Clients

- The right to wear their own clothes.
- The rights to have individual storage space for their private use.
- The right to keep and use their own personal possessions.

- The right to spend a sum of their money for their own expenses.
- The right to have reasonable access to all communication media like phone, net, letter writing and mailing.
- The right to see visitors everyday.
- The right to treatment in the least restricted setting.
- The right to hold civil service status.
- The right to refuse electroconvulsive therapy.
- The right to manage and dispose of property and execute wills.

Role of Psychiatric Nurse

- To protect client's rights, the nurse should be aware of individual's rights as well as patient's rights.
- The nurse should ensure that ward procedures and policies should not violate patient's rights.
- The nurse can protect these rights with the mental health team and including these in care plan helps to protect the patient's rights rightly.

FORENSIC PSYCHIATRY

- The word forensic has many means. Literally, forensic means of the law and is based on the Latin word 'forum' meaning, what is out of doors... The Ancient Romans met outside in... (forums) for public meetings, political debates and public legal hearings to try offenders... (Parker, 1985).
- Forensic psychiatry is a specialized branch of psychiatry where the medical and the legal worlds overlap. It deals with disorders of the mind and their relation to legal principles.

The Forensic Psychiatry comprised of three distinct but overlapping areas that deal with different issues.

- Forensic psychiatry.
- Criminal Areas:
  - Expert witness/testifying.
  - Dangerous or long-term offender applications.
  - Fitness to stand trial.
  - Probation and parole.
  - Review Boards.
- Civil Areas:
  - Divorce and custody evaluations.
  - Negligence and malpractice.
  - Personal injury.
  - Workman's compensation boards.
  - Workplace violence.
- Clinical Criminology
- Interpersonal violence:
  - Major mental illness within the forensic framework (psychosis, schizophrenia, mood disorders, etc.)
  - Paraphilias and sex offending
  - Personality disorders with the forensic mental health framework
  - Psychopathy

- Substance Abuse.
- Risk assessment and risk management.
- Treatment programing.

Psychiatry and Law

- Capacity: To consent to treatment, to manage property, to consent to emergency treatment, etc.
- Community treatment orders
- Consent: Informed, consent to treatment, etc.
- Consent and capacity board
- Confidentiality of patient records
- Duty of care
- Duty to warn
- Involuntary Hospitalization
- Mental health act
- Patient's rights under the Mental Health Act
- Substitute.

RELATION BETWEEN COMMUNITY AND FORENSIC PSYCHIATRY

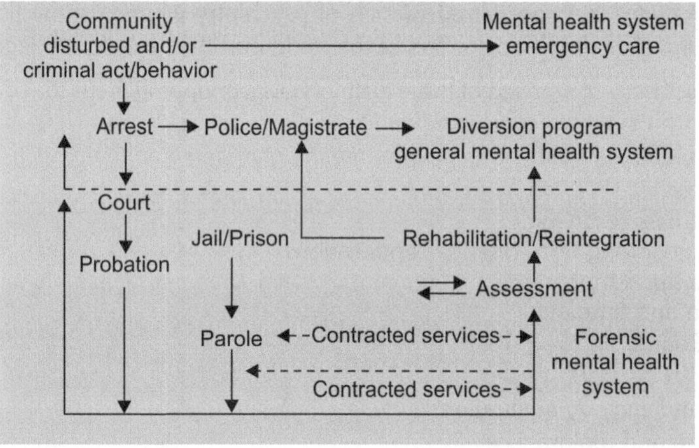

Fig. 14.4: Relationship between Community and Psychiatry. (Stephen, 2003)

The basic forensic psychiatry (Fig. 14.4) includes:

- Crime and psychiatric disorders
- Criminal responsibility
- Civil responsibility
- Laws relating to psychiatric disorders
- Admission procedures of patients in a psychiatric hospital
- Civil rights of the patient
- Psychiatrists and the court.

Crime and Psychiatric Disorders

From the history, we can hypothesize that there are close associations between crime and psychiatric disorders like schizophrenia, psychosis, neurosis, affective disorders, epilepsy, personality disorders including drug addiction.

Mentally ill people may commit offence because:

- They do not understand the implications of their behavior
- Because of positive symptoms
- Abnormal mental states like confusion, excitement, etc.
- Drug related violence.

Criminal Responsibility

- Mentally ill offenders usually stand trial in the same way as their offender, but when sentence is passed, consideration is given to their mental state and diagnosis. In determining whether or not a person is guilty it its necessary to consider his mental state at the time of the act.
- Before anyone can be convicted of a crime, the prosecution must prove;
  - That he carried-out an unlawful act (Actus reus).
  - That he/she had a certain guilty state of mind at the time, namely mens rea (Guilty mind).

When a person is charged with the offence, defence can be made that he is not capable because he/she did not have a sufficient degree of mens rea. This defence can be raised in several ways:

- Not guilty by reason of insanity (under the MC Naughton rules).
- Diminished responsibility (not guilty of murder but guilty of manslaughter, which requires a lesser degree of criminal intent).
- Incapacity to form an intent because of an automation, e.g. if mother kills her child in the first year of its life, she is not usually held legally responsible for murder but only for the less serious crime of infanticide.
  - According to Section 84 of the Indian Penal Code of 1860 'Nothing is an offense which is done by a person who, at the time of doing it, by reason of unsoundness of mind, is incapable of knowing the nature of the act, or that he is doing what is either wrong of contrary to law'. A mentally retarded person is not liable in criminal law:

    Low classifies criminal lunatics into three classes:
    - An under trial, who can not stand trial because of mental illness.
    - Guilty but insane.
    - Criminals who later become mentally ill.

The McNaughton Rules

Daniel McNaughton was 29 years old, son of a Glasgow wood-turner, a man of 'gloomy and reserved social habits' and was suffering from delusions. He decided to murder Sir Robert Peel, the Prime Minister. He made elaborate plans and travelled to London, but in fact mistakenly shot and killed Edward Druminod, Peel's private secretary in daylight in front of numerous witnesses on 20th January 1843. During the trial, McNaughton himself admitted that 'they have accused me of crimes of which I am not guilty, they do everything to harass and persecute me and in fact they wish to murder me. McNaughton knew what he was doing and was aware that he was committing a criminal act but felt compelled to do so because of the delusion he was having at that time.

Psychiatrists were called and it was accepted:
- That he was suffering from persecutory delusion
- That the act was committed under a delusion
  - McNaughton was found 'not guilty on the grounds of insanity'. McNaughton himself was sent to Bethlehem and later Broadmoor asylum where he died in 1865.
  - In McNaughton's case, the Lord Chancellor put to a panel of His Majesty's Judges, five questions designed to classify the legal position. Their replies given on 19th June 1843, constitute the so-called 'McNaughton rules'.

The following are the main points of the McNaughton's rules:
- Every man is to be presumed to be sane, until the contrary be proved.
- An insane person is punishable, if he knew at the time of committing such a crime that he was acting contrary to law.
- To establish a defense on the ground of insanity, it must be clearly proved that at the time of the committing of the act, the accused was suffering under such defect of reason, from disease of the mind, as not to know the nature and quality of the act he was doing; or if he did know it, that he did not know he was doing what was wrong.
- Finally it is the jury's role to decide whether the defendant was insane.

Durham Rule (1954)

'An accused person is not criminally responsible, if his unlawful act is the product of mental disease or mental defect'. In this, the causal connection between the mental abnormality and the alleged crime should be established. This rule is also known as 'Product Rule'.

American Law Institute (ALI) Test

'A person is not responsible for criminal conduct if at the time of such conduct, as a result of mental disease of defect he lacks adequate capacity either to appreciate the criminality of his conduct or to conform his conduct to the requirements of the law'.

The ALI test is similar to the combination of the Mc Naughton rule and the irresistible impulse test. This rule excludes psychopaths. This popular test is used by all courts in USA.

CIVIL RESPONSIBILITY

Before a court of Law, all persons are considered to be same, otherwise it is to be proved. A person has no responsibility in the following conditions, if he is proved to be a lunatic.

Testamentary Capacity (Will)

- As per Section 59 of the Indian Succession Act. 1925. 'Every person of sound mind, not being a minor, may dispose of his property by will'.
- A will can be declared invalid if it is proved that at the time of making the will, the testator.
  - Was of unsound mind.
  - Did not have the mental capacity to understand the consequences of the act.

Marriage

Under the Hindu Marriage Act, 1995 a marriage with a person who was an idiot or a lunatic at the time of marriage, can be declared as null and void on application.

Judicial Separation

If lunacy starts after marriage and continues for two years, even with treatment, the other party can apply for legal separation.

Divorce

It can be decreed if the other party has been incurably of unsound mind for a continuous period of at least three years. But the other party has to pay for the maintenance of the lunatic.

Witness

Under the Indian Evidence Act, 1872 (Section 118) a lunatic is incompetent evidence in a court of law if he is unable to understand the questions asked or to give rational answers to them by virtue of lunacy.

Contract

Under the Indian Contract Act, 1872 (Section 11) every person to be competent to contract, must be a major and of sound mind, i.e. he is capable of understanding the contract and of forming a rational judgment as to its effect upon his interests.

Transfer of Property

Under the Transfer of Property Act, 1882 (Section 7) only persons competent to contract, are authorized to transfer property.

The Right to Vote and the Right to Stand for Election

No person of unsound mind can contest an election or exercise the franchise of voting.

Adoption

Under Hindu Adoptions and Maintenance Act (Act 78 of 1956) any Hindu male who is of sound mind and is not a minor can adopt a child with the consent of his wife unless she has been declared by a court to be of unsound mind. Similarly, any Hindu female 'who is of sound mind' is not a minor and is not married can adopt a child.

Laws Relating to Psychiatric Disorders

Laws Relating to Psychiatry in India

- The care and Treatment Legislation (Mental Health Legislations)
- Criminal responsibilities formulation (criminal laws)
- Civil Status Provisions (civil laws)

Mental Health Related Legislations

- Mental Health Act 1987
- Persons With Disabilities Act 1996
- Rehabilitation Council of India Act 1992
- Juvenile Justice Act 1986
- Consumer Protection Act 1986.

Civil Laws Relating to Mental Ill Persons

- Indian Evidence Act 1925: Section 118
- Law of Contract – Sect. 6, 11, 12
- Right to vote and stand for Election–Act 326, 102 of the Constitution of India
- Law of Torts
- Testamentary Capacity–Section 59 of Indian Succession Act 1925.
- Marriage and Mental Health Legislation
  - Indian Divorce Act–1869
  - Parsi Marriage and Divorce Act 1936
  - Dissolution of Muslim Marriage Act 1939
  - Special Marriage Act 1954
  - The Hindu Marriage Act 1955, 1976
  - The Family Court Act–1984.

Civil Laws Relating to Psychiatry

- Provision as to Accused Person of Unsound Mind—Sec 328–339 Cr.Pc. 1973
- Criminal Responsibility–Sec 84 IPC–1860
- Attempt to Commit Suicide–Sec 309 IPC
- Right to Private Defence against an Insane Person–Sec 98 IPC
- Unnatural offenses–Sec 377 IPC (sexual perversion)
- Affrays (Sec 159 in Mania)
- Misconnect in Public under intoxication (for example, Alcohol Defence–Section 5010 IPC).
- NDPS Act 1985 (Amended 1988).

Suicide and Indian Law

- Suicide is the only criminal act for which a person is punished if he fails in the attempt to do so
- No person shall be deprived of his life. Act 21 is Constitution of India
- Sec 309/IPC–attempt to commit suicide punishable
- Sec. 306–abetment of suicide an offense
- No specific laws for assisted suicide and euthanasia.

The Narcotic Drug and Psychotropic Substances Act. (Act 61 of 1985)

In India, the Opium Act of 1857 was revised first in 1878. In 1950, the Opium Act of 1878 was revised as the Opium and Revenue Laws Act 1950.

On 16th September 1985, both these acts were repeated and Act 61 of NDPSA 1985 was enforced.

The NDPS Act, 1985 and the NDPS (Amendment) Act 1988 provide legislative measures to control operations relating to narcotic drugs and psychotropic substance and to implement the provision of the international convention in the matter.

The NDPS Act, is comprehensive and supersedes all previous acts (Opium Act, 1857) Opium Act 1878, Dangerous Drugs Act 1930. The NDPS Act consist of eight chapters and 122 Sections:

- *Chapter I:* Definition, preliminary note
- *Chapter II:* Powers of officers

- *Chapter III:* Opium poppy cultivation and production of opium and poppy straw
- *Chapter IV:* Manufacture, sale and export of opium
- *Chapter V:* Manufactured drugs
- *Chapter VI:* Import, export and transshipment of narcotic drug and psychotropic substances
- *Chapter VII:* Psychotropic substances
- *Chapter VII A:* Special provision regarding manufacture, possession, transport, import-export, purchase and consumption of narcotic drugs and psychotropic substances for medical and scientific purposes.
- *Chapter VIII:* Miscellaneous.

Main Features of NDPS ACT

- The NDPS Act includes narcotic drugs (opium, poppy, straw, cannabis, cocaine, coca and all related synthesized drugs) and psychotropic substances (76 drugs and their derivatives, for example major tranquilizers, minor tranquilizers, pentazocine, barbiturates, etc).
- In this Act, if any person produces, possesses, transports, imports, sells, purchases or uses any narcotic drugs or psychotropic substances (except 'Ganja') he shall be punishable with.
  - Rigorous imprisonment (RI) for not less than 10 years (which may extend to 20 years) and
  - A fine of not less than 1 lakh rupees (which may extend to 2 lakh rupees).
- For repeat of offense a rigorous imprisonment of not less than 15 years which maybe extended up to 30 years and a fine of not less than 1.5 lakh rupees which may extend up to 3 lakhs.
- Which maybe extended up to 3 lakh rupees.
- For handling 'Ganja' a rigorous imprisonment which may extend to 10 years and a fine up to 1 lakh rupees.
- On carrying 'small quantities' for example, heroin 250 mg, opium 5 mg, cocaine 125 mg, charas 5 mg as were later specified in this act, the punishment may extend to 1 year or a fine or both. For ganja (below 500 gm), imprisonment is up to 6 months.
- Under a specified court order, there is a provision for detoxification of the patient.
- Under a later enactment, the prevention of illicit traffic in Narcotic Drugs and Psychotropic Substances Act (NDPSA), 1988 (Act 46) was passed. Now there is a provision for preventive detention, seizure of property, death penalty if a person is bound to be trafficking more than or equal to 1 kg of pure heroin despite conviction and warning on the first attempt.

ILLEGAL DRUG TRAFFICKING

Introduction

The system of control of Narcotic Drugs in India has been put in place considering the requirement of narcotic drugs and psychotropic substances for medical use and the country's obligations towards the UN conventions. India is a signatory to the UN single convention on Narcotic Drugs 1961, the convention on psychotropic substances, 1971 and the convention on Illicit Traffic in Narcotic Drugs and psychotropic substances, 1988 which prescribe various forms of control aimed to achieve the dual objective of limiting the use of narcotics drugs and psychotropic substances for medical and scientific purposes as well as preventing the abuse of the same.

The administrative and legislative set up in the field of Narcotics has been put in place in the country in accordance with the aforesaid spirit of the UN Conventions. The basic legislative instrument of the Government of India in the regard is the Narcotics Drugs and Psychotropic Substances (NDPS) Act, 1985. Various Ministries and Departments under the Government of India as well as the State Government exercise various functions pertaining to drug demand and supply reduction. The aspect a drug supply reduction is looked after by various enforcement agencies under the Ministry of Finance, Ministry of Home Affairs and State Government. The aspect of drug demand reduction is handled by the ministry of social justice and empowerment and that of treatment of drug addicts and their rehabilitation falls under the domain of the ministry of health.

The majority of the drug trafficking originates from Afghanistan and Pakistan and the revenue is believed to be used to finance terrorism. (Vicky Nanjappa). The illegal drug trade in India is estimated to generate between 10000 to 20000 crore Indian rupees.

Routes of Drug Trafficking

India has been a traditional consumer of opium and various cannabis derivatives (bhang, marijuana/ganja and hashish). These narcotics were mostly consumed for medicinal purposes for recreation or during religious and social ceremonies. Earlier, almost all the demands for these drugs were met locally. Only a small quantity of hashish was suggested in from Nepal and Pakistan. Since 1980, the rise in drug trafficking has become a national concern. In subsequent years, the large scale availability of synthetic and medicinal drugs and their abuse have added new dimensions to the concerns about drug trafficking.

The global pattern of the flow of illegal drug reveals that of all drugs, heroin and cocaine are trafficked for long distances, hashish is smuggled for relatively shorter distances; and marijuana/ganja and psychotropic substance like Amphetamine Type Stimulus (ATS), which are consumed locally travel the shortest distance. Nearly 70% of these narcotics and drugs are trafficked over land using various modes of transportation making the country's borders the first point of contact for drug trafficking. As regards India, depending upon the nature of the border and its milieu as well as the production, demand and supply of drugs, different borders like India–Pakistan border, Indian–Nepal border, India–Bhutan border, India–Myanmar border, India–Bangladesh border, respectively. This route is known as Golden Triangle.

According to UN report 2012—courier and postal services are the means of smuggling drug out of India. Banned pharmaceutical preparations are trafficked through ships and internet.

Admission and Discharge Procedures

The psychiatric clients maybe voluntarily or involuntarily admitted to the mental health hospital. Voluntary admission of generally available to mentally ill adults who are severely ill and dangerous to self or others or property and inpatient setting is only treatment option.

The client admitted under this type can be discharged under certain conditions according to the country of practice.

Admission procedure includes series of tasks and legal health proceedings. A psychiatric nurse practitioner must be aware of all the rules, routines and procedure of the institute regarding the admission.

Consent should be taken from the client or client's significant others (in voluntary admission) which include consent for treatment, certain procedures and investigations. Informing the client about rules and regulations of the institute is a primary function of a nurse. The client is provided bed according to severity of disease condition and situation like client with severe psychotic features should be kept in place where he himself and others are well protected and continuous observation can be possible. Then, the client can be warmly welcomed by the nurse and made comfortable without confrontation and argumentation. It provides opportunity for developing a therapeutic nurse-client relationship. Seclusion and restraining of a psychiatric client maybe needed when the client is dangerous for himself or others, but only after written prescription by the psychiatrist and after consent from the client or significant others.

Discharge Procedure

Discharge of the client also requires certain procedure to follow. At the time of admission of the client, his/her significant others should be told possible stay and projected outcomes. The tentative date of discharge should be intimated to client and significant others. On the day of discharge the psychiatric nurse helps the client in gathering all his/her belongings and all documents related to treatment.

The nurse will also explain about the follow-up and medication which are to be continued after discharge from fellow clients.

The nurse also explains regarding possible adverse effects of medication and early signs of relapse of diseases and routines for follow-ups. The psychiatric nurse also ensures that all the documents are placed in right place and all the dues are paid by the client before discharge. Follow-up time schedule should be intimated.

 CIVIL RIGHTS OF THE MENTALLY ILL

Due to global human right concerns, efforts have been made to safeguard the human rights of the mentally ill. A person who is supported to look after the mentally ill person and who does not take proper care and shows cruelty, maybe summoned by the court, or receipt of such an information either from the public or police. Stringent punishment has also been provided for those who subject the mentally ill person will not be used in research except after obtaining proper consent from him and any communication or correspondence in any form shall not be usually be consumed or intercepted.

In the statement of objects and reasons of the Mental Health Bill, 1981' it has been stated that 'it is now realized no stigma should be attached to such illness as it is curable' and that 'the mentally ill persons are to be treated like other sick persons and the environment around them should be made as normal as possible'.

It has been suggested by WHO (Curren and Harding, 1978) that 'consideration be given to the need to provide effective management policy and whether the institution is publicly or privately owned'.

Informed Consent

A written consent from the patient (on a specified form provided for the purpose), if competent to sign, should always be taken.

If the client is not competent to sign, the form must be signed by his guardian or by both the patients and by a close relative. Before getting the consent of the patient or his legal guardian, a full explanation is necessary in regard to the risks involved in the investigation, treatment and procedures administered to the client.

Informed consent to be obtained for the following conditions:
- Admission of a person to a psychiatric hospital on a voluntary basis.
- Procedures like ECT, psychosurgery and other invasive investigatory procedures like lumbar puncture, sphenoidal EEG, etc.
- Penthanol analysis (Narco-Analysis test).
- Drug treatments like disulfiram therapy and clozapine therapy.
- Admission of any research drugs (Drug trials).

Psychiatrists and the Court

Psychiatry has become established as a medical speciality and psychiatrists now have achieved the status of an expert for the purpose of assisting the law in performing its role. Based on a plea of insanity a psychiatrists can give evidence convincing judges that the crimes were committed as a result of his mental illness. Thus one can see that the psychiatrist owes a peculiar duty to himself and his speciality to create an image of an individual, who is honest, truthful and objective. The rule that an expert's opinion is admissible is to provide scientific information that is outside the experience or knowledge of the judge.

It is not normally permissible for a psychiatrist to comment on the intent of the accused person, that is the role of a judge to decide. Psychiatric evidence about the reactions of normal people to provocation will be inadmissible. Psychiatric evidence maybe given to show that a witness suffers from a disease, defect or abnormality of the mind that affects the reliability of his evidence and despite these basic rules, exemptions and inconsistencies are common in jurisdiction throughout the world.

Psychiatrists would prefer to believe that as experts, they can simply offer an informed independent opinion to the court after careful examination that is unbiased and unprejudiced. It has to be kept in mind that many forensic psychiatrists have had the painful experience of learning that their report is not be used or that another report is to be requested to examine the case or that the report is not to be shown to the court fully but selected aspects will be used to assist in eliciting oral evidence. The psychiatrist must also face cross-examination which may tend to place him in a negative and defensive position. Needel (1980) identified three possibilities for the potential abuse of psychiatric testimony.
- Experts who offer biased opinions based on either calculated or unconscious prejudices
- Physicians lacking in psychiatric sophistication who give psychiatric testimony
- Fully qualified experts who unintentionally or through laziness perform an examination that does not serve as a professionally adequate basis for their conclusions.

There are three types of witness:
- Witness as to fact
- Professional witness
- Expert witness.

The expert witness has special knowledge and experience within a defined field and his opinion is requested rather than his description or recollection of facts which form part of the case itself.

Do's and Don'ts as Expert Evidence

Do's

- The psychiatrist must be punctual
- He must dress appropriately

- Appear confident (but not arrogant)
- Speak clearly and audibly
- Keep to the point
- Evidence should be comprehensible and simple language
- Keeps sentences short.

Don'ts

- Do not use jargon
- Do not use technical expressions not generally understandable by lay person.
- Do not use words of foreign origin (e.g. Cyclothymia instead of 'mood swing').
- Do not use polysyllabic or uncommon words
- Do not lose your temper even if provoked by the council.

Replies to questions although put by the advocate, will be addressed to the judge and head of jury. The conventional appellation to the judge is 'Your Honour' in the lower courts and "Your Lordship' in High Courts. Most often the counsel and judges are courteous and considerate towards the expert witness, but their question will be probing in nature.

In all cases, it is advisable to go over the case-files and documents briefly beforehand to refresh the memory. In criminal cases, it maybe helpful to see the accused again before the proceeding start. This is particularly important where the issue is fitness to plead.

The performance in the witness box and the impression that the witness makes on the court are obviously, important in contributing successfully to the proceedings and their outcome.

ROLE OF PSYCHIATRIC NURSE

Role of a Psychiatric Nurse in Admission Procedure

- Making the psychiatric client to settle in ward
- Welcoming the client to hospital
- Orientation of client
- Though assessment of client
- If client shows suicidal ideas—keeping him/her in observation unit
- Instructing rules and regulations
- Assessing legal procedures
- History Collection and MSE
- Record Monitoring.

Role of Nurse During Patient's Parole

Parole is the permission given to patient's to perform certain rituals or attend family functions.

- Relatives are clearly instructed about the purpose for which the client is being sent home and when he should be brought back to hospital
- Instruct the relatives about 'the changing behaviors' to be adopted
- If the client is on drugs, educate the family members about side effects and follow-up
- Client's relatives be asked to observe communication pattern, sleeping cycle, drugs interactions, socially accepted skills, etc.

Role of Nurse During Discharge of the Client

- Nurse must ensure that the client leaves the hospital unit with all belongings and personal effects has the appropriate medications with him and appointment for follow-up has been made and understood.
- All necessary instructions specially regarding medication regimen, side-effects, etc. must be clearly provided to the client and his/her family members
- Any administrative procedures should be completed such as no dues, procedures, etc.
- The nurse should ascertain his/her travel plan and offer assistance necessarily
- While discharging, keep emotional stability and cope with departure.

Nursing Malpractice

Nursing malpractice involves the failure of professionals to provide proper and competent care that is given by the members of their profession, resulting in harm to the client. Harm includes physical and psychosocial aspects of client's life.

For Malpractice the following should be proved:
- A legal duty of care existed
- The nurse performed the duty negligency
- The damages were suffered by the plaintiff as a result
- Damages were substantial in nature.

Common areas of liability in psychiatric services:
- Suicide of the client
- Failure to diagnose the disease condition
- Problems related to ECT
- Misuse and abuse of psychoactive drug administration
- Breach of confidentiality
- Failure to obtain informed consent
- Failure in reporting and recording.

Steps to avoid liability in psychiatric services:
- The nurse is responsible in reporting information to coworkers involved in client care
- Maintain confidentiality of patient's information
- Practicing according to Law and Nurse Practice Act
- Collaborate with colleagues to determine the best course of action
- Use standard research based protocol during decision making and while providing care
- Always think first about patient's rights and welfare
- Develop effective interpersonal relationship with patients and family
- Document all data accurately.

Record Monitoring

Nurses notes and progress charts as well as notes constitute legal documents and hence should be maintained carefully and safely. While writing, they must be nonjudgmental and in objective manner. Always record with sign and date and time.

Standard of Forensic Mental Health Nursing

Forensic mental health nursing practice is the assessment and formulation, planning, implementation and evaluation of nursing care and treatment with in a therapeutic alliance with people experiencing mental disorder who are involved in criminal justice processes.

Forensic mental health nurses can practice at courts, police departments, jails/prisons, secure hospital and at large community settings.

Standards of Forensic Nursing

Standard 1

The forensic mental health nurse will structure the treatment environment to integrate security with therapeutic goals.

Standard 2

The forensic mental health nurse will apply knowledge of the legal framework to service delivery and individual care.

Standard 3

The forensic mental health nurse will conduct forensic mental health nursing practice ethically.

Standard 4

The forensic mental health nurse will practice within an interdisciplinary team that may include criminal justice staff.

Standard 5

The forensic mental health nurse will establish, maintain and terminate therapeutic relationship with forensic service patients using the nursing process.

Standard 6

The forensic mental health nurse will integrate assessment and management of offence issues into nursing care processes.

Standard 7

The forensic mental health nurse will assess for the impact of trauma and engage in strategies to minimize the effects of trauma.

Standard 8

The forensic mental health nurse will assess and manage risk potential of forensic service patients.

Standard 9

The forensic mental health nurse will manage the containment and transition process of forensic service patients.

Standard 10

The forensic mental health nurse will promote optimal physical health of forensic service patients.

Standard 11

The forensic mental health nurse will minimize potential harm from substance use by forensic service patients.

Standard 12

The forensic mental health nurse will practice respectfully with families/careers of forensic service patients.

Standard 13

The forensic mental health nurse will advocate for the mental health needs of forensic service patients in a prison or police custodial setting.

Standard 14

The forensic mental health nurse will support and encourage optimal functioning of forensic service patients in long-term care.

Standard 15

The forensic mental health nurse will demonstrate professional integrity in response to challenging behaviors.

Standard 16

- The forensic mental health nurse will engage in strategies that minimize the experience of stigma and discrimination for forensic service patients.
- The above mentioned standards will guide and help the nurse to provide comprehensive and holistic care.

Role and Responsibilities of Nurse

Nursing as a profession is influenced in each country by legal acts referred to as the Practice Act. The practice of psychiatric nursing healthy demands an in-depth knowledge of the law, particularly involves the rights of mentally ill and the delivery of quality of care. History provides questionable practices in delivering nursing overcome these, today's psychiatric nurses should follow the legal and ethical context of care because they are accountable for quality of care.

15 Community Mental Health Nursing

HISTORICAL TRENDS OF COMMUNITY MENTAL HEALTH SERVICES IN INDIA

History is a screen through the past lightens the present and the present brightens the future. Psychiatry/mental health by virtue of its ability to deal with human thoughts and emotions and provide a pathway for healthy minds provides an important platform towards being a mentally sound human being in the society as well as community.

The concept generation of community mental health is the third major revolution. Always Indian culture has stressed upon great importance to spiritual life and detachment from material living. Very early description points out the modern concept of community networking.

The new concept of community mental health thought is supposed to be derived from mental hygiene movement of Clifford Beers in 1908 and Adolf Meyer's recommendation of establishment of treatment centers in the community 1913. He advocated management of mentally ill clients outside the four walls and proposed a comprehensive community mental health approach. The period between 1955–1980 was an era of deinstitutionalization in USA and other western countries. This provided an impetus to the development of community psychiatry.

The thought of inspiration for the community mental health movement in India was erupted from three sources:

1. First source is the realization in western countries that the treatment of mentally ill patients should be given in hospitals. In the 1960s American Psychiatrists discussed the 'social breakdown syndrome', which resulted from long-term hospitalization. This prompted the John F Kennedy administration to launch the community mental health programme.
2. The second source is the realization that institution based psychiatric services through trained professional can in fact be very expensive and that countries like India will not have the sufficient resources to deliver services through conventional methods for many years.
3. The third source was discovery that paraprofessional and nonprofessional could deliver reasonable mental health care by undergoing simple and short innovative training.

Till independence, the approach of the Indian Government was to establish custodial centers. In 1920, Dr Berkeley Hill and his colleagues helped to raise the standard of treatment and care at the mental hospital at Ranchi and introduced occupational therapy, psychological therapies and other rehabilitative services.

In 1930, an Association of the Medical Superintendents of Mental Hospitals was established. ECT, Insulin Coma Therapy are practiced at Ranchi hospital. The first psychiatric out patient service, precursor to the present day general hospital psychiatric units, was set-up at RG Kar Medical College, Calcutta in 1933 by Dr GS Bose.

The 1950s saw second phase of development of psychiatric services, when there was a breakthrough in area of delivery of care to the mentally ill. All India Institute of Mental Health (later named NIMHANS) was established in 1954 at Bangalore for training of mental health professionals. NIMHANS, now is a deemed university which has been a World Health Organization collaborating center for research and training psychiatrists and allied professionals. Later, many new mental hospitals were built in different places, such as Amritsar (1947), Hyderabad (1953), Srinagar (1958), Jamnagar (1960) and New Delhi (1966). In 1957 Dr Vidy Sagar, Superintendent of Amritsar Mental Hospital, involved the family members of the mentally ill in the management, by allowing them to stay with their patients in open tents pitched in the hospital campus. He observed that the patients recovered fast and were taken back to their homes. Based on this principle family wards were established at Bangalore and CMC Vellore.

The third phase began in 1960s with the establishment of General Hospital Psychiatric Units (GHPUS). Though the first general hospital psychiatric department was started at Bombay and Calcutta way back in 1933, More units and departments started working in 1970s. Mudaliar Committee, in 1962, envisaged that within the next ten years, psychiatric units would be set-up in all the districts of the country. These had a number of advantages over the mental hospitals.

Advantages of GHPU Over Mental Hospitals

- Shorter periods of hospitalization
- Involvement of family and significant others
- Greater acceptance of services
- Easily approachable without stigma
- Attracted more patients with minor mental health problems
- Integration of mental health into general health system.

The fourth phase of development of psychiatric services in the country saw the extension of care from mental hospitals and general hospitals to the primary health care centers and the community. By the mid 1970s it was realized that the existing mental health services were highly centralized and situated predominantly in urban areas. Catering to the needs of only a small proportion of the population. Indian psychiatric doctors showed their concern for organizing mental health services. Indian psychiatric society conducted seminars and workshop in Madurai 1971, Trivandrum 1985, and Nagpur 1976, WHO/SEARO meetings (1971, 1974) and the presidential addresses in annual conferences of Indian Psychiatric Society emphasized the need to integrate mental health into the general health care and provide the same through primary care approach. An expert committee of the WHO had recommended that developing countries should organize mental health services by integrating these services with their existing system of primary health care. It brought out a technical report in 1974 and paved the way for community mental health programme. Efforts were made to operationalize the primary care approach in the country. The noted ones are community care approach in two-centers-Sakalwara village near Bangalore and Raipur Rani block of Ambala district Haryana state. These programs demonstrated that basic mental health care can be provided by health workers and doctors in primary health care centers, if they are adequately trained. India adopted a National Mental Health Programme in 1982, which has an integration of mental health into general health services as the primary approach for delivering mental health care throughout the country.

During the past decade a wide variety of factors have contributed to the fifth phase of development, which is currently bringing about major changes in mental health services. Many unethical practices at different hospitals (Erwady tragedy) by media exposure has brought major changes in mental health services. Media has stressed more on rights of patients and situation of jail mates. These improvements helped to fund more in mental health care. Many have opened now OPDs, rehabilitation centers, family wards, etc.

In recent years, there has been a perceptible growth of voluntary and nongovernmental organizations (e.g. CRY, LAKHYA, CADABAMS) taking an active interest in various aspects country, are involved in a variety of programs which include the rehabilitation of patients with chronic mental illness, running day care facilities, half-way homes, quarter-way homes and crisis intervention centers, suicide prevention work, training and research. They have the advantage of highly committed volunteers and the potential for initiating innovative programs.

Another visible development during the past few years has been the growth of private sector in psychiatric care services; especially in developed and urban areas. Number of private nursing homes and hospitals for the mentally ill, as well as psychiatry wards in private and general hospital has been on the increase. Private consultant psychiatrists with office based practices have also been growing in number in most large cities. While these facilities have added to the overall availability and quality of psychiatric services, they cater to the needs of only certain sections of society such as urban middle and upper classes.

The public health consequences of mental and psychosocial disorders are now being realized in India more than ever before. An increasing number of persons with various minor mental disorders are beginning to consult mental health care services. The special needs of certain categories of the population such as children, the aged, women and the rural underprivileged have been recognized. Although the availability of a variety of mental health services has steadying increased in India, there is still a wide gap between the existing morbidity and the available services with the current rapid urbanization and economic liberalization in the country and the resultant social change the demand for mental health services is only most likely to increase in number.

MENTAL HEALTH SERVICES AT VARIOUS LEVELS IN INDIA

Central level:
- National level hospitals, NIMHANS, IHBAS, Ranchi hospital.

State level:
- State Level hospital, e.g. Agra, Dharwar, Amritsar, National Mental Health Programme.

District level:
- General Hospital Psychiatric Units.
- Teaching Hospitals
- District Mental Health Programme.

Local level:
- Primary Health Centers
- Community Mental Health Centers
- Subcenters.

Mental health services are delivered through mental hospitals at central, state and district levels.

Innovative Programmes in Mental Health

Crash programs offered at NIMHANS, Bengaluru. Dr RMV Varma, Director and Dr Karan Singh, Minister of Health in the Central Government, jointly introduced Community Based Mental Health Programme at NIMHANS.

A community psychiatry unit was started in October 1975. This community unit launched the following programmes:

- Primary Health Center (PHC) based meal mental health programme. In this, multipurpose workers are trained to recognize severe mental illness cases and follow them up to train PHC doctor to diagnose and treat cases of severe mental disorders.
- *General Practitioner (GP) based urban mental health programme:* Under this programme manual was prepared to teach the General Practitioners methods of treating common mental disorders.
- *School mental health programme:* In this programme school teachers were trained to diagnose children with emotional problems and counsel them.
- *Home based follow-up of psychiatric clients:* Here nurses were trained to follow-up patients in their home settings through monthly visits.
- *Extension programs by 'Satellite Clinics':* Mental health team conducts a weekly or monthly clinic at taluk or district head-quarters. The local medical and nongovernment voluntary organizations are motivated to be the local hosts and help in care. Such satellite clinics are functioning at six centers of Karnataka and a few at other parts of the country.
- *Extensive use of outdoor services:* Family members are encouraged to treat their clients at home and get drugs and instructions from the hospital by regular visits. All types of treatment, including ECT, are given in OPD set-up. Short stay ward (few hours to 48 hours) facility is organized in the out patient building, so that acute problems are managed and the patient is discharged. The hospital also organizes free or subsidized drug supply, so that drug compliance improves.
- Involvement of ICDS personnel in child mental health care.
- Anganwadi workers are trained in basic mental health care, so that they identify and refer children with mental retardation and behavioral problems to medical institutions.
- *Training by volunteers:* Interested and committed 'natural helpers' in the community are given 40 sessions of training in counseling; so as to help individuals in distress.
- Student enrichment program and student volunteers program to educate about mental health.

The Chandigarh Experiment

By seeing the NIMHANS, community psychiatry unit, a rural mental health program was started at PGI, Chandigarh, with the help of WHO. Besides Chandigarh and Bengaluru, similar rural mental health programs were taken up at other psychiatric centers in Baroda, Calcutta, Delhi, Hyderabad, Jaipur, Lucknow, Patiala and Vellore. Some of the states like Haryana, Himachal Pradesh, Punjab, Pondicherry, Uttar Pradesh, Maharashtra, Gujarat, Kerala, Rajasthan, Andhra Pradesh, Assam and West Bengal initiated pilot programmes further.

Other care includes, disaster management, crisis interventions unit were set-up at NIMHANS and PGI to tackle disasters. With this, research is given more importance at PG level and at doctoral level.

NATIONAL MENTAL HEALTH PROGRAMME (NMHP)

Historical Development of NMHP

The Government of India felt the necessity of evolving a plan of action aimed at the mental health component of the National Health Programme. For this; an expert group was formed in 1980, who met a number of times and discussed the issue with many important people concerned with mental health in India as well as the Director, Division of Mental Health, WHO,

Geneva. Finally, in February 1981, a small drafting committee met in Lucknow and prepared the first draft of the NMHP. This was presented at a workshop of experts (over 60 professionals) on mental health, drawn from all over India at New Delhi, on 20–21 July 1981. Following the discussion, the draft was substantially revised and a new one was presented at the second workshop on 2nd August 1982 to a group of experts from not only the psychiatry and medical stream but also education, administration, law and social welfare. The final draft was submitted to the central council of health, Indian's highest health policy making body at its meeting held on 18–20 August 1982, for its adoption as the NMHP for India. The council discussed this program at length and adopted a resolution for its implementation in the States and Union Territories as follows:

'Mental health must form an integral part of the total health programme and as such should be included in all national policies and programs in the field of Health, Education and Social Welfare. Realizing the importance of mental health in the course curricula for various levels of health professionals, suitable action should be taken in consultation with the appropriate authorities to strengthen the Mental Health Education components. While appreciating the efforts of the Central Government in pursuing legislative action on Mental Health Bill, the joint conference expressed its earnestness to see that the bill takes a legal shape at the earliest.'

NEED OF NMHP

The NMHP reviews the mental health situation in terms of needs, facilities and services. A wealth of information is available in India concerning the prevalence of mental disorders. According to most of the surveys; about 10 to 20 per 1000 of the population are affected by a serious mental disorder at any point in time (point prevalence). The main burden of psychiatric morbidity in the adult population consists of acute mental disorder, chronic or frequently recurring mental illnesses, emotional illnesses, such as anxiety, hysteria, neurotic depression, alcohol abuse and alcohol and drug dependence and psychiatric disturbances among children. No factual data are currently available regarding the loss of productivity of income and even of life, due to mental illness. However, it should be pointed out that suffering due to mental illness often is not confined to the affected individual, but causes severe social dysfunction of entire families.

From the available data, it is safe to conclude that not more than 10% of those who need urgent mental health care are receiving the required help with the existing services. The situation is worse in rural areas as the concentration of services and facilities is greater in the cities. Further, a simple extension of the present system of care will not be able to ensure adequate services to the vast majority of the Indian Population in the near foreseeable future.

In view of the gross disparities between needs and available services, there are essentially two approaches for immediate action. They are not alternatives since the difference between them lies mainly in the emphasis and in the level of priority assigned to different levels of service development. The first option would be to direct available resources to the establishment and strengthening of psychiatric units in all district hospitals. It would be hoped that those units would become foci of an expanding mental health service, through setting up out patient clinics and mobile teams. In general terms, the approach would be directed from the center to the periphery. In contrast, an alternative approach would be to train an increasing number of different categories of health personnel in basic psychiatric and mental health skills. There would thus, be a functional infrastructure before completing, in all instances, a physical independent mental health infrastructure.

Most mental health facilities in India actually function as passive recipients of patients. They become operational only where coping mechanisms in the community fail. These institutions have little knowledge and hardly any impact on the coping mechanisms as they exist and operate in the community. It is essential that the role of all mental health institutions in India become more active with the social mechanisms involved, not only in the development of mental illness, but also in the more important issue of maintaining mental health.

OBJECTIVES OF NMHP

- To ensure the availability and accessibility of minimum mental health care for all in the foreseeable future, particularly to the most vulnerable and under privileged sections of the population.
- To encourage the application of mental health knowledge in general health care and in social development.
- To promote community participation in the mental health service development and to stimulate efforts towards self-help in the community.
- Prevention and treatment of mental and neurological disorders and their associated disabilities.
- Use of mental health technology to improve general health services.
- Application of mental health principles in total national development to improve quality of life.
- *Approaches to the statement of program objective were*: Diffusion of mental health skills to the periphery of the health service system, appropriate appointment of tasks in mental health care; and integration of basic mental health care into general health services and linkage to community development and mental health care. The service component will include three sub program treatment, rehabilitation and prevention.

Goals/Targets of NMHP (1982)

Within One Year

- Each state will have adopted the present plan of action in the field of mental health.
- The Government of India will have appointed a focal point within the Ministry of Health specifically for mental health action.
- A National Coordinating Group will be formed comprising representatives of all states, senior health administrators and professionals from psychiatry, education, social welfare and other related professionals.
- A task force will have worked out the outlines of a curriculum of mental health workers identifies in the different states as the most suitable to apply basic mental health skills and for medical officers working at PHC level.

Within Five Years

- At least 5000 of the target nonmedical professional will have undergone two week training in mental health care.
- At least 20% of all psychiatrist working in PHC centers will have undergone two weeks training in mental health.
- The creation of the post of a psychiatrist in at least 50% of the districts within five years.
- A psychiatrist at the district level will visit all PHC settings regularly and at least once in every month for supervision of the mental health program for continuing education. This program

will be fully operational in at least one district in every state and Union Territory and at least 50% of all districts in some states.

- Each state will appoint a program officer responsible for organization and supervision of the mental health program.
- Each state will provide additional support for creating or augmenting community mental health components in the teaching institutions.
- On the recommendation of a task force, appropriate psychotropic drugs to be used at PHC level will be included in the list of essential drugs in India.
- In psychiatric units, beds will be provided inpatients to at medical college hospitals in the country.

Activities Planned for Implementation of NMHP

- Community mental health programs at primary health care level in states and union territories, with a plan to cover a population of about 3–5 lakhs in the 7th five year plan.
- Training of existing PHC personnel for mental health care delivery, with no additional staff.
- Development of a state level Mental Health Advisory Committee and identification of a state level program officer (preferably a psychiatrist).
- Establishment of Regional Centers of Community Mental Health (at least one during the plan period).
- Formation of National Advisory Group on Mental Health.
- Development of a task force for mental hospitals.
- Prevention and promotion of mental health.
- Task force for mental health education for undergraduate medical students.
- Voluntary agencies to be involved in mental health care.
- Priority areas identified as child mental health, public mental health education and drug dependence.
- Mental health training of at least one doctor at every district hospital during the next five years.
- Establishment of a department of, public mental health in all medical colleges and strengthening of existing ones.
- Provision for at least 3 to 4 essential psychotropic drugs in adequate quantity at the PHC level. An important example of the District Mental Health Program is at Bellary district, in Karnataka. Started in 1985, caters to a population of 1.5 million. District hospital psychiatry units have been opened in every district of Kerala and Tamil Nadu.

Following the implementation of National Mental Health Program in India 1982, other neighboring countries soon followed the example by drawing national programs for mental health (Sri Lanka 1982) Bangladesh 1982, Pakistan 1986 Nepal 1987.

Progress between 1982 and 2002

After adoption of NMHP, the following progress is seen:

- Development of models for the integration of mental health with primary health care (Raipur Rani model in North India and Sakalwara in South India).
- In 1984 the district model for mental health care was initiated by NIMHANS, Bengaluru. It identified the practicability of the district mental health team initiating mental health care. This was extended to 25 districts in 20 states between 1995 and 2000.
- Community care alternatives and NGO initiatives are increased.

- Public awareness increased enormously due to community based mental health care.
- Legislations supportings mental health care are developed namely, the Narcotic Drugs and Psychotropic Substance (NDPS) Act 1985, the MHA 1987 and Persons with Disability Act 1995 all of these legislations have changed the mental health care approach.
- Recognition of human rights of the mentally ill by the National Human Rights Commission.
- The National Health Policy 2002 clearly recognized mental health as a part of general health and specified how mental health has to be included as a part of general health services and the importance of human rights of the mentally ill.
- *Growth of mass media:* Both professionals and nonprofessionals participated in discussing mental health issues through the media.
- ICMR, New Delhi gave a big push to mental health research. This research helped to understand the role of cultural context in mental disorders, and also shown to feasibility of developing models involving schools primary health care, general practitioners and working with families.

After in-depth situation analysis and extensive consultations with state authorities the NMHP underwent radical restructuring to have a balance between various components of mental health care delivery system, and clearly specified budget allocations.

The restrategized NMHP was formally launched on 22nd Oct. 2003 by the Honorable Health Secretary at a National Workshop held at Vigyan Bhavan, New Delhi.

The salient features include:

- Redesigning DMHP around a nodal situation, which in most instances will be the zonal medical college.
- Strengthening medical colleges to improve psychiatric treatment facilities with adequate man power.
- Research and development programs in the field of community mental health.
- The restrategized NMHP expected to provide a balanced framework for the provision of comprehensive community based mental health services with a closely networked referral system.
- Promoting intersectoral collaboration and linkages with other national programmes.
- Provision of essential psychotropic drugs; family support.
- Developing self-help group and provision of funds for their activities.
- Human resource development conducting short-term training courses for professional and paraprofessionals.
- Organizing public mental health education.
- Involving private sectors and voluntary organizations in provision of mental health care services at community.
- At district level, mental health team has to be posted to render clinical care and integration of mental health at peripheral institutions.
- Services are focused to special sections of high-risk populations.
- Research and development programs in the field of community mental health.

Barriers to the Implementation of NMHP

- Poor funding
- Limited undergraduate training in psychiatry
- Inadequate mental health human resources
- Limited number of models and their evaluation
- Uneven distribution of resources across states

- Nonimplementation of the MHA 1987
- Privatization of health care in 1990s.

Major Developments During the Past Two Decades

- Increased range of treatments
- Greater recognition of the role of families
- Community mental health care
- Wide variety of care models
- Increased human resources, especially psychiatrists
- Persons with Disability Act 1995
- Judicial activism
- Recognition of stigma and discrimination
- World wide focus on mental health on the occasion of the World Health Day, October 2001, with WHO World health report 2001 being devoted entirely to mental health.

Revised Goals of NMP

- Strengthening families and communities for the care of person suffering from mental disorders.
- Organization of a wide range of mental health initiatives to support individuals and families, with special focus on immediate delivery of the most essential services to the ones with the greater needs.
- Supporting through mental health initiatives rebuilding of social cohesion, community development, promotion of mental health and the rights of the persons with mental disorders.

Plan of Action for Mental Health Care

- Organizing services
- Community mental health care facilities
- Support to families
- Human resource development
- Public mental health education
- Private sector mental health care
- Support to voluntary organizations
- Promotion and preventive interventions
- Administrative support.

Further Plan Priorities

- Family as the focus of care
- Public Mental Health Education
- Intersectoral collaboration
- Role of voluntary organizations
- Integration with general health services
- Human resource development
- Enhancing funding for mental health care
- Emphasis on prevention of disease and promotion
- Administrate structures.

District Mental Health Programme (DMHP)

The District Mental Health Programme (DMHP) was launched under NMHP in 1996 (IX Five year plan). The DMHP was based on 'Bellary Model' with the following components.

- Early detection and treatment.
- Training, imparting short-term training to general physicians for diagnosis and treatment of common mental illnesses with limited number of drugs under guidance of specialist. The health workers are being trained in identifying mentally ill persons.
- IEC: Public awareness generation.

Starting with 4 districts in 1996 the program was expanded to 27 districts by the end of the IX plan.

The NMHP was restrategized in the year 2003 (X five year plan) with the following components.

- Extension of DMHP to 100 districts
- Upgradation of psychiatry wings of Government Medical Colleges/General Hospital
- Modernization of State Mental Hospitals
- IEC
- Monitoring and evaluation.
- *Manpower development schemes:* Centers of excellence and setting up/strengthening of PG training Department of Mental Health Specialities are the new schemes/components.
- Strengthening the Central and State mental authorities to make them effective in monitoring mental health care agencies, ongoing mental health care program and promoting intersectoral collaboration.
- Motivating research and training to generate extensive data regarding epidemiological information of mental illnesses, their course, outcome, therapies needed, burden on family and society. Development of awareness with strengthening information and communication drive by involving nongovernment organizations and mass media.
- In XI five years plan, to address shortage of manpower in mental health in short-term basis for DMHP teams. To support CME, Distance Learning E-mode learning, addressing speciality training areas such as Child Psychiatry, Geriatric Psychiatry, etc. and Operational Research related to NMHP was introduced.

The following list of medicines made mandatory at different levels.

LIST OF MEDICINES	
S. no.	**Name of the drug that should be available at PHC/PHU/CHC/Sub divisional/District Hospital**
1.	Tab: Chlorpromazine – 100 mgs
2.	Tab: Risperidone – 2 mgs
3.	Inj: Promethazine – 50 mgs
4.	Tab: Imipramine – 75 mgs
5.	Inj: Fluphenazine – 25 mgs
6.	Tab: Trihexyphenidyl – 2 mgs
7.	Tab: Diazepam – 5 mgs
8.	Tab: Phenobarbitone – 30 mgs and 60 mgs
9.	Tab: Diphenyl hydantoin – 100 mgs
10.	Tab: Lithium carbonate – 300 mgs

Contd...

Contd...

LIST OF MEDICINES	
S. no.	**Name of the drug that should be available at PHC/PHU/CHC/Sub divisional/District Hospital**
11.	Tab: Carbamazepine – 200 mgs
12.	Inj: Haloperidol – 10 mgs
13.	Cap: Fluoxetine – 20 mgs
14.	Tab: Olanzapine – 5 mgs

The above list is an indicative list. Other drugs for mentally ill could also be procured at competitive rates.

THE MENTAL HEALTH CARE BILL 2012

This bill includes the following data:

Chapter I: Preliminary
- Short title, extent and commencement.
- Definitions.

Chapter II: Mental Illness and Capacity to Make Mental Health Care and Treatment Decisions.
- Determination of mental illness.
- Capacity to make mental health care and treatment decisions.

Chapter III: Advance Directive
- Advance directive
- Manner of making advance directive
- Maintenance of online register
- Revocation, amendment or cancellation of advance
- Advance directive not to apply to emergency treatment
- Duty to follow advance directive
- Power to review, acter, modify or cancel advance directive
- Review of advance directives
- Liability of medical health professional in relation to advance directive.

Chapter IV: Nominated Representative
- Appointment and revocation of nominated representative
- Nominated representative of a minor
- Revocation, alteration cancellation of nominated representative by board.
- Duties of nominated representatives.

Chapter V: Rights of Persons with Mental Illness:
- Rights to access mental health care
- Rights to community living
- Right to protection from cruel, inhuman and degrading treatment
- Right to equality and non discrimination
- Right to information
- Right to confidentiality
- Restriction on release of information in respect to mental illness

- Right to access medical records
- Right to personal contacts and communication
- Right to legal aid
- Right to make complaints about deficiencies in provision of services.

Chapter VI: Duties Appropriate Government

- Promotion of mental health and preventive programs
- Creating awareness about mental health and reducing stigma associated with mental illness
- Appropriate government to take measures as regard to human resource development and training, etc. Coordination within appropriate government.

Chapter VII: Central Mental Health Authority

- Establishment Central Mental Health Authority
- Composition of Central Mental Health Authority
- Term of office, salaries and allowances of Chairperson and Members
- Resignation
- Filling of vacancies
- Vacancies, etc. not to invalidate proceedings of Central Authority
- Member not to participate in meetings in certain cases
- Officers and other employees of Central Authority
- Functions of Chief Executive of Officer of Central Authority
- Transfer of assets, liabilities of Central Authority
- Functions of Central Mental Health Authority
- Meeting of central authority.

Chapter VIII: State Mental Health Authority

- Establishment State Mental Health Authority
- Composition of state mental health authority
- Term of office, salaries and allowances of chairperson and other member.
- Resignation
- Filling of vacancies
- Vacancies, etc. not to invalidate proceedings of state authority
- Member not to particular in meeting in certain cases
- Officers and other employees of State Authority
- Functions of chief executive officer of State Authority
- Transfer of assets, liabilities of State Authority
- Function of State Mental Health Authority
- Meeting of State Authority.

Chapter IX: Finance, Accounts and Audit:

- Grants by Central Government to Central Authority
- Central Mental Health Authority Fund
- Accounts and Audit of Central Authority
- Annual Report of Central Authority
- Grants by State Government
- State Mental Health Authority Fund
- Accounts and Audit of State Authority
- Annual Report of State Authority.

Chapter X: Mental Health Establishment
Chapter XI: Mental Health Renew Commission
Chapter XII: Admission, Treatment and Discharge
Chapter XIII: Responsibilities of other Agencies
Chapter XIV: Restriction to Discharge Functions by Professional not Covered by Profession.
Chapter XV: Offences and Penalties
Chapter XVI: Miscellaneous.

Nurse's Role in NMHP and DMHP

The National Mental Health Programme for India (1982) recommended the formation of a District Mental Health Team (DMHT); in order to decentralize mental health care at the district level; with two qualified psychiatric nurses and one psychiatrist. The role of the psychiatric nurses in the district mental health team include, providing care to the inpatients. The care includes meeting their basic needs, conducting occupational therapy, recreational therapy and individual and group therapy; along with mental health education to families and the public in general. In addition to this, qualified psychiatric nurses will actively participate in decentralized training to professionals and nonprofessionals working at taluk and Primary Health Centers (PHCs). They will also supervise the task of multipurpose workers in mental health care delivery. They assist psychiatrist in research activities in monitoring mental health care at district and PHC level. Their active participation in mental health education to the public will go a long way in creating public awareness in the case of individual with various mental disorders. The other functions include monitoring of records and reports and channelizing the report to higher authority.

INSTITUTIONALIZATION VS DEINSTITUTIONALIZATION

Before 19th century, because of unavailability of drugs and psychiatric care, psychiatric patients were kept in an institutions for the safety and security of patient and society. The nursing care was totally custodial. These institutions provided structure, social contest, food, clothing, and medical services to mentally ill patients.

During 1900, the hospitals were lodged heavily with understaffed health personnel. By now only, recent advances in research given rise to effective medications and other somatic treatments. These large hospitals have taxed the society as well as the government. To overcome this burden and newer laws, resulted in the concept of deinstitutionalization. It was both a historical fact and a set of legal mandates governing the treatment of mentally ill persons. In this policy people who formerly required long hospital stays become more able to leave the institutions return to their communities and homes.

The philosophy of deinstitutionalization, changed health care economics and advances in the treatment of mental illness, especially psychopharmacology developments, significantly influenced the transformation of state mental hospitals.

Merits of Deinstitutionalization

- Involvement of family and social system while care.
- Better care would be provided to mentally ill patients in their home communities surrounded by those who were not mentally ill.
- Early recovery and low cost maintenance.

Demerits of Deinstitutionalization

- Low quality care because of poor coordination between caregivers and community.
- Revolving door syndrome: The psychiatric clients were often returned to hospital, stabilized and discharged again in a cycling pattern.
- Lack of knowledge and modern concepts of psychosocial rehabilitation.
- Low motivation of health personnel to work at community.

Essential Components of a Deinstitutional Process

- Prevention of inappropriate mental hospital admissions though the provision of community facilities.
- Discharge to the community of long-term institutional patients who have received adequate preparation.
- Establishment and maintenance of community support system of noninstitutionalized patients.

Institutionalization of Psychiatric Clients

In recent years the focus of psychiatric care has shifted away from extended care predominantly inpatients settings and toward shorter lengths of inpatient stays and a wider choice among the continuum of care options. Most inpatient psychiatric settings now have and average length of stay of 5 to 10 days when compared to 24 to 30 days during last decades.

Indications

- Prevention of harm to self/others/community at large.
- Management of severe symptoms.
- Need for a rapid, multidisciplinary diagnostic evaluation that requires frequent observation by trained professional.

Treatment Objective

- Rapid evaluation and diagnosis.
- Lowering behavior that is dangerous to self or others.
- Preparing the patient and significant caregivers to manage the patient's care in a least restrictive setting.
- Arranging for effective aftercare to facilitate continued improvement in the patient's condition and functional level.

Community support services programs were developed to meet the needs of persons with mental illness outside the institution. These programs focus on rehabilitation, vocational needs, education and socialization as well as management of symptoms and medications.

In India, alternative community based services are not adequately developed and existing mental hospitals are not fully equipped with therapeutic activities. Now, we require a balanced approach, i.e. inpatient treatment needs to be improved and community based health programs strengthened.

Now, there is an urgent need to sensitize governments on the importance of mental health and clearly define the goals/motto and objectives of community based health programs. Mental health services should be integrated into the overall health system. Innovative community based programs which are culturally and gender appropriate and reach out to all the sect of the population need to be developed. In this time, it is better to involve indigenous system of medicine like Ayurveda, Homeopathy, Siddha, and other holistic systems in community. This significantly enhances the social health fabric and lowers economic burden of an individual as well as nation at a large perceptive. We need, well organized care inspite of human resources are increasing, thinking whole community as a global society.

PREVENTIVE PSYCHIATRY: MODELS, LEVEL AND ROLE OF NURSE

Preventive psychiatry denotes about preventing the disease to occur at first time. Many models describes preventive measures. A model is a theoretical way of understanding a concept or idea. It represents different ways of approaching complex issues in a unified manner.

Models of Preventive Psychiatry

Clinical Model

- It denotes the absence of signs and symptoms of disease indicates health
- Illness would be the presence of conspicuous signs and symptoms of disease. People who use this model of health to guide their use of health care services may not seek preventive health services, or they may wait until they are very ill to seek care. Clinical model is the conventional model of the discipline of medicine.

Role Performance Model

- Health is indicated by the ability to perform social roles
- Role performance includes work, family and social roles, with performance based on societal expectations.
- Illness would be the future to perform a person's roles at the level of others in society
- This model is basis for work and school physical examination and physician excused absences.
- The sick role, in which people can be excused from performing their social roles while they are ill, is a vital component of the role performance model.

Adaptive Model

- The ability to adapt positively to social, mental and physiological changes is indicative of preventive health
- Illness occurs when the person fails to adapt or becomes inadaptive toward these changes.

High Level Wellness Model (Dunn, 1961)

- It recognizes health as an ongoing process toward a person's highest potential of functioning
- This process involves the person, family and the community
- The model describes high-level wellness as the experience of a person alive with the glow of good health, alive to the tips of their fingers with energy to burn, tingling with vitality at times like this the world is a glorious places.
- The wellness illness continuum (Travis and Ryan, 1988) is a visual comparison of high–level wellness and traditional medicines, view of wellness.
- High level wellness according to Ar dell (1977) is a lifestyle focussed approach which you design for the purpose of pursuing the highest level of health within your capability.

Holistic Health Model by Edelman and Mandle (2002)

- Holism represents the interaction of a person's mind, body and spirit within the environment.
- It is based on the belief that people (or their parts) cannot be fully understood if examined solely in pieces apart from their environment.
- Holism sees people as ever changing system of energy.
- In this model, health professionals consider clients the ultimate experts regarding their own health and respect client's.
- Subjective experience as relevant in maintaining health or assisting in healing. Here, the clients are involved in their healing process, thereby assuming some responsibility for health maintenance.

Milio's Framework for Prevention of Illness

- Nancy Milio developed a framework for prevention that includes concepts of community oriented population focused care.
- Milio stated that behavioral patterns of the populations and individuals: who make-up populations are a result of habitual selection from limited choices.
- She challenged the common notion that a main determinant for unhealthful behavioral choice is lack of knowledge.

Tannahill Model of Health Promotion

- *Health education:* Communication activity aimed at enhancing well-being and preventing ill-health through favorably influencing the knowledge, beliefs attitudes and behavior of the community.
- *Health protection:* It refers to the policies and codes of practice aimed at preventing ill-health or positively enhancing well-being, e.g. no smoking in public places. Health protection is responsible for the development and implementation of legislation, policies and programs in the areas of environmental health protection, community care facilities and Emergency Preparedness.

Mental Health Promotion Model

- The purpose of mental health promotion for people with mental illness is to ensure that individuals with mental illness have power, choice and control over their lives and mental health, and that their communities have the strength and capacity to support individual empowerment and recovery.
- The person with mental illness is the central focus, participating in his/her community, involved in decision-making about mental health services and choosing which supports are most appropriate.
- These are four key resources which should be available to the person to support their mental health.
  a. Mental health services.
  b. Family and friends.
  c. Consumer groups and organization.
  d. Genetic community services and groups.

Levels of Prevention Model

- This model advocated by Leavell and Clark in 1975, has influenced both public health practice and ambulatory care delivery worldwide.
- This model suggests that the natural history of any disease exists on a continuum, with health at one end and advanced disease at the other.
- The model delineates three levels of the application of preventive measures that can be used to promote health and arrest the disease process at different points along the continuum.
- The goal is to maintain a healthy state and to prevent disease or injury.

It has been defined in terms of four levels:

1. Primordial prevention
2. Primary prevention
3. Secondary prevention
4. Tertiary prevention.

Primordial Prevention

- Prevention of the emergence or development of risk factors in population or countries in which they have not yet appeared.
- Efforts are directed towards discouraging children from adopting harmful lifestyles.

Primary Prevention

According to Caplan, it is defined as an effort directed towards reducing the incidence of mental disorders in a community. Secondary prevention refers to decreasing the duration of disorder while tertiary prevention refers to reducing the level of impairment.

Primary prevention is to prevent the onset of a disease or disorder and thereby decrease its incidence within the population. The emphasis in primary prevention is mainly on health development and effective coping abilities of individuals.

The factors to be emphasized during primary prevention of mental illness are:

Biological and Physical Factors

Prenatal and postnatal check-ups and care helps to diagnose anomalies such as mental retardation and organic mental disorders. Special follow-up during antenatal period regarding nutrition, immunization/vaccination, avoidance of the use of drugs and alcohol, repeated X-rays, prevention of repeated abortion, genetic counseling of the courple with a high-risk of chromosomal abnormalities like mongolism, family history of mental retardation and AIDS/HIV infection, help in reducing mental illness in the neonate. Encourage safe abortion of a defective fetuses if diagnosed *in utero*.

Physical Factors

For the normal mental growth of child minimum requirements such as nutritious food, shelter, and clothing are required. Parents should provide all these to their children. A couple childless should be guided for investigations and encouraged for adoption.

Psychosocial Factors

The individual should learn to cope with a crisis situation by learning needed competencies.

Physical Competencies

A child must be taught about coordination of muscles, protecting oneself from injuries like head injury which may lead to mental illness.

Intellectual Competencies

Exposure to computers and scholastic activities helps to improve the memory and other functions.

Emotional Competencies

Teaching emotional equilibrium during stress and problem-solving methods.

Social Competencies

Children should be provided opportunities for group interaction. Socialization with guests and friends to chat/accept his/her strengths and weakness. A child should be taught to cope with changes as adolescence, puberty, marriage, pregnancy and childbirth, etc.

Sociocultural Factors

To reduce incidences of mental illnesses, it is very necessary to provide psychoeducation/mental health education to people, to enable them to cope with stress. Education can be provided by multimedia, online and offline services such as TV/Radio, Internet/video, Conferences, exhibitions, role plays and print media. Educating teachers on drug-addiction and identification of learning disorders and other common psychological problems plays a pivotal role. Social empowerment helps to build healthy society.

Secondary Prevention

It aims at early detection and prompt treatment of an illness or disorder. The main emphasis is on minimizing the duration of the illness. It includes early detection and prompt intervention of high-risk individuals such as recently divorced/widowed; failure in exams, heavy loss, etc. Crisis intervention and public education are components of secondary prevention. Crisis intervention theories and services are important attempts at secondary prevention. For crisis intervention partial/short-term hospitalization like day care centers can be utilized. Walk in-clinics where client comes and goes anytime of day/night, to get professional help can be useful for many clients.

Tertiary Prevention

The main goal of tertiary prevention is to reduce the prevalence of residual symptoms, defects and disabilities caused due to illness or a disorder. In mental illnesses, tertiary prevention enables those with chronic mental illness to reach the highest feasible level of functioning. It has a very important role in psychiatry while dealing with most severe and debilitating illness like schizophrenia, severe affective disorders and severe form of personality disorders. Even though these illnesses are cured without any residual functional deficits, these clients will need extensive psychosocial rehabilitation but unfortunately these type of illnesses leave residual deficits in most of the cases like their ability to socialize with others, handle the usual stress of daily life and achieve their potential. Following services should be provided for disability prevention.

Treatment and follow-up: The client should be given prescribed psychotropic drug in right dose, through right route and at right time. These clients are observed for side effects and further complications.

Individual therapy and family therapy: These therapies support the individual as well as her/his family for early recovery.

Occupational therapy/vocational therapy: The clients need to be rehabilitated and helped to become socially and economically productive. His/her areas of interest can be assessed and explored and he/she can be helped to choose a job. Rehabilitation and after care plays an important aspect for mentally ill clients. It helps to empower the client for their independence.

Community facilities for mentally ill clients are:

- Day care centers/hospital
- Half-way homes
- Foster homes
- Group homes
- Sheltered workshops
- Self-help groups
- Mental health emergency care hot lines
- Walk-in-clinics

Mental health services available at primary, secondary, tertiary levels including rehabilitation.

Nurses Role

At Primary Level

In primary prevention, the focus is on lowering the rate of new cases of mental disorders in given population services provided for primary prevention are genetic counseling, early childhood-parent education program early socialization program such as play groups, self-help person for awareness regarding mental illness, etc.

Mental Health Services at the Secondary Level

Secondary prevention includes crisis intervention through hot lines, walk-in-clinics, treatment (medication, physical or psychosocial interventions) in hospitals, hospitalization and psychotherapies.

Mental Health Services Available a Tertiary Level

Psychosocial rehabilitation or tertiary prevention include the following services: Day care hospital, half-way homes, group homes, sheltered workshops, self-help groups and liaison workers.

Nurse Role in Primary Prevention

The role of nurse in primary prevention focuses on the target population/group/high-risk group and the provision of awareness and education.

The community mental health nurse plays an important role in identifying high-risk group and prevention of mental illness in those by education and awareness. The important tasks are:

- Educating parenting skills and child rearing skills to prospective new parents.
- Antenatal care to mother regarding harmful effects of certain things like: radiation, drugs, smoking, drug abuse including alcohol, etc.
- Motivating pregnant mothers for compulsory institutional delivery so that timely and adequate help can be provided during pregnancy to protect the newborn from anoxia and other related birth injuries.
- Educating mother about diet and supplements during pregnancy.
- Teaching the groups/individuals, ways to cope with the changes associated with various maturational life changes.
- Teaching concepts of mental health to various groups within the community.
- Providing crisis counseling to individuals/group in the community.
- Providing crisis intervention strategies.
- Teaching ways of coping and support to unemployed or homeless individuals.
- Providing support and education to specific group like widows, police personnel, just retired employees, adolescents entering puberty, etc.

Nurses Role in Secondary Prevention

Secondary prevention aims at early detection and prompt treatment of the illnesses. The nurse's role in secondary includes the following:

- The community mental health nurse should carry-out ongoing assessment of the clients who are at risk for development of mental disorders.
- Early diagnosis and referral services.
- Early detectation of complications and prompt treatment.
- Assessment for adverse effects of medications.
- Psychoeducation and mental health education.
- Crisis intervention strategies.

Nurses Role in Tertiary Prevention

The goal of tertiary prevention is to reduce the prevalence of residual defects and disabilities caused by an illness or a disorder. Nursing in tertiary prevention focuses on helping clients learn and relearn socially acceptable behavior, so that they can achieve a satisfying role in family and community. The nurse should provide rehabilitation and follow–up services to achieve this goal.

- Consider and assess the rehabilitation services required during initial diagnosis and treatment planning.
- Teaching the client activities of daily living and encouraging independence to her/his maximum ability.
- Referring the client to various community centers after discharge from the hospital.
- Monitor the effectiveness of such centers and help the client in finding vocation independence and job placement services.
- Utilizing the available resources of the family and community for helping the client in long term rehabilitation in diseases like schizophrenia and BPAD.

PSYCHOSOCIAL REHABILITATION

Introduction

Psychosocial rehabilitation (PSR) is a term used to describe services that aim to restore the client's ability to function in the community. It not only includes the medical and psychosocial treatment but also include ways to foster social intervention, to promote independent living to encourage vocational performance (Cook et al 1996). PSR aims to integrate patients back into the community rather than segregating them in separate facilities. The overall goal of PSR is to teach skills and provide community supports so that the individual with mental disabilities can function in social, vocational, educational, and familial roles with the least amount of supervision from the helping health professional. The professionals must involve families in treatment planning and implementation. So, PSR is labor intensive and person-to-person venture in practical way.

Definitions

According to Maxwell Jones (1952): It is an attempt to provide the best possible community role which will enable the patient to achieve the maximum range of activity, interest and of which he is capable.

Rehabilitation is the process of minimizing psychiatric impairments, social disadvantages and adverse personal reactions so that disabled is helped to use her/his abilities and to acquire confidence and self-esteem through experiencing success in social roles.

It is the process designed to bring back the client to a normal stage, to help the handicapped individual to make maximum use of their residual capacities and to enable them to lead a beneficial and meaningful life in the community. It aims at helping the client to re-establish or regain his interest to do useful activities maybe physical, mental, social, recreational or job oriented.

Philosophy of PSR

The overall philosophy of psychiatric rehabilitation in mental disorders comprises two intervention strategies. The first strategy is individual–centered and aims at developing the patient's skills in interacting with a stressful environment. The second strategy is ecological and directed towards developing environmental recourses to reduce potential stressors. Most disabled persons need a combination of both approaches.

Newer Concepts of PSR

Psychiatric rehabilitation cannot be imposed. It concentrates on the individual's rights as a respected partner and endorses his/her involvement and self-determination concerning all aspects of the treatment and rehabilitation process. These values are also used in recovery. Within the concept of recovery engaging the patient in his/her own care planning. It is now essential that the client can rely on his or her therapist's understanding and trust; as most of the chronically ill and disabled persons lose close, intimate and stable relationships in the course of the disease. Recent research on rehabilitation suggests that social support is associated with recovery from chronic diseases, greater life satisfaction and enhanced ability that enhanced ability to cope with life stressors. Corrigan et al have found that the most important factor facilitating recovery is the support of peers. So, it includes network building measures.

Indications of PSR

- Chronic disorders like schizophrenia, OMD, BPAD, etc.
- Mental retardation
- Alcohol and multidrug abusers
- Personality disorders, etc.

Basic Principles of Rehabilitation

- Increasing independence would be the first step in rehabilitation process.
- Primary focus is on improvement of capabilities and competence of patient's with psychiatric problems.
- Maximum use must be made of residual capacities.
- Client's active participation is very essential.
- Skill development, therapeutic environment are fundamental interventions for a successful rehabilitation process.

Areas of Rehabilitation

- *Occupational rehabilitation:* Greatly achieved by providing occupational and individual therapy and providing employment.
- *Domestic rehabilitation:* The chronic mentally ill clients require long-term hospitalization or stay in homes.
- *Social rehabilitation:* Here, more attention is given to the abilities of the client is required for normal social interactions.

Current Approaches to PSR

Generally, people with psychiatric disabilities tent to have the same life aspirations as people without disabilities in their social life. They want to be respected and valued as autonomous individuals and lead a life as normal as possible. They mostly desire:

- Their own housing
- An adequate education and a meaningful work career
- Satisfying social and intimate relationships and
- Participation in community life with full rights.

Housing

Housing for chronically mentally ill have many options. It ranges from 24 hour staffed sheltered homes to partial housing measures.

Work

The beneficial effects of work for mental health is much more. Therefore, vocational rehabilitation has been a core element of rehabilitation. It is based on the assumption that work does not only improve activity, social contacts, etc. but may also promote gains in related areas such as self-esteem and quality of life, as work and employment are a step away from dependency and a step to integration into society.

Vocational rehabilitation programs in the community provide a series of graded steps to promote job entry or reentry. For less disabled persons, brief and focused techniques are used to teach how they can find a job, fill out applications and conduct employment interviews. In transitional employment, a temporary work environment is provided to teach vocational skills, which should enable the affected person to move onto competitive employment.

Today, the most promising vocational rehabilitation model is supported employment (SE). The work of Robert Drake and Deborah Becker influenced the conceptualization of SE. In their individual placement model, disabled persons are placed in competitive employment according to their choices as soon as possible and receive all support needed for them. The support provided is continued indefinitely. Participation in SE programs is followed by an increase in the ability to find and keep employment.

Building Interpersonal Relationships

This involves Social Skills Training (SST). This is promulgated by Robert Liberman, who has designed systematic and structured skill training. They framed modules with different topics. The modules focus on medication management; symptom management, substance abuse management, basic conversational skills, interpersonal problem-solving, friendship and intimacy; recreation and leisure, workplace fundamentals, community reentry and family involvement. Each module is composed of skills areas. The skills areas are taught in exercises with multimedia and mass media including assignments.

Keeping Relationships

Keeping harmony among relationships between clients and family members is a real challenge. Care giving imposes a great burden to family as well as others. Family intervention programs necessary to reduce the burden. It helps to lower the relapse rate and also in improving outcome, e.g. psychosocial functioning.

Developing Environmental Resources

Psychiatric rehabilitation requires individualized and specialized treatment which requires many resources. Developing community support system is necessary to regulate the resources a newer concept known as case management (CM) was evolved. Case management focuses on all aspects of the physical and social environment. The core elements of CM are the assessment of client's needs, the development of comprehensive service plans for the clients and the arrangement of service delivery.

Providing Psychoeducation

It includes diagnosing the problem, telling the person what to expect regarding illness and discussing treatment alternatives.

Group Therapy

The positive aspects of group therapy include an opportunity for ongoing contact with others, validation of their perceptions, sharing their views about problems and problem-solving abilities.

Rehabilitation Team

Psychiatric rehabilitation team include psychiatrist, clinical psychologist, psychiatric social worker, psychiatric nurse, occupational therapist, recreational therapist, counselor and other allied health professionals.

Steps in Psychiatric Rehabilitation

Psychiatric rehabilitation begins when client admits the hospital. It starts with a comprehensive medical psychiatric diagnosis and functional assessment. These are key elements in identifying impairments and disabilities. The steps of rehabilitation include:

Reduction of Impairments

Rehabilitation interventions with psychiatric clients require education or elimination of the symptoms and cognitive impairments that interfere with social and vocational performance. These impairments are reduced and eliminated for the greater part by various psychotropic agents.

Remediation of Disabilities Through Skill Training

Skill training is used to remediate disabilities in social, family and vocational functioning. Clients generally require training in self-care skills, interpersonal skills, vocational and employment pursuits, recreational and leisure skills.

Remediating Disabilities Through Supportive Interventions

When restoration of social and vocational functioning, through skills training is limited by continuing deficits, rehabilitation strategies aim at helping the individual compensate for handicap by learning new skills in living and working environments, adjusting the individual and family expectations to a level of functioning that is realistically attainable.

Remediation of Handicaps

In addition to clinical rehabilitation interventions, the disabled persons can be helped to overcome their handicaps through social rehabilitation interventions, e.g. community support programs.

Role of Nurse in Psychosocial Rehabilitation

Psychosocial rehabilitation is a comprehensive and holistic process which includes client, family and society/community as major core concepts. Actually it is the process of minimizing psychiatric complications. Impairments social disadvantages and adverse personal reactions; so that the disabled individual is helped to empower his residual talents/skill and to live independently. The psychiatric nurse is a key person who helps to coordinate the efforts of members of therapeutic team with family and community in large. For successful rehabilitation, cooperation and coordination of health care personnel, client, his/her family members and community agencies such as self-help groups (SHG's) and various voluntary agencies is needed.

Assessment of the Client

The nurse should assess the individual in the areas of symptoms present, motivation, strengths, interpersonal skills, self-esteem, activities of daily living and drug compliance.

Assessment of Family

- Family structure including family developmental stages, roles, responsibilities, norms and values.

- Family's collaboration and attitude towards client
- Emotional climate of the family
- Past family experiences with mental health services
- The family's understanding of the client's problems and the plan of care
- Assess for economical states and collective approach strategies.

Assessment of Community

It includes assessment of community agencies that provide services to people who have mental illnesses, assessment of attitudes of the people towards the mentally ill, etc.

Planning and Implementation

It focuses on fostering independence by maximizing personal strengths. The nurse and the client work together to find ways for the client to overcome any remaining impaired areas of functioning. Innovative techniques are used to make independent.

Client Centered Interventions

Inpatient/Hospital Rehabilitation

It involves therapeutic community, recreational therapy, social skills training, indigenous therapies and training in basic living skills.

Community Rehabilitation

It includes providing psychiatric care in community settings, like client's home settings, residential care settings, foster homes, half-way homes, etc.

Family Interventions

- Psychoeducation/Mental Health Education to family members regarding the disease process, available resources, communication skills and problem-solving methods.
- Motivating the family members to provide proper care to the client.
- Group therapy and support to family members through self-help groups, nurses are in a favorable position to help families cope with stress and adapt to changes in the family structure.

Community Interventions

Many ways are favorable for nurses to intervene in the community. These may include psychoeducation to the public by mass media, training and educating school teachers, local leaders and other allied health professionals in the rehabilitation of mentally ill clients.

Evaluation

It usually takes place at the level of impact on the client, family and the effectiveness of the community service system.

Vocational Rehabilitation

It is a part of continuous and coordinated process of rehabilitation which involves the provision of those vocational services (e.g. vocational guidance, vocational training and selective placement) designed to enable a disabled person secure and retain suitable job.

- *Examples:* Vocational Rehabilitation Centers in India:
  - Vocational Rehabilitation Center, Chennai.
  - Mithra special school and vocational training center for the mentally retarded, Chennai.
  - Banyan, Chennai.
  - Shristi Center for Psychiatric Rehabilitation, Madurai.
  - VTC (vocational training center) for the physically handicapped run by Ministry of Labor, Govt. of India has opened up its facility for mentally ill in Chennai.
  - Indian Red Cross Society (IRCS) which VTC for the handicapped has offered vocational training for the chronic mentally ill.
  - Indian Council for Child Welfare, an NGO caring for under privileged children.

Phases in Vocational Rehabilitation

- Vocational assessment
- Vocational counseling
- Vocational training
- Job exploration
- Job placement
- Follow-up

Vocational Assessment

It is carried out in four areas, viz clinical, social, psychological and vocational.

- Clinical assessment includes assessing for residual psychiatric symptoms which may affect his ability of function.
- Social assessment includes assessing family support, attitude of family members and economic status of family.
- Psychological assessment includes assessing self-esteem, confidence, patient's level of motivation.
- Vocational assessment includes assessing physical strength, hand-head coordination, attention, concentration, etc.

Vocational Counseling

This includes informing patients and family members regarding the type of training available. Family consent should be taken for rehabilitation training.

Vocational Training

It includes:

- Course content
- Duration of training
- Incentives
- Assessment of the progress
- Imparting skills
- Supervision

Job exploration: It is finding out various jobs available in the community.

Job placement: This includes selecting suitable job, placement of the client in the job, checking the facilities available and evaluating work performance.

Follow-up: It includes evaluation of the four dimensions viz clinical, social, psychological and vocational.

Vocational program: It includes the following things.

Open Competitive Job Placement

Though it is difficult to place the mentally restored in open competitive job placements, it is also possible to provide opportunity for selected groups of clients with the clinical diagnoses of reactive psychoses, bipolor affective disorders and acute psychotic episodes. They can be equipped to function successfully by regular follow-up programs.

Sheltered Employment

It is provided for those disabled persons, who, because of the nature and severity of the disability, cannot cope with ordinary employment. This is suitable for those with the problems of mental retardation, chronic mental illness (e.g. schizophrenia, repeated attacks of affective disorder in spite of regular medication).

Self-Employment

Self-employment is provided for those disabled persons, who, because of the nature and severity of the disability, cannot cope with ordinary employment. This is suitable for those with the problems of mental retardation, chronic mental illness.

Those persons who cannot cope with the demands of vocational adjustment in open competitive job situations, but who have the capacity to do, some work with the help of any family members, maybe considered for self-employment schemes which are usually sponsored by different welfare schemes of nationalized banks and social welfare departments.

Home Bound Work Programs

For those disabled needing total care, work can be given at home, which shall be collected by the center and paid according to the performance.

MENTAL HEALTH SERVICES FOR PSYCHIATRIC CLIENTS

Partial Hospitalization

It is an innovative alternative to hospitalization. It is ideally suited to most of the psychiatric diseases/syndromes, particularly chronic psychotic disorders, neurosis, personality disorders, drug and alcohol dependence and mental retardation. It also includes day care centers, day hospitals and day treatment programs.

Partial hospitalization has the advantages of lesser separation from families, more involvement in the treatment program and a lessening of client's preoccupation with the illness, which maybe intensified by full hospitalization.

Examples of Day Care Centers in India

- Sanjivini day care center, Delhi
- SCAFF (Schizophrenia research foundation) Chennai has started a day care center called Bavishya in 1985
- Anugraha Day Care Center, Chennai
- Association of the friends of mentally ill, Mumbai
- Institute of Mental Health, Ahmedabad
- Psychiatric Center, Kolkata
- NIMHANS, Bengaluru
- The Richmond fellowship society, Bengaluru
- Krupamajie Institute of Mental Health, Miraj

Quarter-Way Homes

This is usually located within the hospital area itself, but not having the regular services of a hospital. There may not be routine nursing staff or routine rounds and most of the activities of the place are taken care of by the clients themselves.

Half-Way Homes

It is a transitory residential center for mentally ill clients who no longer need the full services of a hospital, but are not yet ready for a completely independent living. It attempts to maintain a climate of health rather than of illness, and to develop and strengthen individual capacities. At the same time it enables the recognition of problems that require medial attention and permits the discovery of conditions in the community which are acting adversely on the individual. Thus, half-way homes have a major role in the rehabilitation of the mentally ill individual.

Objectives

- To ensure a smooth transition from hospital to the family
- To integrate the individual into the mainstream of life

Activities at Half-Way Homes

Community mental health nurses play a vital role in monitoring the progress of discharged clients in half-way homes, especially with regular to their medication regimen and coordination of care. The interventions carried out in half-way homes include:

- *Assessment:* Clinical assessment including assessing for residual psychiatric symptoms which may affect his ability to function; social assessment including assessing family support, attitude of family members including assessing self-esteem, confidence, patient's level of motivation; vocational assessment including assessing physical strength, hand-head coordination, attention, concentration, etc.
- Remediating disabilities through supportive services.
- Imparting Activities of Daily Living (ADL), meditation, yoga and physical exercises.

Outcomes

- *Expected outcomes could be:* Successful return of the clients to their homes, prevention of relapses, economic self-sufficiency made possible through vocational counseling and self-employment programs.

- Nurses need to be familiar with the various types of half-way homes available in the community; collaboration with such facilities is absolutely essential for successful rehabilitation.

Examples of Half-Way Homes in India

- *Roshmi:* North Eastern State.
- Richmond Fellowship Society (India) Bengaluru, Delhi.
- Vishwas Half-way Homes, Delhi.
- Medico Pastoral Association, Bengaluru.
- Atmashakti Vidyalaya, Bengaluru.
- Puraskara After Care Home, Bengaluru.
- Cadabam's Homes for the Mentally Disabled, Bengaluru.
- Family Fellowship Society for Psychosocial Rehabilitation, Bengaluru.
- Raju Rehabilitation Foundation, Bengaluru.
- YWCA Half-Way Home for Mentally Ill, Chennai.
- Dr. Boaz's rehabilitation center, Chennai
- Dr. Dhairyan's Psycho Therapy and Rehabilitation Center, Chennai.
- Sky Half-Way Home at Madurai.
- Delhi Psychosocial Rehabilitation society.
- Paripurnata half-way Home, West Bengal.
- Society for Mental Health, Kerala.
- Leena Khurana Day care cum Half-way Home, Delhi.

Self-Help Groups

- Self-help groups for mental health are voluntary associations of people who share a common desire to overcome mental illness or otherwise increase their level of cognitive or emotional well-being.
- They have homogeneity. The members have same disorders and share their experiences good or bad, successful or unsuccessful with one another. The members work together using their strengths to gain control over their lives. By doing so, they educate each other, provide mutual support, and alleviate the sense of alienation usually felt by people drawn to this kind of group. In other words, self-help groups are based on the premise that people who have experienced a particular problems are able to help others who have the same problems.
- One of their most important functions is to demonstrate to individuals that they are not alone in having a particular problem. Sharing each other's experiences not only help the members by providing mutual support, but also by generating alternate ways to view and resolve problems. This they help in overcoming maladaptive patterns of behavior or states of feeling that traditional mental health professionals have not generally dealt with successfully.
- They emphasize cohesion, which is exceptionally strong in these groups. Because the group member have similar problems and symptoms, they develop a strong emotional bond. But each group may have its unique characteristics, to which the members can attribute magical qualities of healing.
- Strategies: The strategies used by group leaders include promotion of dialogue, self-disclosure and encouragement among members. Concepts used in support groups include psychoeducation, self-disclosure and mutual support.

- *Processes:* The processes involved in self-help groups are social affiliation; learning self-control; and modeling methods to cope with stress and acting to change the social environment.
- The end result is that these groups prevent physical, emotional and social problems and breakdowns; improve an individual's or a family's quality of life; and provide the education necessary to develop the member's potential further.

Examples of Self-Help Groups

- Alcoholics Anonymous (AA)
- Association for Mentally Disabled (AMEND)
- TOPS
- Groups of Single Parents
- Emotions Anonymous/Emotional Health Anonymous
- Peer Support Group
- National Association for Mental Health
- Depression and Bipolar Support Alliance (DBSA)
- GROW
- Recovery International

The self-help group movement in India is in its ascendency.

One on the recent developments is the start of AMEND in Bengaluru. People with mental illness suffer from social stigma and discrimination. More so their family members are struck with disbelief, loneliness and sorrow. Families of such people have got together to form an organization in Bengaluru known as AMEND—Association for mentally disabled under the leaders of Dr Nirmala Srinivasan. It has been advocating and practicing family based care. At AMEND, families share experiences, talk about side effects of medication and discuss medication and discuss how they can communicate problems to psychiatrist. It also conducts workshops to train consumers in living skills so that they can look after themselves, tell them what is wrong with one self, why they need to take their medication, and what can happen if they stop and so on so forth. Many of AMEND's consumers have been rehabilitated and are holding jobs as part of their occupational therapy.

Suicide Prevention Centers

Many suicides prevention centers are in India in the voluntary sector doing good work and helping those in need. For example:

- Sneha, Chennai
- Sahara, Mumbai
- Helping Hands and MPA, Bengaluru
- Sanjivini and Sumaitri, New Delhi
- Community Group Homes
- Large Homes for Long-Term Care.

MENTAL HEALTH AGENCIES: GOVERNMENT AND VOLUNTARY: NATIONAL AND INTERNATIONAL

Mental Health Agencies: Government at National Level

There are more than 42 mental hospitals in the country with the bed availability of 20,893 in the government sector. In the private sector there are more 6000 beds. These facilities have to manage an estimated 1.02 crore people with severe mental illness and 5.12 crore people with common mental disorder. Pursuit to the orders of the Honorable Supreme Court in CWP No. 334 of 2001, the Government of India, constituted a number of teams to inspect and report a state the state of mental health services, with special focus on mental hospitals. These teams visited all state capitals and Government run mental hospitals across the country during Nov. 2001–Jan 2002.

Mental Health Agencies: International

- *World Health Organization (WHO):* WHO defines mental health as not simply absence of disease but a positive state of physical, mental and social well-being. WHO's present program now integrates mental health concerns to prevent and control mental disorders. One of the important recommendations of WHO (2001) has been to develop community based mental health care program. WHO's contribution to classify mental disorders has been its international classification of disease (1CD-10) which enables clinicians and researchers in different countries to use a uniform set of diagnostic categories.
- *The United Nations Educational Scientific and Cultural Organization (UNESCO):* UNESCO collaborates among nations through educational, cultural and scientific channels and attempts to foster peace and respect for human rights with fundamental freedom for all. UNESCO initially arranged the use of satellites for educational and mental health purposes. It helps in the training of scientists as well as in the development of scientific research in developing countries.
- *World Federation for Mental Health (WFMH):* WFMH was established in 1948 as an international congress of nongovernment organizations and individuals concerned with mental health. Its purpose is to promote cooperation at the international level between governmental, nongovernmental mental health agencies and its membership has now extended to more than 50 countries. The Federation has been granted consultative status by both WHO and UNESCO and it assists the UN agencies by collecting information on mental health conditions all over the world. The goals of WFMH are as follows:
  - To promote mental health and optimal functioning
  - To prevent mental, neurological and psychosocial disorders
  - To heighten public awareness about the importance of mental health
  - To improve care and treatment of those with mental, neurological and psychosocial disorders
- *The International Society for Mental Health Online:* It is a nonprofit organization formed in 1997 to promote the understanding, use and development of online communication information and technology for the international mental health community. The Achieve serves as a valuable resource for researchers, clinicians and ordinary for the international sources for researcher, clinicians and ordinary people interested in the topic of online mental health.
- *National Alliances for the Mentally Ill.*
  - It is a nonprofit self-help, support and advocacy organization of consumers, families and friends of people with severe mental illnesses. It was founded in 1979.
- *National Resource and Training Center on Homelessness and Mental Illness:* This organization focuses on the effective organization and delivery of services for people who are homeless and have serious mental illness.

- *The National Mental Health Association:* It is situated at US. It works to improve the mental health of all Americans, especially the 54 million people with mental disorders; through advocacy, education, research and service.
- *The Canadian Mental Health Association:* It supports the mental health of all and supports the resilience and recovery of people experiencing mental illness.
- *National Alliance on Mental Illness (NAMI):* NAMI is the largest grassroots mental health organization in the US, dedicated to improving the lives of persons living with serious mental illness and their families.

Mental Health Agencies: Voluntary/Nongovernmental Agencies/Self-help Group in India

Nongovernment organizations or voluntary organizations are a valuable community resource for mental health. They are often more sensitive to the local realities than centrally driven programs and are usually strongly committed toward innovation and change. They often play an extremely important role in society, in the absence of a formal or well functioning mental health system, filling the gap between community needs and available community services and strategies. They help in suicide prevention, crisis support, formation of self-help of families, organizing community based housing facilities for short-term and long-term care of person with chronic illnesses; setting up of facilities like day care center, sheltered employment facilities, living skill management for school dropout children and community mental health education.

NGOs in India

1. Alzheimer and Related Disorders Society of India (ARDSI), Kochi
2. Sangath Society, Goa
3. The Research Society, Mumbai
4. Samadhan, New Delhi
5. Schizophrenia Research Foundation (SCARF)
6. Medico-Pastoral Association (MPA)
7. TT Krishnamachari Foundation, Chennai
8. Total Response to Alcohol and Drug Abuse, Kerala, Karnataka
9. National Addiction Research Center, Mumbai
10. Sneha, Chennai
11. MPA, Bengaluru
12. Prerana, Mumbai
13. AMEND, Bengaluru
14. Narendra Foundation, Karnataka
15. SACRED
16. GASS (Grameena Abyudayg Seva Samiti)
17. ADD, India
18. Vidya, Sagar
19. Nav-Bharat Jagriti Kendra, North India
20. Association of People with Disability (APD)
21. Association for Promoting Social Action (APSA)
22. Paraspara Trust
23. Centre for Advocacy in Mental Health, CAMH

24. M.S. Chellamuthu Foundation
25. The Richmond Fellowship Society
26. Chaitanya Home for Schizophrenics, Pune
27. Snehi Institute for mental health care
28. Ashra, Orissa
29. Antara NGO's for refugees of mental health Kolkata.
30. Institute for Psychological Health, Mumbai

All these organizations are helping the mentally ill in multiple ways including research.

Challenges/Drawbacks of Community Mental Health in India

Considering the concept of NMHP and DMHP, very little progress is achieved in India. Lack of human resources, budget, awareness, political will, innovations, etc. have hampered the status of mental health.

Community Mental Health Psychiatric Nursing

It is the application of specialized knowledge to population and communities to promote and maintain mental health, and to rehabilitate populations at risk that continue to have residual effects of mental illness.

Community mental/psychiatric nursing differs from hospital settings. Community setting requires that the psychiatric nurse possesses knowledge about a broad array of community resources and be flexible in approaching problems related to individual psychiatric symptoms, family and support systems and basic living needs such as housing and financial support.

Objectives of Community Mental Health Nursing

- To provide preventive activities to populations for the purpose of promoting mental health.
- To provide psychosocial interventions immediately as crisis erupts.
- To provide corrective learning experiences for client-group who have deficits and disabilities in the basic competencies needed to cope in society; and to help individual develop a sense of self-worth and independence.
- To anticipate when population become at risk for particular emotional problems and to identify and change social and psychological factors that diversely affect peoples interaction with their environments.
- To develop innovative approaches to preventive activities.
- To assist in providing mental health education to population about mental health and illness and to teach people how to assess their mental health.
- Providing prompt interventions considering holism.
- To help individual develop a sense of self-worth and independence.

Community Psychiatric Nursing Process

Nursing Assessment: It includes:

- Assessment for residual symptoms, impairments due to positive and negative symptoms
- Secondary social disadvantages such as unemployment, poverty and homelessness, as well as stigma attached to psychiatric illness
- Assessment for expressed emotions (EE) such as low self-esteem, poor motivation and capacity for self-management and performance of social roles

- Unpredictable behavior risk of harm to self and others and liability to relapse
- Economic status of the client
- Availability of human and related recourses in the community
- Social situations to which the client is likely to return to
- The expected outcome of the assessment is a detailed outline to the person's present functioning, highest level of functioning and the needed services.

Nursing interventions: According to Carr et al (1984)-roles include; 1984 roles includes:

Consultative role: It includes providing advise to other professional in the community about the type and level of nursing care required for a given client group.

Clinician role: Here, this includes providing direct nursing care to the client in the community setting.

Therapeutic role: Employing psychotherapeutic and behavioral methods for management of clients.

Researcher role: The psychiatric nurse may assess the care given to the client/client group, and may also assess the outcome of ongoing care program. Evaluating the program and finding out newer ways.

Educator: Creating awareness in the community about mental health and mental illness with special focus on vulnerable groups.

Trainer/Manpower Facilitator: Training of paraprofessionals, community leaders, school teachers, police personnel, and other care-giving professionals in the community setting.

Manager/Administrator: Management of resources, planning and coordination.

Domiciliary care: It includes home-visiting. Care includes administration of medicines, assessment for level of functioning, monitoring side effects, assessment for complications and counseling, etc.

Liaison role: Nurses working in the community help the patients and the family members by bridging the gap between the client and the hospital/clinic, client and the employers and also by networking in the community for resource development.

Preventive roles: These include primary, secondary and tertiary roles.

Other roles: Social skills training:

- Stress management program
- Bereavement counseling
- Group meetings
- Out reach services
- Child care services
- Elderly care services
- Drug addictive care services

MENTAL HEALTH NURSING ISSUES FOR SPECIAL POPULATION

Every child will not be good in behavior at childhood times. Some types of mental illness, affects some children. Identifying mental disorders in children can be a difficult task for health personnel. Children differ from adults in that they experience many physical, mental and emotional changes as they progress through their also are in the natural growth and development. They are also in the process of learning how to cope with, adapt and relate to others and the world around them.

Many psychiatric disorders like, anxiety disorders like, ADHD, developmental disorders, learning and communication disorders, schizophrenia, and tics are the main seen disorders symptoms various according to the type of illness.

Multiple etiology contributes for illness. It maybe heredity, biological causes, psychological trauma, and stress may cause illness—if the symptoms interfere the growth and development, then it needs treatment. These are treated with medications and as well as different therapies without treatment, many mental disorders can continue into adulthood and lead to problems in all areas of the person's adult life. Children with untreated are at high-risk of drug abuse, destructive behavior and suicide when treated early. They full recover and can lead a normal life.

Usually the nursing care includes prompt treatment and emphatically dealing with the child. Family education and counseling are also helpful.

ADOLESCENCE

Adolescence is a developmental stage, occurring from age between 10 and 19 years, which marks a child's transition to young adulthood. It is generally a time of self-discovery in which young people aim to define their status and place in the society. During adolescent development, children complete puberty and physical growth. They also develop important social, emotional and intellectual skills, while striving toward independence and autonomy. This time can be a challenging time for teenagers as well as their families. In the quest for independence, many adolescents starts questioning parental authority and often show signs of rebelliousness, which can create family tension. Teenagers also typically struggle with an increasing need to belong in society. As a result, many spend more time with friends than family. This allows teens to develop and practice social skills. However, it is also within this setting that adolescents may face issues regarding peer pressure, sexual intercourse and experimentation with alcohol and drugs.

For some adolescents, these common trials can be aggravated by ongoing factors, such as a dysfunctional family, inadequate education, living in a poverty and or high crime neighborhoods. Feelings of stress, confusion and depression from circumstance related to family, academic and social life can overwhelm many young people. This sometimes can put adolescents at risk for dropping out of school, running away from house, joining gangs/roudy groups, developing substance abuse or dependence, having unprotected sex, committing suicide and other types of self-destructive behaviors.

Mental health problems include all diagnosable emotional, behavioral and mental disorders. Behavioral, mental disorders and or substance abuse issue can create a chain of events contributing to violent or suicidal behavior. Particularly, if not recognized and treated, these problems may affect a young person's self-esteem, ability to maintain relationships and their success in scholastic activities. It is the co-occurrence of behavioral and mental disorders that can be most risky, e.g. antisocial conduct co-existing with depression that may result in violent or suicidal behavior. If not treated early and promptly, these may develop into severe problems in adult years.

The nursing interventions include assessment, treatment by psychosocial therapies, counseling and empowerment.

Women

In recent trends, because of women empowerment, nowadays women are more prone for mental disorders. These are:

Depression: Women are twice as likely as to get depression.

Anxiety and Specific Phobias: Statistics predicts that women are twice as likely as men to have panic disorder, generalized anxiety and specific phobias.

Post Traumatic Stress Syndrome (PTSD): Women are twice as likely to develop PTSD following a traumatic event.

Suicide Attempts: Men die from suicide at four times the rate that women do, but women attempt suicide two or three times more often than men.

Eating Disorders: Women account for at least 85% of all anorexia and bulimia cases and 65% of binge-eating disorders cases.

Mental Health: Women's Symptoms are also Different

Even though when men and women share a common mental health diagnosis, the symptoms and subsequently the treatment can be different. For example, a depressed man likely to report job related problems: while a woman more likely to report physical ailments; like fatigue or appetite and sleep disturbances.

Causes for Gender Differences

Biological Causes

Female hormonal fluctuations are known to play a role in mood and depression. The hormone estrogen can have positive effects on the brain, protecting schizophrenic women from severe symptoms during certain phases of their menstrual cycles and maintaining the structure of neurons in the brain, which protects against some aspects of Alzheimer's on the less positive side, women tend to produce less of the mood stabilizer serotonin and synthesize it more slowly than men; which may account for the higher rates of depression. A woman's genetic make-up is also believed to play a role in the development of neurological disorders such as Alzheimer's disease.

Sociocultural Influences

Despite strides in gender equality, women still face challenges when it comes to socioeconomic power, status, position and dependence; which can contribute to depression and other disorders. Women are still the primary caregivers for children, and it is estimated that they also provide more than 80% of all care giving for chronic ill elders, which adds stress to a woman's life.

Girls tend to become dissatisfied with their bodies at puberty, a reaction that is linked to depression. Girls are also sexually abused more often than boys, and one in five women will experience rape or attempted rape, which can lead to depression and panic disorder.

Behavioral Influences

Usually women are more apt to report mental health disturbances than men and more prone to depression and treat the condition with mood altering drugs.

Psychiatric nurses working in community should be very alert to note and assess these cases keeping the principles of psychiatric nursing.

ELDERS

In recent years, old age population is very fast growing in India as well as globally. Currently the number of people aged 60 and over is more than 800 million in the world. Projections indicate that this figure will increase to over two billion in 2050. People aged 60 can now expect to survive an additional 18.5 to 21.6 years. Soon the world will have a higher number of older adults than children.

Older adults face special health challenges. Many of the very old lose their ability to live independently because of limited mobility, frailty or other physical or mental health problems and require some form of long-term care. Global statistics shows that, more than 25% of adults aged 55–65 suffer from a mental disorder (UNFPA, 2012). Mental health problems of older adults are under, identified by health care professional and older people themselves, and older people are often reluctant to seek help.

Mental Health Problems in Older Adults

A multitude of social, demographic, psychological and biological factors contribute to a person's mental health status. Almost all these factors are particularly pertinent amongst older adults.

The factors such as poverty, social isolation, loss of independence, loneliness and losses of different kinds can affect mental health. Elders are more likely to experience events such as bereavements or physical disability that affect emotional well-being and can result in poorer mental health. They may also be exposed to maltreatment at home and in care institutions. On the other hand, social support and family interactions can boost the dignity of older adults and are likely to have a protective role in the mental health outcomes of this population.

There are more older women worldwide than older men. This difference enhances with advancing age and has been called 'feminization of aging'. Older men and women generally have lower income but better family support networks. On the other hand both depression and alzheimer's disease are more prevalent among women.

Intergenerational solidarity is declining, especially in high-income countries. In some low and middle income countries a grandparent is increasingly more likely to be living with a grandchild. These so called 'skipped generation' living arrangements are becoming more common because of economic migration and in some societies as a consequence of HIV/AIDS related issues.

An important risk factor to the mental health of elders and an important human rights issue are elder maltreatment. WHO defines elder maltreatment as 'a single or repeated act or lack of appropriate action, occurring within any relationship where there is an expectation of trust that causes harm or distress to an older person. This type of abuse includes, physical, sexual, psychological, emotional, financial and material abuse, abandonment; neglect and serious loss of dignity and self-respect. In growing countries, nearly 4–6% of older persons have experience maltreatment at home. This frequency is still higher, as many older adults are too scared or are unable to report maltreatment. Elder maltreatment can lead not only to physical injuries but also to serious, sometimes long-lasting psychological consequences including depression and anxiety.

Role of Nurse

- Nursing assessment looking holistically.
- Promoting active and healthy aging practices.
- *Geriatric networking:* Participating in meaningful activities, strong personal relationships and maintain good physical health care are key factors.
- Deinstitutionalization and close monitoring in home setting.
- Abstaining from alcohol, smoking and intake of narcotic drugs.
- Early identification and prompt treatment of noncommunicable diseases.
- Involving civil society, NGOs and public private partnerships in care.
- Intellectual activation to combat dementia and other disorders.
- Psychoeducation on diet, exercises and facilities available for elder by government and nongovernmental agencies.
- Support and counseling and cognitive behavioral interventions.

VICTIMS OF VIOLENCE AND ABUSE

Violence denotes pain and furor. Violence maybe many types like family violence, sexual assault/rape, and religious violence. Usually, the violence occurs at home within family relations is called domestic violence. Domestic violence has an impact on the mental health of the victims involved and results in long-term negative consequences for all. It maybe social, psychological as well as sexual.

Sexual assault is the forced perpetration of an act of sexual contact with another person without proper consent. Rape is considered a universal crime against women, a violent sexual act committed against a woman's will and involving the threat of force.

Women who experience abuse/assault/rape from a partner are more likely to experience depression, PTSD or anxiety. They are having a large chance to get drugs or alcohol and be addicted.

In elderly, usually they are exploited, abused, neglected by their caregivers, mostly by their spouses or other family members. Abuse in elders, maybe physical, social or economic, violation of rights and neglect. These issues can treated by counseling and psychosocial interventions.

Handicapped People

The handicapped people are having a disability maybe partially or more which affects their day-to-day life. They spend more time acquire new skills or coping. If the handicapped is lost hearing, sight or speech, they need around the clock care and concern. Nursing role includes basic care with counseling and rehabilitation.

HIV/AIDS

AIDS is caused by a virus infection 'human immunodeficiency virus/HIV. It is mainly characterized by profound loss of immune functions with a depletion of CD4 and T lymphocytes.

When any individual(s) are faced with HIV/AIDS, first their physical health deteriorates along with depression, anxiety and sometimes dementia (AIDS dementia complex or ADC). Other psychosocial effects such as social stigma, grief, ongoing struggles with illness, diminished quality of life and medications.

Depression is the most common mental disorder among HIV infected individuals. Symptoms of depression include low self-esteem, anxiety, forgetfulness, sleep disturbances, changes in appetite, weight loss or gain, decreased libido and a sense of hopelessness. Anxiety maybe presented as a sense of numbness, emotional detachment or a dazed state. detachment or a dazed state. Different types of anxiety disorder include panic disorder, obsessive compulsive disorder, post-traumatic stress disorder, generalized anxiety disorder.

Anxiety disorder and phobias. AIDS dementia complex (ADC) or HIV associated dementia is common among people with advanced HIV disease. They have problem thinking clearly, like lack of concentration, loss of memory, social withdrawal, sluggish thinking, short attention span, lethargy, poor coordination, impaired judgment, vision problems and altered personality traits.

Professional counseling involving individual support, interpersonal interaction, group support and cognitive behavioral treatment. It maybe treated with antidepressants, stimulants and anxiolytics. Use of NGO's and Self-Help Groups help the client in maintaining his/her socio-economic support.

Glossary

A

Abandonment: A unilateral withdrawal of professional relationship when there is still a need for continuing health care.
Abreaction: 'Remembering with feeling'; bringing into conscious awareness painful events that have been repressed and re-experiencing the emotions those were associated with the events.
Adaptation: Restoration of the body homeostasis following a psychological/or physiological response to stress.
Affect: A pattern of observable behaviors that is the expression of a subjectively experienced feeling state (emotion).
Apathy: Lack of feeling, emotion, interest or concern.
Aggression: Behavior that defends an individual's own basic rights by violating the basic rights of others.
Attachment: Refers to the quality of the emotional relationship between the two people.
Atypical: An adjective used to describe unusual or uncharacteristic variations of a disorder.
Agoraphobia: The fear of being in places or situations from which escape might be difficult or in which help might not be available in the event of a panic attack.
Akinesia: Muscular weakness or a loss or partial loss of muscle movement: a type of extra pyramidal symptom associated with antipsychotics.
Alcoholic anonymous: A self-help organization for the treatment of alcoholism.
Alternative medicine: Practices that differ from usual allopathic medicine.
Altruism: Providing assistance and support to others creates a positive self-image and promotes self-growth.
Amnesia: An inability to recall important personal information that is too difficult to explain by ordinary forgetfulness.
Anhedonia: Inability to experience or imagine any pleasant emotion.
Anorgasmia: Inability to achieve orgasm.
Anosmia: Inability to smell.
Aphasia: Inability to communicate through speech, writing or signs, caused by dysfunction of brain enters.
Aphonia: Inability to speak.
Apraxia: Inability to carry out motor activities despite intact motor function.
Assault: An act that results in a person's genuine fear and apprehension that he or she will be touched without consent.

Assertiveness: Behavior that enables individuals to act in their own best interests.
Associate looseness/loose associations: A thinking process characterized by speech in which ideas shift from one unrelated subject to another.
Ataxia: Muscular incoordination.
Attitude: A frame of reference around which an individual organizes knowledge about his or her world.
Autism: A focus inward on a fantasy world while distorting or excluding the external environment, common in schizophrenia.
Automatic thoughts: Thoughts that occur rapidly in response to a situation and without rational analysis.
Autonomy: Independence; self-governance.
Aversive stimulus: A stimulus that follows a behavioral response and decreases the probability that the behavior will occur; also called punishment.
Avolition: An inability to initiate and persist in goal directed activities.

B

Behavior disorder: Any aberrant or maladaptive pattern of behavior.
Battery: The unconsented touching of another person.
Behavior modification: A treatment modality aimed at changing undesirable behaviors, using behavioral theory.
Bereavement: Psychological, physiological or behavioral responses associated with loss of death.
Binge and purge: Consuming high calories and vomiting.
Bioethics: Ethical principles of medicine.
Biofeedback: Use of instrument to become aware of processes in the body that usually go unnoticed and to bring them under voluntary control.
Bipolar disorders: Characterized by mood swings from profound depression to extreme euphoria.
Body image: One's sense of the self and one's body.
Borderline personality disorder: A disorder characterized by a pattern of intense and chaotic relationships with affective instability, fluctuating and extreme attitudes, regarding other people, impulsivity direct or indirect self-destructive behavior and lack of clear or certain sense of identity, life span or values.
Boundaries: The level of participation and interaction between individuals and between subsystems.
Bonding: Attachment or emotional ties between caregiver and infant.

C

Cachexia: A state of ill health, malnutrition and wasting, extreme emancipation.
Cannabis: The dried flowers of hemp plant, when taken produce euphoric effects.
Catalepsy: Waxy flexibility—rigid maintenance of body position over an extended period.
Cataplexy: Episodes of sudden bilateral loss of muscle tone result in the individual collapse, often associated with intense emotions such as anger, fear or guilt.
Catatonia: A type of schizophrenia that is characterized by stupor or excitement, stupor characterized by extreme psychomotor retardation, mutism, negativism and posturing, excitement characterized by psychomotor agitation in which the movements are purposeless.

Catharsis: It is one of the steps of group therapy in which members in a group can express both positive and negative feelings in a nonthreatening atmosphere.
Clang associations: A pattern of speech in which the choice of words is governed by sounds.
Concrete thinking: Thought processes that are focused on specifies rather than on generalities and immediate issues rather than eventual outcomes.
Confidentiality: The right of an individual to the assurance that his or her case will not be discussed outside the boundaries of health care team.
Conduct disorder: It is a persistent pattern of behavior that involves violation of rights of others.
Confusion: Inability of a person to make sense of the environment, reflected in agitated behavior, disorganized language, incorrect memories or poor memories.
Coping: Ways in which individuals deal with anxiety, stress, illness or other forms of tension and adversity.
Coping strategies: Behaviors, cognition and perceptions employed by a person to maintain (functioning) when faced with stress/illness.
Coping styles: Relatively enduring and characteristic ways in which individuals respond to stressful situations, such as illness.
Crisis: Psychological disequilibrium in a person who confronts a hazardous circumstance that constitutes an important problem which for the time he or she can neither escape nor solve with usual problem solving resources.
Crisis intervention: A brief form of treatment, whereby techniques to reduce the emotional distress brought on by a traumatic or stressful event are employed.
Cyclothymia: A chronic mood disturbance involving numerous episodes of hypomania and depressed mood, of insufficient severity or duration to meet the criteria for bipolar disorder.

D

Day care center: A hospital for day setting.
Deinstitutionalization: Detaching psychiatric patients from hospital setting to live in community.
Delirium: A state of mental confusion and excitement characterized by disorientation of time, and place, including hallucinations, incoherence of speech, and a continual state of aimless physical activity.
Delusion: False personal beliefs, not consistent with a person's intelligence or cultural background or a fixed false belief.
Dependence: It refers to when a person is reliant on a day- to- day level.
Dementia: Impairment in cognitive functioning that is progressive and interferes with social and occupational abilities.
Depersonalization: An alteration in the perception or experience of the self so that the feeling of one's own reality is temporarily lost.
Displacement: Feelings are transferred from one target to another that is considered less threatening or neutral.
Dyspareunia: Pain during sexual intercourse.
Dysthymic disorder: A depressive neurosis.
Dystonia: Involuntary muscular movements of the face, arms, legs, and neck, maybe due to side effects of antipsychotics.

E

Echolalia: Repetition of words of an examiner.
Echopraxia: Imitating the movements of the examiner.
Ego defense mechanisms: Strategies employed by the ego for protection in the face of threat to biological or psychological integrity.

F

Fetishism: A paraphilic disorder characterized by recurrent sexual and sexually arousing fantasies involving the use of nonliving objects.
Flight of Ideas: Changing thoughts from one topic to another.
Flooding: Also called as implosive therapy. It is used to desensitize individuals to phobic stimuli.
Free association: A technique used to help patients bring to consciousness material that has been repressed.
Frotteurism: A paraphilic disorder characterized by the recurrent preoccupation with intense sexual urges or fantasies involving touching or rubbing against a nonconsenting person.
Fugue: A sudden unexpected travel away from home or customary work locale with assumption of a new identity.
Flashback: A recurrence of a memory, feeling or perceptual experience from the past.
Foster homes: A home where psychiatric patient stays in a recovery stage.

G

Generalized anxiety disorder: A disorder characterized by chronic, unrealistic, and excessive anxiety and worry.
Gender identity disorder: A sense of discomfort associated with an incongruence between biologically assigned gender and subjectively experienced gender.
Genogram: A graphical representation of family generation with health aspects.
Geriatrics: The branch of clinical medicine deals with old age people.
Gerontology: The study of normal aging.
Grief: A subjective state of emotional, physical, and social responses to the real or perceived loss of a valued entity.
Granny-bashing: Media-generated term for elder abuse.
Granny-dumping: Abandoning elder people.
Gustatory hallucinations: Hallucinations involving the perception of taste.

H

Hallucinations: False sensory perception not associated with reality.
Homosexuality: A sexual preference for persons of the same gender.
Hyperkinesis: Over activity, distractibility, excitability and impulsivity seen mainly in children.
Hypersomnia: Excessive sleep.
Hypochondriasis: A unrealistic fear of having a chronic disease.
Hysteria: A dramatic symptoms characterized by recurrent, multiple somatic complaints.

 I

Id: It acts on 'pleasurable principle' which identified by Freud.

Identification: An attempt to increase self-worth by acquiring certain attributes and characteristics of an individual one admires.

Illusion: A misperception of a real external stimulus.

Incoherence: Unrelated speech or thinking without any logical connection.

Insomnia: A subjective complaint of difficulty falling or staying asleep or poor sleep quality.

Insight: Conscious awareness and understanding of one's own psychodynamics and symptoms of maladaptive behavior.

Intellectualization: A defense to avoid stress by using logic, reasoning and analysis.

Interdisciplinary: Providing care with various disciplines work to gather with common goal.

Introjection: Defense mechanism in which attitudes and behavior of another are internalized to help the person to cope with separation.

Introversion: Preoccupation with oneself and accompanying reduction of interest in the outside world.

Isolation: The separation of a thought or a memory from the feeling tone or emotions associated with it.

 J

Jamis vu: Illusion of failure to recognize a familiar situation.

Jargon aphasia: Incoherent, meaningless, neologistic speech.

Justice: An ethical principle reflecting that all individuals should be treated equally and fairly.

 K

Kleptomania: A recurrent failure to resist impulses to steal objects not needed for personal use or monetary value.

Korsakoff's psychosis: A syndrome of confusion, loss of recent memory and confabulation in alcoholics, caused by a deficiency of thiamine.

L

La belle indifference: A symptom of conversion disorder in which there is a relative lack of concern that is out of keeping with the severity of the impairment.

Laissezfaire: A leadership type in which the leader lets group members do as they like.

Labile affect: Affect repeatedly and rapidly shifts from one extreme to another e.g. from despair to elation.

Libido: The psychic drive or energy usually associated with the sexual intact.

Loosening of associations: A disturbance of speech in which ideas change from one subject to another.

Lesbian: A female homosexual.

Long-term memory: Memory for remote events or those that occurred many years ago. The type of memory that is preserved in the elderly individual.

 M

Magical thinking: A primitive form of thinking in which an individual believes that thinking about a possible occurrence can make it happen.

Mania: A type of bipolar disorder in which the predominant mood is elevated, expensive or irritable .

Masochism: Sexual stimulation derived from being humiliated, beaten, bound or otherwise made to suffer.

Melancholia: A severe form of severe depressive disorder.

Mental health: The successful adaptation to stressors from the internal or external environment, evidenced by thoughts, feelings, and behavior that are age-appropriate and congruent with local and cultural norms.

Mental illness: Maladaptive responses to stressors from the internal or external environment, evidenced by thoughts, feelings and behaviors that are incongruent with the local and cultural norms, and interfere with the individual's social, occupational, and/or physical functioning.

Mood: A pervasive and sustained emotion that colors the perception of the world.

Mourning: The psychological process (or stages) through which individual disciplines passes on the way to successful adaptation to the loss of a valued object.

Multidisciplinary team: A concept of providing care for a client in which individual disciplines provide specific services for the client without formal arrangement for interaction between the disciplines.

 N

Negative symptoms: It includes neurotic symptoms.

Neurosis: A disorder in which the individual has insight into the illness and they can distinguish between subjective experience and external reality.

Nihilistic delusion: Delusional belief that oneself, or others or the world does not exist or is about to cease to exit.

Neurotic disorder: A psychiatric disturbance, characterized by excessive anxiety and/or depression, disrupted bodily functions, unsatisfying interpersonal relationships, and behaviors that interfere with routine functioning.

Nonmaleficence: The ethical that espouses abstaining from negative acts toward another, including acting carefully to avoid harm.

Nursing process: It is a dynamic, systemic by which nurses assess, diagnose, identify outcomes, plan, implement and evaluate nursing care.

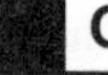 O

Obsessive-compulsive disorder: Recurrent thoughts or ideas (obsessions) that an individual is unable to put out of his/her mind, and actions that an individual is unable to refrain from performing (compulsions).

Oculogyric crisis: Occurs in dystonia which is a sign of extrapyramidal symptom, eyes look upward, head is turned to one side.

Occupational therapy: It uses goal directed activities appropriate to a persons' age and social role, to restore, develop and maintain the ability for individual living.

Operant conditioning: The learning of a particular action or type of behavior that is followed by a reinforcement.
Orientation: Awareness of one's self in relation to time, place and person.
Orgasm: A heightened sexual response or pleasure.
Overcompensation: A conscious or unconscious process in which a real or imagined physical or psychological deficit generates exaggerated correction.
Overt sensitization: A type of aversion therapy that produces unpleasant consequences for undesirable behavior.
Overvalued idea: A sustained preoccupation that is unreasonable given the evidence available, that is held strongly but not to a delusional degree.

 P

Panic attack: Acute, episodic attacks of extreme anxiety may occur with or without physiological symptoms.
Paramnesia: Distorted recall leading to falsification of memory.
Paranoid schizophrenia: A type of schizophrenia where paranoid delusions and illusions are prominent.
Parasomnia: Abnormal behavior or physiological events occur during sleep or sleep wake transitions.
Passivity phenomena: Delusional belief that an external agency is controlling that aspects of oneself that are usually under own's control.
Phobia: Exaggerated psychological irrational fear of a specific type.
Positive symptoms: Presence of hallucinations, illusions, disorganized speech and grossly disorganized speech.
Posturing: Inappropriate or bizarre bodily posture adopted continuously over a sustained period.
Pressured speech: Speech that is increased in amount, accelerated and difficult or impossible to interrupt.
Poverty of speech: Decreased speech in quantity and quality.
Psychalgia: Severe prolong pain without pathology.
Psychiatric emergency: It is a sudden onset of unusual disordered or socially inappropriate behavior caused by an emotional or physiological situation.
Psychogenic fugue: Amnesia associated state in which the person flees from home, forgets his entire past but not the basic skills.
Psychosis: Very severe type of personality which involves impairment of ego functions. Impaired reality is mostly seen.
Primary gain: The relief from emotional conflict and the freedom from anxiety achieved by a defense mechanism.
Presenile: Pertaining to premature old age as judged by mental or physical condition.
Projection: A defense mechanism, operating unconsciously, in which what is emotionally unacceptable in the self is unconsciously rejected and attributed (projected) to others.
Pseudo dementia: Symptoms of depression that mimic those of dementia.
Psychodrama: A specialized type of group therapy that employs a dramatic approach in which 'patients' become' actors' in life situation scenarios.
Psychoimmunology: The study of the implications of immune system in psychiatry.

Psychotherapy: Therapy involving psychological instead of medical treatment of mental disorders.
Pyromania: An inability to resist the impulse to set fires.

S

Sadism: Recurrent urges and sexually arousing fantasies involving acts in which the psychological or physical suffering of the victim is sexually exciting.
Self-concept: The composite of beliefs and feelings that one holds about oneself at a given time, formed from perceptions of other's reactions.
Self-consistency: The component of the personal identity that strives to maintain a stable self image.
Senile: It means old age.
Shaping: In learning process, one shapes the behavior of another by giving reinforcements for increasingly closer approximations to the desired behavior.
Slander: An action with which an individual may be charged for orally sharing information that is detrimental to a person's reputation.
Social skills training: It is learning of social interactions, functional skills that are relevant for daily living.
Somatization: A method of coping with psychosocial stress by developing physical symptoms.
Splitting: A primitive ego defense mechanism in which the person is unable to integrate and accept both positive and negative feelings.

T

Tangentiality: The inability to get to the point of a story. The speaker introduces many unrelated topics, until the original topic of discussion is lost.
Tardive dyskinesia: Syndrome of symptoms characterized by bizarre facial and tongue movements, a stiff neck, and difficulty swallowing. It may occur as an adverse effect of long term therapy with some antipsychotics.
Temperament: A set of inborn personality characteristics that influences an individuals' manner of reacting to the environment and ultimately influence on interpersonal communication.
Territoriality: The innate tendency of individuals to own space. Individuals lay claim to areas around them as their own. This can have an influence on interpersonal communication.
Tertiary prevention: Health care that is directed toward reduction of the residual effects associated with severe or chronic physical or mental illness.
Time out: An aversive stimulus or punishment during which the individual is removed from the environment where the unacceptable behavior is being exhibited.
Token economy: In behavior modification, a type of contracting in which the reinforces for desired behaviors are presented in the form of tokens, which may then be exchanged for designated privileges.
Tolerance: Tolerance refers the body's capacity to endure levels of medication over periods of time. It can also be used to refer to an addict's capacity to consume levels of either alcohol or illegal drugs due to repeated use or exposure.
Tort: The violation of a civil law in which an individual has been wronged. In a tort action, one party asserts that wronged conduct on the part of the other has caused harm, and compensation for harm suffered is sought.

Tourette's disorder: A stereotyped movement disorder characterized by repeated, involuntary rapid movements of various muscle. Groups involving vocal tics such as grunts, barks, sniffs etc.

Transsexualism: A disorder of gender identity or gender dysphoria of the most extreme variety. The individual, despite having the anatomical characteristics of a given gender, has the self-perception of being of the opposite gender, and may seek to have gender changed through surgical intervention.

Transvestic fetishism: Recurrent urges and sexually arousing fantasies involving dressing in the clothes of the opposite gender.

Trichotillomania: The recurrent failure to resist impulses to pull out one's own hair.

Truancy: Absence from school without permission.

U

Unconscious: The part of mind which the content is only rarely subject to awareness.

Undoing: A mechanism used to symbolically negate or cancel out a previous action or experience that one finds intolerable.

Universality: One curative factor of groups in which individuals realize that they are not alone in a problem and in the thoughts and feelings they are experiencing . Anxiety is relieved by the support and understanding of others in the group who share similar experiences.

Utilitarianism: The lethal theory that espouses 'the greatest happiness for the greatest number'. Under this theory, action would be taken based on the end results that will produce the most good (happiness) for the most people.

V

Vandalism: Willful defacement or destruction of property.

Vegetative state: State of deterioration in which the patient is immobile, out of contact with the environment, unresponsive to questioning and ultimately has to be fed and toileted.

Verbigeration: Stereotyped and seemingly meaningless repetition of words or sentences.

Visual asymbolia: Words can be transcribed but not read.

Visual hallucinations: A hallucination involving sight, which may consist of formed images, such as of people, or of unformed images, such as flashes of light.

Voyeurism: Peeping; one of the paraphilias, characterized by marked distress over, or acting on, urges to observe unsuspecting people, usually strangers, who are naked or in the process of disrobing, or who are engaging in sexual activity.

W

Walk-in-clinics: Patient/client can walk in any time of the day or night for professional help.

Waxy flexibility: A patient's movements have the feeling of a plastic resistance, as if the person was made of wax.

Wernicke's aphasia: Loss of the ability to comprehend language coupled with production of inappropriate language.

Withdrawal symptom: It is an organic mental disorder following stopping or reduction in the intake of a substance such as alcohol, opioids, etc.

Withdrawn behavior: It is an attempt in which the patient tries to avoid social interaction.

Word salad: A mixture of words and phrases that lack comprehensive meaning or logical coherence; commonly seen in schizophrenic states.
Whistle blowing: This is the act of informing a relevant person in an organization of instances or services in which patients are at risk.

Y

Yoga: A system of beliefs and practices, the ultimate goal of which is to unite the human soul with the universal spirit.

Z

Zoophilia: One of the paraphilias, characterized by marked distress over, or acting on, urges to indulge in sexual activity that involves animals.

Index

Page numbers followed by *f* refer to figure and *t* refer to table, respectively.

R

S

NOTES

NOTES